Health, United States, 2000
with Adolescent Health Chartbook

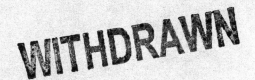
U.S. DEPARTMENT OF HEALTH AND HUMAN SERVICES
Centers for Disease Control and Prevention
National Center for Health Statistics
6525 Belcrest Road
Hyattsville, Maryland 20782-2003

July 2000
DHHS Pub. No. 00-1232

U.S. Department of Health and Human Services (DHHS)

Donna E. Shalala
Secretary

Office of Public Health and Science, DHHS

David Satcher, M.D., Ph.D.
Assistant Secretary for Health and Surgeon General

Centers for Disease Control and Prevention (CDC)

Jeffrey P. Koplan, M.D., M.P.H.
Director

National Center for Health Statistics, CDC

Edward J. Sondik, Ph.D.
Director

Health, United States, 2000 is the 24th report on the health status of the Nation. This report was compiled by the Centers for Disease Control and Prevention (CDC), National Center for Health Statistics (NCHS). The National Committee on Vital and Health Statistics served in a review capacity.

Health, United States presents national trends in health statistics. Major findings are presented in the highlights. The report includes a chartbook on adolescent health and trend tables.

Adolescent Health Chartbook

In each edition of *Health, United States*, a chartbook focuses on a major health topic. This year the Adolescent Health Chartbook describes the health of the adolescent population, 10–19 years of age. Adolescence is a period of accelerated growth and change, bridging the complex transition from childhood to adulthood. Young people experience profound biological, emotional, intellectual, and social changes, and the patterns of behavior they adopt may have long-term consequences for their health and quality of life. The chartbook presents data on the current status of adolescent health, with a focus on the transitions in adolescent health status by single year of age. The 32 figures and accompanying text show differences in health status, injury, mortality, reproductive health, health care utilization, and risk behaviors by age and gender. Many charts also describe racial, ethnic, and sociodemographic differences.

Trend Tables

The chartbook is followed by 146 trend tables organized around four major subject areas: health status and determinants, health care utilization, health care resources, and health care expenditures. A major criterion used in selecting the trend tables is the availability of comparable national data over a period of several years. The tables report data for selected years to highlight major trends in health statistics. Earlier editions of *Health, United States* may present data for additional years that are not included in the current printed report. Where possible, these additional data are available in Lotus 1–2–3 and Excel spreadsheet files as listed in Appendix III.

Racial and Ethnic Data

Several tables in *Health, United States* present data according to race and Hispanic origin consistent with Department-wide emphasis on expanding racial and ethnic detail in presenting health data. Trend data on race and ethnicity are usually in the greatest detail possible, after taking into account the quality of data, the amount of missing data, and the number of observations. The large differences in health status by race and Hispanic origin that are documented in this report may be explained by several factors including socioeconomic status, health practices, psychosocial stress and resources, environmental exposures, discrimination, and access to health care. New standards for presenting Federal data on race and ethnicity are described in Appendix II under Race.

Changes in This Edition

Similar tables appear in each volume of *Health, United States* to enhance the use of this publication as a standard reference source. However, each year new tables are added to reflect emerging topics in public health and changes in the content of ongoing tables are made to enhance their usefulness. New to *Health, United States, 2000* are data on early prenatal care for States (table 7) based on vital statistics; use of ambulatory health care as measured by visits to doctor's offices, clinics, and emergency departments, as well as home visits from nurses and other health professionals (table 71) based on the National Health Interview Survey (NHIS); access to care by children under 18 years of age as measured by no health care contacts within the past 12 months (table 75), hospital emergency department use by children (table 77) and by adults (table 79) based on NHIS; injury-related visits to hospital emergency departments based on the National Hospital Ambulatory Medical Care Survey (NHAMCS) (table 84); fee-for-service Medicare enrollees and payments based on data from the Health Care Financing Administration (table 134); and health

Preface

care use and expenditures by Medicare beneficiaries based on the Medicare Current Beneficiary Survey (table 135).

Data for racial and ethnic groups are expanded in tables showing contraceptive use (table 18), infant and neonatal mortality rates by State (tables 24 and 25), limitation of activity (table 57), interval since the last health care contact (table 72), and Medicaid recipients (table 136). In addition, new tables 7, 71, 75, 77, 79, and 135 also present data for racial and ethnic groups.

In other changes, death rates for lung cancer (ICD 162) replace death rates for respiratory cancer (ICD 160–165) in tables 30, 31, and 40; the age range of data on dental visits (table 80) and untreated dental caries (table 81) is expanded to encompass children, adults, and the elderly; Medicare expenditures for managed care and fee-for-service care are added to table 133. Tables that present NHIS, NAMCS, NHAMCS, National Nursing Home Survey, and National Home and Hospice Care Survey data are age adjusted using a new population standard, the year 2000 population (see Appendix II, Age adjustment). A newly designed brochure features representative charts and tables from the report.

Appendixes

Appendix I describes each data source used in the report and the limitations of the data and provides references for further information about the sources.

Appendix II is an alphabetical listing of terms used in the report. It also contains standard populations used for age adjustment, *International Classification of Diseases* (ICD) codes for cause of death and diagnostic and procedure categories.

Appendix III lists tables with additional years of trend data that are available electronically in Lotus 1–2–3 and Excel spreadsheet files on the NCHS home page and CD-ROM.

The Index to Trend Tables is a useful tool for locating data by topic. Tables are cross-referenced by such topics as Child and adolescent health, Women's health, Elderly population, Nutrition related, State data, American Indian, Asian, Black, and Hispanic origin populations, Education, and Poverty status.

Electronic Access

Health, United States has its own home page on the NCHS web site at www.cdc.gov/nchs. Click on "Top 10 Downloads". The direct Uniform Resource Locator (URL) address for the *Health, United States* home page is:

www.cdc.gov/nchs/products/pubs/pubd/hus/hus.htm.

Health, United States, 2000, the Adolescent Health Chartbook, and each of the 146 individual trend tables are available as separate Acrobat .pdf files on the *Health, United States* home page. In addition individual tables are downloadable as Lotus 1–2–3 and Excel spreadsheet files. Previous editions of *Health, United States* and chartbooks, starting with the 1993 edition, also may be accessed from the *Health, United States* home page.

Health, United States is also available, along with other NCHS reports, on a CD-ROM entitled "Publications from the National Center for Health Statistics, featuring *Health, United States, 2000,*" vol 1 no 6, 2000. These publications can be viewed, searched, printed, and saved using Adobe Acrobat software on the CD-ROM. The CD-ROM may be purchased from the Government Printing Office.

Questions?

For answers to questions about this report, contact:
Data Dissemination Branch
National Center for Health Statistics
Centers for Disease Control and Prevention
6525 Belcrest Road, Room 1064
Hyattsville, Maryland 20782–2003
phone: 301–458–INFO
E-mail: nchsquery@cdc.gov
Internet: www.cdc.gov/nchs

Overall responsibility for planning and coordinating the content of this volume rested with the Office of Analysis, Epidemiology, and Health Promotion, National Center for Health Statistics (NCHS), under the general direction of Diane M. Makuc and Jennifer H. Madans.

Health, United States, 2000 highlights, trend tables, and appendixes were prepared under the leadership of Kate Prager. Trend tables were prepared by Alan J. Cohen, Margaret A. Cooke, La-Tonya D. Curl, Catherine Duran, Virginia M. Freid, Karen E. Fujii, Andrea P. MacKay, Mitchell B. Pierre, Jr., Rebecca A. Placek, Anita L. Powell, Kate Prager, Laura A. Pratt, and Henry Xia of NOVA Research Company with assistance from Amy M. Branum, Patricia A. Knapp, Brenda E. Mitchell and Jennie Wald. Production planning and coordination of appendixes and index to trend tables were managed by Anita L. Powell. The *Health, United States* brochure was designed by Brenda E. Mitchell. Production planning and coordination of trend tables were managed by Rebecca A. Placek. Administrative and word processing assistance were provided by Carole J. Hunt, Camille A. Miller, and Anne E. Cromwell.

The **Adolescent Health Chartbook** was prepared by Andrea P. MacKay, Lois A. Fingerhut, and Catherine Duran, under the general direction of Kenneth C. Schoendorf and Diane M. Makuc. Data and analysis for specific charts were provided by Lara Akinbami, Christine S. Cox, Alisa M. Jenny, Clemencia M. Vargas, Stephanie J. Ventura, and Margaret Warner of NCHS; Melinda L. Flock and Joseph M. Posid of the National Center for HIV, STD, and TB Prevention, CDC; Laura Kann and Sherry C. Everett of the National Center for Chronic Disease Prevention and Health Promotion, CDC; Laura Lippman of the National Center for Education Statistics; and Michael R. Rand of the Bureau of Justice Statistics. Advice on the content of the chartbook was provided by Charles E. Irwin, Jr., of the National Adolescent Health Information Center, University of California, San Francisco; John L. Kiely and Elizabeth Goodman of Children's Hospital Medical Center of Cincinnati; and Trina Anglin of the Health Resources and Services Administration.

Publications management and editorial review were provided by Thelma W. Sanders and Rolfe W. Larson. The designer was Sarah M. Hinkle. Graphics were supervised by Stephen L. Sloan. Production was done by Jacqueline M. Davis and Annette F. Holman. Printing was managed by Joan D. Burton and Patricia L. Wilson.

Electronic access through CD-ROM and the NCHS internet site was provided by Christine J. Brown, Michelle L. Bysheim, Jacqueline M. Davis, Annette F. Holman, Gail V. Johnson, Demarius V. Miller, Sharon L. Ramirez, Thelma W. Sanders, Julia A. Sothoron, and Tammy M. Stewart-Prather.

Data and technical assistance were provided by Charles A. Adams, Robert N. Anderson, Margaret C. Avery, Linda E. Biggar, Viona I. Brown, Catharine W. Burt, Margaret D. Carroll, Pei-Lu Chiu, Robin A. Cohen, Richard H. Coles, Thomas D. Dunn, Lois A. Fingerhut, Katherine M. Flegal, Nancy G. Gagne, Cathy Hao, Ann M. Hardy, Barbara J. Haupt, Kristina Kotulak-Hays, Rosemarie Hirsch, Donna L. Hoyert, Deborah D. Ingram, Susan S. Jack, Clifford L. Johnson, Kenneth D. Kochanek, Lola Jean Kozak, Robert J. Kuczmarski, Linda S. Lawrence, Karen L. Lipkind, Marian F. MacDorman, Joyce A. Martin, Jeffrey D. Maurer, Linda F. McCaig, Geraldine M. McQuillen, William D. Mosher, Sherry L. Murphy, Cheryl R. Nelson, Francis C. Notzon, Maria F. Owings, Jane Page, Jennifer D. Parker, Gail A. Parr, Linda J. Piccinino, Harry M. Rosenberg, Susan M. Schappert, Charlotte A. Schoenborn, J. Fred Seitz, Mira Shanks, Manju Sharma, Alvin J. Sirrocco, Betty L. Smith, Genevieve W. Strahan, Anne K. Stratton, Luong Tonthat, Clemencia M. Vargas, Stephanie J. Ventura, and David A. Woodwell of NCHS; Tim Bush, Andrea Gates, and Luetta Schneider of the National Center for HIV, STD, and TB Prevention, CDC; Samuel L. Groseclose and Patsy A. Hall of the Epidemiology Program Office, CDC; Lisa M. Koonin and Lilo T. Strauss of the National Center for Chronic Disease Prevention and Health Promotion, CDC; Monina Klevens of the National Immunization Program, CDC; Evelyn Christian of the Health Resources and Services Administration; Mitchell Goldstein of the Office of the Secretary,

Acknowledgments

DHHS; Joanne Atay, Judy Ball, Joseph C. Gfroerer, Janet Greenblatt, Patricia Royston, Richard Thoreson, and Deborah Trunzo of the Substance Abuse and Mental Health Services Administration; Ken Allison, Lynn A. G. Ries, Arthur L. Hughes, and Deborah Dawson of the National Institutes of Health; Gerald S. Adler, Cathy A. Cowan, Janice D. Drexler, David A. Gibson, Leslie Greenwald, Helen C. Lazenby, Katharine R. Levit, Anna Long, Anthony C. Parker, and Madie W. Stewart of the Health Care Financing Administration; Joseph Dalaker of the Census Bureau; James Barnhardt, Alan Blostin, Kay Ford, Daniel Ginsburg, and Janice Windau of the Bureau of Labor Statistics; Elizabeth Ahuja and Laura O'Shea of the Department of Veterans Affairs; Susan Tew of the Alan Guttmacher Institute; Wendy Katz of the Association of Schools of Public Health; Richard Hamer of InterStudy; Patrick O'Malley of the University of Michigan; C. McKeen Cowles of Cowles Research Group; and Gerald D. Williams of CSR Incorporated.

Contents

Contents ....

Population Characteristics

Health Status

Reproductive Health

Risk Behaviors

List of Figures ....

Health Care Access

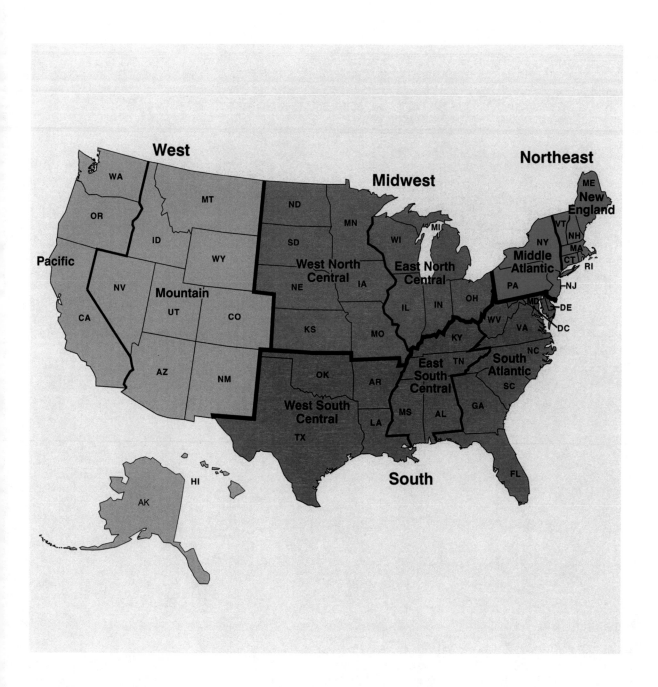

Adolescent Population Characteristics

In 1999, 40 million residents of the United States were adolescents 10–19 years of age, comprising approximately 14 percent of the U.S. population. The racial and ethnic composition of the adolescent population of the United States is changing and will be increasingly diverse in the 21st century. Social determinants and educational achievement play an important role in the health of these adolescents.

■ In 1999 two-thirds of the adolescent **population** was non-Hispanic white and one-third was of other racial and ethnic groups. By the year 2050, projections of the population indicate that Hispanic, black, American Indian, and Asian adolescents will constitute 56 percent of the adolescent population (figure 1).

■ **Poverty** during adolescence has immediate and lasting negative consequences. In 1998, 17 percent of all adolescents lived in families with incomes below the poverty level. One-parent households headed by women experience the highest rates of poverty. Forty percent of adolescents in female-headed families were living in poverty, compared with 8 percent of adolescents in two-parent families (figure 2).

■ **Employment** during the adolescent years can have beneficial or negative effects on the health and well-being of youth. In 1999 approximately two-fifths of adolescents 16–19 years of age were employed during the school year and over one-half worked during the summer months. The proportion of adolescents employed during the school year and during the summer increased with age (figure 3).

■ Although most adolescents complete high school, in 1998 the **dropout rate** among students 15–19 years of age in grades 10–12 was 4 per 100 students. The proportion of adolescents who dropped out without completing high school increased from 2 percent of students 15–16 years of age to almost 11 percent of those 19 years of age. Students from low-income families dropped out of high school about four times as frequently as students from middle-income and high-income families (figure 4).

Adolescent Health Status

Indicators of adolescent health status include activity limitation, dental health, suicide ideation and attempts, as well as emergency department visit rates, hospital discharge rates, and death rates. The health of adolescents varies by age, gender, race and Hispanic origin.

■ **Activity limitation** due to a physical, mental, or emotional health problem is one indicator of adolescent health status. The vast majority of adolescents do not have any activity limitation. In 1997 approximately 8 percent of adolescents 10–17 years of age were reported to have some activity limitation. Receipt of special education services was the only activity limitation identified for about 5 percent of adolescents (figure 5).

■ During 1988–94 one-fifth of adolescents 10–19 years of age had at least one **untreated dental caries** or active tooth infection. Three times as many adolescents in families living below the poverty level had untreated caries as did adolescents in families with incomes twice the poverty level or higher (figure 6).

■ **Suicidal ideation or attempting suicide** is one indicator of mental or emotional health. In 1999, 25 percent of female adolescents and 14 percent of male adolescents in grades 9–12 reported seriously considering or attempting suicide (figure 7).

■ Adolescents may be **victims of violent crimes**, including rape or sexual assault, aggravated and simple assault, and robbery. During the period 1992–97 an average of approximately 3.4 million adolescents 12–19 years of age were reported to be victims of violent crimes each year. The rates of violent crime victimization for adolescents 12–19 years of age were lower in 1997 than in 1992, with declines in each of the major categories of victimization (figure 15).

Emergency Department Visits by Adolescents

■ In 1995–97 adolescents 10–19 years of age made about 11.6 million **emergency department visits** each year. Approximately one-half of these visits were for injuries. Injury-related and noninjury-related visit rates increased with age. Among female adolescents pregnancy-related emergency department visit rates increased almost sevenfold between 14 and 19 years (figures 8 and 9).

■ In 1995–97 four **causes of injury**—being struck, falls, cuts, and motor vehicle traffic-related injuries—accounted for nearly 60 percent of all injury-related emergency department (ED) visits. ED visit rates for cuts and motor vehicle traffic-related injuries increased with age, while ED visit rates for falls decreased with age (figure 10).

■ The most common **emergency department injury diagnoses** include fractures, sprains and strains, open wounds, and contusions. In 1995–97 these four injury diagnoses accounted for 80 percent of first-listed injury diagnoses in emergency department visits for adolescents 10–19 years of age (figure 11).

■ Asthma, upper respiratory conditions, and abdominal or gastrointestinal (GI) conditions are among the leading **emergency department (ED) noninjury diagnoses** for adolescents 10–19 years of age. Among female adolescents, the ED visit rate for abdominal and GI conditions, as well as ED visits for sexually transmitted diseases, urinary tract infections, and pregnancy-related conditions, increased markedly with age (figure 12).

Adolescent Hospitalizations

■ In 1995–97 adolescents 10–19 years of age had 1.6 million hospitalizations annually. **Hospital discharge rates** increased with age across the adolescent years, but the pattern varied by gender and diagnosis (figure 8).

■ In 1995–97 noninjury-related causes accounted for 72 percent of all **hospital discharges** among male adolescents and 39 percent (excluding pregnancy) among female adolescents. Injuries accounted for 26 percent of discharges among males and 8 percent among females. Among female adolescents, pregnancy-related causes (including deliveries and diagnoses associated with pregnancy) accounted for 53 percent of discharges (figure 13).

■ Asthma, psychoses, fractures, poisoning, and appendicitis were among the leading first-listed **hospital discharge diagnoses** for adolescents in 1995–97. These five diagnoses accounted for 20 percent of all hospital discharges (figure 14).

Adolescent Mortality

■ In 1996–97 about 19,000 adolescents died each year. Nearly 14,000 adolescents died annually from injury-related causes; in contrast 5,000 adolescents died from natural causes. The proportion of all **deaths** from injuries increased with age from 47 percent among adolescents 10 years of age to 81 percent among adolescents 18 years of age (figure 16).

■ **Motor vehicle traffic-related injuries and firearm-related injuries** are the two leading causes of injury death among adolescents 10–19 years of age. In 1996–97 these two causes accounted for 55 percent of all deaths and 75 percent of all injury deaths. Motor vehicle traffic death rates increased markedly with age, with the greatest increase occurring between ages 15 years and 16 years for male and female adolescents (figure 17).

■ In 1996–97 **motor vehicle traffic-related and firearm-related death rates** among adolescents varied by urbanization of residence, although marked increases with age were apparent in all three urbanization categories. Adolescents living in the most densely populated counties had higher death rates associated with interpersonal violence (firearm homicide), while adolescents living in more rural counties had higher rates of motor vehicle fatalities (figure 18).

Adolescent Reproductive Health

As adolescents develop sexually, they face issues and decisions about their own sexuality. The majority of today's adolescents are becoming sexually active during their teen years and experience many of the health consequences associated with sexual activity, such as pregnancy and sexually transmitted diseases. Disparities by age, race, and Hispanic origin were observed in all measures of reproductive health.

.... Highlights

Adolescent Health

■ More than 900,000 adolescents become pregnant each year. In 1996 the **pregnancy rate** was 98.7 pregnancies per 1,000 adolescent women aged 15–19, a decrease of 15 percent since 1991. Pregnancy rates increased with age from 67.8 for adolescents 15–17 years of age to 146.4 for adolescents 18–19 years (figure 19).

■ In 1997–98 there were approximately 493,600 births annually to adolescents 13–19 years of age, accounting for 13 percent of all births in each year. There was a consistent pattern of increasing **birth rates** by maternal age. Overall, 19-year-old adolescents were nearly seven times as likely to have a birth as their 15-year-old counterparts (figure 20).

■ Infants of adolescent mothers are more likely to be **low birthweight** than infants of mothers in their twenties and thirties. In 1997–98, 13.2 percent of infants born to adolescents under the age of 15 years and 9.5 percent of infants born to adolescents 15–19 years of age were low birthweight. In contrast 7.2 percent of infants born to women in their twenties and thirties were low birthweight (figure 21).

■ The **infant mortality** rate is an important indicator of the health and well-being of infants and their adolescent mothers. During 1995–97 there were 10.6 infant deaths per 1,000 live births to adolescent mothers. Among the youngest adolescent mothers (13–14 years of age) the infant mortality rate was 1.8 times that of mothers 19 years of age (figure 22).

■ **Sexually transmitted diseases** (STD's) are the most commonly reported infectious diseases among sexually active adolescents; chlamydia and gonorrhea are the most common bacterial causes of STD's. Reported rates for chlamydial and gonococcal infections are higher among female adolescents 15–19 years of age than among male adolescents and adults of either gender (figure 23).

■ Although the overall prevalence of **acquired immunodeficiency syndrome** (AIDS) is relatively low among adolescents, adolescents in some minority and racial groups are disproportionately affected by HIV and AIDS (figure 24).

Adolescent Risk Behavior

Many adolescents are engaging in risk behaviors that are harmful or dangerous to themselves and others, with consequences to their health and well-being that may be immediate or long-term. There were distinct differences in the percentage of students engaging in risk behaviors by grade level, gender, race, and Hispanic origin.

■ In 1999 one-half of all high school students reported that they had ever been **sexually active**. Sixty-six percent of female students and 64 percent of male students in the 12th grade had ever had sexual intercourse, compared with 33 percent of female students and 45 percent of male students in the 9th grade. Between 1991 and 1999 the proportion of high school students reporting sexual experience decreased by 8 percent (figure 25).

■ In 1999 more than one-third of high school students reported **smoking cigarettes** in the previous 30 days, and 17 percent reported smoking frequently (20 or more days). The prevalence of cigarette smoking among high school students in 1999 was 27 percent higher than in 1991. (figure 26).

■ In 1999 about one-half of all high school students (48 percent of female and 52 percent of male students) reported **alcohol use** in the previous 30 days. Binge drinking, that is, having 5 or more drinks on 1 occasion, was reported by 28 percent of female students and 35 percent of male students during the same 30-day period (figure 27).

■ **Marijuana** is the most commonly used illicit drug among high school students. In 1999 almost one-half (47 percent) of high school students had ever used marijuana, and more than one-fourth had used marijuana one or more times in the past 30 days (figure 28).

■ **Weapon carrying** is associated with violence and serious injury. In 1999, 6 percent of female and 29 percent of male high school students reported carrying a gun or other weapon in the past 30 days. Between 1991 and 1999 the percent of students who reported carrying a weapon decreased by 35 percent (figure 29).

■ **Physical activity** provides important health benefits for adolescents. In 1999 more than two-thirds of all high school students participated in moderate to vigorous physical activity. Male and female students were more likely to participate in 9th grade than in higher grades (figure 30).

Adolescent Health Care Access

Adolescents have lower rates of health care utilization than younger and older persons, despite the health problems that affect the adolescent population, such as sexually transmitted diseases, emotional and behavioral problems, unintended pregnancy, drug and alcohol abuse, and injuries and violence. Access to and use of health care services is dependent in part on health insurance coverage or the ability to pay for services.

■ In 1997, 17 percent of adolescents had no **health care coverage**. One-third of adolescents in families with incomes below the poverty level were uninsured compared with 8 percent of adolescents in families with incomes greater than two times the poverty level. The proportion of adolescents without health care coverage increased with age in every income category (figure 31).

■ Lack of health insurance coverage has a significant impact on adolescents' access to routine health care. In 1997 the percent of adolescents who had not had a **health care visit** in the past year was 2.6 times as high for those without health insurance as for those with health insurance. The percent of adolescents without a health care visit declined with age among females and increased with age among males (figure 32).

Mortality Trends

In 1998 life expectancy at birth increased to an all-time high and life expectancy for black males increased for the fifth consecutive year. Infant mortality was unchanged from 1997. The death rate for HIV infection declined for the third straight year. Death rates for heart disease, cancer, stroke, homicide, and suicide also decreased in 1998.

■ In 1998 **life expectancy** at birth reached an all-time high of 76.7 years and **infant mortality** remained at a record low 7.2 deaths per 1,000 live births (tables 23 and 28).

■ Between 1993 and 1998 **life expectancy** at birth for black males increased 3.0 years to a record high of 67.6 years, due in large part to continuing declines in mortality from HIV infection and homicide. However, life expectancy was still 6.9 years shorter for black males than for white males in 1998 (table 28).

■ Mortality from **heart disease**, the leading cause of death, declined 3 percent in 1998, continuing a long-term downward trend. The 1998 age-adjusted death rate for heart disease was about one-half the rate in 1970 (tables 30, 32, and 37).

■ Mortality from **cancer**, the second leading cause of death, decreased 1.6 percent in 1998, continuing the decline that began in 1990. Over the preceding 20-year period, 1970–90, age-adjusted cancer death rates steadily increased (tables 30, 32, and 39).

■ Mortality from **stroke**, the third leading cause of death, appears to have resumed a downward trend. In 1998 the age-adjusted death rate fell 3.1 percent, declining for the third straight year following a leveling off earlier in the decade. Between 1980 and 1992 stroke mortality declined at an average rate of 3.6 percent per year (tables 30, 32, and 38).

■ Mortality from **unintentional injuries,** the fifth leading cause of death, was unchanged between 1997 and 1998. Since the 1970's the trend in injury mortality has been generally downward (tables 30 and 32).

■ The age-adjusted death rate for **suicide**, the eighth leading cause of death, has been edging downward during the 1990's. The age-adjusted suicide rate was 10.4 deaths per 100,000 population in 1998, compared with 11.5 in 1990 (tables 30, 32, and 47).

■ The age-adjusted **homicide** rate fell almost 9 percent in 1998, continuing a downward trend that began in the early 1990's. At 7.3 homicides per 100,000 population in 1998, this was the lowest rate in about three decades. Despite the overall decline in homicide mortality, this cause is still the leading cause of death for young black males 15–24 years of age (tables 30 and 46).

■ Mortality from **HIV infection** declined 21 percent in 1998, following a 48-percent decline in 1997 and a 29-percent decline in 1996. This 3-year decline contrasts sharply with the period 1987–94, when HIV mortality increased at an average rate of 16 percent per year (tables 30 and 43).

Disparities in Mortality

Despite overall declines in mortality, disparities among racial and ethnic groups, for many causes of death, are substantial. Disparities among persons of different education levels continue. Persons with less than a high school education have death rates at least double those with education beyond high school.

■ In 1997 **infant mortality** rates were highest among infants of black, Hawaiian, and American-Indian mothers (13.7, 9.0, and 8.7 deaths per 1,000 live births). Infant mortality was lowest for infants of Chinese-American mothers (3.1 per 1,000). Mortality rates for infants of Hispanic mothers and non-Hispanic white mothers were the same (6.0 per 1,000 live births) (table 20).

■ **Infant mortality** decreases as the mother's level of education increases and this disparity is greater for white mothers than for mothers in other racial and ethnic groups. In 1997 mortality for infants of non-Hispanic white mothers with less than 12 years of education was more than double that for infants whose mothers had 13 or more years of education. The

Health Status and Determinants

disparity in infant mortality by mother's education was 29 percent for non-Hispanic black mothers and 12 percent for Mexican-American mothers (table 21).

■ **Homicide among young black males** 15–24 years of age declined 10.4 percent per year on average between 1993, the year the rate peaked, and 1998. Despite the decline, the rate in 1998 (96.5 deaths per 100,000 population) was still almost 8 times the rate for young white males. Among adults 25–44 years of age, the homicide rate for black males was nearly 7 times the rate for white males, and the **HIV infection** death rate for adult black males 25–44 years of age was 6 times the rate for white males in this age group (tables 43 and 46).

■ In 1998 the **homicide rate among young Hispanic males** 15–24 years of age (41.1 deaths per 100,000 population) was about 7 times the rate for non-Hispanic white males. Among adults 25–44 years of age, the homicide rate for Hispanic males was more than 3 times the rate, and the **HIV infection** death rate for Hispanic males 25–44 years of age was more than 2 times the rate for non-Hispanic white males (tables 43 and 46).

■ The risk of suicide is higher for elderly white males than for other groups. In 1998 the **suicide rate among white males** 85 years of age and over (62.7 deaths per 100,000 population) was more than 3 times that for young white males 15–24 years (table 47).

■ In 1998 among **American Indians** the age-adjusted death rates for **motor vehicle-related injuries** (31.8 deaths per 100,000 population) and **diabetes** (29.6) were 2 and 2.5 times the rates for white persons and the death rate for **cirrhosis** (22.0) was 3 times the rate for white persons. Death rates for the American-Indian population are known to be underestimated (table 30).

■ In 1998 overall mortality was 53 percent higher for **black Americans** than for white Americans. In 1998 the age-adjusted death rates for the black population exceeded those for the white population by 78 percent for **stroke**, 50 percent for **heart disease**, 33 percent for **cancer**, and almost 700 percent for **HIV infection** (table 30).

■ In 1998 the overall age-adjusted death rate for **Asian-American** males was 40 percent lower than the rate for white males. However the **homicide** rate among Asian males was 14 percent lower than for white males and the death rate for **stroke** was 8 percent higher for Asian males than for white males. Death rates for Asian Americans are known to be underestimated somewhat (tables 36, 38, and 46).

■ In 1998 the age-adjusted death rate for **chronic obstructive pulmonary diseases (COPD)**, the fourth leading cause of death, was 43 percent higher for males than females. Between 1990 and 1998 age-adjusted death rates for males were relatively stable while death rates for females increased at an average annual rate of almost 3 percent (tables 30 and 32).

■ Death rates are higher among persons with less **education**. In 1998 the age-adjusted death rate for chronic diseases among adults with fewer than 12 years of education was more than twice the rate among those with more than 12 years of education. The death rate for injuries for the least educated was 3 times the rate for the most educated adults (table 35).

■ Between 1992 and 1998 the **occupational injury** death rate decreased 13 percent to 4.5 deaths per 100,000 employed workers. The two industries with the highest death rates were mining and agriculture, forestry, and fishing (23–24 deaths per 100,000). Construction with a death rate of 14.5 per 100,000 accounted for the largest number of deaths, nearly 20 percent of all occupational injury deaths (table 50).

Natality

Although birth rates for teens continued the downward trend that began in 1992, birth rates for women in their principal childbearing ages (twenties) increased in 1998 and overall fertility increased for the first time since 1990. The number of births to unmarried women increased 3 percent in 1998, the highest number ever reported. The proportion of babies born with low birthweight continued to edge upward.

■ In 1998 the **birth rate for teenagers** (15–19 years) declined for the seventh consecutive year, to 51.1 births per 1,000 women aged 15–19 years. Between 1991 and 1998 the teen birth rate declined more for 15–17 year-olds than for 18–19 year-olds (21 percent compared with 13 percent) (table 3).

■ In 1998 the **birth rate for unmarried women** increased slightly to 44.3 births per 1,000 unmarried women aged 15–44 years, but was still below its highest level, 46.9 in 1994. Between 1994 and 1998 birth rates for unmarried black women and unmarried Hispanic women each declined about 11 percent (table 9).

■ **Low birthweight** is associated with elevated risk of death and disability in infants. In 1998 the rate of low birthweight (infants weighing less than 2,500 grams at birth) increased to 7.6 percent overall, up from 7.0 percent in 1990. Since 1990 the low-birthweight rate increased for most racial and ethnic groups, except for black infants. The rise in multiple births has influenced the upward trend in low birthweight (table 12).

■ **Cigarette smoking during pregnancy** is a risk factor for poor birth outcomes such as low birthweight and infant death. In 1998 the proportion of mothers who smoked cigarettes during pregnancy declined to a record low of 12.9 percent, down from 19.5 percent in 1989. However the percent of teenage mothers 15–19 years who smoked increased between 1994 and 1998 (table 11).

Morbidity

Activity limitation and health status (self- or family member-assessed) are two summary measures of morbidity presented in this report. Additional measures of morbidity that are presented include the incidence of specific diseases.

■ **Activity limitation** due to a chronic condition is substantially higher among those with lower family incomes. In 1997 non-Hispanic white and non-Hispanic black persons who were poor were nearly three times as likely to report activity limitation

as were those with family income at least twice the poverty threshold (29–30 percent compared with 11 percent of the noninstitutionalized population, age adjusted) (table 57).

■ In 1998 the percent of persons reporting **fair or poor health** was 3.9 times as high for persons living below the poverty threshold as for those with family income at least twice the poverty threshold (22.2 percent and 5.7 percent, age adjusted) (table 58).

■ The continuing decline in the number of newly reported **AIDS cases** is evidence of the beneficial effects of new treatment regimens. In 1998, 20 percent fewer cases were reported than in the previous year. Despite the declines, AIDS incidence continues to disproportionately affect the non-Hispanic black and Hispanic populations (table 53).

■ In 1998 **tuberculosis (TB)** incidence declined for the sixth consecutive year to 6.8 cases per 100,000 population, a reflection of the apparent strengthening of TB-control programs nationwide. Despite the progress in controlling TB, the 1998 rate remained above the national objective for 2000 of 3.5 cases per 100,000 (table 52).

■ Between 1990 and 1998 the incidence of primary and secondary **syphilis** declined 87 percent to 2.6 cases per 100,000 population, below the national objective for 2000 of 4 per 100,000 (table 52).

■ The decline in **gonorrhea** incidence that characterized the 1980's slowed in the 1990's. In 1998, gonorrhea incidence increased for the first time since 1980, to 133 cases per 100,000 population, well below the rate when national reporting began in the mid-1970's, but still above the 2000 objective of 100 per 100,000 (table 52).

■ Overall **cancer incidence** has been declining in the 1990's, more so for males than for females. Between 1992 and 1996 cancer incidence rates declined 15 percent for males and 2 percent for females. Despite these declines, cancer incidence is one-third higher among males than females (table 55).

■ **Prostate cancer and lung cancer** are the two most frequently diagnosed cancers in men. In 1996

Health Status and Determinants

incidence of prostate cancer was 65 percent higher in black men than in white men, and lung cancer incidence, 48 percent higher (table 55).

■ **Breast cancer** incidence in 1996 was 11 percent lower for black women than for white women. However survival was lower for black women than for white women. The 5-year relative survival rate for breast cancer diagnosed in 1989–95 was 71 percent for black women and 86 percent for white women (tables 55 and 56).

■ Between 1980 and 1998 the **injuries with lost workdays** rate decreased 26 percent to 2.9 per 100 full-time equivalents (FTE's) in the private sector. Within the goods-producing industries, manufacturing had the highest injury rate (4.2 injuries with lost workdays per 100 FTE's) and within the service-producing sector, the highest injury rate was reported for transportation, communication, and public utilities (4.2) (table 51).

Health Behaviors

Cigarette smoking is the single leading preventable cause of death in the United States. It increases the risk of lung cancer, heart disease, emphysema, and other respiratory diseases. Cigarette smoking by adults has remained stable at about 25 percent since 1990. Heavy and chronic use of alcohol and use of illicit drugs increase the risk of disease and injuries.

■ **Cigarette smoking** is more prevalent among American-Indian men and non-Hispanic black men than among other men. In 1995–98, 41 percent of American-Indian men and 31 percent of non-Hispanic black men were current smokers compared with 27 percent of non-Hispanic white men, 24 percent of Hispanic men, and 18 percent of Asian men. Among women, the prevalence of smoking was highest among American-Indian women (29 percent) and lowest among Hispanic women (14 percent) and Asian women (11 percent) (percents are age adjusted and are for persons 18 years of age and over) (table 61).

■ In 1998, 62 percent of adults 18 years of age and over reported they were **current drinkers**, 22 percent

reported they were lifetime abstainers, and 16 percent were former drinkers. Women were about twice as likely as men to be lifetime abstainers (29 percent compared with 15 percent) (table 65).

■ **Binge drinking**, having five or more alcoholic drinks on at least one occasion in the past month, is more common among young people 18–25 years of age than among younger or older persons. In 1998 among young adults, binge drinking was 1.5–2.4 times as likely for non-Hispanic white persons (38 percent) as for Hispanic and non-Hispanic black persons (25 and 16 percent). In 1998 rates of binge drinking in these populations were higher than in 1997 but similar to rates observed in 1996 (table 62).

■ In 1997 there were more than 161,000 **cocaine-related emergency department visits**, twice as many as in 1990. The greatest increases occurred for persons 35 years and over, reflecting an aging population of drug abusers being treated in emergency departments. However, the proportion of adults aged 35 years and over who reported using cocaine in the past month has remained stable during this period at less than 1 percent (tables 62 and 64).

Health Care Utilization

Prevention Services

Use of preventive health services has substantial positive effects on the long-term health status of those who receive the services. The use of several different types of preventive services has been increasing. However, disparities in use of preventive health care by family income and by race and ethnicity remain in evidence.

■ Between 1990 and 1998 the percent of mothers receiving **prenatal care** in the first trimester of pregnancy increased from 76 to 83 percent. The largest increases in receipt of early prenatal care have occurred for racial and ethnic groups with the lowest levels of use, thereby reducing disparities in use of early care. However in 1998 the percent of mothers with early prenatal care still varied substantially among racial and ethnic groups from 69 percent for American-Indian mothers to 92 percent for Cuban mothers (table 6).

■ In 1998, 79 percent of children 19–35 months of age received the combined **vaccination** series of 4 doses of DTP (diphtheria-tetanus-pertussis) vaccine, 3 doses of polio vaccine, 1 dose of measles-containing vaccine, and 3 doses of Hib (Haemophilus influenzae type b) vaccine, up from 69 percent in 1994. Children living below the poverty threshold were less likely to have received the combined vaccination series than were children living at or above poverty (74 compared with 82 percent) (table 73).

■ In 1998 only 100 cases of **measles** were reported, down from 28,000 cases in 1990, providing evidence of the success of vaccination efforts to increase population immunity to measles (table 52).

■ Regular **mammography** screening for women aged 50 years and over has been shown to be effective in reducing deaths from breast cancer. In 1998, 69 percent of women aged 50 years and over reported mammography screening in the previous 2-year period, up from 61 percent in 1994. Among women living below the poverty threshold in 1998, 53 percent reported recent screening compared with 72 percent of women with family income at or above poverty (table 82).

Access to Care

Access to health care is important for preventive care and for prompt treatment of illness and injuries. Some indicators of access to health care services include having a usual source of health care, having a recent health care contact, use of the emergency department, and treatment of health problems such as dental caries. Access to health care varies by health insurance status, poverty status, race, and ethnicity.

■ In 1997, 14 percent of children under 18 years of age had no **health insurance coverage**. More than one-quarter of children with family income of 1–1.5 times the poverty level were without coverage compared with only 6 percent of those with income above twice the poverty level (table 128).

■ In 1997–98, 13 percent of children under 18 years of age did not have a **health care visit to an office or clinic** within the previous 12-month period. Uninsured children were nearly three times as likely as those with health insurance to be without a recent visit (29 percent compared with 10 percent) (table 75).

■ In 1997–98, about 7 percent of children under 18 years of age had **no usual source of health care**. More than one-quarter of children without health insurance coverage had no usual source of health care (table 76).

■ In 1998, 20 percent of children under 18 years of age had an **emergency department visit** within the past 12 months. Children living below the poverty threshold were 50 percent more likely than nonpoor children to have a recent emergency department visit (27 percent compared with 18 percent) (table 77).

■ In 1998, three-quarters of children under 18 years of age had a **dental visit** in the past year. Hispanic and non-Hispanic black children were less likely than non-Hispanic white children to have a recent dental visit (62 percent, 70 percent, and 77 percent, respectively) (table 80).

■ In 1998 one in five adults 18 years of age and over had an **emergency department visit** within the past 12 months. Emergency department visits were more common among young adults 18–24 years of age and elderly persons 75 years of age and over (25 and 24 percent) than among adults 25–64 years (17–19 percent) (table 79).

■ In 1988–94, 28 percent of adults 18–64 years of age had at least one untreated **dental cavity**, down from 48 percent in 1971–74. Although substantial declines in untreated dental cavities have occurred for adults at all income levels, nearly one-half of adults living in poverty compared with one in five nonpoor adults had an untreated cavity in 1988–94 (table 81).

Outpatient Care

Major changes continue to occur in the delivery of health care in the United States, driven in large part by the need to rein in rising costs. One significant change has been a decline in use of inpatient services and an increase in outpatient services such as outpatient surgery and home health care.

■ In 1997, 61 percent of all **surgical operations** in community hospitals were performed on outpatients, up from 51 percent in 1990, 35 percent in 1985, and 16 percent in 1980 (table 95).

■ Among the elderly, use of **home health care** grew by more than 70 percent during the period from 1992 to 1996, while the use of **hospice** services remained fairly stable over the same period (data are age adjusted) (table 88).

Inpatient Care and Resources

Utilization of hospital inpatient services has declined, as has the number of beds in community hospitals. Utilization of nursing home care has also declined.

■ **Hospital discharge rates** are higher among poor persons than among those with higher family incomes. In 1998 among persons under 65 years of age, hospital discharge rates for the poor were double those for persons with family income above twice the poverty level (175 and 87 per 1,000 population). Average length of stay was 1.5 days longer for the poor than for the nonpoor (5.3 and 3.8 days) (data are age adjusted) (table 89).

■ Between 1985 and 1998 the **hospital discharge rate** declined by one-quarter from 138 discharges per 1,000 population to 103 per 1,000, while **average length of stay** declined by almost 1.5 days, from 6.3 to 4.9 days (data are age adjusted) (table 90).

■ Between 1990 and 1998 the number of **community hospital beds** declined from 927,000 to 840,000. Community hospital occupancy, estimated at 63 percent in 1998, has been relatively stable since the mid-1990's, after declining from 67 percent in 1990 and 76 percent in 1980 (table 109).

■ In 1997 there were almost 1.5 million elderly **nursing home residents** 65 years of age and over. One-half of the elderly residents were 85 years of age and over and three-fourths were female. Between the mid-1970's and 1997, nursing home utilization rates increased for the black population and decreased for the white population (table 96).

■ In 1998 there were 1.8 million **nursing home beds** in facilities certified for use by Medicare and Medicaid beneficiaries. Between 1995 and 1998 nursing home bed occupancy in those facilities was relatively stable, estimated at 84 percent in 1998 (table 113).

■ Between 1984 and 1994 the supply of beds in inpatient and residential **mental health organizations** declined 14 percent to 98 beds per 100,000 population. The decline was greatest for state and county mental hospitals with a reduction of 45 percent to 31 beds per 100,000 population (table 110).

National Health Expenditures

After 25 years of double-digit annual growth in national health expenditures, the rate of growth slowed during the 1990's. However the United States continues to spend more on health than any other industrialized country.

■ In 1998 **national health care expenditures** in the United States totaled almost $1.15 trillion, increasing less than 6 percent from the previous year and continuing the slowdown in growth of the 1990's. During the 1980's national health expenditures grew at an average annual rate of 11 percent (table 115).

■ This slowdown in growth is also reflected in the **Consumer Price Index (CPI)**. The rate of increase in the medical care component of the CPI declined from 6.3 percent in 1990–95 to 3.3 percent in 1995–99 (table 116).

■ The combination of strong economic growth and the slowdown in the rate of increase in health spending over the last few years has stabilized **health expenditures as a percent of the gross domestic product (GPD)** at 13.4–13.7 percent between 1995 and 1998, after increasing steadily from 8.9 percent in 1980 (table 115).

■ Despite the slowdown in the growth of health spending, the United States continues to spend a larger share of **GDP** on health than any other major industrialized country. The United States devoted 13.4 percent of GDP to health in 1997 compared with about 10–11 percent each in Germany, Switzerland, and France, the countries with the next highest shares. (table 114).

Expenditures by Type of Care and Source of Funds

Expenditures for hospital care as a percent of national health expenditures continue to decline. The sources of funds for medical care differ substantially according to the type of medical care being provided.

■ **Expenditures for hospital care** continued to decline as a percent of national health expenditures

from 42 percent in 1980 to 33 percent in 1998. Physician services accounted for 20 percent of the total in 1998, drugs for 11 percent, and nursing home care for 8 percent (table 118).

■ **Home health care expenditures** declined 6 percent between 1996 and 1998 as Medicare's new cost controls and fraud-and-abuse activities restrained growth in spending (table 118).

■ Between 1995 and 1998 **drug expenditures** increased at an average annual rate of 11 percent. The rate of increase for drug expenditures during this period was more than double the rate of increase for total national health expenditures. In 1999 prescription drugs posted one of the highest rates of increase in the Consumer Price Index, 5.7 percent (tables 116 and 118).

■ Between 1993 and 1998 the average annual increase in **total expenses in community hospitals** was 3.7 percent, following a period of higher growth that averaged 9.3 percent per year from 1985 to 1993 (table 122).

■ In 1998, 34 percent of **personal health care expenditures** were paid by the Federal Government and 10 percent by State and local government; private health insurance paid 33 percent and 20 percent was paid out-of-pocket (table 119).

■ In 1998 the major **sources of funds** for hospital care were Medicare (32 percent) and private health insurance (31 percent). Physician services were also primarily funded by private health insurance (51 percent) and Medicare (22 percent). In contrast, nursing home care was financed primarily by Medicaid (46 percent) and out-of-pocket payments (33 percent) (table 119).

■ In 1997 the average monthly charge per **nursing home** resident was $3,609. Residents for whom the source of payment was private insurance, family support, or their own income paid close to the average charge compared with an average monthly charge of over $6,000 when Medicare was the payor and $3,100 when Medicaid was the source of payment (table 124).

Health Care Expenditures

■   **The National Institutes of Health (NIH)** account for about 80 percent of Federal funding for health research and development. In 1997 the National Cancer Institute accounted for 20 percent of NIH's research and development budget, the National Heart, Lung and Blood Institute for 12 percent, and the National Institute of Allergy and Infectious Diseases for 10 percent. The Department of Defense accounted for 7 percent of Federal funding for health research and development (table 126).

■   In 1999 **Federal expenditures for HIV-related activities** increased 12 percent to $10 billion, compared with a 7-percent increase the previous year. Of the total Federal HIV-related spending in 1999, 58 percent was for medical care, 20 percent for research, 14 percent for cash assistance, and 8 percent for education and prevention (table 127).

Publicly Funded Health Programs

The two major publicly-funded health programs are Medicare and Medicaid. Medicare is funded by the Federal government and reimburses the elderly and the disabled for their health care. Medicaid is funded jointly by the Federal and State governments to provide health care for the poor. Medicaid benefits and eligibility vary by State. Medicare and Medicaid health care utilization and costs vary considerably by State.

■   In 1998 the **Medicare** program had 38.8 million enrollees and expenditures of $213 billion (table 133).

■   In 1996, 82 percent of **Medicare** beneficiaries were non-Hispanic white, 9 percent were non-Hispanic black, and 6 percent were Hispanic. Some 22–24 percent of Hispanic and non-Hispanic black beneficiaries were persons under 65 entitled to Medicare through disability compared with 10 percent of non-Hispanic white beneficiaries (table 135).

■   In 1996, 10 percent of non-Hispanic white **Medicare** beneficiaries had a nursing home stay compared with 8 percent of non-Hispanic black beneficiaries and 5 percent of Hispanic beneficiaries. White beneficiaries were also more likely to have received dental care than non-Hispanic black or

Hispanic beneficiaries (44 percent compared with 19 percent and 28 percent) (table 135).

■   Total health expenditures per **Medicare** beneficiary (including non-Medicare health expenditures) varied from $7,800 for Hispanic beneficiaries to $8,900 for non-Hispanic white and $10,670 for non-Hispanic black beneficiaries in 1996 (table 135).

■   In 1998 **hospital insurance (HI)** accounted for 64 percent of Medicare expenditures. Expenditures for home health agency care decreased to 9 percent of the HI expenditures in 1998, down from 13 percent in 1997. Expenditures for skilled nursing facilities continued to climb as a percent of the HI expenditures (10 percent in 1998) (table 133).

■   In 1998 **supplementary medical insurance (SMI)** accounted for 36 percent of Medicare expenditures. Payments to managed care organizations increased from 6 percent of the SMI expenditures in 1990 to 20 percent in 1998 (table 133).

■   Of the 33 million **Medicare enrollees** in the fee-for-service program in 1997, 11 percent were 85 years of age and over and 14 percent were under 65 years of age. Among elderly fee-for-service Medicare enrollees, payments increase with age from an average of $4,000 per enrollee for those aged 65–74 years to $7,900 for those 85 years and over (table 134).

■   In 1997 **Medicare payments per enrollee** averaged $5,416 in the United States, ranging from $3,700–$3,800 in North Dakota, South Dakota, Vermont, and Montana to more than $6,700 in Massachusetts, the District of Columbia, and Louisiana (table 143).

■   In 1998 **Medicaid** vendor payments totaled $142 billion for 40.6 million recipients (table 136).

■   In 1998 children under the age of 21 years comprised 47 percent of **Medicaid** recipients but accounted for only 16 percent of expenditures. The aged, blind, and disabled accounted for 26 percent of recipients and 71 percent of expenditures (table 136).

■ Of the 40.6 million **Medicaid** recipients in 1998, 41 percent were white, 24 percent black, 16 percent Hispanic, and 16 percent were of unknown race and ethnicity (table 136).

■ In 1998, 22 percent of **Medicaid** payments went to nursing facilities, 15 percent to general hospitals, 14 percent to prepaid health care, and 10 percent to prescribed drugs (table 137).

■ In 1998, 50 percent of **Medicaid** recipients used prepaid health care at a cost averaging $955 per recipient. One-fifth of recipients used early and periodic screening and family planning services but these services received just over 1 percent of Medicaid funds in 1998. The annual cost per recipient for screening and family planning averaged about $220 for each service (table 137).

■ In 1998 the percent of **Medicaid recipients enrolled in managed care** varied substantially among the States from 0 in Alaska and Wyoming to 98–100 percent in Montana, Colorado, and Tennessee (table 144).

■ Between 1997 and 1998 spending on health care by the **Department of Veterans Affairs** increased by less than 2 percent to $17.4 billion. In 1998, 38 percent of the total was for inpatient hospital care, down from 58 percent in 1990; 42 percent for outpatient care, up from 25 percent in 1990; and 10 percent for nursing home care, unchanged since 1990. In 1998, 55 percent of inpatients and 41 percent of outpatients were low-income veterans without service-connected disability (table 138).

■ In 1997 **State mental health agency per capita expenditures** for mental health services ranged from $23 in Tennessee and West Virginia to $113 in New York and averaged $64 per capita for the total United States (table 142).

Privately Funded Health Care

About 70 percent of the population has private health insurance, most of which is obtained through the workplace. The share of employees' total compensation devoted to health insurance has declined in recent years. The health insurance market continues to change rapidly as new types of managed care products are introduced. The use of traditional fee-for-service medical care continues to decline.

■ Between 1994 and 1997 the age-adjusted proportion of the population under 65 years of age with **private health insurance** has remained stable at 71–72 percent after declining from 76 percent in 1989. Some 92 percent of private coverage was obtained through the workplace (a current or former employer or union) in 1997 (table 128).

■ In 1999 **private employers' health insurance costs** per employee-hour worked increased from $1.00 to $1.03 after declining from $1.14 in 1994. Among private employers the share of total compensation devoted to health insurance declined from 6.7 percent in 1994 to 5.4 percent in 1998 and 1999 (table 121).

■ The average monthly contribution by full-time employees for family **medical care benefits** was 40 percent higher in small companies ($182 in 1996) than in medium and large companies ($130 in 1997) (table 132).

■ During the 1990's the use of **traditional fee-for-service** medical care benefits by full-time employees in private companies declined sharply. In 1996 in small companies, 36 percent of full-time employees who participated in medical care benefits were in fee-for-service plans, down from 74 percent in 1990. In 1997 in medium and large companies, 27 percent of participating full-time employees were in fee-for-service plans, down from 67 percent in 1991. In 1996–97 full-time employees in private companies who participated in medical care benefits were more likely to be enrolled in preferred provider organizations (PPO's) than in health maintenance organizations (HMO's) (table 132).

■ In 1999, 30 percent of the U.S. population was enrolled in **health maintenance organizations (HMO's)**, ranging from 23–24 percent in the Midwest and South to 37 percent in the Northeast and 41 percent in the West. HMO enrollment has been steadily increasing. Enrollment in 1999 was 81 million persons, more than double the enrollment in 1993 (table 131).

■ In 1997 non-Hispanic black and Hispanic persons were less likely to have private health insurance than were non-Hispanic white persons. However among those with private health insurance coverage, non-Hispanic black and Hispanic persons were more likely than their non-Hispanic white counterparts to enroll in **HMO's**. The elderly were less likely to be enrolled in private HMO's than were younger adults and children (table 130).

■ In 1999 the percent of the population enrolled in **HMO's** varied among the States from 0 in Alaska to 52–53 percent in California and Massachusetts. Other States with more than 40 percent of the population enrolled in HMO's in 1999 included Rhode Island, Delaware, Maryland, and Oregon (table 145).

■ In 1998 the proportion of the population without **health care coverage** (either public or private) was 16.3 percent, compared with 16.1 percent the previous year and 12.9 percent in 1987. In 1998 the proportion of the population without health care coverage varied from 10 percent or less in Hawaii, Rhode Island, Vermont, Minnesota, Iowa, and Nebraska, to 20 percent or more in Mississippi, Texas, New Mexico, Arizona, Nevada, and California (table 146).

The Adolescent Health Chartbook describes the health of the adolescent population, 10–19 years of age. Adolescence is a period of accelerated growth and change, bridging the complex transition from childhood to adulthood. Young people experience profound biological, emotional, intellectual, and social changes, and the patterns of behavior they adopt may have long-term consequences for their health and quality of life.

Definitions of adolescence, and the years encompassed, vary. Adolescence is generally regarded as the period of life from puberty to maturity; the meaning of "puberty" and "maturity" are often debated by health professionals. Many adolescents begin puberty by age 10, although there is significant individual variation in the developmental and maturation time line. By age 19, most adolescents have completed high school and are embarking on widely divergent paths and living situations—from college to military service to employment. They are completing their teen years and entering the young adult realm, with new legal standing, responsibilities and independence.

The population commonly referred to as "teenagers" constitutes a unique cohort in American population and society. This second decade of life is often a turbulent period, in which adolescents experience hormonal changes, physical maturation, and frequently, opportunities to engage in risk behaviors. During this period adolescents experience special vulnerabilities, health concerns, and barriers to accessing health care.

The teenage years are also a time of exploration, idealism, and cynicism. Adolescents have remarkable creativity, energy, and potential. This period offers adolescents an opportunity to begin planning for their futures, to adopt healthy attitudes about risk behaviors, and to develop meaningful roles in their communities. More teens than ever before are making committments to community service through volunteer activities.

Organization of the Chartbook

The chartbook presents data on the current status of adolescent health, with a focus on the changes in health status during the adolescent period. Many of the health status measures are shown by single year of age or by two- or three-year age intervals to highlight the changes that occur in health as adolescents move through this important developmental period. Summary measures combining 5- or 10-year age groups (the norm for analyses of childhood health events) do not adequately capture the wide variation in health status and the vast developmental differences between younger and older adolescents.

Race and ethnic variation in adolescent health is discussed when the data sources allow for such analysis. Gender differences in some aspects of health status among adolescents become more apparent with age. These are presented when the data allow for such analysis and the differences are notable.

Socioeconomic status, as measured by family income, poverty status, or level of parents' education, is strongly associated with the health of adolescents as well as the health of persons of all ages in the United States (1). Differences in the life circumstances of high- and low-socioeconomic status adolescents and their families influence health and health risk behavior through a number of pathways. Low family income decreases the ability to afford comfortable housing, healthy food, and appropriate health care, and to live in a safe and healthy environment. To fully assess the impact of socioeconomic factors in the health of adolescents, it is important to include examination of their school and family environments, as well as their broader sociostructural environments (2). A comprehensive presentation on socioeconomic status and adolescent health is beyond the scope of this chartbook. However, information on selected social determinants of health (figures 2–4) and the strong relationship between socioeconomic status and adolescent health has been documented in charts based on data sources that allow such analysis (figures 5, 6, 31, 32).

Characterizing the health of adolescents requires not only measuring mortality and morbidity but also describing other indicators of adolescent health. Risk behaviors, including behaviors that contribute to unintentional and intentional injuries, tobacco use, alcohol and other drug use, sexual behavior, physical inactivity, and unhealthy dietary behaviors may have a profound impact on current and future health. Reproductive health is a key element in adolescent health. The decision to become sexually active can have long-term and lasting consequences for some adolescents.

Healthy People 2010, a nationwide health promotion and disease prevention agenda that sets specific health objectives for the year 2010, also encompasses adolescent health (3). Twenty objectives have been designated as "critical adolescent objectives". Several of these objectives are included as leading Health Indicators in *Healthy People 2010*. Leading Health Indicators have been identified as major public health concerns of the U.S. and will be used to spotlight health achievements and challenges in the next decade. Throughout this chartbook, data that relate to either the 20 critical adolescent objectives or the Leading Health Indiators are noted as such.

This chartbook is divided into sections on population characteristics, health status, reproductive health, risk behaviors, and health care access. References are made to related tables in *Health, United States*. The 32 figures and accompanying text are followed by technical notes and data tables for each figure. Data tables include points graphed and for some charts additional related data are presented. The technical notes describe in further detail information about data sources and methods used that are not covered in the *Health, United States* Appendixes.

Population Characteristics

The first section of the chartbook describes selected sociodemographic characteristics of the adolescent population. One of the most notable characteristics is the changing distribution in the racial and ethnic composition of the adolescent population (figure 1). Today approximately 66 percent of adolescents are non-Hispanic white. It is estimated that in 2050, this proportion will decrease to 44 percent.

Other sociodemographic measures, including family structure, poverty status, employment, and dropout rates, describe the economic circumstances of adolescents (figures 2–4). Family structure affects adolescents' economic well-being (figure 2).

Educational achievement is one of the most important indicators of lifetime economic opportunity and is associated with health status. Adolescents who drop out of high school will have fewer opportunities to succeed in the work force than their peers who complete high school (figure 4).

Health Status

The second section of the chartbook presents selected measures of physical, dental, and mental health status. Although adolescents do have physical health problems, they are at a greatly reduced risk from life-threatening illnesses that affect the very young or very old. Some adolescents experience a disability or chronic health condition that limits their activity or requires special education services (figure 5). The negative effects of poverty on dental health status as measured by untreated dental caries are apparent in figure 6.

Many of the normal transitions of life, such as the adjustment to the physical and biological changes to their bodies and new levels of independence and responsibility can be stressful for teenagers. Although mood swings are a common feature of adolescence, more serious suicidal thoughts or suicide attempts are indicators of a mental or emotional health problem (figure 7).

Adolescents are the victims of violent acts in their homes, schools, and communities. During the period 1992–97 an average of 3.4 million adolescents each year were victims of violent crime, including rape or sexual assault, aggravated and simple assault, and robbery (figure 15).

To further assess adolescent health status, data on emergency department visits and hospital discharges were analyzed (figures 8–14). These sources identify health events for which emergency department care or inpatient hospital care was received and provide information on leading diagnoses for injury and noninjury among adolescents.

Injuries are a major cause of emergency department visits among adolescents. In 1995–97 four external causes of injury accounted for nearly 60 percent of all injury-related visits: falls, being struck by or against an object or person, cuts, and motor-vehicle crashes (figure 10). The most common injury diagnoses were fractures, sprains and strains, open wounds, and contusions (figure 11). Asthma, upper respiratory conditions and abdominal or gastrointestinal conditions were among the leading noninjury-related diagnoses for adolescents' visits to emergency departments in 1995–97 (figure 12).

Hospital discharge rates for both injury and noninjury diagnoses increased with age for male and female adolescents (figure 13). Asthma, psychoses, appendicitis, fractures, and poisoning were among the leading first-listed diagnoses for hospitalized adolescents in 1995–97, accounting for 20 percent of all hospital discharges (figure 14).

Mortality rates are a measure of the most serious adolescent health events. Leading causes of injury mortality are presented in figures 16–18. Motor vehicle traffic-related injuries and firearm-related injuries are the two leading causes of death among adolescents 10–19 years of age, accounting for 55 percent of all deaths (figure 17). Changes in mortality by single year of age across the adolescent period are significant and striking. Where adolescents reside, that is, in urban, suburban, or rural settings, influences mortality risks. In 1996–97 adolescents living in the most densely populated metropolitan counties had higher death rates associated with interpersonal violence, while those in rural counties had higher rates of motor vehicle-related fatalities (figure 18).

Reproductive Health

The onset of puberty is one of the benchmarks of adolescence. For the first time in their lives, adolescents are facing issues and decisions about their own sexuality. The majority of today's adolescents are becoming sexually active during their teen years and experiencing many of the health consequences associated with sexual activity, such as pregnancy or sexually transmitted disease. More than 900,000 adolescents become pregnant each year (figure 19). Sexually transmitted diseases are the most commonly reported infectious diseases among sexually active adolescents (figure 23). Although the overall incidence of AIDS in adolescents is relatively low, the rate of HIV infection is higher. Sexual activity and drug use

among adolescents place them at high risk for HIV transmission (figure 24) (4). Disparities by age, race and Hispanic origin were observed in all the measures of reproductive health.

In 1997–98 there were approximately 493,600 births each year to adolescent mothers, 13–19 years of age. Birth rates increased with age among all race and ethnicity groups, but varied widely by group (figure 20). Adolescent mothers have a higher risk of low-birthweight infants than mothers in their twenties and thirties (figure 21). Preterm or low-birthweight infants have a markedly increased risk of death or lifelong morbidity. The infant mortality rate among infants of adolescent mothers declines with increasing maternal age (figure 22). The infant mortality rate is an important indictor of the well-being of infants and their adolescent mothers.

Risk Behavior

Adolescents today are confronting societal and peer-related pressures to use tobacco, alcohol, or other drugs and to have sex at earlier ages. Many adolescents are engaging in risk behaviors that are harmful or dangerous to themselves and others, with consequences to their health and well-being that may be immediate or long term. Many of the patterns of behavior initiated during the adolescent years are associated with adult morbidity and mortality.

In 1999 one-half of all high school students had been sexually active; the proportion of students who reported ever having sexual intercourse and those who reported having multiple sex partners increased significantly with age (figure 25).

More than one-third of high school students reported smoking in the previous 30 days (figure 26). Although adolescents cannot legally purchase alcohol, drinking is commonplace among many high school students. One-half of all high school students reported drinking in the past 30 days (figure 27). Marijuana is the most commonly used illicit drug among high school students. In 1999 almost one-half of high school students used marijuana in their lifetime (figure 28).

Weapon carrying is associated with the most serious injuries resulting from violence. In 1999,

6 percent of female high school students and 29 percent of male students reported carrying a gun or other weapon (for example, a knife or club) in the previous 30 days (figure 29).

Although physical activity provides important health benefits for adolescents, the proportion of high school students who participate in physical activity was higher among students in 9th grade than in grades 10–12 (figure 30).

Health Care Access

Lack of health insurance is associated with diminished access to and use of preventive health services. Adolescents from poor and near poor families are morely likely to be uninsured than those from nonpoor families (figure 31). In 1997 adolescents without health insurance were more than twice as likely to not have visited a physician or other health professional in the past year as adolescents with health insurance (figure 32).

Chartbook Data Sources

The data presented in the chartbook are from nationally representative health surveys or vital statistics. One of the data sources, the Youth Risk Behavior Survey (YRBS), is a survey of high school students in grades 9–12. Figures based on the YRBS present data for adolescents by grade level rather than by age. Measures of risk behavior in YRBS are limited to the population of adolescents enrolled and attending high school. Consequently, the measures of risk behaviors in the chartbook may be slightly lower than if all high school-aged adolescents were included in the survey. In 1996, 5 percent of adolescents 14–17 years of age were not enrolled in school. These adolescents are at increased risk of alcohol, drug, and tobacco use, and are more likely to engage in violence-related behavior (5).

For data from the following systems, multiple years are combined to increase the reliability of estimates: the National Hospital Ambulatory Medical Care Survey (1995–97), the National Hospital Discharge Survey (1995–97), the National Crime Victimization Survey (1992–97), the National Vital

Statistics System, Mortality (1996–97), the National Vital Statistics System, Natality (1997–98), the National Linked File of Live Births and Infant Deaths (1995–97), and the AIDS Surveillance System (1996–98). The Third National Health and Nutrition Examination Survey was designed to provide estimates for the period 1988–94. See Technical Notes and Appendix I for descriptions of data sources.

In national surveys that are not specifically designed to study adolescents, the number of observations may not be large enough to analyze differences among age, sex, and race/ethnicity groups. For certain topics, data are presented for all races combined in the chart, and significant race differences (if they exist) are discussed in the accompanying text.

Other Sources of Data

In addition to the data sources used in this chartbook, we would like to acknowledge other sources of available data on adolescent health. Each of the following sources makes a unique contribution to the collective body of knowledge on adolescent health. The National Longitudinal Study of Adolescent Health (National Institutes of Health) was designed to study the influences on health and health behaviors in adolescence, with an emphasis on the social contexts in which adolescents live (6). Monitoring the Future (National Institute on Drug Abuse) is a nationally representative, annual survey of 8th-, 10th-, and 12th-grade students' values, behaviors, and lifestyle orientations (7). The 1998 National Alternative High School Youth Risk Behavior Survey (Centers for Disease Control and Prevention) collected information on health-risk behaviors among students who are at high risk for failing or dropping out of regular high school or who have been expelled from regular high school because of illegal activity or behavioral problems (8). *Great Transitions: Preparing Adolescents for a New Century*, is a report from the Carnegie Council on Adolescent Development about the nature and scope of adolescent problems (9). The National Adolescent Health Information Center at the University of California, San Francisco, with funding from Health Resources and Services Administration (HRSA) compiled data from a wide range of sources in their report *America's Adolescents: Are They Healthy?* (10). In 1997 the Commonwealth Fund conducted surveys of the health of adolescent girls and boys (11, 12). The Kaiser Family Foundation/YM Magazine National Survey of Teens: Teens Talk about Dating, Intimacy, and Their Sexual Experiences reports on a national survey of teens concerning the kinds of sexual situations they face (13). The U.S. Department of Health and Human Services (DHHS) has developed a website to provide information about America's adolescents (http://youth.hhs.gov/).

Data Gaps

Available data sources present several limitations for studying adolescent health. In some sources of data adolescents may not be considered as a separate group. They may be included in tabulations for children under age 15 or under age 18, or they may be included with young adults, ages 15–24. In such cases, trends pertaining specifically to adolescents cannot be separated from those pertaining to children or young adults. In data sources that do categorize adolescents separately, there are inconsistencies in the age ranges employed, making comparisons of data sources difficult. Furthermore, data for adolescents are often not available by single year of age. A major focus of this chartbook has been to address this limitation by presenting data by single year of age when possible.

Another obstacle in assessing the health status of the adolescent population is the lack of information on detailed racial and ethnic minority groups. The socioeconomic status and cultures of ethnic and racial groups may vary widely with important health consequences. Adolescents who are not white or black may be categorized as "other", masking notable health differences. In the chartbook, we presented the most detailed race and ethnic categories available given the constraints of numbers of observations.

For many data sources on adolescent health information on the socioeconomic status of the adolescents is not available. Educational attainment is often used as a measure of socioeconomic status for adults, but this is not a useful measure for an age group that has not yet completed their education. School-based surveys may collect health information

directly from adolescents who are not knowledgeable about their family's income or other measures of socioeconomic status.

There are also important preventive measures for which data are not available, such as the percent of adolescents who are routinely up to date on all their vaccinations.

Several areas exist in which the special needs or problems of adolescents have been recognized. But national data are not available to more fully explore these areas. Some of those issues are briefly discussed here.

■ Adolescents have unique needs in health care services and to meet these health care needs, routine health services must be available in a wide range of settings. While these needs have been recognized by researchers and health policy planners, information about the health services sought by and provided for adolescents is limited (10).

■ Female adolescents have an increased sensitivity about their bodies and the changes in shape and weight that accompany maturation. Some adolescents may develop eating disorders, such as anorexia or bulimia. Eating disorders may have potentially serious medical complications, yet they often go undetected and untreated. The prevalence of eating disorders is particularly difficult to measure because of the underlying denial and secretive nature of the behavior.

■ Although adolescent sexual activity has been well-documented, the extent to which sex is consensual has not been fully evaluated. Because many myths concerning rape persist among adolescents, acquaintance rape and date rape are often unreported and untreated (14, 15).

Conclusion

The health and risk behaviors of adolescents have consequences for their current and long term well-being as well as consequences for society. Today's adolescents are the future adults, parents, leaders, and work force of the Nation.

This chartbook examines a variety of current measures of health status, risk behavior, and health care from national data sources. The differences in health status between younger and older adolescents are documented. The health of the adolescent population also varies by sex, race and ethnicity, and socioeconomic status. Understanding patterns of health among adolescents requires attention to differences in the population and recognition of the economic and racial disparities that exist.

Overall, the majority of adolescents are healthy when assessed by traditional measures of morbidity and mortality. Many of the health threats for adolescents are primarily social and behavioral. Health-risk behaviors often are established during youth, extend into adulthood, and are interrelated (16). Adolescent risk behaviors have been linked to subsequent morbidity or mortality. Motor vehicle and firearm-related injuries are the leading causes of death for adolescents. Intervention and prevention strategies targeting risk behaviors during adolescence may prevent or reduce adolescent and adult morbidity and mortality and promote a healthier transition from childhood to adulthood.

References

1. Pamuk E, Makuc D, Heck K, Reuben C, Lochner K. Socioeconomic Status and Health Chartbook. Health, United States, 1998. Hyattsville, Maryland: National Center for Health Statistics. 1998.

2. E. Goodman. The role of socioeconomic status gradients in explaining differences in US Adolescents' Health. AJPH 89:1522–28. 1999.

3. U.S. Department of Health and Human Services. Healthy People 2010 (Conference Edition, in Two Volumes). Washington: January 2000.

4. Boyers DB, Kegeles SM. AIDS risk and prevention among adolescents. Soc sci Med 33(1):11–23. 1991.

5. Centers for Disease Control and Prevention. Health risk behaviors among adolescents who do and do not attend school: United States, 1992. Morb Mortal Wkly Rep;43:129–132.1994.

6. Resnick MD, Bearman PS, Blum RW, et al. Protecting adolescents from harm. Findings from the National Longitudinal Study on Adolescent Health. JAMA 278(10):823–32. 1997.

7. Wallace JM Jr, Forman TA, Guthrie BJ, Bachman JG, O'Malley PM, Johnston LD. The epidemiology of alcohol, tobacco and other drug use among black youth. J Stud Alcohol. 60(6):800–9. 1999.

8. Centers for Disease Control and Prevention. Youth Risk Behavior Surveillance—National Alternative High School Youth Risk Behavior Survey, United States, 1998. Mor Mortal Wkly Rep CDC Surveill Summ 48(7):1—44.1999.

9. Cohen MI. Great transitions, preparing adolescents for a new century: A commentary on the health component of the concluding report of the Carnegie Council on Adolescent Development. J Adolesc Health 19(1):2–5. 1996.

10. Ozer EM, Brindis CD, Millstein SG, Knopf DK, Irwin CE. America's adolescents: Are they healthy? San Francisco, California: University of California, San Francisco, National Adolescent Health Information Center. 1998.

11. Schoen C, Davis K, Collins KS, et al. The Commonwealth Fund Survey of the Health of Adolescent Girls. NewYork: The Commonwealth Fund. 1998.

12. Schoen C, Davis K, DesRoches C, Shekhdar A. The Health of Adolescent Boys: Commonwealth Fund Survey Findings. NewYork: The Commonwealth Fund. 1998.

13. Kaiser Family Foundation/YM Magazine. National Survey of Teens: Teens Talk about Dating, Intimacy, and their Sexual Experiences. Menlo Park, California: Kaiser Family Foundation. 1998.

14. Ellis GM. Acquaintance rape. Perspect Psychiatr Care 30(1):11–16. 1994.

15. Kershner R. Adolescent attitudes about rape. Adolescence 31(121):29–33. 1996.

16. Centers for Disease Control and Prevention. Youth Risk Behavior Surveillance—United States, 1997. Morb Mortal Wkly Rep 47(SS-3);1–89.1998.

Population

Race and Ethnicity

■ In 1999 almost 40 million residents of the United States were adolescents 10–19 years of age, comprising approximately 14 percent of the U.S. population. Two-thirds of the adolescent population were non-Hispanic white and one-third were of other racial and ethnic groups.

■ The race and Hispanic-origin distribution of the adolescent population, like the general population, changed significantly in the past 20 years, and is projected to continue to change. Projections of the population indicate that Hispanic, black, American Indian, and Asian adolescents will constitute 56 percent of the adolescent population by the year 2050.

■ Increasing racial and ethnic diversity in the general population is reflected in changes in the adolescent population. Although black adolescents are currently the largest minority group of adolescents, Hispanic adolescents will soon become the largest group. The proportion of adolescents who are of Asian or Pacific Islander origin nearly tripled between 1980 and 1999, from 1.6 percent to 4.2 percent. In contrast, there has been little change in the proportion of the adolescent population who are American Indians or Alaska Natives.

■ A large influx of immigrants contributed to changes in the population distribution. In 1990, 19 percent of adolescents lived in immigrant families—that is, the adolescent was an immigrant or had immigrant parents (1). Most future growth in the U.S. population is expected to occur primarily through immigration and higher fertility rates among minority populations (1, 2).

References
1. Hernandez DJ, Charney C, eds. From generation to generation: The health and well-being of children in immigrant families. National Academy Press. Washington: 1998.
2. Council of Economic Advisers for the President's Initiative on Race. Changing America: Indicators of social and economic well-being by race and Hispanic origin. Washington: 1998.

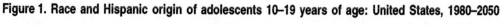

Figure 1. Race and Hispanic origin of adolescents 10–19 years of age: United States, 1980–2050

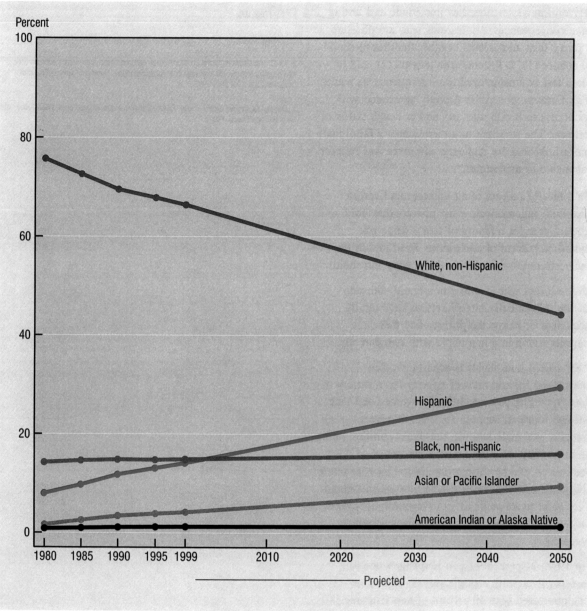

NOTES: Persons of Hispanic origin may be of any race. See Data Table for data points graphed.

SOURCE: U.S. Bureau of the Census, Population Estimates and Projections. See Technical Notes for population estimate methods. See related *Health, United States, 2000*, table 1.

Poverty and Family Structure

Poverty during adolescence has immediate and lasting negative consequences. Adolescents who are poor are more likely than adolescents in other families to drop out of school (1), to become teen parents (2), and to earn less and be unemployed more frequently as adults (3). Furthermore, poverty is strongly associated with poorer access to health care and poorer health status of adolescents. The structure of an adolescent's family is generally linked to the economic resources and support available to that adolescent.

▓ In 1998, 17 percent of all adolescents lived in families with incomes below the poverty threshold ($16,660 a year for a family of four), while an additional 20 percent of adolescents lived in families near poverty (one to two times the poverty threshold).

▓ Adolescents who live in a household with one parent are substantially more likely to have family incomes near or below the poverty line than adolescents living in a household with two parents.

▓ One-parent households headed by women experience the highest rates of poverty for a variety of reasons, including pay inequities for women and lack of paternal financial support. In 1998, 40 percent of all adolescents in female head-of-household families were living in poverty, compared with 8 percent of adolescents in two-parent families. Non-Hispanic black and Hispanic adolescents in female head-of-household families were twice as likely to have family incomes below the poverty line as their non-Hispanic white counterparts.

▓ In 1998, 24 percent of non-Hispanic white adolescents lived with a single parent (mother or father), compared with 59 percent of non-Hispanic black adolescents and 37 percent of adolescents of Hispanic origin.

▓ In contrast to many measures of adolescent health, no age differences were observed in family structure and poverty for adolescents.

References

1. National Center for Education Statistics. The condition of education. 1998.

2. An C, Haveman R, Wolfe B. Teen out-of-wedlock births and welfare receipt: The role of childhood events and economic circumstances. Review of Economics and Statistics 75(2):195–208. 1993.

3. Duncan G, Brooks-Gunn J, eds. Consequences of growing up poor. New York: Russell Sage Press. 1997.

Figure 2. Poverty by family structure, race, and Hispanic origin among adolescents 10–17 years of age: United States, 1998

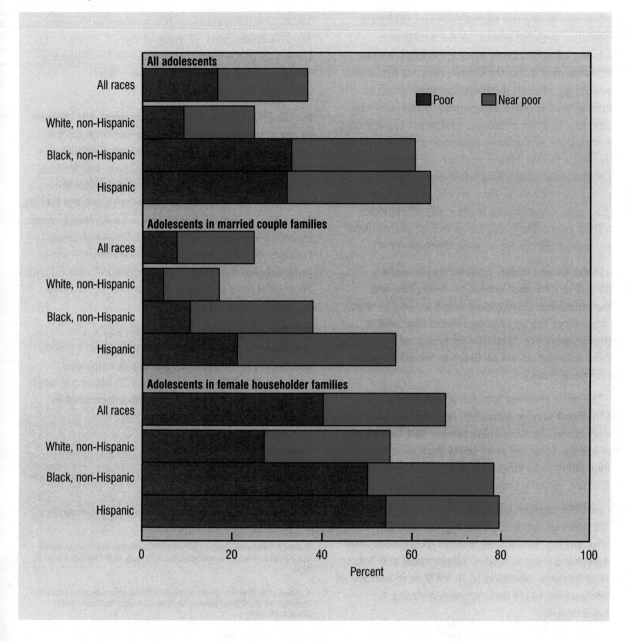

NOTES: Poverty status is derived from the ratio of the family's income to the Federal poverty threshold, given family size. Poor is less than 100 percent of the poverty threshold; near poor is between 100 and 199 percent of the poverty threshold. See Technical Notes for further discussion of poverty threshold. See Data Table for data points graphed.

SOURCE: U.S. Bureau of the Census, Current Population Survey, March Supplement 1999.

Population

Employment

Employment during the adolescent years may have beneficial or negative effects on the health and well-being of youth. Early work experience among adolescents may aid in the development of personal responsibility, smooth the transition from youth to adulthood, and improve occupational attainment and income (1). In some instances, adolescent employment may contribute to the basic economic resources of the adolescent's family. However, there are health and safety concerns for working adolescents. Working teens are more likely to have problems in school and are less able to participate in after school activities than their peers. They also are at risk of occupational injury and of illness due to toxic exposure (2–4).

■ In the United States, adolescents are often employed in jobs after school, on weekends, and during vacations. Employment refers to jobs in which the adolescent has an ongoing relationship with a particular employer. Freelance jobs such as babysitting or lawn mowing are not included in the adolescent employment statistics.

■ The most common jobs for adolescents are in fast-food and service industries, restaurants, retail and grocery stores, farms, nursing homes, and factories. Low-income teens are more likely than their higher income peers to be employed in high-risk jobs such as agriculture, manufacturing, and construction (2).

■ In 1999 approximately two-fifths of all adolescents 16–19 years of age worked during the school year (April). During the summer months (July) when most adolescents are not in school, employment and hours worked increase substantially. In 1999 over one-half of all adolescents 16–19 were employed during the summer months.

■ The proportion of teens who worked increased with age. For example, in 1999 the proportion of teens working during the school year increased from 26 percent of 16-year olds to 56 percent of 19-year olds. Overall, adolescent males and females were equally likely to be employed.

■ Hazardous work environments put adolescents at risk of serious injury or death. During the period 1992–97 there were over 400 fatalities in the work place to adolescents 17 years of age or younger (5). Causes of death included highway and nonhighway vehicle-related incidents, homicides, falls, electrocutions, and fires.

■ In 1998 almost 260,000 adolescents 15–19 years of age were treated in emergency departments for occupational injuries (6). Common nonfatal injuries include sprains and strains, burns, cuts, and bruises. Most persons less than 18 years of age enter the workplace with minimal prior experience for a job (3). More than one-half of adolescents 14–16 years of age treated in emergency departments for work injuries reported that they had received no training in the prevention of the injury they sustained. Healthy People 2010 objectives call for a reduction in the incidence of adolescent work injuries (7).

■ Teens who work more than 20 hours a week are considered to be at a higher risk of negative health outcomes (3). In 1999, 43 percent of employed adolescents worked for more than 20 hours per week during the school year. That number increased to 68 percent during the summer.

References

1. Ruhm C. High school employment: Consumption or investment. Bureau of Labor Statistics. Report NLS94–19. 1994.

2. Landrigan PJ, McCammon JB. Child labor—still with us. Public Health Rep 112:467–73. 1997.

3. Centers for Disease Control and Prevention. Work-related injuries and illnesses associated with child labor—United States, 1993. Morb Mort Wkly Rep 45:464–68. 1996.

4. Resnick MD, Bearman PS, Blum RW, et al. Protecting adolescents from harm. Findings from the National Longitudinal Study on Adolescent Health. JAMA 278:823–32. 1997.

5. Windau J, Sygnatur E, Toscano G. Profile of work injuries incurred by young workers. Monthly Labor Review June 1999.

6. U.S. Consumer Product Safety Commission. National Electronic Injury Surveillance System. 1998.

7. U.S. Department of Health and Human Services. Healthy People 2010 (Conference Edition, in Two Volumes). Washington: January 2000.

Population

Figure 3. Employment during April and July among adolescents 16–19 years of age, by age, race, and Hispanic origin: United States, 1999

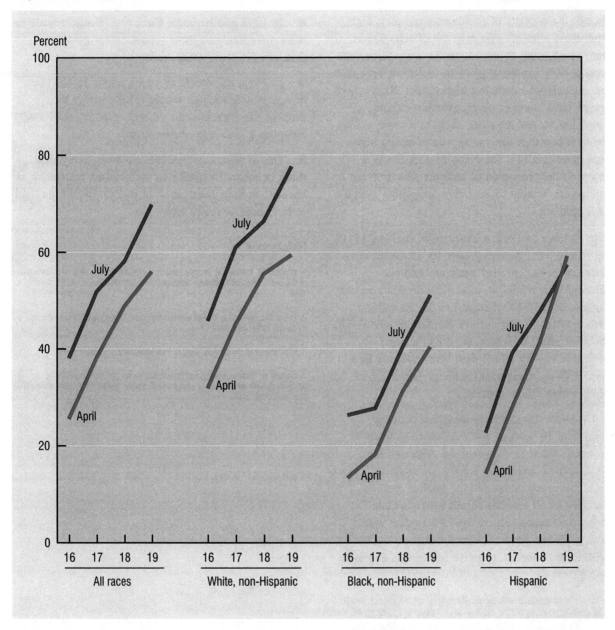

NOTES: Employment is defined as a job in which the adolescent has an ongoing relationship with a particular employer for any number of hours per week. The Bureau of Labor Statistics uses April as representative of school year employment and July as representative of summer employment. See Data Table for data points graphed.

SOURCE: Bureau of Labor Statistics, Current Population Survey, Basic Monthly Survey, April and July 1999.

Population

Dropout Rates

Although the majority of adolescents complete high school, those students who drop out of school have fewer opportunities to succeed in the work force or to assume a fully functional place in society at large than those students who complete high school. High school dropouts have lower earnings, experience more unemployment, and are more likely to receive welfare or be in prison than their peers who complete high school or college (1). The event dropout rate is a measure of the proportion of students who drop out in a single year without successfully completing a high school program.

■ In October of 1998, 4.2 percent of students 15–19 years of age, who were in grades 10–12 the previous October, were not enrolled again and had not completed high school. In total these dropouts account for approximately 400 thousand of the 9.8 million adolescents 15–19 years of age enrolled in school. The cumulative effect of several hundred thousand adolescents leaving school each year translates into several million young adults who are out of school, but lacking a high school credential.

■ The event dropout rates increased with age. Adolescents 18 years of age were twice as likely to drop out as those 15–17 years old. Although the highest dropout rates were among adolescents 19 years of age, this group comprised the smallest portion (8 percent) of all students enrolled the previous October. Increasing relative age of a student within school grade has been associated with behavioral problems, absenteeism, negative self-image, and high dropout rates (2).

■ Socioeconomic status is strongly associated with the decision to stay in school. Students from low income families (lowest 20 percent of family incomes) dropped out of high school at a rate over 3 times that of adolescents from middle income families, and over 4 times the rate of adolescents from high income families (highest 20 percent of family incomes).

■ In 1998 non-Hispanic black and Hispanic students were more likely to leave school before graduating than non-Hispanic white students.

■ In 1998, 85 percent of young adults 18–24 years of age completed high school (3). Reducing the dropout rate increases the percent of young adults who complete a high school education.

■ Out of school adolescents are more likely than those in school to smoke, to use alcohol, marijuana, or cocaine, to have been involved in a physical fight, and to have been sexually active (4).

References

1. McMillen M, Kaufman P. Dropout rates in the United States: 1996. U.S. Department of Education, National Center for Education Statistics. Washington: NCES 98–250. 1997.

2. Hayes DN, Hemenway D. Age-within-school-class and adolescent gun-carrying. Pediatrics 103(5):e64. 1999.

3. U.S. Bureau of the Census. Current Population Survey. October 1998.

4. Centers for Disease Control and Prevention. Health risk behaviors among adolescents who do and do not attend school: United States, 1992. Morb Mortal Wkly Rep 43:129–32. 1994.

Figure 4. Event dropout rates among adolescents 15–19 years of age, by age, race, Hispanic origin, and family income: United States, 1998

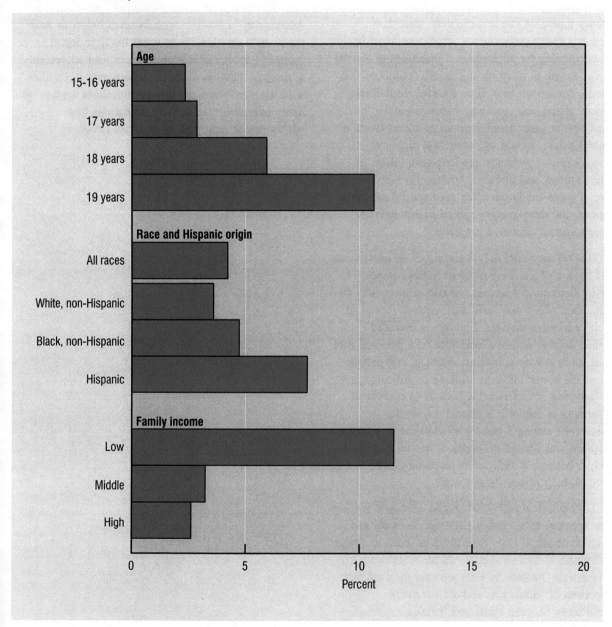

NOTES: The event dropout rate is the percent of those in grades 10–12, ages 15–19, who were enrolled the previous October, but who were not enrolled and had not graduated the following October. Low income is the bottom 20 percent of all family incomes; high income is the top 20 percent of all family incomes; middle income is the 60 percent in between. Age when a person dropped out may be one year younger because the dropout event can occur at any time over a 12-month period. See Data Table for data points graphed.

SOURCE: U.S. Bureau of the Census, Current Population Survey, October 1998.

Activity Limitation

Activity limitation due to a physical, mental, or emotional health problem is a broad measure of health and functioning for adolescents. Limitations in activity are due to one or more chronic health conditions that include, but are not limited to, learning disabilities; hearing, visual, and speech problems; mental retardation or other developmental problems (such as cerebral palsy); mental and emotional problems; musculoskeletal problems; the long-term effects of injury; asthma; and diabetes. Adolescents with one or more of these conditions often need special education services, and many receive special health services through special education programs.

■ In 1997 approximately 8 percent of all adolescents 10–17 years of age were reported to have some activity limitation; 3 percent had one or more activity limitations, which may have also required receipt of special education services. Limitations included needing another person's assistance with personal care needs, such as eating, bathing, dressing, and getting around the home; difficulty walking or difficulty remembering or experiencing periods of confusion. Performing in school is a normal activity for adolescents; among 5 percent of adolescents, activity limitation was limited to receipt of special education services because of difficulty understanding or accomplishing routine school work.

■ Differences in receipt of special education services were apparent by gender, but not age. In every age group, male adolescents were twice as likely as female adolescents to receive special education services. All other activity limitations were reported for a smaller proportion of adolescents and did not differ significantly between males and females.

■ Non-Hispanic white and non-Hispanic black adolescents were more likely to report enrollment in special education services or other activity limitations than their Hispanic peers.

■ The proportion of adolescents with health-related activity limitations varied by poverty status.

Adolescents in families with incomes below or near the poverty threshold were more likely to report receipt of special education services than adolescents in nonpoor families in 1997. Adolescents in families with incomes below the poverty threshold were more likely to report other activity limitations than adolescents in near poor or nonpoor families.

Figure 5. Activity limitation among adolescents 10–17 years of age, by sex, age, race, Hispanic origin, and poverty status: United States, 1997

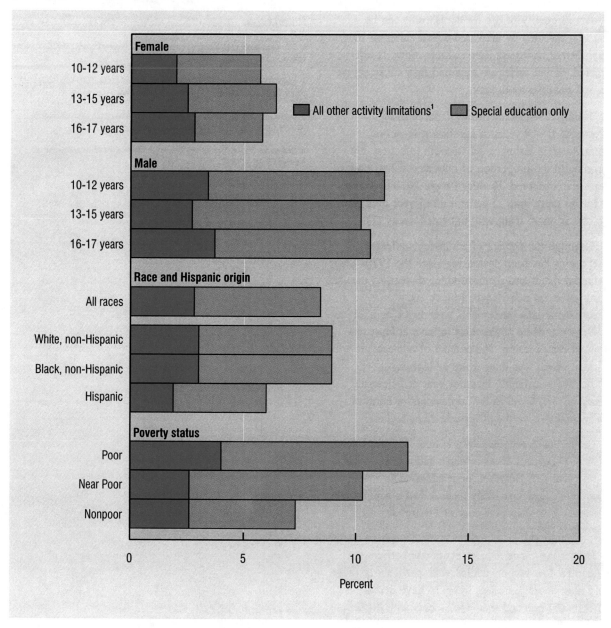

[1]This category may include adolescents receiving special education.

NOTES: Poverty status is derived from the ratio of the family's income to the Federal poverty threshold, given family size. Poor is less than 100 percent of the poverty threshold; near poor is between 100 and 199 percent of the poverty threshold; nonpoor is 200 percent of the poverty threshold or more. See Technical Notes for discussion of activity limitation. See Data Table for data points graphed.

SOURCE: Centers for Disease Control and Prevention, National Center for Health Statistics. National Health Interview Survey. See related *Health, United States, 2000*, table 57.

Untreated Dental Caries

The overall quality of life for adolescents can be negatively affected by untreated dental caries or tooth decay. Dental caries are bacterial infections. If left untreated, dental caries advance and may cause severe pain and possible tooth loss.

■ During 1988–94 one-fifth (19 percent) of adolescents 10–19 years of age had at least one untreated caries lesion or active tooth infection. No difference in the proportion of untreated dental caries by age was observed. Healthy People 2010 objectives call for no more than 15 percent of 15-year olds to have one or more teeth with untreated decay (1).

■ Although the percent of adolescents affected by dental caries has been decreasing since the 1970s (2), substantial racial and socioeconomic disparities persist. During 1988–94 non-Hispanic black and Mexican-American adolescents were twice as likely as non-Hispanic white adolescents to have at least one untreated caries lesion. The percent of adolescents with untreated caries was three times as high for adolescents with family incomes near or below the Federal poverty level as for adolescents in families with incomes twice the poverty level or higher.

■ Dental visits are necessary to treat decayed teeth. In 1997, 77 percent of adolescents had a dental visit in the past year (3). However, poor adolescents (64 percent) were less likely to have had a dental visit in the past year than near-poor and nonpoor adolescents (80 percent).

■ Dental insurance reduces economic barriers to dental care; low-income adolescents, particularly those living near poverty are less likely to have dental insurance (51 percent) than adolescents with higher family incomes (65 percent) or those living below the poverty level (60 percent) (4).

References

1. U.S. Department of Health and Human Services. Healthy People 2010 (Conference Edition, in Two Volumes). Washington: 2000.

2. National Center for Health Statistics. Health, United States, 2000 With Adolescent Health Chartbook. Hyattsville, Maryland: Table 72. 2000.

3. Centers for Disease Control and Prevention. National Health Interview Survey. National Center for Health Statistics. 1997.

4. Centers for Disease Control and Prevention. National Health Interview Survey. National Center for Health Statistics. 1995.

Figure 6. Untreated dental caries among adolescents 10–19 years of age, by family income, race, and Hispanic origin: United States, 1988–94

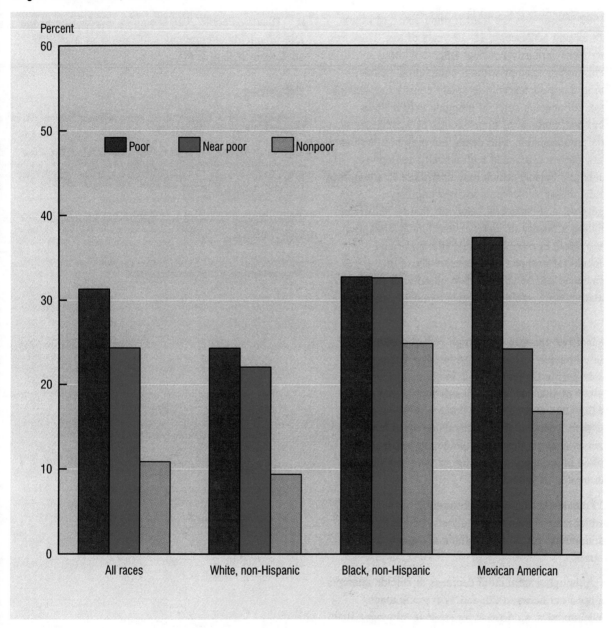

NOTES: Data are based on dental examinations of a sample of the civilian noninstitutionalized population. The income groups are derived from the ratio of the family's income to the Federal poverty threshold, given family size. Poor is less than 100 percent of the poverty threshold; near poor is between 100 and 199 percent of the poverty threshold; nonpoor is 200 percent of the poverty threshold or more. See Data Table for data points graphed.

SOURCE: Centers for Disease Control and Prevention, National Center for Health Statistics, The Third National Health and Nutrition Examination Survey (NHANES III). See related *Health, United States, 2000*, table 81.

Suicide Ideation and Attempts

In 1997 suicide was the third leading cause of injury death among adolescents 13–19 years of age. However, many teens seriously consider suicide without attempting, or attempt without completing suicide. Among those adolescents seriously considering suicide, factors influencing suicidal thoughts may include depression, feelings of hopelessness or worthlessness, and a preoccupation with death, but may not be related to risk factors associated with actually attempting suicide (1). Factors which may contribute to attempting suicide among adolescents include impulsive, aggressive, and antisocial behavior; family influences, including a history of violence and family disruption; severe stress in school or social life; and rapid sociocultural change (2). Substance abuse or dependence can be an important contributor in the escalation from suicidal thoughts to suicide attempts (3).

■ In 1999 one-fifth of all high school students reported having seriously considered or attempted suicide during the previous 12 months. Less than one-half of students who seriously considered suicide actually attempted suicide (8 percent of all students). Less than 3 percent of all students reported having an injurious attempt, that is, a suicide attempt that resulted in an injury, poisoning, or overdose that had been treated by a doctor.

■ Female students were substantially more likely to consider suicide than male students. This difference was identified for all racial/ethnic and grade level subgroups.

■ Although a substantial decrease in suicide attempts was apparent between 9th and 12th grade among female students, a decrease by grade level among male students was not significant. Suicide attempts among non-Hispanic white and Hispanic female students were significantly higher than among their male counterparts; among non-Hispanic black students there was no difference by gender. In contrast, the rate of completed suicides is higher among male adolescents than female adolescents (figure 16).

■ Healthy People 2010 identifies a reduction in the rate of suicide attempts by adolescents as a critical adolescent objective (4).

References

1. Behrman RE, Kliegman RM, Arvin AM, eds. Nelson Textbook of Pediatrics. 15th ed. Philadelphia: W.B. Saunders Company. 1996.

2. Goodwin FK, Brown GL. Risk factors for youth suicide. In: Alcohol, Drug Abuse, and Mental Health Administration. Report of the Secretary's Task Force on Youth Suicide. Vol 2. Washington: U.S. Department of Health and Human Services, Public Health Service, Alcohol, Drug Abuse, and Mental Health Administration; DHHS publication no. (ADM)89–1622. 1989.

3. Gould MS, King R, Greenwald S, et al. Psychopathology associated with suicidal ideation and attempts among children and adolescents. J Am Acad Child Adolesc Psychiatry 37(9):915–23. 1998.

4. U.S. Department of Health and Human Services. Healthy People 2010 (Conference Edition, in Two Volumes). Washington: January 2000.

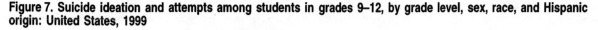

Figure 7. Suicide ideation and attempts among students in grades 9–12, by grade level, sex, race, and Hispanic origin: United States, 1999

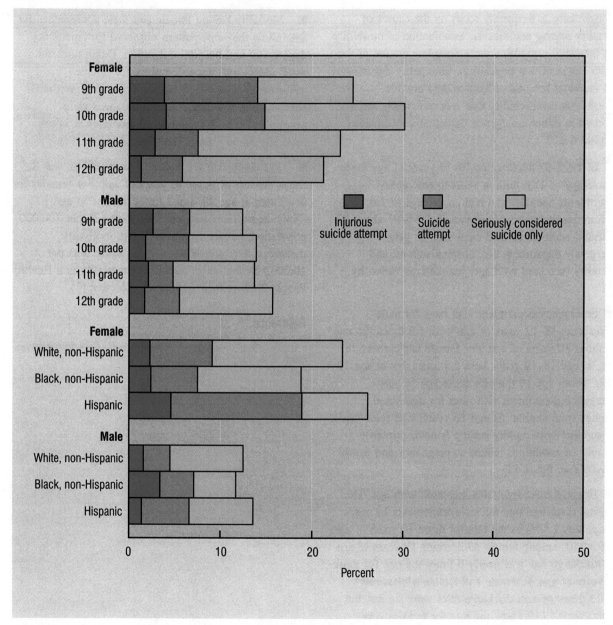

NOTES: Response is for the 12 months preceding the survey. Among students attempting suicide, 6 percent did not report seriously considering suicide. See Technical Notes for survey methods. See Data Table for data points graphed.

SOURCE: Centers for Disease Control and Prevention, National Center for Chronic Disease Prevention and Health Promotion, National Youth Risk Behavior Survey (YRBS).

Emergency Department Visits, Hospital Discharges, and Death Rates

Though there is frequently focus on the causes of mortality among adolescents, examination of morbidity and mortality provides a more complete picture of the health status of that population. Emergency department and inpatient hospital utilization data provide information on morbidity that was sufficiently serious to result in either emergency department or inpatient hospital use.

■ In 1995–97 adolescents 10–19 years of age made an average of 11.6 million visits to emergency departments annually and had an average of 1.6 million hospitalizations per year. In 1996–97 about 19 thousand adolescents died each year. In general, emergency department use, hospitalizations, and mortality increased with age, but patterns varied by sex.

■ Emergency department visit rates for male adolescents 18–19 years of age were 1.6 times the rate for those 10 years of age. For female adolescents, the rates at age 18–19 years were 2.5 times that at age 10 years. From age 10 through about age 16 years, emergency department visit rates for males and females were similar. At age 16 years, visit rates began to increase more rapidly among females primarily because of conditions related to pregnancy and sexual activity (see figure 12).

■ Hospital discharge rates increased with age. The hospital discharge rate for male adolescents 19 years of age was 1.5 times the rate for those 10 years of age. In contrast, among female adolescents 19 years of age the discharge rate was nearly 9 times the rate for those 10 years of age. For male and female adolescents 11–13 years of age, discharge rates were similar, but from ages 14 –19 years, the rate for females was higher than that for males with differences increasing with age. Hospitalization for pregnancy and delivery was the cause of those differences (see figure 13).

■ Mortality among female and male adolescents did not follow the same pattern observed for emergency department and hospital utilization. Death rates for male adolescents exceeded those for female adolescents at each age and the difference increased substantially with age. These differences were primarily due to the age-related increases in injury mortality among males (see figures 16 and 17).

■ The death rate for males 19 years of age was 8 times the rate of those 10 years of age. For females the death rate at age 19 was 3 times the rate at age 10. (Note: death rates are generally shown as per 100,000 population, but for comparability to morbidity measures, they are shown only in figure 8 as per 10,000.) Reduction of adolescent mortality is a Healthy People 2010 critical adolescent objective (1).

Reference

1. U.S. Department of Health and Human Services. Healthy People 2010 (Conference Edition, in Two Volumes). Washington: 2000.

Figure 8. Emergency department visit rates, hospital discharge rates, and death rates among adolescents 10–19 years of age, by age and sex: United States, average annual 1995–97

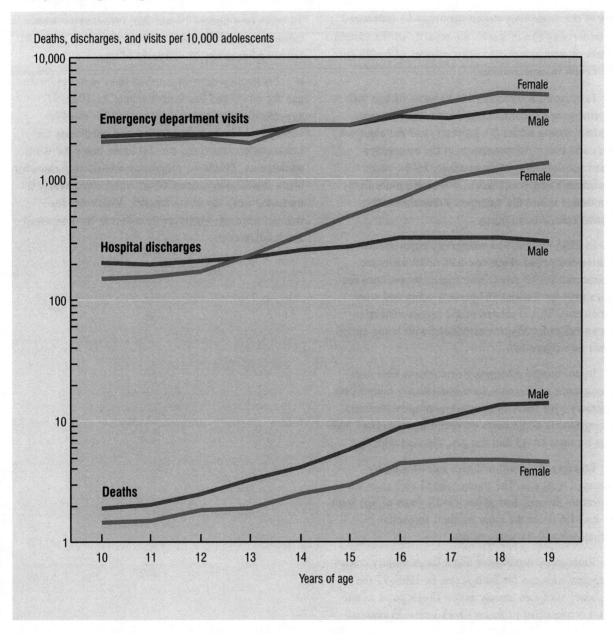

Deaths, discharges, and visits per 10,000 adolescents

NOTES: Death rates are for 1996–97 only. See Appendix I, National Hospital Ambulatory Medical Care Survey and National Hospital Discharge Survey; Appendix II, Cause of Death, and Rate: Death. See Data Table for data points graphed.

SOURCE: Centers for Disease Control and Prevention, National Center for Health Statistics, National Hospital Ambulatory Medical Care Survey (NHAMCS); National Hospital Discharge Survey (NHDS); National Vital Statistics System.

Health Status

Emergency Department Visits

Use of the emergency department may be influenced by underlying health status, the severity of the current illness or injury, access to other sources of health care, and health insurance status.

■ In general, adolescents 10–19 years of age visit the emergency department less often than younger children, young adults 20–24 years, and the elderly 65 years and older. Adolescents visit the emergency department about as often as adults 25–64 years. Adolescents and young adults 20–24 are more likely than others to use the emergency department for reasons related to an injury.

■ In 1995–97 visits to emergency departments for injuries comprised about one-half of all visits for adolescents 10–19 years, with higher proportions for males than for females (63 percent compared with 41 percent). This is related to the higher visit rates among males for injuries associated with being struck or cut (see figure 10).

■ Injury-related emergency department visit rates among male adolescents were consistently higher than noninjury visit rates. In contrast, noninjury visit rates among female adolescents exceeded injury-related visit rates by ages 14–15 and the gap widened with age.

■ Emergency department visit rates for injury increased with age. The injury-related visit rates for adolescent females and males 18–19 years of age were 1.5 and 1.6 times the rates for their respective counterparts 10–11 years of age.

■ Emergency department visits for noninjury causes increased with age for both sexes. In 1995–97 the noninjury visit rate among males 18–19 years of age was 1.6 times that of those 10–11 years. In contrast, among female adolescents 18–19 years of age, the noninjury (and nonpregnancy-related) visit rate was triple that of adolescents 10–13 years of age.

■ Pregnancy-related emergency department visit rates increased almost sevenfold between ages 14 and 19 years (see figures 19 and 20). Pregnancy-related causes accounted for about 11 percent of all visits for female adolescents 18–19 years of age.

■ Emergency department visit rates increased with age for white and black adolescents. In 1995–97 age-specific emergency department visit rates for noninjury and nonpregnancy-related conditions for black adolescents were 1.6–2.0 times those for white adolescents. Similarly, pregnancy-related visit rates for black female adolescents 16–19 years were nearly 3 times the rates for white females. Visit rates for injuries were not significantly different for white and black adolescents.

Figure 9. Emergency department visit rates for injury, noninjury, and pregnancy-related diagnoses among adolescents 10–19 years of age, by age and sex: United States, average annual 1995–97

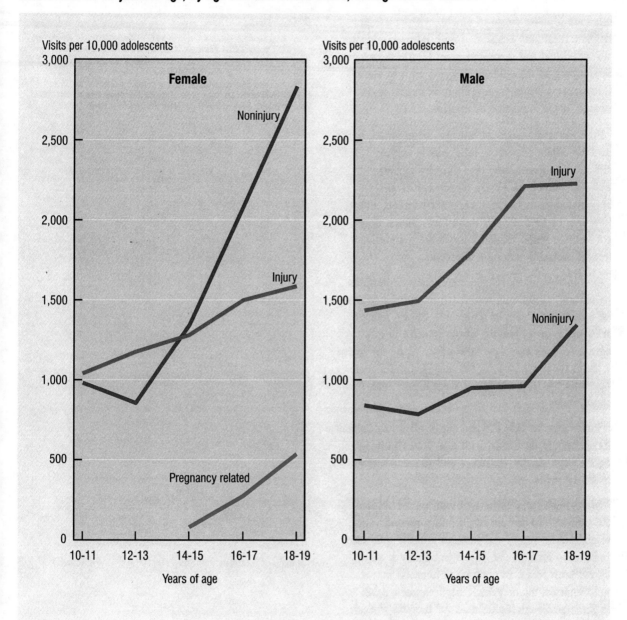

NOTES: See Technical Notes for discussion of emergency department visits. See also Appendix I, National Hospital Ambulatory Medical Care Survey. See Data Table for data points graphed.

SOURCE: Centers for Disease Control and Prevention, National Center for Health Statistics, National Hospital Ambulatory Medical Care Survey (NHAMCS).

Health Status

Injury-Related Visits to Emergency Departments

Injuries are a major cause of emergency department visits. The morbidity associated with injuries is costly on an individual and a societal level (1, 2). A greater understanding of the epidemiology of injuries should lead to improved injury prevention strategies and decreases in the incidence of injuries.

■ Four external causes of injury—being struck by or against an object or person, falls, motor vehicle traffic-related injuries, and being cut by a sharp object—accounted for nearly 60 percent of all injury-related visits to emergency departments among adolescents in 1995–97. Of these four causes, only motor vehicle traffic-related injuries are a significant source of mortality among adolescents.

■ One in five injury-related emergency department visits among adolescents resulted from "being struck by or against an object or a person". Sports-related injuries made up 41 percent of the injuries in this category. At each age, the "struck by..." rate for males was about twice the rate for females. Rates for male adolescents 14–19 years of age were higher than for younger males.

■ Visit rates for falls (16 percent of all injury-related visits) generally decreased with age. Rates in this category were similar for males and females across ages 10–19 years.

■ Injury visit rates associated with motor vehicle traffic injuries (14 percent of all injury-related visits) were similar for males and females at each age, with large relative increases at 14–15 years and at 16–17 years for both sexes. In contrast to nonfatal motor vehicle injuries, motor vehicle traffic-related death rates for males were higher than for females at each age from 10–19 years (see figure 17).

■ Visits for injuries from being cut (9 percent of all injury-related visits) also increased with age, especially from ages 12–13 years to 16–19 years.

References

1. Rice DP, Mackenzie EJ, Associates. Cost of injury in the United States: A report to Congress. San Francisco, California: Institute for Health and Aging, University of California and Injury Prevention Center. The Johns Hopkins University. 1989.

2. Burt CW, Fingerhut LA. Injury visits to hospital emergency departments: United States, 1992–95. National Center for Health Statistics. Vital Health Stat 13(131). 1998.

Figure 10. Emergency department visit rates for selected external causes of injury among adolescents 10–19 years of age, by age and sex: United States, average annual 1995–97

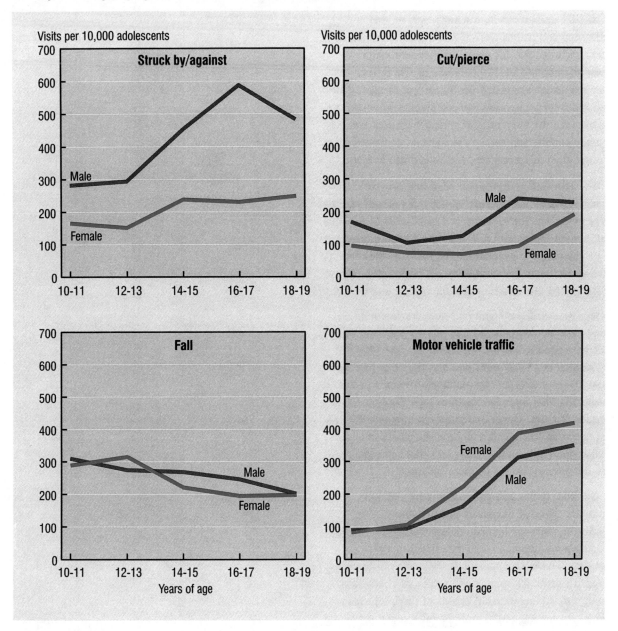

NOTES: See Technical Notes for discussion of emergency department visits. See also Appendix I, National Hospital Ambulatory Medical Care Survey. See Data Table for data points graphed.

SOURCE: Centers for Disease Control and Prevention, National Center for Health Statistics, National Hospital Ambulatory Medical Care Survey (NHAMCS). See related *Health, United States, 2000*, table 84.

Adolescent Health ....

Health, United States, 2000

Health Status

Injury-Related Visits to Emergency Departments

In 1995–97 open wounds, fractures, sprains and strains, and contusions were the four most common injury diagnoses for emergency department visits among adolescents 10–19 years of age. These four injury diagnoses accounted for 80 percent of all first-listed injury diagnoses for adolescents. Open wound injuries were the most often reported diagnoses for male adolescents and sprains, strains and contusions were the most often reported for female adolescents.

■   The emergency department visit rate for open wounds for male adolescents 18–19 years of age was nearly twice that for adolescents 12–15 years of age. Open wound injury visit rates for female adolescents 10–19 years of age were about one-half the rates for males at each age. These injuries are caused primarily by knives and other instruments for cutting or piercing.

■   Emergency department visit rates for fractures among male adolescents did not vary by age. The rates for female adolescents declined with age; the visit rate for fractures at 18–19 years was less than one-half the rate at 10–11 years. Among males 14–19 years of age, age-specific visit rates for fractures were about 3 times those for females. Upper extremity fracture was the most common fracture site reported for males and females. Injuries resulting from falls and being struck were the primary causes of these fractures.

■   Sprains, strains and contusions were the most commonly reported diagnoses in emergency department visits for female adolescents 10–19 years, accounting for one-half of all first-listed injury diagnoses. There were no significant gender differences by age for visits for sprains and strains or contusions. Among the leading external causes of these injuries were motor vehicle traffic crashes, falls, being struck and overexertion.

Figure 11. Emergency department visit rates for selected injury diagnoses among adolescents 10–19 years of age, by age and sex: United States, average annual 1995–97

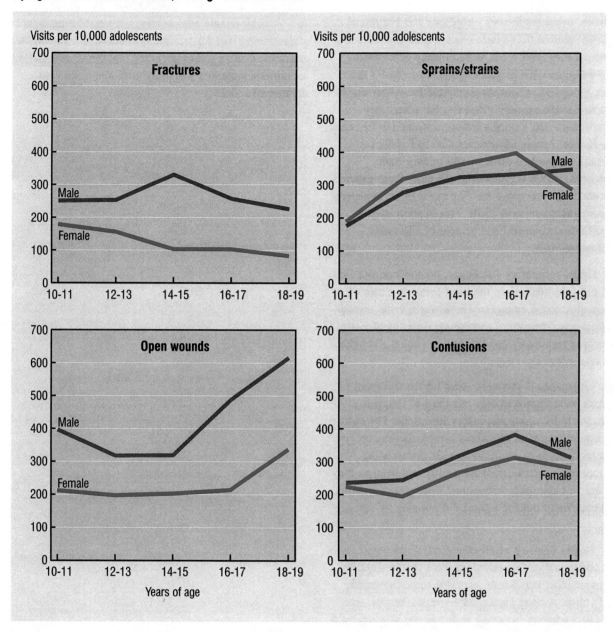

NOTES: See Technical Notes for discussion of emergency department visits. See also Appendix I, National Hospital Ambulatory Medical Care Survey. See Data Table for data points graphed.

SOURCE: Centers for Disease Control and Prevention, National Center for Health Statistics, National Hospital Ambulatory Medical Care Survey (NHAMCS).

Noninjury Visits to Emergency Departments

Asthma, upper respiratory conditions and abdominal or gastro-intestinal (GI) conditions are among the leading principal diagnoses made in emergency departments for adolescents 10–19 years of age. In 1995–97 these three groups of conditions accounted for 40 percent of all first-listed noninjury diagnoses for emergency department visits among adolescent males 10–19 years. In addition, female adolescents also had visits for sexually transmitted diseases and urinary tract infections, which together with the other three groups of conditions accounted for 50 percent of all noninjury (nonpregnancy-related) visits. Pregnancy-related conditions accounted for 5 percent of all female adolescent visits.

■ Upper respiratory conditions, predominantly colds, and ear infections, were the most common cause of noninjury-related emergency department visits among adolescents. The rate of emergency department visits for upper respiratory conditions was similar throughout the adolescent age range.

■ Emergency department visits for the treatment of asthma were approximately one-third as frequent as were visits for upper respiratory infections. The need for urgent treatment of asthma symptoms may be related to acute exposure to specific precipitating factors (for example, poor air quality and pets) or may be due to chronically suboptimal treatment of existing asthma. Visit rates for asthma did not vary by age or sex.

■ Nearly one-half of all emergency department visits for abdominal or GI conditions were due to stomach pains; another one-fourth were due to gastroenteritis and colitis. Among female adolescents, the visit rate for GI conditions increased with age and was almost 5 times as high for those 18–19 years of age as those 10–11 years. Visit rates among female adolescents were approximately twice the rate of their male counterparts, with the difference increasing with age.

■ Among female adolescents, the rate of emergency department visits for treatment of sexually transmitted diseases, urinary tract infections, and pregnancy-related conditions increased markedly with age. (See also figures 19 and 23.)

Figure 12. Emergency department visit rates for selected noninjury diagnoses among adolescents 10–19 years of age, by age and sex: United States, average annual 1995–97

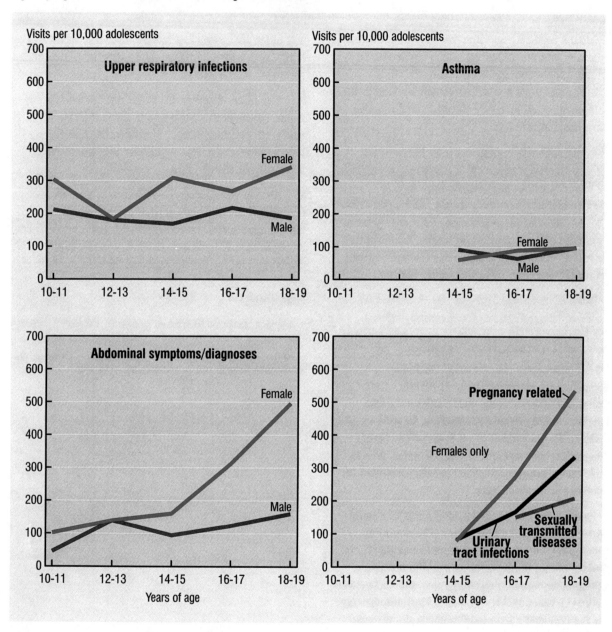

NOTES: Data points are not shown in figure when rates are unreliable. See Technical Notes for discussion of emergency department visits. See also Appendix I, National Hospital Ambulatory Medical Care Survey. See Data Table for data points graphed.

SOURCE: Centers for Disease Control and Prevention, National Center for Health Statistics, National Hospital Ambulatory Medical Care Survey (NHAMCS).

Health Status

Hospital Discharge Rates

Hospitalization is dependent not only on an individual's medical condition, but also on ambulatory care access and utilization (1). Delaying or not receiving timely and appropriate care for chronic conditions and other health problems may lead to the development of more serious health conditions that require hospitalization.

■ Adolescents are among the least likely of all persons to be hospitalized (2). Only younger children have lower inpatient hospitalization rates. For noninjury and nonpregnancy causes, adolescents have the lowest rates of hospitalization, followed by those for younger children and young adults. Adolescents have higher hospital discharge rates for injuries than younger children but lower than older persons.

■ Hospital discharges vary by sex, in large part because of hospitalizations for pregnancy-related causes (including deliveries and diagnoses associated with pregnancy) among female adolescents. In 1995–97 noninjury-related causes, excluding pregnancy, accounted for about 72 percent of all hospital discharges among male adolescents and 39 percent among female adolescents. Injuries accounted for 26 percent of all hospital discharges among males and 8 percent among females. Among female teens, pregnancy-related causes accounted for 53 percent of all discharges.

■ Hospitalizations for injury and noninjury causes increased with age for both sexes. The noninjury discharge rate among males increased marginally. In contrast, among female adolescents, the noninjury (nonpregnancy related) discharge rate doubled between ages 10–11 years and 18–19 years. Hospital discharge rates for pregnancy increased dramatically between ages 12–13 years and 18–19 years (see also figures 19 and 20).

■ As a proportion of all discharges for females, pregnancy-related causes ranged from about 3 percent at 12–13 years to about 73 percent of all hospital

discharges at 19 years. For adolescents 17 years of age and older, the pregnancy-related discharge rate for females exceeded the injury and other noninjury rates for males and females.

■ The injury hospital discharge rate for adolescent males 18–19 years of age was 3 times the rate for males 10–11 years of age. Similarly, the rate for female adolescents 16–19 years of age was 3 times that of those 10–13 years.

■ Among adolescents 14–19 years of age, the noninjury/not pregnancy-related discharge rate for female adolescents exceeded that for male adolescents by more than 25 percent. At each age, the injury discharge rate for males exceeded the rate for females.

References

1. Weisman JS, Epstein AM. Falling through the safety net. Johns Hopkins University Press. 1994.

2. Kozak LJ, Lawrence L. National Hospital Discharge Survey: Annual summary, 1997. National Center for Health Statistics. Vital Health Stat 13(144). 1999.

Figure 13. Short-stay hospital discharge rates for injury, noninjury, and pregnancy-related diagnoses among adolescents 10–19 years of age, by age and sex: United States, average annual 1995–97

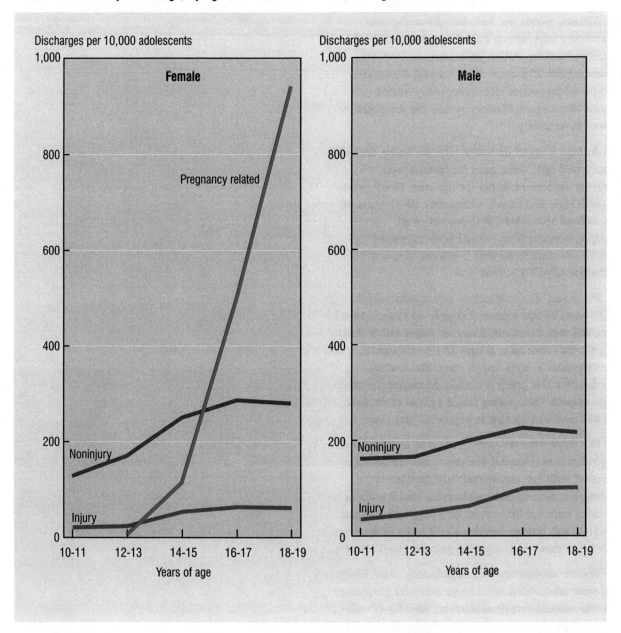

NOTES: See Technical Notes for discussion of hospital diagnoses. See also Appendix I, National Hospital Discharge Survey. See Data Table for data points graphed.

SOURCE: Centers for Disease Control and Prevention, National Center for Health Statistics, National Hospital Discharge Survey (NHDS).

Adolescent Health ....

Health, United States, 2000

Hospital Discharge Rates

■ Asthma, psychoses, fractures, poisoning, and appendicitis were among the leading first-listed diagnoses for hospitalized adolescents in 1995–97, accounting for 20 percent of all hospital discharges (and for 27 percent of all nonpregnancy-related hospital discharges). Patterns by age and sex differ for each of these causes.

■ Asthma hospital discharge rates for males declined sharply with age, while rates for females were relatively unchanged across the age span 10–19 years. For both male and female adolescents 10–11 years of age, asthma accounted for 13 percent of all noninjury/nonpregnancy-related hospitalizations; by ages 18–19 years fewer than 5 percent of these discharges were for asthma.

■ Psychoses[1] hospitalizations among adolescents 10–19 years of age increased sharply up to ages 14–15 years and then plateaued. Rates for males and females were similar, with rates at ages 14–19 years about twice the rates at ages 12–13 years. The leading diagnosis for this group is "major depressive disorder, single episode" accounting for 33 percent of all male and 47 percent of all female psychoses diagnoses.

■ Fractures were the leading cause of injury-related hospitalizations. Hospital discharge rates for fractures increased with age among male and female adolescents. Among male adolescents 16–19 years of age rates were 2.5 times those of younger adolescents (10–11 years); among females 16–19 years of age rates were twice those of younger adolescents (10–11 years).

■ Female adolescents were significantly more likely than male adolescents to be hospitalized for poisoning. The rates among female adolescents 14–17 years of age were 3 times those of female adolescents 12–13 years, with a slight decline among female adolescents 18–19 years. The rates among male adolescents 14–19 years of age remained fairly constant.

[1]ICD-9 CM codes include those for all psychoses, ICD 290–299.

Figure 14. Short-stay hospital discharge rates for selected diagnoses among adolescents 10–19 years of age, by age and sex: United States, average annual 1995–97

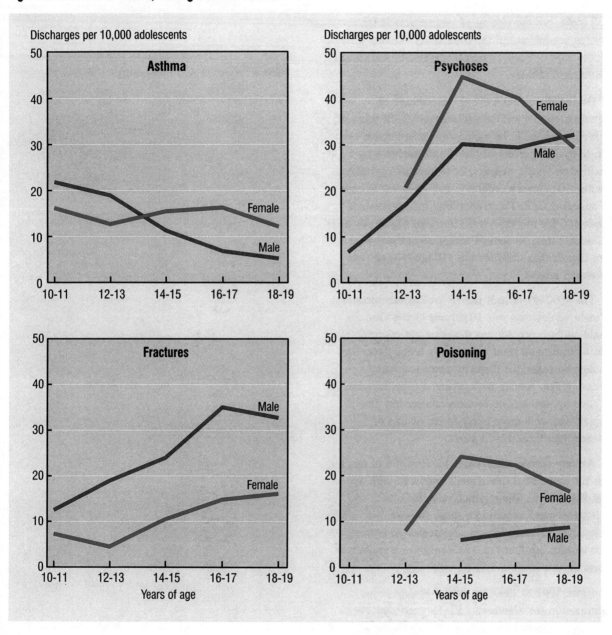

Discharges per 10,000 adolescents

Asthma

Discharges per 10,000 adolescents

Psychoses

Fractures

Poisoning

Years of age

Years of age

NOTES: Data points are not shown in figure when rates are unreliable. See Technical Notes for discussion of hospital diagnoses. See also Appendix I, National Hospital Discharge Survey. See Data Table for data points graphed.

SOURCE: Centers for Disease Control and Prevention, National Center for Health Statistics, National Hospital Discharge Survey (NHDS). See related *Health, United States, 2000*, tables 92 and 93.

Violent Crime Victimization

Adolescents are the victims of violent acts in the home, at school, and in the community. Violent crime includes rape or sexual assault, aggravated and simple assaults, and robbery.

■ During the period 1992–97 an average of approximately 3.4 million adolescents 12–19 years of age were reported to be victims of violent crime each year. Sixty-five percent of the victimizations were classified as simple assaults, 21 percent as aggravated assaults, 10 percent as robbery, and 4 percent as rape and sexual assault. The proportions for aggravated assault and for robbery were somewhat higher for male adolescents than for female adolescents; there were more female than male victims (10 percent) of rape and sexual assault.

■ The 1992–97 overall rate of violent victimizations for male adolescents was 50 percent higher than for female adolescents. Among the youngest adolescents, male victimization rates were nearly twice those for females; however, the disparity narrowed with increasing age. Among males there was no variation in the rates by age; among females adolescents 18–19 years of age were more likely to be victims of violence than those 12–13 years.

■ Among female adolescents 12–19 years of age the rates for rape and sexual assault increased with age (data not shown). The reported rates for older adolescents were about twice those for younger adolescents. Overall, female adolescents and young adult women are four times as likely to be victims of sexual assault as women in all other age groups (1).

■ From 1992 to 1997 the rate of violent crime victimization for adolescents 12–15 years and 16–19 years decreased. Declines were noted for each of the major categories of victimization.

Reference

1. Rickert VI, et al. Date rape among adolescents and young adults. J Pediatr Adolesc Gynecol 11(4):167–75. 1998.

Figure 15. Violent crime victimization rates among adolescents 12–19 years of age, by age and sex: United States, 1992–97

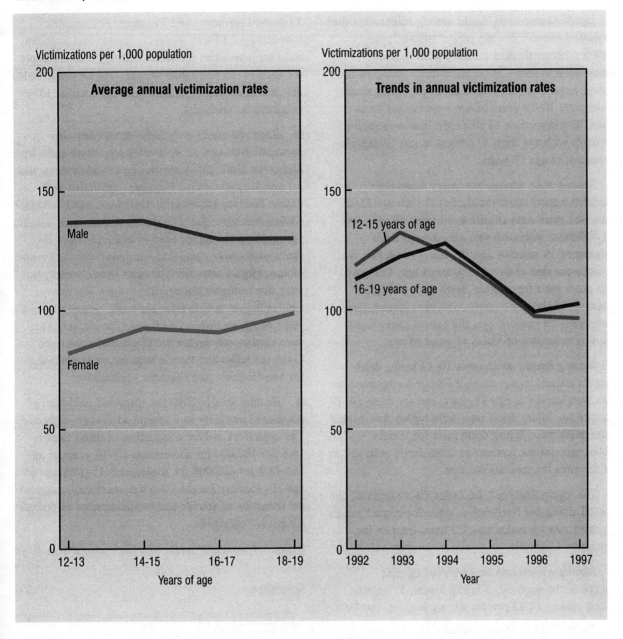

NOTES: See Technical Notes for survey methods. See Data Table for data points graphed.

SOURCE: Bureau of Justice Statistics, Department of Justice. National Crime Victimization Survey.

Death Rates

■ Injuries cause more deaths among adolescents than do natural causes[1]. For the period 1996–97, nearly 14,000 adolescents died annually from injuries compared with about 5,000 adolescents who died from natural causes; that is, 73 percent of all deaths among adolescents 10–19 years of age were caused by an injury. The proportion of all deaths that were injuries increases with age from 47 percent at age 10 years to 81 percent at age 18 years.

■ Among male adolescents injury death rates exceeded natural cause death rates at each age 11–19 years (the rates were similar at 10 years of age), and the difference increased with age. Among male adolescents 19 years of age, the injury death rate was 12 times the rate of those 10 years of age. Compared with death rates for injuries, death rates for natural causes increased more slowly with age. Among male adolescents 19 years of age, the natural cause death rate was twice that of males 10 years of age.

■ Among female adolescents 10–12 years, death rates for natural causes exceeded those for injuries; the rates were similar at age 13 years, and for those 14–19 years of age injury death rates were higher than natural cause death rates. Injury death rates for female adolescents did not increase as consistently with age as did the rates for male adolescents.

■ The injury death rate for males 10–19 years of age was 2.7 times that for females, while for natural causes the death rate for males was 1.3 times the rate for females.

■ Among adolescents unintentional injuries comprised the majority of injury deaths, 57 percent among males and 74 percent among females. For both sexes, the proportion of unintended injury deaths declined with age, as homicide and suicide deaths increased with age.

■ The unintentional injury death rates increased with age, with a particularly large relative increase,

73 percent for males and 79 percent for females, between ages 15 and 16 years. Suicide and homicide rates for males also increased with age, more sharply for ages 10–15 years than for ages 16–19 years. Unlike the pattern for males, suicide rates for females 15–19 years did not increase.

■ Race and ethnicity specific death rates also increased with age. In 1996–97 injury death rates were higher for black and American Indian adolescents than for non-Hispanic white, Hispanic, and Asian and Pacific Islander adolescents. The higher rates for black adolescents were due to higher homicide rates at each age; striking disparities exist in homicide rates for black adolescents compared with other race and ethnic groups. Higher rates for American Indian adolescents were due to higher unintentional injury mortality as well as higher suicide rates especially among those 15 years of age and over. Death rates for natural causes were consistently higher for black adolescents and lower for Asian and Pacific Islander adolescents than for non-Hispanic and Hispanic adolescents.

■ Healthy People 2010 has identified reduction of adolescent mortality as a critical adolescent objective. The objectives call for a reduction of death rates to 16.8 per 100,000 for adolescents 10–14 years of age and 43.2 per 100,000 for adolescents 15–19 years of age (1). Healthy People 2010 has specifically targeted the reduction of suicide and homicide rates as critical adolescent objectives.

[1] "Natural" is a term similar to "noninjury" that is used to categorize causes of death.

Reference

1. U.S. Department of Health and Human Services. Healthy People 2010 (Conference Edition, in Two Volumes). Washington: 2000.

Figure 16. Death rates for injury, by intent of injury, and natural causes among adolescents 10–19 years of age, by age and sex: United States, average annual 1996–97

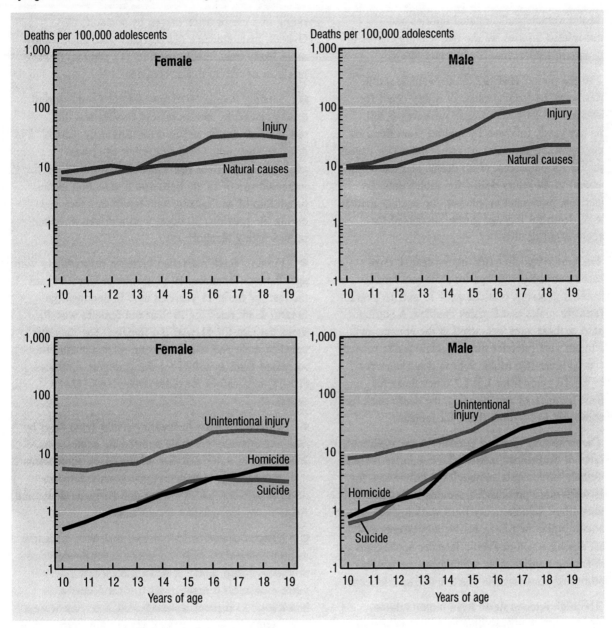

NOTES: Suicide rates for females 10–12 years of age are unreliable and are not shown. Death rates are graphed on a log scale to clearly illustrate how rates change across the entire age span 10–19 years. See Technical Notes for discussion of cause of death coding. See also Appendix II, Cause of Death. See Data Table for data points graphed.

SOURCE: Centers for Disease Control and Prevention, National Center for Health Statistics, National Vital Statistics System. See related *Health, United States, 2000*, tables 33, 45, 46, 47, and 48.

Motor Vehicle and Firearm-Related Deaths

■ Motor vehicle traffic-related injuries and firearm-related injuries are the two leading causes of death among adolescents 10–19 years of age.

■ For the period 1996–97, motor vehicle traffic injuries were the leading cause of injury death for adolescents 10–19 years of age (averaging 6,260 deaths per year), followed by injuries from firearms (averaging 4,250 per year). Together these two causes accounted for 55 percent of all deaths and for 75 percent of all injury deaths for adolescents. By comparison, malignant neoplasms, the leading natural cause of death for this age group, accounted for 6 percent of all deaths.

■ For motor vehicle traffic injury deaths, rates increased markedly with age for male and female adolescents. Notably, between ages 15 and 16 years the rates for males and females doubled. A similar increase at these ages was noted in the emergency department visit rates for motor vehicle traffic-related injuries. (Figure 10). Motor vehicle death rates for males 10–17 years were 1.3–1.7 times those for females; by ages 18 and 19 years, the death rates for males were 2.1–2.5 times those for females.

■ Disparities by race and ethnicity were apparent in the rates of death from motor vehicle injuries for male and female adolescents, although the differences for males were more pronounced. Among males and females motor vehicle injury rates were highest among American Indian or Alaska Native adolescents and lowest among Asian or Pacific Islander adolescents. Rates among non-Hispanic white teens were higher than those of non-Hispanic black and Hispanic teens.

■ The high rates of death from motor vehicle injuries are partially attributable to risk behavior among adolescents. In 1999, 33 percent of high school students reported that in the previous 30 days they rode in a car with a driver who had been drinking alcohol, and 13 percent reported that they drove after drinking alcohol (1). Sixteen percent of students surveyed had rarely or never worn seat belts when riding in a car or truck driven by someone else. Overall, male students (21 percent) were significantly more likely than female students (12 percent) to have rarely or never worn seat belts (1).

■ Healthy People 2010 has identified reduction of deaths caused by motor vehicle crashes and the reduction of deaths and injuries caused by alcohol- and drug- related motor vehicle crashes as critical adolescent objectives (2). The objectives also call for increased use of safety belts and a reduction in the proportion of adolescents who report that they rode, during the previous 30 days, with a driver who had been drinking alcohol.

■ Firearm death rates also increase substantially with age; the rate for males 19 years of age was 28 times the rate for those 11 years of age. In contrast, the firearm death rates for 19 year old females was 10 times the rate for 11 year old females. The disparity between male and female firearm-related death rates increased from threefold for the youngest adolescents (10–11) to ninefold for older adolescents (18–19 years).

■ Differences exist in firearm-related death rates by race and ethnicity for male and female adolescents. Rates were strikingly higher among black adolescents than among other race and ethnic groups. Firearm death rates were lowest among non-Hispanic white and Asian or Pacific Islander adolescents.

■ Firearm deaths include deaths that were classified as unintentional, suicide, homicide, legal intervention, or undetermined intent. Among adolescents 10–19 years of age, 60 percent of all firearm deaths were homicides, 31 percent were suicides, 6 percent were unintentional and 2 percent were of undetermined intent.

References

1. Centers for Disease Control and Prevention. Youth Risk Behavior Survey. 1999.

2. U.S. Department of Health and Human Services. Healthy People 2010 (Conference Edition, in Two Volumes). Washington: January 2000.

Figure 17. Death rates for motor vehicle traffic-related and firearm-related injuries among adolescents 10–19 years of age, by age and sex: United States, average annual 1996–97

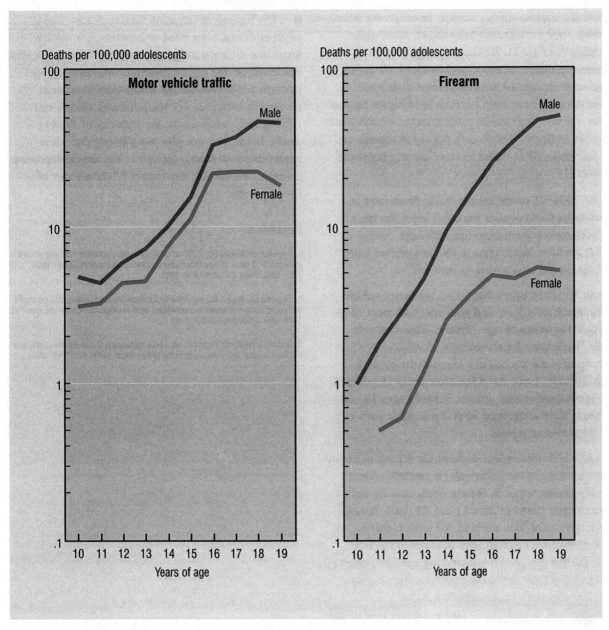

NOTES: The firearm death rate for females 10 years of age is unreliable and is not shown. Death rates are graphed on a log scale to clearly illustrate how rates change across the entire age span 10–19 years. See Technical Notes for discussion of cause of death coding. See also Appendix II, Cause of Death. See Data Table for data points graphed.

SOURCE: Centers for Disease Control and Prevention, National Center for Health Statistics, National Vital Statistics System. See related *Health, United States, 2000*, tables 45 and 48.

Motor Vehicle and Firearm-Related Deaths

Where adolescents reside, whether in urban, suburban, or more rural settings, has been shown to influence mortality risks (1–3). Teenagers living in the most densely populated metropolitan counties have higher death rates associated with interpersonal violence, while those in more rural counties have higher rates of motor vehicle fatalities. In general, motor vehicle death rates are higher in less densely populated settings and firearm homicide is higher in more densely populated settings (1).

■ In 1996–97 motor vehicle traffic death rates in nonmetropolitan counties were 2–3 times the rates in the core metropolitan (counties with large central cities) counties, while rates in the noncore but still metropolitan counties were in between.

■ In all urbanization categories, the motor vehicle traffic death rates increased with age, with most of the increase occurring by age 17 years. Motor vehicle traffic death rates for adolescents 16 years of age (when many adolescents can begin to drive) were approximately twice those for adolescents 15 years of age in all three county groups. Between ages 18 and 19 years the rate declined by 5–7 percent in each of the three county groups.

■ Age and urbanization patterns for firearm mortality differ from those for motor vehicle mortality. Most notably, the increases in firearm death rates by age were steeper. Between ages 11 and 13 years, firearm death rates more than doubled and were higher in nonmetropolitan counties than in either of the two metropolitan groups. With increasing age, the pattern changed and rates in the core counties were higher than those in noncore metropolitan and nonmetropolitan counties. With each single year of age between 13 and 16 years, firearm death rates in the core counties doubled or nearly doubled. Between 16 and 19 years, the rate came close to doubling again. Core county firearm death rates for 15–19 year olds were more than twice the rates in the other two county groups.

■ The manner or intent of firearm deaths, that is, whether deaths were ruled unintentional, a suicide, or a homicide, differs significantly by urbanization category. For example, the higher firearm death rates among younger adolescents in the nonmetropolitan areas resulted from higher unintentional and suicide rates. Among older adolescents, the majority of firearm deaths in the core counties were homicides while among adolescent who resided in the nonmetropolitan counties, suicide was the mostly likely manner of firearm death.

References

1. Fingerhut LA, Ingram DD, Feldman JJ. Firearm and nonfirearm homicide among persons 15–19 years of age: Differences by level of urbanization, United States, 1979–1989. JAMA, 267;3048–3053. 1992.

2. Fingerhut LA, Ingram DD and Feldman JJ. Homicide rates among U.S. teenagers and young adults-differences by mechanism, level of urbanization, race and sex, 1987–1995. JAMA 280(5):423–7. 1998.

3. Cubbin C, Pickle LW, Fingerhut, LA. Social context and the geographic patterns of homicide in black and white males in the United States. AJPH 90:579–87. 2000.

Figure 18. Death rates for motor vehicle traffic-related and firearm-related injuries among adolescents 10–19 years of age, by age and urbanization: United States, average annual 1996–97

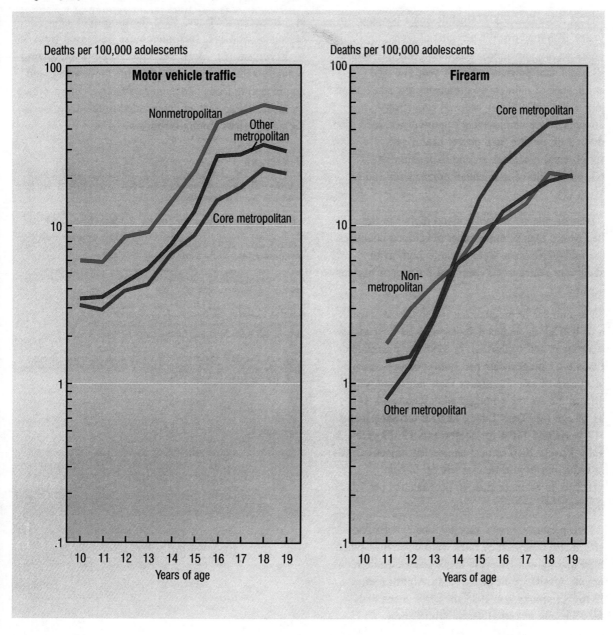

NOTES: Death rates are graphed on a log scale to clearly illustrate how rates change across the entire age span 10–19 years. See Technical Notes for discussion of cause of death coding. See also Appendix II, Cause of Death and Appendix II, Urbanization. See Data Table for data points graphed.

SOURCE: Centers for Disease Control and Prevention, National Center for Health Statistics, National Vital Statistics System. See related *Health, United States, 2000*, tables 45 and 48.

Reproductive Health

Pregnancy Rates

Annually, more than 900,000 adolescents become pregnant. The majority (78 percent) of teen pregnancies are unplanned, accounting for one-fourth of all accidental pregnancies each year (1). The consequences of unintended pregnancy for adolescents include unintended births, reduced educational attainment, fewer employment opportunities, increased likelihood of welfare, and poorer health and developmental outcomes among their infants (2). About one-fourth of unintended pregnancies end in abortion (1).

■ Teen pregnancy rates are much higher in the United States than in many other developed countries. In the mid-1990s rates were twice as high as in England and Wales or Canada, and 8 times as high as in Japan (3).

■ The number of pregnancies is estimated as the sum of live births, induced abortions, and fetal losses (miscarriages and stillbirths). In 1996 the pregnancy rate was 98.7 pregnancies per 1,000 young women 15–19 years of age. Pregnancy rates increased with age, from 2.8 for the youngest adolescents, 10–14 years of age (see Data Table), to 67.8 for adolescents 15–17 years and 146.4 for adolescents 18–19 years. A Healthy People 2010 critical adolescent objective calls for a reduction in pregnancies among female adolescents to no more than 46 pregnancies per 1,000 adolescents (4).

■ Teen pregnancy rates vary by race and Hispanic origin. In 1996 pregnancy rates were more than twice as high among non-Hispanic black and Hispanic teens as among non-Hispanic white teens. Abortion rates were higher among non-Hispanic black teens than either Hispanic or non-Hispanic white teens.

■ The teenage pregnancy rate for young women 15–19 years of age decreased 15 percent since reaching a peak of 116.5 per 1,000 in 1991 (5). Birth rates and abortion rates for adolescents declined in recent years. Fetal losses also declined as the number of young women becoming pregnant declined.

■ Between 1990 and 1995 the proportion of teenagers who ever had intercourse decreased from 55 to 50 percent (6). Moreover, contraceptive use among sexually active teens increased over those years, and contracepting teens chose more effective contraceptive methods. These factors contributed to the decrease in pregnancy rates among teenagers.

References

1. Henshaw, SK. Unintended pregnancy in the United States: 1982–1995. Fam Plann Perspect 30(1):24—9 and 46. 1998.

2. Sex and America's Teenagers. New York: Alan Guttmacher Institute. 1994.

3. Singh S, Darroch JE. Adolescent pregnancy and childbearing: levels and trends in developed countries. Fam Plann Perspec 32(1):14–23. 2000.

4. U.S. Department of Health and Human Services. Healthy People 2010 (Conference Edition, in Two Volumes). Washington: 2000.

5. Ventura ST, Mosher WD, Curtin SC, Abma JC, Hendershot S. Trends in pregnancies and pregnancy rates by outcome: Estimates for the United States, 1976–96. Vital Health Stat 21(56). National Center for Health Statistics. 2000.

6. Abma JC, Chandra A, Mosher WD, et al. Fertility, family planning and women's health: New data from the 1995 National Survey of Family Growth. Vital Health Stat 23(19). National Center for Health Statistics. 1997.

Figure 19. Pregnancy rates according to outcome of pregnancy among adolescents 15–19 years of age, by age, race, and Hispanic origin: United States, 1996

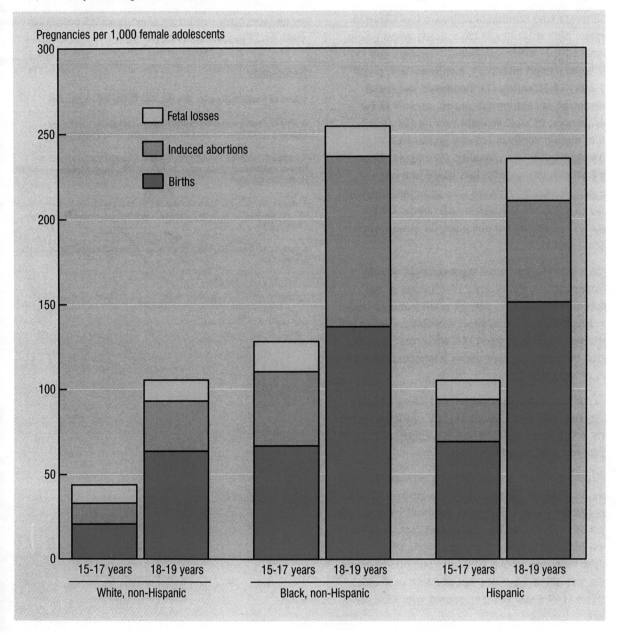

NOTES: Persons of Hispanic origin may be of any race. See Technical Notes for discussion of pregnancy rate estimation. See Data Table for data points graphed.

SOURCE: Ventura SJ, Mosher WD, Curtin SC, Abma JC, Henshaw SK. Trends in pregnancies and pregnancy rates by outcome: Estimates for the United States, 1976–96. Vital Health Stat 21(56). Hyattsville, Maryland: National Center for Health Statistics. 2000. See related *Health, United States, 2000*, tables 3, 8, 16, and 17.

Reproductive Health

Birth Rates

Adolescents who become mothers are less likely to complete high school or to have steady employment, and more likely to receive public assistance and to experience marital instability, compared with peers who delay childbearing (1). Economic and social disadvantage are among the causes, as well as the consequences, of teenage child bearing (2). Infants born to teenage mothers are at a greater risk of low birthweight and infant mortality. (See figures 21 and 22.) Teen mothers are also less likely to receive adequate and timely prenatal care and more likely to smoke (3). Second and higher order births further increase the risk of poor outcomes for young women and their children.

■ In 1997–98 there were approximately 493,600 births annually to adolescents 13–19 years of age, accounting for nearly 13 percent of all births in each year. The birth rate for adolescent women 15–19 years of age was 51.5 births per 1,000 adolescent women, and the birth rate for very young adolescents (13–14 years of age) was 2.6.

■ There is a consistent pattern of increasing birth rate by maternal age. Overall 19-year old teens were nearly seven times as likely to have a birth as their 15-year old counterparts.

■ Birth rates vary considerably by race and Hispanic origin. In 1997–98 Hispanic and non-Hispanic black teens had the highest birth rates followed by American Indian teens; Asian or Pacific Islander teens had the lowest birth rates. Among young women 19 years of age, the birth rate among Hispanics and non-Hispanic blacks was about 3.5 times that of Asian or Pacific Islanders (149.3 and 141.0 compared with 42.6 per 1,000).

■ Teenage birth rates have steadily declined in the 1990's and have fallen almost 18 percent among adolescents 15–19 years of age since 1991 (4). There has also been a 21-percent decrease in the rates of second and higher order births to teens in the 1990's, while the proportion of births to teenagers that were

second and higher order declined from 25 percent in 1991 to 22 percent in 1998 (4, 5).

References

1. Sex and America's Teenagers. New York: Alan Guttmacher Institute. 1994.

2. Kirby D. No easy answers: Research findings on programs to reduce teen pregnancy. Washington: National Campaign to Prevent Teen Pregnancy. 1997.

3. Ventura SJ, Mathews TJ, Curtin SC. Declines in teenage birth rates 1991–97: National vital statistics reports; vol 47 no 12. Hyattsville, Maryland: National Center for Health Statistics. 1998.

4. Ventura SJ, Martin JA, Curtin SC, Mathews TJ. Births: Final data for 1998. National vital statistics reports; vol 48 no 3. Hyattsville, Maryland: National Center for Health Statistics. 2000.

5. Ventura, SJ, Curtin, SC. Recent trends in teen births in the United States. Stat Bull. Jan–Mar 1999.

Figure 20. Birth rates among adolescents 13–19 years of age, by birth order, age, race, and Hispanic origin: United States, average annual 1997–98

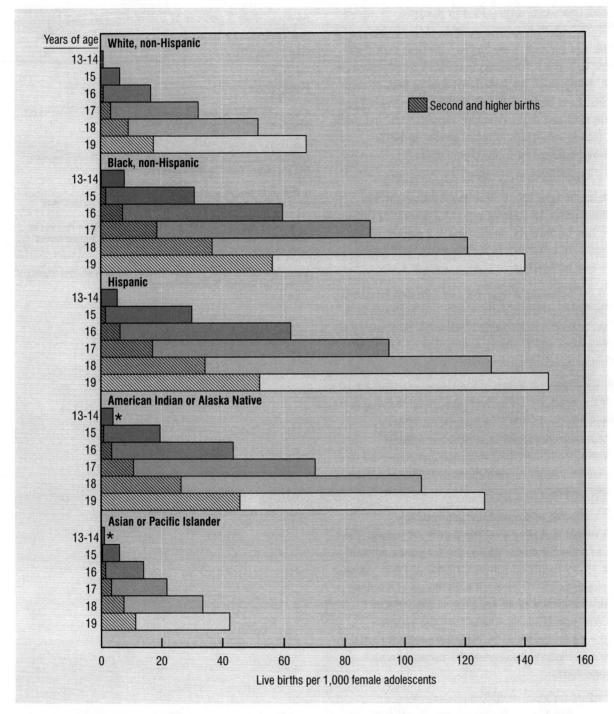

Live births per 1,000 female adolescents

* Second and higher live births were too few to be considered reliable and are not shown separately.

NOTES: Excludes live births with unknown birth order. See Appendix II, Rates, birth. See Data Table for data points graphed.

SOURCE: Centers for Disease Control and Prevention, National Center for Health Statistics, National Vital Statistics System. See related *Health, United States, 2000*, table 3.

Reproductive Health

Low Birthweight

Birthweight, along with period of gestation, is one of the most important predictors of an infant's subsequent health and survival. Low birthweight (less than 2,500 grams or about 5.5 pounds) may result from premature birth, being small for gestational age, or both of these factors. Low-birthweight infants face an increased risk of physical and developmental complications and death (1). Nearly two-thirds of infant deaths in 1997 occurred among low-birthweight babies (2).

■ In 1997–98, 9.5 percent of infants born to adolescents ages 15–19 were low birthweight. For mothers under 15 years of age, 13.2 percent of infants were low birthweight. In contrast, 7.2 percent of infants born to women in their twenties and thirties were low birthweight.

■ Low-birthweight rates vary by race and Hispanic origin. The percent of infants with low birthweight is higher among non-Hispanic black teens than among all other groups and is almost double that of American Indian or Alaska Native teens.

■ Very low-birthweight infants, those weighing less than 1,500 grams, are at the highest risk of dying in their first year. In 1997–98 the percent of very low-birthweight infants of adolescent mothers decreased with increasing maternal age among all race and ethnic groups except American Indian or Alaska Native infants.

■ A number of factors may influence low birthweight including smoking during pregnancy. The rate of smoking during pregnancy for young women ages 15–19 increased between 1994 and 1998. Young women ages 15–19 have the highest rate of smoking during pregnancy of all age groups. Among teen mothers, non-Hispanic whites have the highest smoking rates followed by Native Americans (3, 4). Very low birthweight is primarily associate with preterm birth.

■ Healthy People 2010 objectives call for a reduction in low-birthweight births for all women to no more than 5 percent of live births and very low-birthweight births to no more than 1 percent of live births (5).

References

1. Ventura SJ, Peters KD, Martin JA, Maurer JD. Births and Deaths: United States, 1996. National Center for Health Statistics. 1997.

2. MacDorman MF, Atkinson JO. Infant mortality statistics from the 1997 period linked birth/infant death data set. National vital statistics reports; vol 47 no 23. Hyattsville, Maryland: National Center for Health Statistics. 1999.

3. Mathews TJ. Smoking during pregnancy, 1990–96. National vital statistics reports; vol 47 no 10. Hyattsville, Maryland: National Center for Health Statistics. 1998.

4. Ventura SJ, Martin JA, Curtin SC, Matthews TJ, Park MM. Births: Final data for 1998. National vital statistics reports; vol 48 no 3. Hyattsville, Maryland: National Center for Health Statistics. 2000.

5. U.S. Department of Health and Human Services. Healthy People 2010 (Conference Edition, in Two Volumes). Washington: January 2000.

Figure 21. Low-birthweight live births among adolescent mothers 13–19 years of age, by maternal age, race, and Hispanic origin: United States, average annual 1997–98

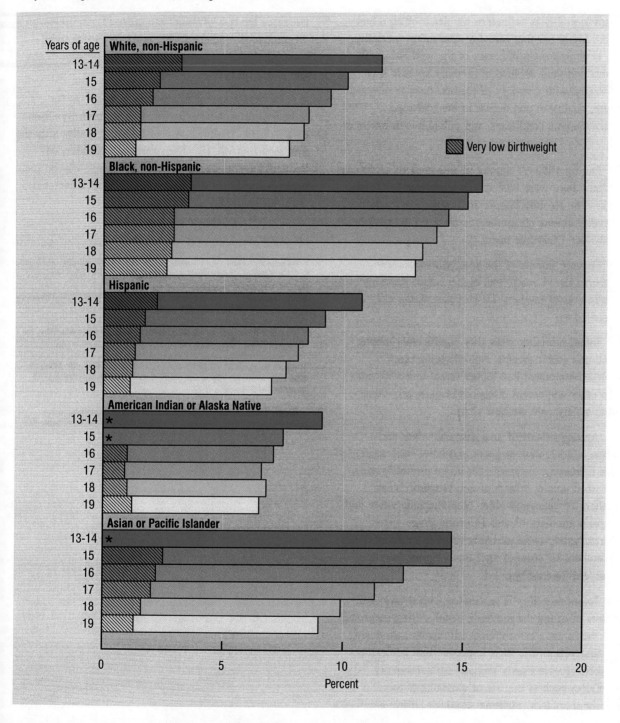

* Very low-birthweight live births were too few to be considered reliable, and are not shown separately. See Data Table for data points graphed.

NOTES: Low birthweight is less than 2,500 grams; very low birthweight is less than 1,500 grams. Excludes live births with unknown birthweight.

SOURCE: Centers for Disease Control and Prevention, National Center for Health Statistics, National Vital Statistics System. See related *Health, United States, 2000*, table 12.

Infant Mortality

Infant mortality is defined as the death of an infant before his or her first birthday. The infant mortality rate is an important indicator of the well-being of infants and their adolescent mothers because it is associated with a variety of factors, such as maternal health, quality of and access to medical care, socioeconomic conditions, and public health practices (1).

■ During 1995–97 among infants born to adolescent mothers there were 10.6 infant deaths per 1,000 live births. The Healthy People 2010 objective for infant mortality among all mothers is no more than 4.5 infant deaths per 1,000 live births (2).

■ Overall, infants of the youngest adolescent mothers (13–14 years) had higher infant mortality rates than infants of mothers 15–19 years of age (17.1 versus 10.4).

■ Infant mortality rates vary significantly among racial and ethnic groups. Non-Hispanic black adolescent mothers had higher infant mortality rates than other adolescent mothers (14.4), nearly twice those of Hispanic mothers (7.6).

■ Among infants of non-Hispanic white and Hispanic adolescent mothers, mortality rates decreased with increasing maternal age; infant mortality rates plateaued among infants of non-Hispanic black mothers 16 years and older. Non-Hispanic white and Hispanic mothers 13 and 14 years of age were approximately twice as likely to have an infant death as mothers 19 years of age; for black mothers this relative difference was 1.4.

■ Infant mortality is associated with a variety of factors affecting the mother's health during pregnancy and the infant's environment and health care during the first year of life. It is important that adolescent mothers receive timely prenatal care and avoid risky behaviors such as the use of alcohol and tobacco during pregnancy. Maternal smoking during pregnancy increases the risk of infant mortality (3). In 1998, 18 percent of mothers 15–19 years of age reported smoking during pregnancy, the highest percent of any age group (4).

■ Among infants of adolescent mothers, as for infants of all mothers, Sudden Infant Death Syndrome (SIDS) is the leading cause of infant mortality after the first month of life (5). The American Academy of Pediatrics recommends putting infants to sleep on their backs because of the lower risk for SIDS associated with this position.

References

1. Kleinman JC, Kiely JL. Infant mortality. Healthy People 2000 statistical notes; vol 1 no 2. Hyattsville, Maryland: National Center for Health Statistics. 1991.

2. U.S. Department of Health and Human Services. Healthy People 2010 (Conference Edition, in Two Volumes). Washington: 2000.

3. Wilcox AJ. Birthweight and perinatal mortality: the effect of maternal smoking. Am J Epidemiol 137:1098–1104. 1993.

4. Ventura SJ, Martin JA, Curtin SC, Mathews TJ, Park MM. Births: Final Data for 1998. National vital statistics reports; vol 48 no. 3. Hyattsville, Maryland: National Center for Health Statistics. 2000.

5. Centers for Disease Control and Prevention. Assessment of infant sleeping position—selected States, 1996. Morb Mortal Wkly Rep 47(41):873–7. October 1998.

Figure 22. Infant mortality rates among infants of adolescent mothers 13–19 years of age, by maternal age, race, and Hispanic origin: United States, average annual 1995–97

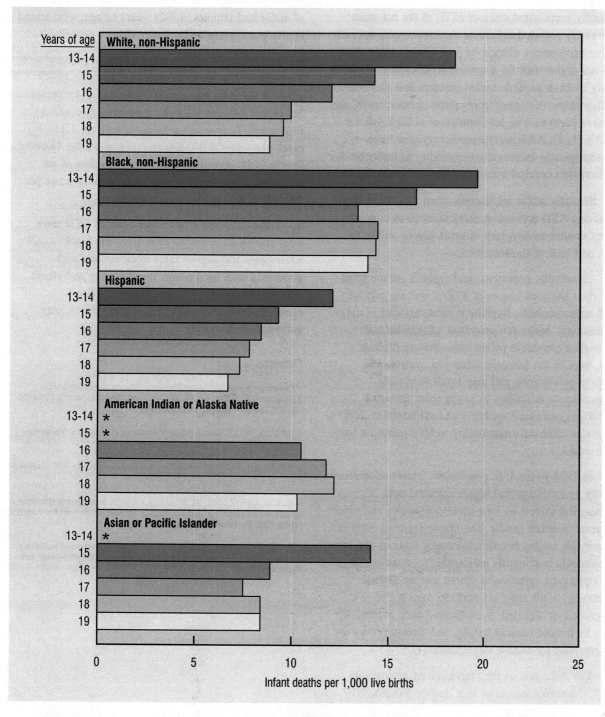

* Infant deaths in this age and race group were too few to be considered reliable and are not shown.

NOTES: See Data Table for data points graphed. For further discussion, see Appendix I, National Linked File of Live Births and Infant Deaths.

SOURCE: Centers for Disease Control and Prevention, National Center for Health Statistics, National Linked Files of Live Births and Infant Deaths. See related *Health, United States, 2000*, tables 20–25.

Reproductive Health

Sexually Transmitted Diseases

Sexually transmitted diseases (STD's) are the most commonly reported infectious diseases among sexually active adolescents. Compared with adults, adolescents are at a higher risk for acquiring STD's: they are more likely to have multiple sexual partners and short-term relationships, to engage in unprotected intercourse, and to have partners who are themselves at high risk for STD's (1, 2). Adolescent women may also have physiologically increased susceptibility to infection due to increased cervical ectopy and lack of immunity (1).

■ Sexually active adolescents often face barriers to receiving STD prevention services, such as concern about confidentiality, lack of insurance or ability to pay, and lack of transportation.

■ Chlamydia, gonorrhea, and syphilis are the most common bacterial causes of STD's, and are curable with antimicrobials. Syphilis is relatively rare among adolescents. When left untreated, chlamydia and gonorrhea can cause pelvic inflammatory disease, abscesses in the fallopian tubes and ovaries, and chronic pelvic pain, and may result in ectopic pregnancy or infertility. In young men untreated infections can cause urethritis and epididymitis. STD's may also increase susceptibility to HIV infection two- to fivefold.

■ In 1998 in the U.S. population, female adolescents 15–19 years of age had higher reported rates of chlamydial infections than adolescent males and older persons of either gender. The higher reported rates of chlamydia among female adolescents than among male adolescents is primarily attributable to detection of asymptomatic infection in young women through screening, while their sex partners may not be diagnosed or reported. Symptomatic male adolescents may be treated without testing, and therefore may not be captured by disease surveillance (1).

■ The reduction of the proportion of adolescents with chlamydia infections is a Healthy People 2010 critical adolescent objective, with a target of 3 percent of males and females, 15–24 years of age, who attend family planning or STD clinics (3).

■ In 1998 rates of gonorrhea in the U.S. population were also higher among female adolescents 15–19 years of age than adolescent males and older persons. Between 1990 and 1998 the gonorrhea rate among adolescents decreased by 50 percent (from 1,114.4 cases per 100,000 in 1990 to 560.6 in 1998). Healthy People 2010 objectives call for a reduction of the incidence of gonorrhea to no more than 19 cases per 100,000 people in the total population (3).

■ Large race and ethnic disparities in STD rates exist among adolescents. Non-Hispanic black adolescents had higher rates of chlamydia and gonorrhea than adolescents in other race and ethnic groups. Differences in socioeconomic status, contraceptive use, and sexual risk behaviors, may influence the disparity in rates (4, 5).

References

1. Centers for Disease Control and Prevention. Sexually Transmitted Disease Surveillance 1998. Centers for Disease Control and Prevention, National Center for HIV, STD, and TB Prevention. September 1999.

2. Gittes EB, Irwin CE. Sexually transmitted diseases in adolescents. Pediatr Rev 14(5):180–9. 1993.

3. U.S. Department of Health and Human Services. Healthy People 2010 (Conference Edition, in Two Volumes). Washington: January 2000.

4. Ellen JM, Kohn RP, Bolan GA, Shiboski S, Krieger N. Socioeconomic differences in sexually transmitted disease rates among black and white adolescents, San Francisco, 1990 to 1992. Am J Public Health. 85:1546–8. 1995.

5. Sieving R, Resnick MD, Bearinger L, et al. Cognitive and behavioral predictors of sexually transmitted disease risk behavior among sexually active adolescents. Arch Pediatr Adolesc Med. 151:243–51. 1997.

Figure 23. Sexually transmitted disease rates reported for adolescents 10–19 years of age, by age, sex, race, and Hispanic origin: United States, 1998

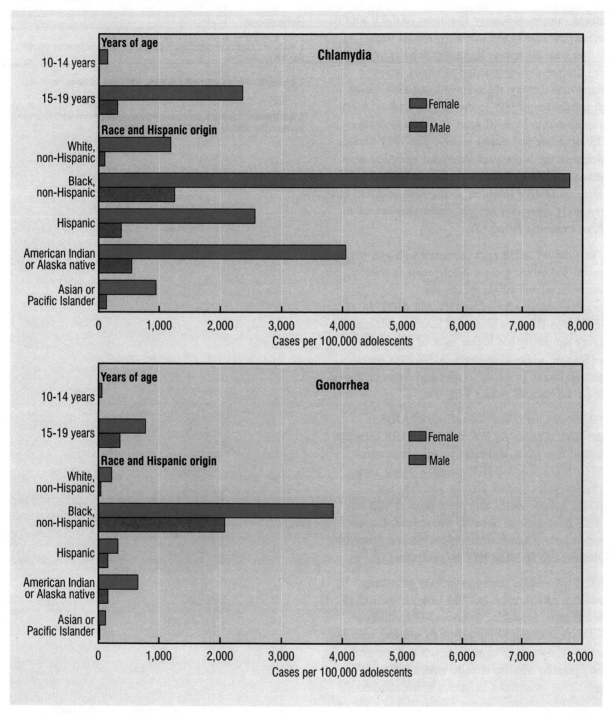

NOTES: Data for States not reporting race/ethnicity and age for the majority of cases were excluded. See Technical Notes for further discussion. See Data Table for data points graphed.

SOURCE: Centers for Disease Control and Prevention, National Center for STD, HIV, and TB Prevention: Sexually Transmitted Disease Surveillance, 1998. See related *Health, United States, 2000*, table 52.

Acquired Immunodeficiency Syndrome (AIDS)

Acquired immunodeficiency syndrome (AIDS), with its associated morbidity and mortality, results from infection with the human immunodeficiency virus (HIV). Before the introduction of highly active antiretroviral therapy, the average incubation period from acquisition of HIV to the development of AIDS was estimated to be 8–10 years (1). Overall declines in AIDS incidence and deaths in 1996 and 1997 provide evidence of the widespread beneficial effects of new treatment regimens. Rather than an inevitable progression of HIV infection, a diagnosis of AIDS now increasingly represents late diagnosis, poor access to care, or treatment failure (2).

■ In 1996–98 AIDS rates increased with age among all racial and ethnic groups. Adolescents in some minority racial and ethnic groups are disproportionately affected by HIV and AIDS. In 1996–98 non-Hispanic black and Hispanic adolescents in every age group had higher rates of AIDS than non-Hispanic white adolescents. AIDS rates among American Indian or Alaska Native and Asian or Pacific Islander adolescents remain very low.

■ Although the overall prevalence of AIDS in adolescents is relatively low, the rate of HIV infection is higher. It is likely that most young adults who develop AIDS acquired HIV infection during their adolescent years. Sexual activity and drug use activities among adolescents place them at high risk for HIV transmission. Sexually transmitted diseases common among adolescents, chlamydia and gonorrhea, are believed to facilitate HIV transmission (1).

■ HIV prevention strategies include promoting knowledge of risk behaviors that increase the risk of HIV infection, increasing awareness of methods to reduce risk, and improving access to effective care and treatment programs to improve health and survival among persons who are already infected. Healthy People 2010 identified a reduction in the number of cases of HIV infection among adolescents as a critical adolescent objective (3).

References

1. Boyers DB, Kegeles SM. AIDS risk and prevention among adolescents. Soc Sci Med 33(1):11–23. 1991.

2. Centers for Disease Control and Prevention. HIV/AIDS Surveillance Report. 9(1). 1997.

3. U.S. Department of Health and Human Services. Healthy People 2010 (Conference Edition, in Two Volumes). Washington: January 2000.

Figure 24. Acquired immunodeficiency syndrome (AIDS) rates reported for adolescents 11–19 years of age, by age, sex, race, and Hispanic origin: United States, average annual 1996–98

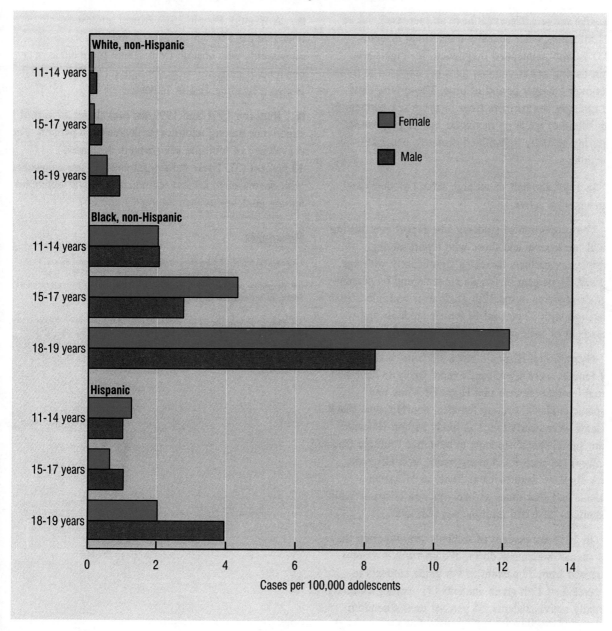

Cases per 100,000 adolescents

NOTES: States not reporting race/ethnicity and age for the majority of cases were excluded from the analysis. See Technical Notes for further discussion. See Data Table for data points graphed.

SOURCE: Centers for Disease Control and Prevention, National Center for STD, HIV, and TB Prevention. See related *Health, United States, 2000*, tables 53 and 54.

Sexual Activity

Sexually active adolescents have an increased risk of HIV infection, other sexually transmitted diseases (STD's), and unintended pregnancy. Teenagers who begin having sex at younger ages are exposed to these risks over a longer period of time. Those who have had multiple sex partners (four or more sex partners in their lifetime) are at an increased risk of pregnancy, acquiring sexually transmitted diseases, and HIV infection.

■ In 1999 one-half of all high school students had been sexually active.

■ The proportion of students who report ever having sexual intercourse and those who report having multiple sex partners increases significantly with age. In 1999, 66 percent of female students and 64 percent of male students in the 12th grade ever had intercourse compared with 33 percent of female students and 45 percent of male students in the 9th grade.

■ Overall, non-Hispanic black students, both male and female, were significantly more likely to have had sexual intercourse than non-Hispanic white and Hispanic students. Among females, non-Hispanic black students were nearly twice as likely as non-Hispanic white and Hispanic students to have had multiple (four or more) sex partners. Among males, non-Hispanic black students were twice as likely as Hispanic students and four times as likely as non-Hispanic white students to have had multiple sex partners.

■ In 1999 the percent of students who reported they had sexual intercourse during the previous 3 months increased from 27 percent of 9th grade students to 51 percent of 12th grade students (1). Among currently sexually active students, 58 percent used a condom during their last sexual intercourse. The proportion of students using condoms decreased with grade level, from 67 percent of 9th grade students to 48 percent of those in 12th grade (1). Condoms are very effective at preventing the transmission of STDs and HIV, but are less effective than some other contraceptive methods at preventing pregnancy.

■ A Healthy People 2010 critical adolescent objective calls for an increase in the proportion of adolescents who abstain from sexual intercourse or use condoms if currently sexually active (2). This measure is also a Leading Health Indicator.

■ Between 1991 and 1999 the prevalence of sexual experience among adolescents decreased 8 percent. The prevalence of multiple sex partners decreased 13 percent (3). These behavioral changes are consistent with decreases in related reproductive health outcomes among adolescents (see figures 19 and 23).

References

1. Centers for Disease Control and Prevention. Youth Risk Behavior Survey. 1999.

U.S. Department of Health and Human Services. Healthy People 2010 (Conference Edition, in Two Volumes). Washington: January 2000.

3. Centers for Disease Control and Prevention. Trends in sexual risk behaviors among high school students—United States, 1991–1997. Morb Mortal Wkly Rep 47:749–51. 1998.

Figure 25. Lifetime sexual activity among students in grades 9–12, by sex, grade level, race, and Hispanic origin: United States, 1999

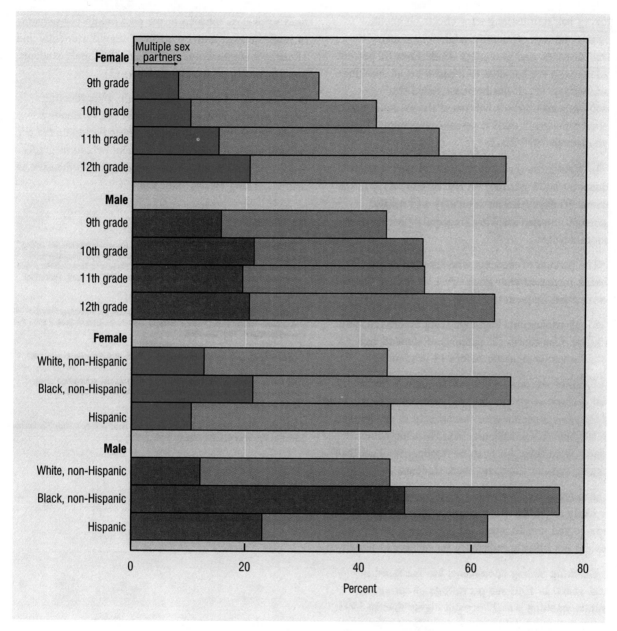

NOTES: Multiple sex partners is defined as four or more sex partners in the student's lifetime. See Technical Notes for survey methods. See Data Table for data points graphed.

SOURCE: Centers for Disease Control and Prevention, National Center for Chronic Disease Prevention and Health Promotion, Youth Risk Behavior Survey (YRBS).

Cigarette Smoking

Smoking has serious long-term effects on health, including the risk of nicotine addiction, smoking-related diseases, and premature death. Over 80 percent of adults who are addicted to tobacco began smoking as adolescents (1). It has been estimated that tobacco-related illnesses will cause the premature death of approximately 5 million persons who were 17 years or younger in 1995 (2).

■ In 1999 more than one-third of all high school students reported smoking on one or more days in the previous 30 days (current smoking), and nearly 17 percent reported smoking frequently (that is, on 20 or more days).

■ The percent of students who reported current smoking increased with grade level, as did the percent who reported frequent smoking.

■ Many adolescents begin smoking before reaching 9th grade. One-fourth (25 percent) of students had smoked a whole cigarette before 13 years of age.

■ Rates of smoking differ substantially between racial and ethnic groups. In 1999 non-Hispanic white and Hispanic students were more likely to smoke than non-Hispanic black students. Non-Hispanic white students were more likely to be frequent smokers than Hispanic and non-Hispanic black students.

■ Among non-Hispanic black students, females were less likely to smoke than males. In contrast, among Hispanic and non-Hispanic white students smoking rates did not differ significantly for males and females.

■ Smoking among adolescents has increased in recent years. In 1999 the prevalence of current cigarette smoking was 27 percent higher than in 1991; current cigarette smoking increased 56 percent among black students, 29 percent among Hispanic students, and 25 percent among white students (3, 4).

■ Adolescents are at risk from other forms of tobacco use as well. In 1999, 8 percent of students used smokeless tobacco in the past month (14 percent of male students and 1 percent of female students) and 18 percent smoked cigars (25 percent of male students and 10 percent of female students) (3).

■ Tobacco use is the single leading preventable cause of death in the United States (1). A Healthy People 2010 critical adolescent objectives calls for a reduction in the proportion of young people in grades 9–12 who have used tobacco products; this measure is also a Leading Health Indicator (5).

References

1. U.S. Department of Health and Human Services. Preventing tobacco use among young people: A report of the Surgeon General. Atlanta, Georgia: Department of Health and Human Services, Public Health Service, Centers for Disease Control and Prevention, National Center for Chronic Disease Prevention and Health Promotion, Office on Smoking and Health. 1994.

2. Centers for Disease Control and Prevention. Projected smoking-related deaths among youth—United States. Atlanta, Georgia: Centers for Disease Control and Prevention. MMWR 45:971–4. 1996.

3. Centers for Disease Control and Prevention. Youth Risk Behavior Survey. 1999.

4. Centers for Disease Control and Prevention. Tobacco use among high school students—United States. Atlanta, Georgia: Centers for Disease Control and Prevention. MMWR 47: 229–33. 1998.

5. U.S. Department of Health and Human Services. Healthy People 2010 (Conference Edition, in Two Volumes). Washington: January 2000.

Figure 26. Current cigarette smoking among students in grades 9–12 by sex, grade level, race, and Hispanic origin: United States, 1999

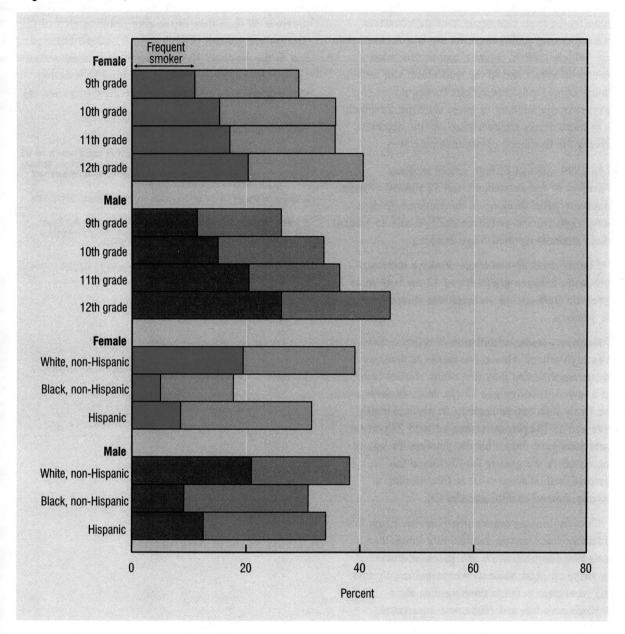

NOTES: Current cigarette smoking is defined as having smoked cigarettes on one or more days of the 30 days preceding the survey; frequent cigarette smoking is defined as having smoked cigarettes on 20 or more days of the 30 days preceding the survey. See Technical Notes for survey methods. See Data Table for data points graphed.

SOURCE: Centers for Disease Control and Prevention, National Center for Chronic Disease Prevention and Health Promotion, Youth Risk Behavior Survey (YRBS).

Alcohol Use

Alcohol is the most commonly used psychoactive substance during adolescence. Its use is associated with motor vehicle crashes, injuries, and deaths; with problems in school and in the workplace; and with fighting, crime, and other serious consequences (1). Heavy, episodic drinking or binge drinking, in which five or more drinks are consumed on one occasion, increases the likelihood of negative outcomes.

■ In 1999 one-half of high school students (48 percent of female students and 52 percent of male students) reported drinking in the previous 30 days. Twenty-eight percent of female students and 35 percent of male students reported binge drinking.

■ Current drinking and binge drinking increased significantly between grades 9 and 12 for both male and female students; the increase was sharper among male students.

■ For many students, initiation of drinking began before high school. Almost one-third (32 percent) of students reported that they first drank alcohol (more than a few sips) before age 13 (2). Male students were more likely than female students to begin drinking before age 13 (37 percent compared with 27 percent). Researchers have found that the younger the age of drinking onset, the greater the likelihood that an individual will, at some point in life, develop a clinically defined alcohol disorder (3).

■ Current drinking among non-Hispanic black male and female students was substantially lower than among non-Hispanic white and Hispanic students. Non-Hispanic black students were significantly less likely to engage in binge drinking than their non-Hispanic white and Hispanic counterparts.

■ Reduction in the proportion of adolescents engaging in binge drinking of alcoholic beverages is a Healthy People 2010 critical adolescent objective. This measure is also a Leading Health Indicator (4).

■ Adolescents who combine drinking and driving are at an increased risk of injury or death. In 1999, 13 percent of high school students reported that in the previous 30 days they drove after drinking alcohol (2). Thirty-three percent of high school students reported that in the previous 30 days they rode in a car with a driver who had been drinking alcohol (2); reducing this proportion is a Healthy People 2010 objective (4).

References

1. National Institute on Alcohol Abuse and Alcoholism. Ninth special report to the U.S. Congress on alcohol and health. Secretary of Health and Human Services. Bethesda, Maryland: National Institutes of Health. (NIH Publication No. 97–4017). June 1997.

2. Centers for Disease Control and Prevention. Youth Risk Behavior Survey. 1999.

3. Grant BR, Dawson DA. Age at onset of alcohol use and its association with DSM-IV alcohol abuse and dependence: Results from the National Longitudinal Alcohol Epidemiologic Survey. J Subst Abuse 9:103–10. 1998.

4. U.S. Department of Health and Human Services. Healthy People 2010 (Conference Edition, in Two Volumes). Washington: January 2000.

Figure 27. Current alcohol use among students in grades 9–12, by sex, grade level, race, and Hispanic origin: United States, 1999

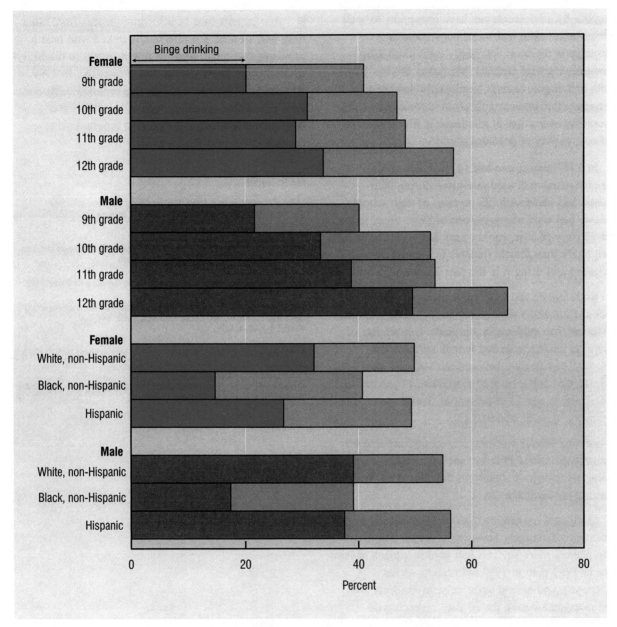

NOTES: Current alcohol use is defined as having 1 or more drinks on 1 or more days of the 30 days preceding the survey; binge alcohol use is defined as having 5 or more drinks on at least one occasion in the 30 days preceding the survey. See Technical Notes for survey methods. See Data Table for data points graphed.

SOURCE: Centers for Disease Control and Prevention, National Center for Chronic Disease Prevention and Health Promotion, Youth Risk Behavior Survey (YRBS).

Risk Behaviors

Marijuana Use

Drug use by adolescents can have immediate as well as long-term health and social consequences. Marijuana is the most commonly used illicit drug among high school students. Marijuana use has both health and cognitive risks, particularly damage to pulmonary functions as a result of chronic use (1, 2). Possession and/or use of marijuana is illegal and can lead to a variety of penalties.

■ In 1999 almost one-half (47 percent) of high school students had used marijuana during their lifetime and one-fourth (27 percent) of high school students had used marijuana one or more times in the past 30 days (that is, current use). Male students were more likely than female students to report ever using marijuana and using it in the past 30 days.

■ Both female and male students in the higher grades (10th–12th) were more likely to have ever used marijuana than students in 9th grade. Current use of marijuana among male and female students also increased significantly between 9th and 12th grade. Of students who had ever used marijuana, 11 percent first tried it before age 13 (8 percent of female students and 15 percent of male students) (3).

■ Among female students, current and lifetime use of marijuana varied little by race and ethnicity. Among males there were no significant differences by race and ethnicity in marijuana use.

■ Marijuana use among high school students increased substantially between 1990 and 1999 (4). Fifty percent more students had used marijuana at least once in 1999 than in 1990 (47 percent versus 31 percent), and almost twice as many students had used marijuana during the 30 days preceding the survey (27 percent versus 14 percent).

■ A Healthy People 2010 critical adolescent objective calls for a reduction in the proportion of adolescents reporting use of marijuana and other illicit substances in the past 30 days (5).

■ Adolescents face health consequences from other drug use, as well. Cocaine use is linked with health problems that range from eating disorders to disability to death from heart attacks and strokes (6). In 1999, 10 percent of high school students reported using some form of cocaine (powder, "crack," or "freebase") during their lifetime and 4 percent reported using cocaine in the past 30 days (3).

References

1. National Institute on Drug Abuse. Marijuana: Facts parents need to know. Washington: U.S. Department of Health and Human Services. (NCADI Publication No. PHD712). 1995.

2. Pope HG Jr., Yurgelun-Todd D. The residual cognitive effects of heavy marijuana use in college students. J Am Med Assoc 275(7). 1996.

3. Centers for Disease Control and Prevention. Youth Risk Behavior Survey. 1999.

4. Centers for Disease Control and Prevention. Alcohol and other drug use among high school students—United States, 1990. Morb Mortal Wkly Rep 40(45);776–7,783–4. 1991.

5. U.S. Department of Health and Human Services. Healthy People 2010 (Conference Edition, in Two Volumes). Washington: January 2000.

6. Blanken AJ. Measuring use of alcohol and other drugs among adolescents. Public Health Rep 108(Supplement 1). 1993.

Figure 28. Lifetime marijuana use among students in grades 9–12, by sex, grade level, race, and Hispanic origin: United States, 1999

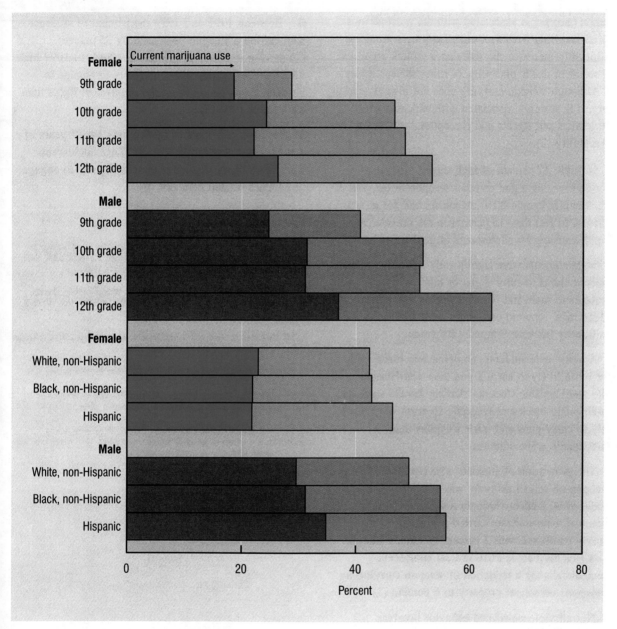

NOTES: Lifetime marijuana use is defined as having ever used marijuana. Current marijuana use is defined as having used marijuana 1 or more times in the 30 days preceding the survey. See Technical Notes for survey methods. See Data Table for data points graphed.

SOURCE: Centers for Disease Control and Prevention, National Center for Chronic Disease Prevention and Health Promotion, Youth Risk Behavior Survey (YRBS).

Weapon Carrying

Weapon carrying is associated with the most serious injuries resulting from violence. Carrying a weapon significantly increases the risk that a violent argument will result in death, disability, or other serious injury (1). Although weapon carrying does not always lead to injury, it is strongly associated with exposure to intimidation and threats and perceptions of fear and vulnerability (2).

■ In 1999, 17 percent of high school students reported carrying a gun or other weapon in the past 30 days. Healthy People 2010 objectives call for a reduction to less than 15 percent in the prevalence of weapon carrying by adolescents in grades 9–12 (3).

■ Male students were significantly more likely than female students to carry a gun or other weapon. Among both male and female students, the percent of students who reported carrying a weapon did not differ significantly between 9th and 12th grade.

■ Among male students, non-Hispanic black students were more likely to carry a gun than non-Hispanic white and Hispanic students. Among female students, non-Hispanic black and Hispanic students were more likely to carry guns and other weapons than non-Hispanic white students.

■ The proportion of students who reported carrying a weapon on school property was smaller. In 1999, 7 percent of all students brought a weapon to school; 11 percent of male students carried a weapon on school property compared with 3 percent of female students (4). A Healthy People 2010 critical adolescent objective calls for a reduction of weapon carrying by adolescents on school property to 6 percent (3).

■ Not all violence-related behavior involves weapons. In 1999, 27 percent of female students and 44 percent of male students were involved in one or more physical fights (4). Reduction in physical fighting among adolescents is a Healthy People 2010 critical adolescent objective (3).

■ Between 1991 and 1999 the percent of students who carried a weapon decreased by 35 percent (26 percent in 1991, 17 percent in 1999). In 1999 high school students were also less likely to engage in physical fights or to be injured in physical fights than students in 1991 (5).

■ In 1996, 5 percent of adolescents 14–17 years of age were not enrolled in school. These adolescents were more likely than their in-school peers to engage in violence-related behavior (6).

References

1. Centers for Disease Control and Prevention. Measuring the health behavior of adolescents: The Youth Risk Behavior Surveillance System and recent public health reports on high-risk adolescents. Public Health Rep 108(1). 1993.

2. Lowry R, Powell KE, Kann L, Collins JL, Kolbe LJ. Weapon-carrying, physical fighting and fight related injury among U.S. adolescents. Am J Prev Med 14:122–9. 1998.

3. U.S. Department of Health and Human Services. Healthy People 2010 (Conference Edition, in Two Volumes). Washington: January 2000.

4. Centers for Disease Control and Prevention. Youth Risk Behavior Survey. 1999.

5. Brener ND, Simon TR, Krug EG, Lowry R. Recent trends in violence-related behaviors among high school students in the United States. JAMA 282:440–46. 1999.

6. Centers for Disease Control and Prevention. Health risk behaviors among adolescents who do and do not attend school: United States, 1992. Morb Mortal Wkly Rep 43:129–32. 1994.

Figure 29. Weapon carrying in the past 30 days among students in grades 9–12, by sex, grade level, race, and Hispanic origin: United States, 1999

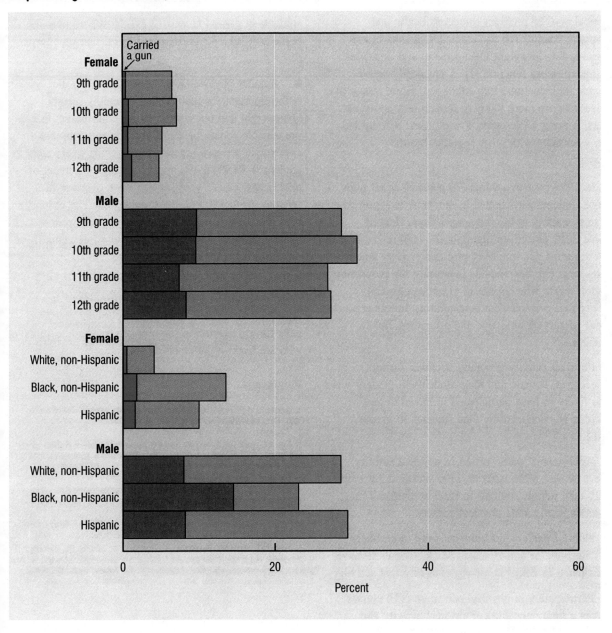

Percent

NOTES: Weapons include a gun, knife, or club. See Technical Notes for survey methods. See Data Table for data points graphed.

SOURCE: Centers for Disease Control and Prevention, National Center for Chronic Disease Prevention and Health Promotion, Youth Risk Behavior Survey (YRBS).

Physical Activity

Physical activity provides important health and emotional benefits for adolescents. It lowers blood pressure, aids in weight management, and improves cardiorespiratory function (1). A physically active lifestyle may continue into adulthood, while less active adolescents are more likely to remain less active as adults. Among adolescents, low physical activity has been associated with other negative health behaviors (2).

■ In 1999 over two-thirds (70 percent) of all high school students participated in moderate to vigorous physical activity in the previous 7 days. Healthy People 2010 objectives highlight the importance of both vigorous and moderate physical activity among adolescents (3). Specifically, increasing the proportion of adolescents who engage in vigorous physical activity that promotes cardiorespiratory fitness is a critcal adolescent objective and a Leading Health Indicator.

■ Physical activity generally declines during adolescence. Female and male students in grade 9 were more likely to have participated in moderate or vigorous physical activity than students in grades 10–12.

■ Adolescents' participation in physical activity differs by sex. Male students were substantially more likely than female students to have participated in moderate or vigorous physical activity.

■ Non-Hispanic white students were more likely than Hispanic or non-Hispanic black students to have participated in moderate or vigorous physical activity.

■ Participation in physical education (PE) classes assures a minimum level of physical activity and provides a forum to teach physical activity strategies and activities that can be continued into adulthood. In 1999 over one-half (56 percent) of all high school students were enrolled in PE class. Students in grade 9 were twice as likely to be enrolled in PE class as students in grades 11 and 12 (4). However, only 29 percent of students participated in PE classes every day.

■ Regular physical activity and a healthy diet are both important for maintaining a healthy weight. Overweight and obesity are major contributors to many preventable causes of death. Adolescents who are overweight are at a greater risk of being overweight as adults (5). In 1988–94, approximately 11 percent of adolescents 12–17 years of age were overweight (*Health, United States, 2000*, table 69). The proportion of adolescents from poor households who were overweight was almost twice that of adolescents from middle-and high-income households.

■ The prevelance of overweight and obesity has been identified as a Leading Health Indicator in Healthy People 2010; a critical adolescent objective calls for a reduction in the proportion of adolescents who are overweight or obese (3).

References

1. Centers for Disease Control and Prevention. Mortality patterns—United States, 1997. Morb Mortal Wkly Rep 48(30):664–8. August 1999.

2. Pate RR, Heath GW, Dowda M, Trost SG. Associations between physical activity and other health behaviors in a representative sample of U.S. adolescents. Am J Public Health 86(11):1577–81. 1996.

3. U.S. Department of Health and Human Services. Healthy People 2010 (Conference Edition, in Two Volumes). Washington: January 2000.

4. Centers for Disease Control and Prevention. Youth Risk Behavior Survey. 1999.

5. Troiano RP, Flegal KM, Kuczmarski RJ, Campbell SM, Johnson CL. Overweight prevalence and trends for children and adolescents: The National Health and Nutrition Examination Surveys, 1963–1991. Archives of Pediatr Adolesc Med. 149. 1995.

Figure 30. Participation in moderate to vigorous physical activity among students in grades 9–12, by sex, grade level, race, and Hispanic origin: United States, 1999

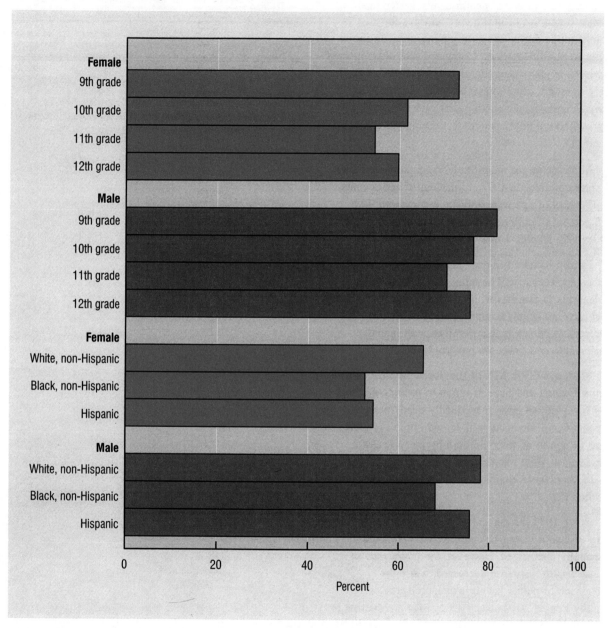

NOTES: Moderate to vigorous physical activity is defined as activity which caused the person to sweat or breathe hard for at least 20 minutes on 3 or more of the previous 7 days or walking or biking for at least 30 minutes on 5 or more of the previous 7 days. See Technical Notes for survey methods. See Data Table for data points graphed.

SOURCE: Centers for Disease Control and Prevention, National Center for Chronic Disease Prevention and Health Promotion, Youth Risk Behavior Survey (YRBS).

Health Care Access

Health Care Coverage

Access to and use of health care services for adolescents is dependent, to a great degree, on the ability to pay for services. Compared with their insured counterparts, uninsured adolescents are five times as likely to lack a usual source of care, four times as likely to have unmet health needs, and twice as likely to go without a physician contact during the course of a year (1).

■ Adolescents are more likely to be uninsured than younger children. In 1997, 17 percent of adolescents 10–19 years of age were uninsured compared with 12.5 percent of children under 6 years of age (tables 128, *Health, United States, 2000*).

■ Family income is a key factor in the likelihood that an adolescent will be uninsured. One-third of adolescents in families with incomes below the poverty level have no health insurance, compared with 8 percent of adolescents in families with incomes greater than two times the poverty level.

■ Medicaid (Title XIX of the Social Security Act) is a joint Federal and State program to provide medical care for qualified poor or medically needy persons. Expansions in Medicaid will extend eligibility until 19 years of age to all poor children by the year 2002. However, in 1996 one-third of uninsured adolescents 13–18 years were eligible for Medicaid but were not enrolled (2).

■ Since 1984 the percent of adolescents with some form of health insurance coverage has remained essentially unchanged. However, the prevalence of private health insurance decreased, while the prevalence of public health insurance increased (1). Healthy People 2010 objectives call for a reduction to 0 percent in the proportion of children (including adolescents) and adults under 65 years of age without health care coverage (3).

References

1. Newacheck PW, Brindis CD, Cart CU, et al. Adolescent health insurance coverage: recent changes and access to care. Pediatrics 104(2 Pt 1):195–202. August 1999.

2. Selden TM, Banthin JS, Cohen JW. Medicaid's problem children: Eligible but not enrolled. Health Aff 17:192–200. May/June 1998.

3. U.S. Department of Health and Human Services. Healthy People 2010 (Conference Edition, in Two Volumes). Washington: January 2000.

Figure 31. Health care coverage of adolescents 10–19 years of age, by type of health care coverage, age, and poverty status: United States, 1997

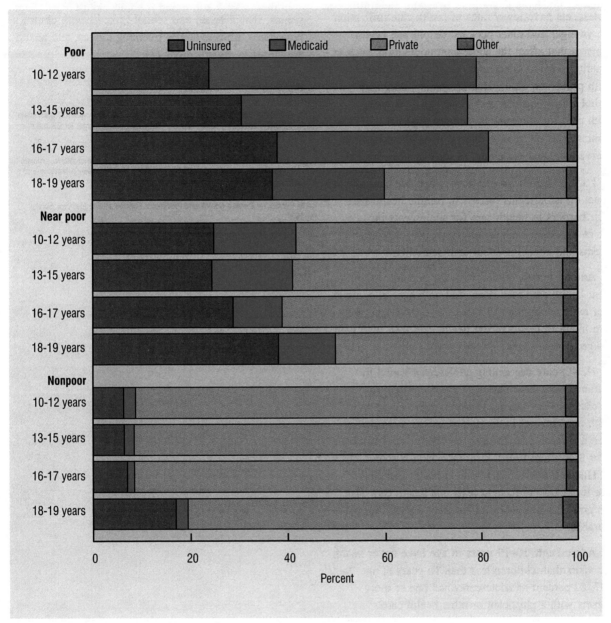

NOTES: Poverty status is derived from the ratio of the family's income to the Federal poverty threshold, given family size. Poor is less than 100 percent of the poverty threshold; near poor is between 100 and 199 percent of the poverty threshold; nonpoor is 200 percent of the poverty threshold or more. See Data Table for data points graphed.

SOURCE: Centers for Disease Control and Prevention, National Center for Health Statistics, National Health Interview Survey. See related *Health, United States, 2000*, table 128.

Health Care Visits

Adolescents have lower rates of health care utilization than younger and older persons, despite the health problems that affect the adolescent population, such as sexually transmitted diseases, emotional and behavioral health problems, unintended pregnancy, drug and alcohol abuse, injuries, and violence (1). Routine health care for adolescents includes physical examinations, preventive interventions and education, observations, and screening, as well as sick care (2).

■ Lack of health insurance coverage has a significant impact on adolescents' access to routine health care. Other barriers to health care for adolescents include lack of experience negotiating complex medical systems and concerns about confidentiality.

■ Among female adolescents, the percent without a recent health care visit decreased with age. In contrast, older male adolescents (18 and 19 years of age) were more likely to lack a recent health care visit than their younger counterparts.

■ Health care use among adolescents varied by insurance status and race. In 1997 the proportion of adolescents who had not visited a physician or other health professional in the past year was more than twice as high for adolescents without health insurance as for those with health insurance. Non-Hispanic black and Hispanic adolescents without health insurance were less likely to have at least one health care visit than non-Hispanic white adolescents without health insurance.

■ Adolescents 10–19 years of age have fewer health care visits than children less than 10 years of age. In 1997, 82 percent of adolescents had one or more contacts with a physician or other health care professional compared with 91 percent of children less than 10 years of age (3).

■ To meet the health care needs of adolescents, routine health care services need to be available in a wide range of settings, including community-based clinics, school-based and school-linked health clinics, physicians' offices, family planning clinics, and health maintenance organizations (1).

References

1. Irwin CE, Brindis C, Holt KA, Langlykke K, eds. Health care reform: Opportunities for improving adolescent health. Arlington, Virginia: National Center for Education in Maternal and Child Health. 1994.

2. Green M ed. Bright futures: Guidelines for health supervision of infants, children, and adolescents. Arlington, Virginia: National Center for Education in Maternal and Child Health. 1994.

3. Centers for Disease Control and Prevention. National Health Interview Survey. 1997.

Figure 32. Lack of a health care visit in the past 12 months among adolescents 10–19 years of age, by age, sex, health care coverage, race, and Hispanic origin: United States, 1997

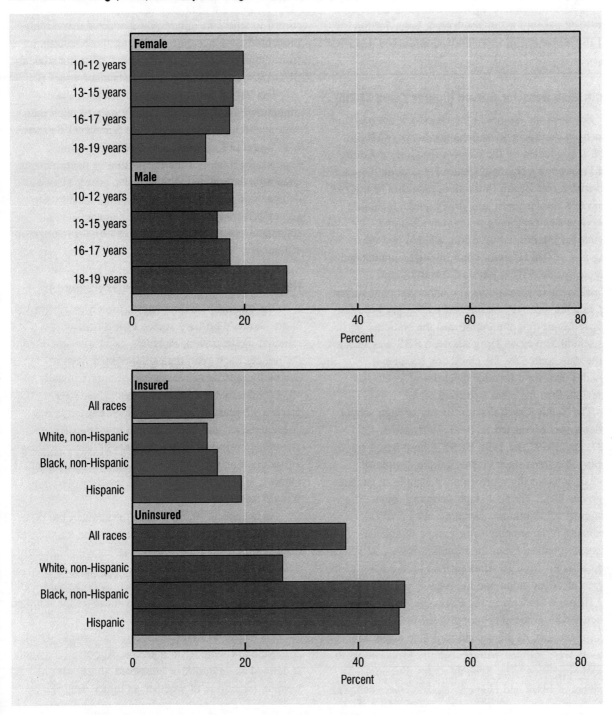

NOTE: Health care visit is defined as being seen by a physician or other health professional in a doctor's office, clinic, or some other place. Excluded are visits to emergency rooms, hospitalizations, home visits, and telephone calls. See Data Table for data points graphed.

SOURCE: Centers for Disease Control and Prevention, National Center for Health Statistics, National Health Interview Survey.

Technical Notes

Data Sources

Appendix I describes the data sources used in the chartbook except for the Youth Risk Behavior Survey and the National Crime Victimization Survey described below.

Youth Risk Behavior Survey (figures 7 and 25–30)

Seven of the figures in the chartbook are based on data from the Youth Risk Behavior Survey (YRBS). YRBS, conducted by the Centers for Disease Control and Prevention's National Center for Chronic Disease Prevention and Health Promotion, monitors health-risk behaviors among youth and young adults including behaviors that contribute to unintentional and intentional injuries, tobacco use, alcohol and other drug use, sexual behavior contributing to unintended pregnancy and STD's, physical inactivity and unhealthy dietary behaviors (1). Other national surveys that monitor various measures of adolescent behavior include Monitoring the Future and the National Household Survey on Drug Abuse. YRBS was selected as the data source for the chartbook because it provides data for a broader spectrum of youth risk behaviors than the other two sources.

The Youth Risk Behavior Survey of high school students was conducted in 1990, 1991, 1993, 1995, 1997, and 1999. The 1999 YRBS school-based survey employed a three-stage cluster sample design to produce a nationally representative sample of students in grades 9–12. The first-stage sampling frame contained 1,270 primary sampling units (PSU's), consisting of large counties or groups of smaller, adjacent counties. From the sampling frame, 52 PSU's were selected from 16 strata formed on the basis of the degree of urbanization and the relative percent of black and Hispanic students in the PSU. The PSU's were selected with probability proportional to school enrollment size. At the second sampling stage, 187 schools were selected with probability proportional to school enrollment size. Schools with substantial numbers of black and Hispanic students were sampled at higher rates than all other schools. The third stage of sampling consisted of randomly selecting one or two intact classes of required subjects from grades

9–12 at each chosen school. All students in the selected classes were eligible to participate in the survey. A weighting factor was applied to each student record to adjust for nonresponse and for the varying probabilities of selection, including those resulting from the oversampling of black and Hispanic students. SUDAAN was used to compute standard errors (2).

The YRBS data are subject to at least three limitations. First, these data apply only to adolescents who attend high school. In 1996, 5 percent of persons 14–17 years of age were not enrolled in school. Second, the extent of underreporting or overreporting cannot be determined, although the survey questions demonstrate good test-retest reliability. Finally, the survey provides no information on socioeconomic status and other variables that might explain subgroup differences.

National Crime Victimization Survey (figure 15)

The National Crime Victimization Survey (NCVS) is the Nation's primary source of information on criminal victimization, including crimes not reported to the police. Each year, data are obtained from a nationally representative sample of approximately 43,000 households comprising more than 80,000 persons 12 years of age and over on the frequency, characteristics, and consequences of criminal victimization in the United States. The survey collects information on victimization by rape, sexual assault, robbery, assault, theft, household burglary, and motor vehicle theft.

As defined in NCVS, violent crime can be classified into three categories: simple and aggravated assault; rape/sexual assault; and robbery. Violent crime does not include personal theft, such as purse snatching, or property crimes, such as household theft. Crime victimization rates are calculated as the number of events per 1,000 population.

An assault is an unlawful physical attack, whether aggravated or simple, on a person. Aggravated assault is defined as an attack or attempted attack with a weapon regardless of whether an injury occurred as well as an attack without a weapon when serious injury results. Serious injury includes broken bones, loss of teeth, internal injuries, loss of consciousness, and any injury requiring 2 or more days of hospitalization. Simple assault is an attack without a weapon, resulting in either minor injury or in undetermined injury and requiring less than 2 days of hospitalization. It also includes attempted assault without a weapon and verbal threats of assault. Robbery is a theft, completed or attempted, directly from a person, of property or cash by force or threat of force, with or without a weapon. Rape or sexual assault is a completed or attempted attack generally involving unwanted sexual contact between the victim and offender.

NCVS uses a generalized variance function (GVF) to calculate standard errors for their estimates. GVF represents the curve fitted to the individual crime measures. Standard errors were calculated using the jackknife repeated replication technique. For more information about NCVS, see /www.ojp.usdoj.gov/bjs/.

Measures and Methods

Demographic Measures

The chartbook focuses on the changes that occur in the health status of adolescents, by single year of age. For this chartbook adolescents are defined as individuals 10–19 years of age. Some data sources did not have sufficient numbers of observations to allow calculation of reliable estimates by single year of age, and so age was grouped in 2- or 3-year categories. For some measures there were no differences by age; in those charts, data were presented for variables that did show variation within the adolescent population, such as gender, race and ethnicity, and poverty status. Data from YRBS were presented for grades 9, 10, 11, and 12, rather than by age because of the sample design of that survey.

When race and ethnicity differences are presented, data are shown for non-Hispanic white, non-Hispanic black, and Hispanic adolescents except for the figure on untreated dental caries (figure 6), which includes data for Mexican Americans. Hispanic persons may be of any race. The race and ethnicity distribution (figure 1), birth rates (figure 20), and low- and very low-birthweight percents (figure 21) are shown for five groups: non-Hispanic white, non-Hispanic black,

American Indian or Alaska Native, Asian or Pacific Islander, and Hispanic adolescents. For those charts, data for white and black adolescents are also included in the data table. Depending on the variable of interest, some data sources did not have sufficient numbers of observations to allow calculation of reliable estimates of the adolescent population by race and ethnicity within age categories.

Population (figure 1)

Population figures for 1980 and 1990 are based on decennial censuses, figures for 1985 are based on intercensal estimates of resident population, and figures for 1991–99 are based on postcensal estimates of resident population. Estimates for 2000–50 are middle series population projections of the U.S. Bureau of the Census. (U.S. population estimates by age, sex, race, and Hispanic origin: 1980 to 1991. Current Population Reports. Series P-25, No. 1095. Washington: U.S. Government Printing Office, Feb 1993; unpublished estimates tables for 1995–99 that are available on the Census Bureau Web site, for data years 1995–99; U.S. Bureau of the Census, Day JC. Population projections of the United States by age, sex, race, and Hispanic origin: 1995 to 2050. Current population reports; Series P-25, No. 1130. Washington: U.S. Department of Commerce. 1996, for data years 2000–50.)

Poverty (figures 2, 5, 6, and 31) and Family Income (figure 4)

The Federal poverty threshold is used as the measure of poverty status in figures 2, 5, 6, and 31. The income classes are derived from the ratio of the family's income to the family's Federal poverty threshold, given family size. In 1997 a family of four with an annual income below $16,400 was below the Federal poverty line. Poor is defined as less than 100 percent of the poverty threshold. Near poor is between 100 and 199 percent of the poverty threshold (that is, between $16,400 and $32,799 for a family of four in 1997), and nonpoor is 200 percent of the poverty threshold or more. In 1998 the poverty threshold for a family of four increased to $16,660 a year. (www.census.gov/hhes/poverty/threshld.html).

Estimates of poverty by family structure (figure 2) are for adolescents who are related to the householder and who are under age 18. The data do not include adolescents who are in foster care or institutional care.

Family income level is used as the measure of socioeconomic status in figure 4. Low income is the bottom 20 percent of all family incomes; high income is the top 20 percent of all family incomes; and middle incomes is the 60 percent in between.

Activity Limitation (figure 5)

The prevalence of activity limitation among adolescents, 10–17 years of age, is based on parent responses in the 1997 National Health Interview Survey family core questionnaire. The adolescent was considered to have an activity limitation if the parent gave a positive response to any of the following questions about the adolescent:

■ Because of a physical, mental, or emotional problem, does ____ need the help of other persons with personal care needs, such as eating, bathing, dressing, or getting around inside the home?

■ Because of a health problem does ____ have difficulty walking without any special equipment?

■ Is ____ limited in any way because of difficulty remembering or because of periods of confusion? . . . in any activities because of physical, mental, or emotional problems?

■ Does ____ receive Special Education?

Suicide Ideation and Attempts (figure 7)

In 1999 estimates of suicide ideation and attempts among high school students are based on positive responses to questions on YRBS that asked if the student "seriously considered suicide" or "actually attempted suicide" in the past 12 months. Some students (6 percent) who reported attempting suicide did not report seriously considering suicide, suggesting that these attempts might have been unplanned.

Emergency Department Visits (figures 9–12)

An injury-related visit in the National Hospital Ambulatory Medical Care Survey, Emergency Department Component, is defined as follows: "yes" was checked on the patient record form in response to the question, "Is visit related to injury or poisoning?" or a cause of injury or a nature of injury diagnosis was provided, or an injury-related reason for visit was reported (3). All other diagnoses are for noninjury visits except those that are pregnancy related. See table I for a listing of the code numbers used to define the diagnostic categories.

Table I. Codes for diagnostic categories from the *International Classification of Diseases, Ninth Revision, Clinical Modification* (ICD–9–CM)

Diagnostic category	ICD–9–CM code numbers
Noninjury:	
Psychoses	290–299
Upper respiratory infection. . .	460–465, 381, 382, 34.0
Asthma	493
STD's	54.1, 77.98, 78.10, 78.11, 78.19, 78.88, 79.4, 90–92, 94, 98.10, 98.16–.17, 98.30, 98.36–.39, 98.86, 99.0–.2, 99.40–.41, 99.5, 112.1, 131.0, 131.8–.9, 614.0–.5, 614.7–.9, 615.0–.9, 616.10, 623.5, 628.2, 647.0–.2, 980–988.
Urinary tract infection.	595.0, 595.9, 599.0, 590.1, 590.8, 590.9
Abdominal/gastrointestinal. . .	789.0, 558.9, 535.0, 535.5–9, 540, 541, 531–534
Pregnancy related	630–677 or V22, V23, V27
Injury:	
Fractures[1].	800.0, 800.5, 801.0, 800.5, 803.0, 803.5, 804.0, 804.5, 807–829
Sprains and Strains.	840–848
Open Wounds[2]	870–873, 874.8, 874.9, 875–884, 888–894
Contusions	920–924
Poisoning	960–989
External cause of injury:	
Motor vehicle traffic	E810–E819, E958.5, E988.5
Fall.	E880–E886, E888, E957, E968.1, E987
Struck by, against	E916–E917, E960.0, E968.2, E973, E975
Cut/pierce.	E920, E956, E966, E974, E986

[1]This set of ICD codes differs from the traditional categorization of fractures that has generally included ICD codes 800–829. ICD codes for skull fracture with intracranial injuries and spinal fractures with spinal cord injuries are excluded. Those codes are categorized with internal organ injuries.

[2]This set of codes differs from the traditional grouping of ICD codes 870–897. Omitted are injuries to the larynx, trachea, pharynx, and thyroid, which would be categorized with internal organ injuries. In addition, codes for traumatic amputations are grouped separately.

The external cause of injury is defined using only the first-listed cause. The category "being struck by or against an object or a person" is a broad one that includes a specific code for sports-related injuries.

It should be noted that principal diagnoses based on emergency department (ED) data are not as detailed as discharge diagnoses from in-patient settings. Thus, when one compares ED data for adolescents 10–19 years using the traditional fracture category (ICD–9–CM codes 800–829) with the new categorization for fractures, the correspondence is over 99 percent. On the other hand, comparing fractures groupings using data from the National Hospital Discharge Survey, about 6 percent of discharges had a principal diagnosis of skull fracture with intracranial injury and about 2 percent had a spinal fracture with spinal cord injury.

Hospital Discharge Rates (figures 13 and 14)

Cause-specific hospital discharge data from the National Hospital Discharge Survey are defined based on the first-listed diagnosis. See table I for a listing of the code numbers used to define the diagnostic categories.

Mortality (figures 16–18)

See Appendix I, National Center for Health Statistics, National Vital Statistics System for a description of the data source. External cause of injury codes (E-codes) are assigned for all deaths for which the underlying cause of death as listed on the death certificate was an injury. See table II for code numbers used to define cause of death categories. The E-codes are designed to classify environmental events, circumstances, and conditions that contributed to the injury. E-codes have two dimensions: cause or mechanism of injury (for example, firearm, motor vehicle, and poisoning) and intent or manner of death (including unintentional, suicide, homicide, intent undetermined, and other.) For a discussion of the urbanization strata, see Appendix II, Urbanization.

Mortality data are graphed on a log scale because of the large variation in death rates from different causes and for different ages. Use of a log scale

Table II. Codes for cause of death categories from the *International Classification of Diseases, Ninth Revision (ICD-9)*

Cause of death	ICD-9 Code numbers
Natural causes	001–799
Injury[1]	E800–E869, E880–E929, E950–E999
Motor vehicle traffic	E810–E819, E958.5, E988.5
Fall	E880–E886, E888, E957, E968.1, E987
Struck	E916–E917, E968.2, E960.0, E973, E975
Cut	E920, E956, E966, E974, E986
Firearm	E922, E955.0–E955.4, E965.0–E965.4, E970, E985.0–E985.4
Unintentional injury	E800–E869, E880–E929
Suicide	E950–E959
Homicide	E960–E969

[1]Injury codes exclude adverse effects and complications of medical care.facilitates presentation and comparison of

facilitates presentation and comparison of mortality from causes or ages with disparate rates. The log scale also emphasizes relative rather than absolute change.

Pregnancy Rates (figure 19)

Pregnancies are estimated as the sum of the three outcomes: live births, induced abortions, and fetal losses (miscarriages and stillbirths). The birth data are complete counts of all live births. See Appendix I, National Center for Health Statistics, National Vital Statistics System for a description of the data sources for live births.

Abortion estimates in this report are based on national estimates compiled by the Alan Guttmacher Institute (AGI) from their surveys of all known abortion providers. The AGI estimates are distributed by age, race, and Hispanic origin, according to estimates prepared by the CDC's National Center for Chronic Disease Prevention and Health Promotion based on reports from State health departments. See Appendix I, Alan Guttmacher Institute and National Center for Chronic Disease Prevention and Health Promotion, Abortion Surveillance for a description of data sources for abortion estimates.

Information on fetal losses is based on the 1995 National Survey of Family Growth (NSFG). See Appendix I, National Center for Health Statistics, National Survey of Family Growth for a description of

Adolescent Health

this data source. The proportion of pregnancies ending in fetal loss (excluding induced abortions) in the 5 years preceding the 1995 survey are used. The rate of pregnancy loss depends on the degree to which losses at very early gestations are detected.

Information on abortion and fetal losses, needed to calculate pregnancy rates, was not available for American Indian or Alaska Native and Asian or Pacific Islander adolescents.

Sexually Transmitted Diseases (figure 23)

Sexually transmitted disease surveillance is conducted by the Division of STD Prevention, National Center for HIV, STD, and TB Prevention, CDC, based on cases reported to State health departments.

In 1998, 49 States and the District of Columbia reported cases of chlamydial infection; for the State of New York, only cases from New York City were reported. While case reporting of chlamydial infections is improving, it remains incomplete in many areas. A combination of factors limit the documentation of the incidence of chlamydia: variable compliance with public health laws and regulations that require health care providers and laboratories to report cases to local health authorities, large numbers of asymptomatic persons who can be identified only through screening, limited resources to support screening activities, and incomplete management systems for collecting, maintaining, and analyzing case reporting (4).

In 1998 cases of gonorrhea were reported by all 50 States, the District of Columbia, and selected cities. Reporting of gonococcal infections has likely been biased toward reporting of infections in persons of minority race or ethnicity who attend public STD clinics (5).

In 1998 incidence rates for chlamydia and gonorrhea were calculated as the number of cases per 100,000 adolescents based on the 1997 postcensal population estimates from the Bureau of the Census data (U.S. Bureau of the Census: 1991–97 Estimates of the Population of Counties by Age, Sex and Race/Hispanic origin 1991 to 1997; machine-readable data files). The cited rates are not adjusted for sexual

activity rates, and therefore underestimate the actual prevalence in the sexually active adolescent population.

The percent of cases for which race/ethnicity and age were unknown or unspecified differed considerably by area. States were excluded from analysis if race/ethnicity and age were not reported for the majority of cases. For 1998 Colorado, District of Columbia, Michigan, New Jersey, New York, Ohio, and South Carolina were excluded. Otherwise, if race/ethnicity or age was unknown or unspecified, cases were distributed according to the distribution of cases for which these data were available.

AIDS (figure 24)

AIDS rates are calculated as AIDS cases per 100,000 adolescents, for the year reported and the age at diagnosis. Population denominators for the 50 States and District of Columbia are based on official postcensus estimates from the U.S. Bureau of Census. Age-, sex-, and race/ethnicity-specific rates are based on year-specific additional detail files on "Monthly Population Estimates, 1990 to 1999" found on the U.S. Bureau of Census Web page (www.census.gov/population/www/estimates/uspop.html). The pooled 3-year rate from 1996–1998 is the number of cases reported during that 36-month period for each age, sex, and race/ethnicity category divided by the sum of the 1996, 1997, and 1998 age, sex, and race/ethnicity category population, multiplied by 100,000. See Appendix I, National Center for HIV, STD, and TB Prevention, AIDS Surveillance for a description of the AIDS surveillance system.

Health Care Visit (figure 32)

The estimates of the proportion of adolescents without a health care visit in the past 12 months were based on the 1997 National Health Interview Survey. Information was reported by the adolescent's parent for adolescents 10–17 years of age and self-response for those 18–19 years of age. A health care visit was defined as being seen by a physician or other health professional, in a doctor's office, clinic, or other setting. Emergency department visits were excluded.

References

1. Centers for Disease Control and Prevention. Youth risk behavior surveillance, United States 1999. CDC Surveillance Summaries, MMWR (in press).

2. Shah BV, Barnwell BG, Bieler GS. SUDAAN user's manual, release 7, first edition. Research Triangle Park, North Carolina: Research Triangle Institute. 1996.

3. Nourjah P. National Hospital Ambulatory Medical Care Survey: 1997 emergency department summary. Advance data from vital and health statistics; no 304. Hyattsville, Maryland: National Center for Health Statistics. 1999.

4. Division of STD Prevention. Sexually Transmitted Disease Surveillance 1998. Department of Health and Human Services, Atlanta: Centers for Disease Control and Prevention (CDC). September 1999.

5. Fox KK, Whittington W, Levine WC, et al. Gonorrhea in the United States, 1981–1996: demographic and geographic trends. Sex Transm Dis 25(7):386–93. 1998.

Data Tables for Figures 1–32 ....

Figure 1. Percent of adolescents 10–19 years of age

Year	White, non-Hispanic	Black, non-Hispanic	Hispanic	White	Black	American Indian/ Alaska Native	Asian/Pacific Islander
1980	75.6	14.2	7.9	83.1	14.5	0.8	1.6
1985	72.5	14.5	9.7	81.5	15.0	1.0	2.6
1990	69.4	14.7	11.7	80.1	15.3	1.1	3.4
1995	67.7	14.7	13.0	79.5	15.4	1.2	3.9
1999	66.3	14.8	14.0	79.0	15.6	1.2	4.2
Projected							
2000	65.9	14.7	14.1	78.7	15.6	1.2	4.5
2010	60.5	15.1	17.9	76.7	16.3	1.2	5.9
2020	55.7	15.7	20.8	74.5	17.1	1.3	7.1
2030	52.0	15.7	23.8	73.4	17.4	1.3	7.9
2040	48.0	15.9	26.6	71.9	17.8	1.3	8.9
2050	44.2	16.1	29.5	70.7	18.3	1.4	9.6

Figure 2. Poverty by family structure among adolescents 10–17 years of age

Family structure, race, and Hispanic origin	Poor	Near poor
	Percent	
All adolescents:		
All races.	16.7	20.0
White, non-Hispanic.	9.2	15.6
Black, non-Hispanic.	33.1	27.5
Hispanic.	32.0	31.9
Adolescents in married couple families:		
All races.	7.7	17.1
White, non-Hispanic.	4.7	12.3
Black, non-Hispanic.	10.6	27.2
Hispanic.	21.0	35.3
Adolescents in female householder families:		
All races.	40.2	27.2
White, non-Hispanic.	27.1	28.0
Black, non-Hispanic.	50.1	28.2
Hispanic.	54.2	25.3

Figure 3. Employment in April and July among adolescents 16–19 years of age

Race and Hispanic origin	Age in years				
	16	17	18	19	16–19
	Percent				
All races:					
April.	25.6	38.2	48.9	56.0	42.1
July	38.1	51.9	58.0	69.8	54.5
White, non-Hispanic:					
April.	31.9	45.2	55.5	59.5	48.1
July	45.8	61.0	66.4	77.7	62.9
Black, non-Hispanic:					
April.	13.4	18.3	31.2	40.4	25.5
July	26.3	27.7	40.3	51.1	35.9
Hispanic:					
April.	14.2	27.9	41.2	59.1	36.0
July	22.6	39.1	47.6	57.3	41.5

Figure 4. Event dropout rates among adolescents 15–19 years of age

	Age				Race and Hispanic origin				Family income		
	15–16 years	17 years	18 years	19 years	All races	White, non-Hispanic	Black, non-Hispanic	Hispanic	Low	Middle	High
Percent	2.3	2.8	5.9	10.6	4.2	3.6	4.7	7.7	11.5	3.2	2.6
SE	0.4	0.4	0.7	1.7	0.3	0.4	0.9	1.4	1.3	0.4	0.5

SE Standard error.

Figure 5. Activity limitations among adolescents 10–17 years of age

	Special education only		All other limitations[1]		Total limitations	
Age, sex, race, and income	Percent	SE	Percent	SE	Percent	SE
Female						
10–17 years.	3.6	0.3	2.4	0.2	5.9	0.3
10–12 years.	3.7	0.4	2.0	0.3	5.7	0.5
13–15 years.	3.9	0.5	2.5	0.3	6.4	0.6
16–17 years.	3.0	0.5	2.8	0.4	5.7	0.6
Male						
10–17 years.	7.4	0.4	3.2	0.3	10.7	0.5
10–12 years.	7.8	0.6	3.4	0.4	11.2	0.7
13–15 years.	7.5	0.6	2.7	0.4	10.3	0.7
16–17 years.	6.9	0.7	3.7	0.5	10.6	0.8
Race and Hispanic origin						
All races	5.6	0.2	2.8	0.2	8.4	0.3
White, non-Hispanic	5.9	0.3	3.0	0.2	9.0	0.4
Black, non-Hispanic	5.9	0.6	3.0	0.4	8.9	0.7
Hispanic	4.1	0.4	1.9	0.3	6.1	0.5
Poverty status						
Poor	8.3	0.8	4.0	0.5	12.3	0.9
Near poor	7.7	0.7	2.6	0.4	10.2	0.8
Nonpoor	4.7	0.3	2.6	0.2	7.4	0.4

[1]May include special education.
SE Standard error.

Figure 6. Untreated dental caries among adolescents 10–19 years of age

	Poverty status					
	Poor		Near poor		Nonpoor	
Race and Hispanic origin	Percent	SE	Percent	SE	Percent	SE
All races	31.3	2.3	24.3	2.9	10.9	1.0
White, non-Hispanic	24.3	4.3	22.1	3.7	9.4	1.0
Black, non-Hispanic	32.8	2.9	32.7	3.5	24.9	3.2
Mexican American	37.4	3.2	24.3	2.6	16.9	3.9

SE Standard error.

Data Tables for Figures 1–32 ....

Figure 7. Suicide ideation and attempts among students in grades 9–12

Grade level, race, and Hispanic origin	Female						Male					
	Seriously considered suicide[1]		All suicide attempts[2]		Injurious suicide attempts		Seriously considered suicide[1]		All suicide attempts[2]		Injurious suicide attempts	
	Percent	SE	Percent	SE	Percent	SE	Percent	SE	Percent	SE	Percent	SE
9th	24.4	2.0	14.0	1.3	3.8	0.7	11.9	1.4	6.1	1.2	2.6	0.8
10th	30.1	1.6	14.8	1.7	4.0	0.9	13.7	1.9	6.3	1.2	1.8	0.6
11th...................	23.0	1.9	7.5	1.2	2.8	0.8	13.7	1.8	4.8	0.9	2.1	0.7
12th	21.2	1.9	5.8	1.2	1.3	0.4	15.6	1.8	5.4	1.3	1.7	0.6
Total	24.9	1.1	10.9	0.8	3.1	0.4	13.7	0.8	5.7	0.6	2.1	0.3
White, non-Hispanic	23.2	1.2	9.0	1.2	2.3	0.6	12.5	0.7	4.5	0.6	1.6	0.4
Black, non-Hispanic	18.8	1.2	7.5	1.3	2.4	0.7	11.7	1.4	7.1	2.7	3.4	2.0
Hispanic	26.1	1.5	18.9	2.0	4.6	1.0	13.6	1.5	6.6	1.3	1.4	0.4

SE Standard error.

[1]Includes students who attempted suicide.

[2]Six percent of students attempting suicide did not report seriously considering suicide.

Injurious suicide attempt - an injury, poisoning or overdose that was treated by a doctor or nurse.

Figure 8. Emergency department visit, hospital discharge, and death rates among adolescents 10–19 years of age

Age	Female Rate	Female SE	Male Rate	Male SE
Emergency department visits	Events per 10,000 adolescents			
10 years	2,071.0	160.6	2,302.3	172.7
11 years	2,110.1	180.0	2,393.7	203.8
12 years	2,219.3	172.7	2,358.3	180.7
13 years	2,028.7	190.3	2,345.6	181.4
14 years	2,781.3	218.5	2,828.0	182.7
15 years	2,786.6	187.1	2,825.2	194.5
16 years	3,515.3	252.6	3,326.6	221.4
17 years	4,431.4	225.4	3,164.1	232.2
18 years	5,082.7	305.5	3,657.2	253.5
19 years	5,076.3	362.1	3,686.0	290.8
Hospital discharges				
10 years	152.8	13.1	205.1	16.4
11 years	156.9	13.4	199.3	19.1
12 years	177.2	15.8	211.4	15.6
13 years	234.8	17.3	227.3	16.6
14 years	343.5	21.5	259.3	18.2
15 years	502.9	25.9	280.3	18.0
16 years	712.6	31.0	336.1	21.4
17 years	1,000.6	43.6	328.0	19.1
18 years	1,222.5	48.7	334.7	20.7
19 years	1,357.5	54.9	312.2	19.8
Deaths				
10 years	1.5	0.1	1.9	0.1
11 years	1.5	0.1	2.1	0.1
12 years	1.8	0.1	2.5	0.1
13 years	1.9	0.1	3.3	0.1
14 years	2.5	0.1	4.3	0.1
15 years	3.0	0.1	5.8	0.1
16 years	4.5	0.1	9.0	0.2
17 years	4.8	0.1	10.9	0.2
18 years	4.9	0.1	14.0	0.2
19 years	4.7	0.1	14.4	0.2

SE Standard error.

Data Tables for Figures 1–32 ....

Figure 9. Injury, noninjury, and pregnancy-related emergency department visit rates among adolescents 10–19 years of age

	Injury		Noninjury		Pregnancy related	
Sex and age	Rate	SE	Rate	SE	Rate	SE
Female			Visits per 10,000 adolescents			
10–11 years....................	1,038.0	77.4	981.4	88.8	*	*
12–13 years....................	1,173.2	99.3	854.4	76.0	*	*
14–15 years....................	1,277.9	94.0	1,340.6	102.0	78.9	21.6
16–17 years....................	1,496.9	110.8	2,082.9	122.5	274.3	39.2
18–19 years....................	1,584.2	111.1	2,831.8	200.6	536.2	79.9
Male						
10–11 years....................	1,432.8	108.7	839.0	76.2	...	...
12–13 years....................	1,491.3	94.6	782.7	69.4	...	...
14–15 years....................	1,799.0	108.8	948.0	88.8	...	...
16–17 years....................	2,209.9	151.6	959.2	88.5	...	...
18–19 years....................	2,225.0	150.9	1,342.6	122.7	...	...

SE Standard error.
* Number in this category is too small to calculate reliable rates; relative standard error greater than 30 percent.
... Category not applicable.

Figure 10. Emergency department visit rates for selected external causes of injury among adolescents 10–19 years of age

	Female		Male	
Age and external cause	Rate	SE	Rate	SE
Struck by or against		Visits per 10,000 adolescents		
10–11 years....................	164.9	30.2	282.4	45.2
12–13 years....................	150.8	31.9	294.1	37.7
14–15 years....................	237.1	38.2	452.3	51.9
16–17 years....................	229.4	39.7	588.4	68.9
18–19 years....................	247.5	38.9	483.1	59.7
Cut or pierce				
10–11 years....................	94.1	21.3	168.5	28.3
12–13 years....................	71.7	17.2	103.7	20.5
14–15 years....................	67.9	18.0	124.2	24.2
16–17 years....................	91.5	25.0	238.2	33.9
18–19 years....................	189.0	34.4	226.9	36.1
Fall				
10–11 years....................	288.1	39.7	310.4	47.0
12–13 years....................	314.6	51.5	275.1	41.5
14–15 years....................	220.1	39.0	268.7	46.5
16–17 years....................	194.4	30.6	246.3	45.3
18–19 years....................	197.4	32.2	202.1	33.4
Motor vehicle traffic				
10–11 years....................	81.7	28.7	90.1	25.4
12–13 years....................	105.1	25.2	94.3	23.7
14–15 years....................	221.1	38.2	161.6	33.4
16–17 years....................	385.3	50.4	311.9	49.1
18–19 years....................	416.6	48.4	349.2	50.3

SE Standard error.

Figure 11. Emergency department visit rates for selected injury diagnoses among adolescents 10–19 years of age

Age and injury diagnosis	Female		Male	
	Rate	SE	Rate	SE
Fractures	Visits per 10,000 adolescents			
10–11 years....................	179.1	32.8	250.7	38.7
12–13 years....................	156.2	34.0	253.2	30.9
14–15 years....................	103.7	22.4	330.9	44.1
16–17 years....................	103.8	27.3	257.7	41.9
18–19 years....................	83.0	21.2	225.7	40.8
Sprains and strains				
10–11 years....................	189.0	39.1	175.9	31.9
12–13 years....................	319.1	46.7	277.9	39.9
14–15 years....................	362.3	46.9	325.2	42.3
16–17 years....................	398.3	50.3	334.1	44.1
18–19 years....................	286.9	43.1	348.8	43.2
Open wounds				
10–11 years....................	212.4	31.0	396.7	51.9
12–13 years....................	198.0	41.3	318.0	40.6
14–15 years....................	203.5	33.6	319.5	33.7
16–17 years....................	214.7	30.6	488.0	52.4
18–19 years....................	338.2	57.4	616.2	76.4
Contusions				
10–11 years....................	223.9	37.4	235.9	37.6
12–13 years....................	194.8	34.9	244.0	36.2
14–15 years....................	267.6	40.4	318.5	41.6
16–17 years....................	313.3	48.3	382.7	54.0
18–19 years....................	282.2	34.6	313.6	40.4

SE Standard error.

Data Tables for Figures 1–32 ....

Figure 12. Emergency department visit rates for selected noninjury diagnoses among adolescents 10–19 years of age

Age and noninjury diagnosis	Female		Male	
	Rate	SE	Rate	SE
Upper respiratory infections	Visits per 10,000 adolescents			
10–11 years..........................	303.8	46.5	211.4	36.2
12–13 years..........................	183.1	36.0	179.1	32.6
14–15 years..........................	308.3	52.4	168.4	31.4
16–17 years..........................	268.0	31.6	216.7	36.9
18–19 years..........................	342.0	44.9	186.3	34.7
Asthma				
10–11 years..........................	*	*	96.7	17.8
12–13 years..........................	*	*	*	*
14–15 years..........................	59.3	14.7	91.6	26.6
16–17 years..........................	89.9	19.5	64.2	17.3
18–19 years..........................	97.6	24.4	98.6	25.8
Abdominal symptoms				
10–11 years..........................	101.7	24.6	45.0	13.2
12–13 years..........................	138.8	26.3	138.5	27.0
14–15 years..........................	160.5	30.0	93.9	23.0
16–17 years..........................	311.9	47.6	122.9	27.4
18–19 years..........................	495.9	59.7	159.6	29.7
Sexually transmitted diseases				
10–11 years..........................	*	*	*	*
12–13 years..........................	*	*	*	*
14–15 years..........................	*	*	*	*
16–17 years..........................	151.8	31.2	*	*
18–19 years..........................	210.4	39.1	*	*
Urinary tract infections				
10–11 years..........................	*	*	*	*
12–13 years..........................	*	*	*	*
14–15 years..........................	83.1	23.5	*	*
16–17 years..........................	168.7	39.0	*	*
18–19 years..........................	335.3	49.4	*	*
Pregnancy-related diagnoses				
10–11 years..........................	*	*	...	...
12–13 years..........................	*	*	...	...
14–15 years..........................	78.9	21.6	...	...
16–17 years..........................	274.3	39.2	...	...
18–19 years..........................	536.2	79.9	...	...

* Number in this category is too small to calculate reliable rates; relative standard error greater than 30 percent.
... Category not applicable.

Figure 13. Injury, noninjury, and pregnancy-related hospital discharge rates among adolescents 10–19 years of age

Sex and age	Injury		Noninjury		Pregnancy related	
	Rate	SE	Rate	SE	Rate	SE
Female	Discharges per 10,000 adolescents					
10–11 years................................	21.2	2.5	128.4	10.1	*	*
12–13 years................................	23.8	2.7	170.9	12.9	5.9	1.2
14–15 years................................	53.8	5.0	250.6	15.6	114.7	7.8
16–17 years................................	63.5	5.2	286.8	15.6	501.0	21.8
18–19 years................................	61.9	5.3	280.1	14.7	942.3	36.9
Male						
10–11 years................................	34.7	3.8	161.9	13.6	...	...
12–13 years................................	46.7	4.2	165.9	11.2	...	...
14–15 years................................	63.2	5.1	199.4	13.1	...	...
16–17 years................................	99.3	7.1	225.9	14.6	...	...
18–19 years................................	101.1	7.4	216.7	13.3	...	...

SE Standard error.
* Number in this category is too small to calculate reliable rates; relative standard error greater than 30 percent.
... Category not applicable.

Figure 14. Hospital discharge rates for selected diagnoses among adolescents 10–19 years of age

Age and diagnoses	Female		Male	
	Rate	SE	Rate	SE
Asthma	Discharges per 10,000 adolescents			
10–11 years...................	16.2	2.4	21.8	2.8
12–13 years...................	12.7	1.7	18.9	2.4
14–15 years...................	15.5	2.8	11.3	1.5
16–17 years...................	16.3	2.4	6.8	1.2
18–19 years...................	12.2	1.7	5.2	2.1
Psychoses				
10–11 years...................	*	*	6.6	1.4
12–13 years...................	20.7	3.7	17.0	2.9
14–15 years...................	44.8	6.9	30.2	4.5
16–17 years...................	40.2	5.9	29.5	4.0
18–19 years...................	29.5	3.3	32.3	4.6
Poisoning				
10–11 years...................	*	*	*	*
12–13 years...................	8.0	1.8	*	*
14–15 years...................	24.2	3.6	6.0	1.3
16–17 years...................	22.3	2.9	7.6	1.3
18–19 years...................	16.6	2.5	8.8	1.8
Fractures				
10–11 years...................	7.3	1.2	12.5	1.8
12–13 years...................	4.5	1.0	18.9	2.0
14–15 years...................	10.5	2.2	23.9	2.8
16–17 years...................	14.8	2.5	35.0	3.9
18–19 years...................	16.1	2.4	32.7	4.1

SE Standard error.
* Number in this category is too small to calculate reliable rates; relative standard error greater than 30 percent.

Data Tables for Figures 1–32 ....

Figure 15. Violent crime victimization rates among adolescents 12–19 years of age

	Female		Male	
Age	Rate	SE	Rate	SE
	Victimizations per 1,000 adolescents			
12–13 years.....................	82.0	4.8	137.0	6.0
14–15 years.....................	92.4	5.1	137.5	6.1
16–17 years.....................	90.6	5.1	129.8	5.9
18–19 years.....................	98.6	5.4	129.9	6.1

	12–15 years of age		16–19 years of age	
Year	Rate	SE	Rate	SE
1992........................	118.3	7.9	112.6	7.8
1993........................	132.1	6.3	122.1	6.2
1994........................	123.9	5.4	127.6	5.6
1995........................	111.3	5.1	113.7	4.8
1996........................	96.8	4.9	98.9	5.1
1997........................	95.9	5.2	102.2	5.4

SE Standard error.

Figure 16. Injury and natural cause death rates among adolescents 10–19 years of age

	Injury								Natural cause	
	All injury		Unintentional		Suicide		Homicide			
Sex and age	Rate	SE	Rate	SE	Rate•	SE	Rate	SE	Rate	SE
Female	Deaths per 100,000 adolescents									
10 years..............................	6.3	0.4	5.6	0.4	*	*	0.5	0.1	8.4	0.5
11 years........................	6.0	0.4	5.1	0.4	*	*	0.7	0.1	9.1	0.5
12 years..............................	7.8	0.5	6.4	0.4	*	*	1.0	0.2	10.6	0.5
13 years..............................	9.6	0.5	6.9	0.4	1.4	0.2	1.3	0.2	9.5	0.5
14 years..............................	14.4	0.6	10.4	0.5	2.1	0.2	1.9	0.2	11.0	0.5
15 years..............................	19.6	0.7	13.5	0.6	3.3	0.3	2.6	0.3	10.6	0.5
16 years..............................	32.0	0.9	24.1	0.8	3.8	0.3	3.8	0.3	12.5	0.6
17 years..............................	33.8	1.0	25.7	0.8	3.5	0.3	4.3	0.3	14.1	0.6
18 years..............................	34.3	1.0	24.9	0.8	3.5	0.3	5.5	0.4	14.8	0.6
19 years..............................	30.7	0.9	21.5	0.8	3.3	0.3	5.6	0.4	16.0	0.7
Male										
10 years..............................	9.8	0.5	8.3	0.5	0.6	0.1	0.8	0.1	9.6	0.5
11 years..............................	11.1	0.5	9.0	0.5	0.8	0.1	1.2	0.2	9.6	0.5
12 years..............................	15.2	0.6	11.6	0.6	1.6	0.2	1.5	0.2	10.3	0.5
13 years..............................	19.9	0.7	14.3	0.6	3.1	0.3	2.0	0.2	13.2	0.6
14 years..............................	28.6	0.9	17.7	0.7	5.4	0.4	5.1	0.4	14.0	0.6
15 years..............................	44.0	1.1	25.1	0.8	8.4	0.5	9.6	0.5	14.3	0.6
16 years..............................	73.2	1.4	43.4	1.0	12.4	0.6	16.3	0.6	16.8	0.7
17 years..............................	90.5	1.5	49.0	1.1	14.7	0.6	25.6	0.8	18.0	0.7
18 years..............................	117.6	1.8	61.5	1.3	19.7	0.7	34.0	1.0	22.0	0.8
19 years..............................	121.6	1.8	61.3	1.3	21.9	0.8	36.1	1.0	22.3	0.8

SE Standard error.
* Number in this category is too small to calculate reliable rates; fewer than 20 deaths.

Figure 17. Death rates for motor vehicle traffic-related and firearm-related injuries among adolescents 10–19 years of age

| | Motor vehicle deaths | | | | Firearm-related deaths | | | |
| | Female | | Male | | Female | | Male | |
Age	Rate	SE	Rate	SE	Rate	SE	Rate	SE
	Deaths per 100,000 adolescents							
10 years	3.1	0.3	4.8	0.3	*	*	1.0	0.2
11 years	3.3	0.3	4.4	0.3	0.5	0.1	1.8	0.2
12 years	4.4	0.3	5.9	0.4	0.6	0.1	2.8	0.3
13 years	4.5	0.3	7.3	0.4	1.2	0.2	4.6	0.3
14 years	7.5	0.4	10.0	0.5	2.5	0.3	9.4	0.5
15 years	11.3	0.6	15.5	0.6	3.6	0.3	15.9	0.6
16 years	21.7	0.8	33.0	0.9	4.9	0.4	25.6	0.8
17 years	22.6	0.8	37.3	1.0	4.7	0.4	34.5	0.9
18 years	22.2	0.8	46.7	1.1	5.5	0.4	46.7	1.1
19 years	18.4	0.7	45.5	1.1	5.2	0.4	49.8	1.1

SE Standard error.
* Number in this category is too small to calculate reliable rates; fewer than 20 deaths.

Figure 18. Death rates for motor vehicle traffic-related and firearm-related injuries among adolescents 10–19 years of age

| | Core | | Other metropolitan | | Nonmetropolitan | |
Age	Rate	SE	Rate	SE	Rate	SE
Motor vehicle	Deaths per 100,000 adolescents					
10 years	3.2	0.4	3.5	0.3	6.0	0.6
11 years	3.0	0.4	3.6	0.3	5.9	0.6
12 years	3.9	0.4	4.4	0.3	8.5	0.7
13 years	4.3	0.5	5.4	0.4	9.2	0.8
14 years	6.7	0.6	7.7	0.5	14.0	0.9
15 years	8.7	0.6	12.3	0.6	22.2	1.2
16 years	14.4	0.8	27.4	0.9	44.7	1.6
17 years	17.4	0.9	28.1	0.9	51.1	1.7
18 years	23.0	1.1	32.0	0.9	56.6	1.9
19 years	21.5	1.0	29.7	0.9	53.8	1.9
Firearm						
10 years	*	*	*	*	*	*
11 years	1.4	0.3	0.8	0.1	1.8	0.3
12 years	1.5	0.3	1.3	0.2	3.0	0.4
13 years	2.7	0.4	2.5	0.3	4.3	0.5
14 years	6.7	0.6	5.8	0.4	5.7	0.6
15 years	14.9	0.8	7.4	0.4	9.3	0.7
16 years	24.8	1.1	12.4	0.6	11.1	0.8
17 years	33.4	1.2	15.4	0.6	13.8	0.9
18 years	44.5	1.5	19.1	0.7	21.5	1.2
19 years	46.1	1.5	21.1	0.7	20.5	1.1

SE Standard error.
* Number in this category is too small to calculate reliable rates; fewer than 20 deaths.

Data Tables for Figures 1–32 ....

Figure 19. Pregnancy rates for adolescents 10–19 years of age

Age, race, and Hispanic origin	Birth	Abortion	Fetal loss	Pregnancy
Age 10–14 years	Outcomes per 1,000 female adolescents			
All races	1.2	1.1	0.5	2.8
White, non-Hispanic	0.4	0.5	0.2	1.1
Black, non-Hispanic	3.8	3.9	1.0	8.7
Hispanic	2.6	1.3	0.4	4.3
American Indian/Alaska Native.......................................	1.7	- - -	- - -	- - -
Asian/Pacific Islander	0.6	- - -	- - -	- - -
Age 15–17 years				
All races	33.8	19.0	15.0	67.8
White, non-Hispanic	20.6	12.5	10.8	43.9
Black, non-Hispanic	66.6	43.7	17.7	128.1
Hispanic	69.0	24.7	11.3	105.0
American Indian/Alaska Native.......................................	46.4	- - -	- - -	- - -
Asian/Pacific Islander	14.9	- - -	- - -	- - -
Age 18–19 years				
All races	86.0	44.9	15.5	146.4
White, non-Hispanic	63.7	29.4	12.4	105.6
Black, non-Hispanic	136.6	100.1	17.7	254.4
Hispanic	151.1	59.5	24.8	235.4
American Indian/Alaska Native.......................................	122.3	- - -	- - -	- - -
Asian/Pacific Islander	40.4	- - -	- - -	- - -
Age 15–19 years				
All races	54.4	29.2	15.2	98.7
White, non-Hispanic	37.6	19.1	11.4	68.1
Black, non-Hispanic	94.2	65.9	17.7	177.8
Hispanic	101.8	38.6	16.7	157.1
American Indian/Alaska Native.......................................	73.9	- - -	- - -	- - -
Asian/Pacific Islander	24.6	- - -	- - -	- - -

- - - Data not available.

Figure 20. Birth rates for adolescents 13–19 years of age

Race and Hispanic origin	Age					
	13–14	15	16	17	18	19
	Births per 1,000 female adolescents					
All Races						
Total.	2.6	13.5	29.8	50.0	73.9	91.0
First birth	2.5	12.8	27.0	42.1	56.3	61.8
Second and higher	0.1	0.6	2.6	7.6	17.0	28.5
White, non-Hispanic						
Total.	0.9	6.3	16.7	32.5	52.1	68.0
First birth	0.9	6.2	15.7	29.0	42.7	50.1
Second and higher	*0.0	0.1	0.9	3.3	9.1	17.5
Black, non-Hispanic						
Total.	7.9	31.3	60.2	89.4	121.7	141.0
First birth	7.6	29.3	52.6	70.2	84.2	83.8
Second and higher	0.2	1.7	7.2	18.6	36.8	56.4
Hispanic						
Total.	5.5	30.3	63.1	95.8	130.0	149.3
First birth	5.3	28.6	56.1	77.7	94.3	95.8
Second and higher	0.1	1.5	6.3	17.1	34.4	52.2
White						
Total.	1.6	10.5	24.8	43.9	66.3	83.5
First birth	1.6	10.0	22.8	37.8	52.3	59.0
Second and higher	0.0	0.4	1.8	5.7	13.6	23.9
Black						
Total.	7.6	30.4	58.7	87.1	118.7	137.5
First birth	7.4	28.6	51.3	68.6	82.2	81.9
Second and higher	0.2	1.7	7.0	18.0	35.8	54.7
American Indian or Alaska Native						
Total.	4.0	19.8	44.4	71.3	107.1	127.9
First birth	3.8	18.7	40.1	59.7	79.1	80.7
Second and higher	*	*0.9	3.5	10.7	26.5	45.7
Asian or Pacific Islander						
Total.	1.1	6.0	14.0	21.8	33.7	42.6
First birth	1.0	5.6	12.6	18.4	26.1	31.0
Second and higher	*	0.4	1.4	3.3	7.4	11.3

* Rates based on fewer than 50 events are considered unreliable. Rates based on fewer than 20 events are considered highly unreliable and are not shown.

Data Tables for Figures 1–32 ....

Figure 21. Low-birthweight live births among adolescent mothers 13–19 years of age

Race and Hispanic origin	Maternal age in years					
	13–14	15	16	17	18	19
	Percent of live births					
All races						
All low birthweight	13.2	11.6	10.7	9.8	9.4	8.8
Moderately low birthweight	10.1	9.1	8.5	8.0	7.6	7.2
Very low birthweight	3.1	2.5	2.1	1.8	1.8	1.6
White, non-Hispanic						
All low birthweight	11.5	10.0	9.5	8.6	8.3	7.7
Moderately low birthweight	8.3	7.8	7.4	7.0	6.8	6.4
Very low birthweight	3.2	2.3	2.0	1.5	1.5	1.3
Black, non-Hispanic						
All low birthweight	15.7	15.0	14.4	13.8	13.3	12.9
Moderately low birthweight	12.1	11.6	11.4	10.9	10.4	10.3
Very low birthweight	3.6	3.5	2.9	2.9	2.8	2.6
Hispanic						
All low birthweight	10.7	9.2	8.4	8.0	7.6	7.0
Moderately low birthweight	8.5	7.5	7.0	6.8	6.4	5.9
Very low birthweight	2.2	1.7	1.5	1.3	1.2	1.1
White						
All low birthweight	11.1	9.7	9.0	8.4	8.1	7.5
Moderately low birthweight	8.4	7.7	7.2	6.9	6.7	6.2
Very low birthweight	2.7	2.0	1.8	1.4	1.4	1.2
Black						
All low birthweight	15.8	14.9	14.3	13.7	13.2	12.9
Moderately low birthweight	12.1	11.5	11.4	10.8	10.4	10.2
Very low birthweight	3.6	3.4	2.9	2.9	2.8	2.6
American Indian or Alaska Native						
All low birthweight	9.1	7.5	7.1	6.6	6.9	6.5
Moderately low birthweight	*8.0	6.4	6.1	5.7	5.8	5.3
Very low birthweight	*	*	*1.0	*0.9	*1.0	1.2
Asian or Pacific Islander						
All low birthweight	14.5	14.4	12.5	11.3	9.9	9.0
Moderately low birthweight	*9.9	12.0	10.3	9.3	8.3	7.7
Very low birthweight	*	*2.5	*2.2	2.0	1.6	1.3

* Rates based on fewer than 50 events are considered unreliable. Rates based on fewer than 20 events are considered highly unreliable and are not shown.
Low birthweight - less than 2,500 grams.
Moderately low birthweight - 1,500–2,499 grams.
Very low birthweight - less than 1,500 grams.

Figure 22. Infant mortality rates among infants of adolescent mothers 13–19 years of age

Race and Hispanic origin	Maternal age in years						
	13–14	15	16	17	18	19	13–19
	Infant deaths per 1,000 live births						
All races	17.1	13.7	11.4	10.6	10.3	9.5	10.6
White, non-Hispanic	18.4	14.2	12	9.9	9.5	8.8	9.9
Black, non-Hispanic	19.6	16.4	13.4	14.4	14.3	13.9	14.4
Hispanic	12.1	9.3	8.4	7.8	7.3	6.7	7.6
White	15.2	12.1	10.6	9.1	8.8	8.2	9.1
Black	19.6	16.3	13.3	14.3	14.3	13.8	14.4
American Indian or Alaska Native	*	*	*10.5	11.8	12.2	10.3	11.2
Asian or Pacific Islander	*	*14.1	*8.9	*7.5	8.4	8.4	8.7

* Rates based on fewer than 50 events are considered unreliable. Rates based on fewer than 20 events are considered highly unreliable and are not shown.

Figure 23. Sexually transmitted disease rates reported for adolescents 10–19 years of age

Age, race, and Hispanic origin	Chlamydia		Gonorrhea	
	Female	Male	Female	Male
	Reported cases per 100,000 adolescents			
10–14 years	142.5	7.9	58.0	8.5
15–19 years	2,359.4	308.4	779.7	354.6
White, non-Hispanic	1,190.8	100.6	218.2	41.7
Black, non-Hispanic	7,786.3	1,256.2	3,851.7	2,075.9
Hispanic	2,564.2	371.2	320.8	155.5
American Indian or Alaska Native	4,056.7	547.1	654.4	156.7
Asian or Pacific Islander	949.8	126.6	119.4	24.8

Figure 24. Acquired immunodeficiency syndrome reported rates for adolescents 11–19 years of age

Age, race, and Hispanic origin	Female	Male
	Reported cases per 100,000 adolescents	
White, non-Hispanic		
11–14 years	0.11	0.21
15–17 years	0.14	0.36
18–19 years	0.52	0.89
Black, non-Hispanic		
11–14 years	2.02	2.04
15–17 years	4.31	2.76
18–19 years	12.16	8.28
Hispanic		
11–14 years	1.26	1.01
15–17 years	0.63	1.03
18–19 years	2.03	3.95

Data Tables for Figures 1–32 ....

Figure 25. Lifetime sexual activity among students in grades 9–12

	Female				Male			
	Ever had sexual intercourse		Multiple sex partners		Ever had sexual intercourse		Multiple sex partners	
Grade level and race and Hispanic origin	Percent	SE	Percent	SE	Percent	SE	Percent	SE
9th	32.5	3.9	7.9	1.2	44.5	3.1	15.6	1.7
10th	42.6	2.6	10.1	1.4	51.1	3.9	21.4	4.2
11th..............................	53.8	2.3	15.1	2.4	51.4	2.9	19.4	2.8
12th..............................	65.8	3.9	20.6	2.7	63.9	3.2	20.6	2.0
Total	47.7	2.2	13.1	1.2	52.2	2.3	19.3	2.0
White, non-Hispanic	44.8	2.3	12.7	1.2	45.4	2.4	12.1	1.5
Black, non-Hispanic	66.9	5.8	21.3	4.5	75.7	3.3	48.1	6.5
Hispanic	45.5	3.2	10.5	1.9	62.9	2.8	23.0	3.2

SE Standard error.
Multiple sex partners - 4 or more partners in lifetime.

Figure 26. Cigarette smoking in the past 30 days among students in grades 9–12

	Female				Male			
	Current smoker		Frequent smoker		Current smoker		Frequent smoker	
Grade level, race, and Hispanic origin	Percent	SE	Percent	SE	Percent	SE	Percent	SE
9th	29.2	2.5	11.0	1.4	26.1	3.1	11.4	1.6
10th	35.7	2.1	15.3	2.0	33.6	1.5	15.0	2.0
11th..............................	35.6	2.7	17.1	1.6	36.4	3.0	20.4	2.9
12th..............................	40.5	3.0	20.3	3.1	45.2	3.4	26.1	5.2
Total	34.9	1.3	15.6	1.3	34.7	1.5	17.9	1.6
White, non-Hispanic	39.1	1.8	19.4	1.9	38.2	1.9	20.9	1.7
Black, non-Hispanic	17.7	1.8	5.0	1.6	21.8	3.6	9.1	2.2
Hispanic	31.5	2.4	8.5	1.6	34.0	2.3	12.5	2.3

SE Standard error.
Current smoker - smoked 1 or more days.
Frequent smoker- smoked 20 or more days.

Figure 27. Alcohol use in the past 30 days among students in grades 9–12

Grade level and race and Hispanic origin	Female				Male			
	Current drinking		Binge drinking		Current drinking		Binge drinking	
	Percent	SE	Percent	SE	Percent	SE	Percent	SE
9th	41.0	3.0	20.2	1.6	40.2	2.3	21.7	2.0
10th . , ...	46.8	1.7	31.1	1.9	52.7	3.0	33.4	2.8
11th.	48.3	2.6	29.0	2.4	53.5	3.0	38.8	3.0
12th	56.9	3.0	33.9	2.9	66.6	2.3	49.5	2.8
Total	47.7	1.4	28.1	1.1	52.3	1.5	34.9	1.4
White, non-Hispanic	49.8	2.4	32.2	1.6	54.9	2.1	39.1	1.7
Black, non-Hispanic	40.7	3.9	14.7	2.8	39.1	4.7	17.4	2.7
Hispanic	49.3	2.8	26.8	2.3	56.3	2.9	37.5	2.5

SE Standard error.
Current drinking - alcohol use on 1 or more days.
Binge drinking - 5 or more drinks on 1 occasion.

Figure 28. Lifetime and current Marijuana use among students in grades 9–12

Grade level, race, and Hispanic origin	Female				Male			
	Ever used		Current use		Ever used		Current used	
	Percent	SE	Percent	SE	Percent	SE	Percent	SE
9th	28.7	2.8	18.6	2.0	40.7	3.4	24.7	2.6
10th	46.7	2.1	24.3	2.2	51.6	4.2	31.4	3.3
11th.	48.5	2.1	22.1	2.3	51.0	3.2	31.1	3.3
12th	53.2	3.4	26.3	2.9	63.8	2.4	36.9	3.6
Total	43.4	1.2	22.6	0.9	51.0	2.1	30.8	1.9
White, non-Hispanic	42.3	1.6	22.9	1.3	49.2	3.0	29.6	2.5
Black, non-Hispanic	42.7	2.7	21.9	2.9	54.8	5.9	31.2	4.8
Hispanic	46.4	2.9	21.8	2.0	55.8	3.1	34.8	3.5

SE Standard error.
Current use - used marijuana 1 or more times in the past 30 days.

Data Tables for Figures 1–32 ....

Figure 29. Weapon carrying in the past 30 days among students in grades 9–12

	Female				Male			
	Carried a weapon		Carried a gun		Carried a weapon		Carried a gun	
Grade level, race, and Hispanic origin	Percent	SE	Percent	SE	Percent	SE	Percent	SE
9th	6.5	1.1	0.4	0.1	28.7	2.9	9.7	2.0
10th	7.1	1.1	0.8	0.2	30.7	2.2	9.6	1.4
11th............................	5.2	0.8	0.7	0.2	26.9	2.5	7.4	1.2
12th	4.8	1.1	1.2	0.5	27.3	2.7	8.3	1.6
Total	6.0	0.6	0.8	0.1	28.6	1.8	9.0	1.2
White, non-Hispanic	3.6	0.4	0.5	0.1	28.6	2.5	8.0	1.4
Black, non-Hispanic	11.7	2.1	1.8	0.6	23.1	3.7	14.5	3.5
Hispanic	8.4	1.4	1.6	0.5	29.5	1.6	8.2	1.0

SE Standard error.
Weapon - such as a knife, gun, or club.

Figure 30. Participation in moderate to vigorous physical activity among students in grades 9–12

	Female		Male		All students	
Grade level, race, and Hispanic origin	Percent	SE	Percent	SE	Percent	SE
9th	72.9	2.9	81.6	2.2	77.3	2.1
10th	61.6	3.7	76.3	2.1	68.9	2.4
11th............................	54.4	2.2	70.5	2.3	62.6	1.4
12th	59.7	2.7	75.6	1.9	67.6	2.0
Total	62.7	1.2	76.4	1.4	69.5	1.0
White, non-Hispanic	65.3	1.4	78.1	2.0	71.9	1.2
Black, non-Hispanic	52.5	1.7	68.1	4.2	60.0	2.4
Hispanic	54.3	2.6	75.7	2.3	64.9	2.2

SE Standard error.

Figure 31. Health care coverage of adolescents 10–19 years of age

	Uninsured		Medicaid		Private		Other	
Family income and age	Percent	SE	Percent	SE	Percent	SE	Percent	SE
Poor								
10–19 years................	31.4	1.4	42.9	1.6	23.9	1.6	1.9	0.4
10–12 years	23.9	1.8	55.2	2.2	19.0	1.8	2.0	0.7
13–15 years	30.6	2.1	46.6	2.3	21.5	2.0	1.3	0.5
16–17 years	38.0	2.8	43.6	3.0	16.4	2.2	2.1	0.9
18–19 years	37.0	2.9	22.8	2.4	37.9	3.9	2.2	0.8
Near poor								
10–19 years................	28.0	1.2	14.6	0.9	54.7	1.4	2.7	0.5
10–12 years	24.8	1.7	17.0	1.5	56.1	2.0	2.1	0.5
13–15 years	24.4	1.8	16.6	1.5	55.9	2.1	3.1	0.7
16–17 years	28.8	2.2	10.1	1.4	58.1	2.4	3.0	0.9
18–19 years	38.2	2.5	11.6	1.6	47.2	2.7	3.1	0.8
Nonpoor								
10–19 years................	8.2	0.5	2.1	0.2	87.0	0.6	2.6	0.3
10–12 years	6.3	0.6	2.5	0.3	88.7	0.8	2.5	0.4
13–15 years	6.4	0.6	2.1	0.3	89.0	0.8	2.1	0.3
16–17 years	7.0	0.7	1.5	0.4	89.1	0.9	2.4	0.4
18–19 years	17.0	1.3	2.4	0.5	77.5	1.5	3.1	0.6

SE Standard error.

Figure 32. No health care visits among adolescents 10–19 years of age

	Female		Male	
Age	Percent	SE	Percent	SE
10–19 years.....................................	17.7	0.8	18.9	0.8
10–12 years	20.0	1.5	18.0	1.4
13–15 years	18.2	1.3	15.3	1.2
16–17 years	17.5	1.7	17.5	1.4
18–19 years	13.3	1.8	27.5	2.5

	Insured		Uninsured	
Race and Hispanic origin	Percent	SE	Percent	SE
All races	14.5	0.6	37.8	1.8
White, non-Hispanic	13.4	0.7	26.6	2.5
Black, non-Hispanic	15.1	1.5	48.2	4.2
Hispanic	19.4	1.5	47.3	2.7

SE Standard error.

Trend Tables

Health Status and Determinants

Population

Fertility and Natality

Mortality

List of Trend Tables ....

Utilization of Health Resources

Ambulatory Care

List of Trend Tables ....

List of Trend Tables ....

Table 1 (page 1 of 2). Resident population, according to age, sex, detailed race, and Hispanic origin: United States, selected years 1950–98

[Data are based on decennial census updated by data from multiple sources]

Sex, race, Hispanic origin, and year	Total resident population	Under 1 year	1–4 years	5–14 years	15–24 years	25–34 years	35–44 years	45–54 years	55–64 years	65–74 years	75–84 years	85 years and over
All persons						Number in thousands						
1950	150,697	3,147	13,017	24,319	22,098	23,759	21,450	17,343	13,370	8,340	3,278	577
1960	179,323	4,112	16,209	35,465	24,020	22,818	24,081	20,485	15,572	10,997	4,633	929
1970	203,212	3,485	13,669	40,746	35,441	24,907	23,088	23,220	18,590	12,435	6,119	1,511
1980	226,546	3,534	12,815	34,942	42,487	37,082	25,634	22,800	21,703	15,580	7,729	2,240
1990	248,710	3,946	14,812	35,095	37,013	43,161	37,435	25,057	21,113	18,045	10,012	3,021
1997	267,636	3,797	15,353	38,778	36,580	39,610	43,998	33,633	21,813	18,499	11,706	3,871
1998	270,299	3,776	15,190	39,163	37,213	38,774	44,520	34,585	22,676	18,395	11,952	4,054
Male												
1950	74,833	1,602	6,634	12,375	10,918	11,597	10,588	8,655	6,697	4,024	1,507	237
1960	88,331	2,090	8,240	18,029	11,906	11,179	11,755	10,093	7,537	5,116	2,025	362
1970	98,912	1,778	6,968	20,759	17,551	12,217	11,231	11,199	8,793	5,437	2,436	542
1980	110,053	1,806	6,556	17,855	21,418	18,382	12,570	11,009	10,152	6,757	2,867	682
1990	121,239	2,018	7,581	17,971	18,915	21,564	18,510	12,232	9,955	7,907	3,745	841
1997	131,018	1,943	7,858	19,861	18,806	19,810	21,883	16,457	10,390	8,269	4,629	1,112
1998	132,046	1,929	7,767	20,050	19,042	19,254	22,101	16,900	10,806	8,250	4,761	1,187
Female												
1950	75,864	1,545	6,383	11,944	11,181	12,162	10,863	8,688	6,672	4,316	1,771	340
1960	90,992	2,022	7,969	17,437	12,114	11,639	12,326	10,393	8,036	5,881	2,609	567
1970	104,300	1,707	6,701	19,986	17,890	12,690	11,857	12,021	9,797	6,998	3,683	969
1980	116,493	1,727	6,259	17,087	21,068	18,700	13,065	11,791	11,551	8,825	4,862	1,559
1990	127,471	1,928	7,231	17,124	18,098	21,596	18,925	12,824	11,158	10,139	6,267	2,180
1997	136,618	1,854	7,495	18,917	17,774	19,799	22,115	17,176	11,422	10,230	7,077	2,759
1998	138,252	1,847	7,423	19,113	18,172	19,521	22,419	17,685	11,870	10,146	7,191	2,866
White male												
1950	67,129	1,400	5,845	10,860	9,689	10,430	9,529	7,836	6,180	3,736	1,406	218
1960	78,367	1,784	7,065	15,659	10,483	9,940	10,564	9,114	6,850	4,702	1,875	331
1970	86,721	1,501	5,873	17,667	15,232	10,775	9,979	10,090	7,958	4,916	2,243	487
1980	94,924	1,485	5,397	14,764	18,110	15,928	11,005	9,771	9,149	6,095	2,600	621
1990	102,143	1,604	6,071	14,467	15,389	18,071	15,819	10,624	8,813	7,127	3,397	760
1997	108,893	1,549	6,240	15,727	15,057	16,209	18,355	14,158	9,047	7,349	4,204	998
1998	109,489	1,533	6,179	15,837	15,216	15,675	18,463	14,483	9,413	7,309	4,316	1,066
White female												
1950	67,813	1,341	5,599	10,431	9,821	10,851	9,719	7,868	6,168	4,031	1,669	314
1960	80,465	1,714	6,795	15,068	10,596	10,204	11,000	9,364	7,327	5,428	2,441	527
1970	91,028	1,434	5,615	16,912	15,420	11,004	10,349	10,756	8,853	6,366	3,429	890
1980	99,788	1,410	5,121	14,048	17,643	15,887	11,227	10,282	10,324	7,950	4,457	1,440
1990	106,561	1,524	5,762	13,706	14,599	17,757	15,834	10,946	9,698	9,048	5,687	2,001
1997	112,441	1,472	5,924	14,926	14,064	15,857	18,161	14,456	9,728	8,961	6,388	2,507
1998	113,511	1,461	5,879	15,051	14,369	15,540	18,341	14,822	10,113	8,853	6,480	2,600
Black male												
1950	7,300	- - -	- - -	1,442	1,162	1,105	1,003	772	460	299	- - -	- - -
1960	9,114	281	1,082	2,185	1,305	1,120	1,086	891	617	382	137	29
1970	10,748	245	975	2,784	2,041	1,226	1,084	979	739	461	169	46
1980	12,612	270	970	2,618	2,813	1,974	1,238	1,026	855	568	228	53
1990	14,420	322	1,164	2,700	2,669	2,592	1,962	1,175	878	614	277	66
1997	16,121	282	1,185	3,090	2,790	2,551	2,548	1,622	960	690	319	86
1998	16,340	284	1,149	3,130	2,838	2,533	2,606	1,696	987	699	329	90
Black female												
1950	7,745	- - -	- - -	1,446	1,300	1,260	1,112	796	443	322	- - -	- - -
1960	9,758	283	1,085	2,191	1,404	1,300	1,229	974	663	430	160	38
1970	11,832	243	970	2,773	2,196	1,456	1,309	1,134	868	582	230	71
1980	14,071	267	953	2,583	2,942	2,272	1,490	1,260	1,061	777	360	106
1990	16,063	316	1,137	2,641	2,700	2,905	2,279	1,416	1,135	884	495	156
1997	17,826	274	1,151	2,995	2,771	2,827	2,892	1,956	1,253	958	544	207
1998	18,090	276	1,118	3,033	2,820	2,818	2,954	2,045	1,291	966	552	216

See notes at end of table.

[Data are based on decennial census updated by data from multiple sources]

Sex, race, Hispanic origin, and year	Total resident population	Under 1 year	1–4 years	5–14 years	15–24 years	25–34 years	35–44 years	45–54 years	55–64 years	65–74 years	75–84 years	85 years and over
American Indian or Alaska Native male						Number in thousands						
1980	702	17	60	153	164	114	75	53	37	22	9	2
1990	1,024	24	88	206	192	183	140	86	55	32	13	3
1997	1,153	21	81	237	206	193	172	115	65	39	19	6
1998	1,168	21	80	237	210	191	175	119	67	40	20	6
American Indian or Alaska Native female												
1980	718	16	57	149	158	118	79	57	41	26	12	4
1990	1,041	24	85	200	178	186	148	92	61	41	21	6
1997	1,169	20	79	229	200	181	177	122	73	48	27	12
1998	1,192	20	78	230	207	183	179	127	76	49	28	13
Asian or Pacific Islander male												
1980	1,814	35	129	321	334	367	252	159	110	72	29	6
1990	3,652	68	258	598	665	718	588	347	208	133	57	12
1997	4,851	91	352	808	753	858	808	562	319	190	87	23
1998	5,049	92	358	845	777	855	857	602	339	201	97	26
Asian or Pacific Islander female												
1980	1,915	34	127	307	325	423	269	193	126	70	33	9
1990	3,805	65	247	578	621	749	664	371	264	166	65	17
1997	5,182	88	340	767	740	934	886	642	369	264	118	33
1998	5,459	89	347	798	775	980	944	690	390	277	130	37
Hispanic male												
1980	7,280	187	661	1,530	1,646	1,255	761	570	364	201	86	19
1990	11,388	279	980	2,128	2,376	2,310	1,471	818	551	312	131	32
1997	15,074	354	1,363	2,786	2,764	2,824	2,281	1,292	711	454	192	54
1998	15,233	357	1,376	2,926	2,751	2,682	2,320	1,339	741	470	211	59
Hispanic female												
1980	7,329	181	634	1,482	1,547	1,249	805	615	411	257	116	30
1990	10,966	268	939	2,039	2,028	2,073	1,448	868	632	403	209	59
1997	14,274	336	1,294	2,657	2,387	2,408	2,111	1,319	801	567	289	106
1998	15,017	343	1,317	2,805	2,547	2,494	2,228	1,405	856	595	310	118
White, non-Hispanic male												
1980	88,035	1,308	4,773	13,318	16,555	14,739	10,285	9,229	8,802	5,906	2,519	603
1990	91,743	1,351	5,181	12,525	13,219	15,967	14,481	9,875	8,303	6,837	3,275	729
1997	95,127	1,225	4,995	13,202	12,522	13,628	16,280	12,979	8,394	6,930	4,025	947
1998	95,601	1,206	4,922	13,183	12,699	13,230	16,358	13,265	8,733	6,876	4,118	1,010
White, non-Hispanic female												
1980	92,872	1,240	4,522	12,647	16,185	14,711	10,468	9,700	9,935	7,708	4,345	1,411
1990	96,557	1,280	4,909	11,846	12,749	15,872	14,520	10,153	9,116	8,674	5,491	1,945
1997	99,444	1,165	4,742	12,517	11,889	13,669	16,246	13,256	8,996	8,439	6,119	2,407
1998	99,839	1,147	4,675	12,505	12,048	13,276	16,322	13,544	9,332	8,307	6,193	2,489

- - - Data not available.

NOTES: The race groups, white, black, American Indian or Alaska Native, and Asian or Pacific Islander, include persons of Hispanic and non-Hispanic origin. Conversely, persons of Hispanic origin may be of any race. Population figures are census counts as of April 1 for 1950, 1960, 1970, 1980, and 1990 and estimates as of July 1 for other years. See Appendix I, Department of Commerce. Populations for age groups may not sum to the total due to rounding. Although population figures are shown rounded to the nearest 1,000, calculations of birth rates and death rates shown in this volume are based on unrounded population figures for decennial years and starting with data year 1992. See Appendix II, Rate. Data for additional years are available (see Appendix III).

SOURCES: U.S. Bureau of the Census: 1950 Nonwhite Population by Race. Special Report P-E, No. 3B. Washington. U.S. Government Printing Office, 1951; U.S. Census of Population: 1960, Number of Inhabitants, PC(1)-A1, United States Summary, 1964; 1970, Number of Inhabitants, Final Report PC(1)-A1, United States Summary, 1971; U.S. population estimates, by age, sex, race, and Hispanic origin: 1980 to 1991. Current Population Reports. Series P–25, No. 1095. Washington. U.S. Government Printing Office, Feb. 1993; U.S. resident population—estimates by age, sex, race, and Hispanic origin (consistent with the 1990 Census, as enumerated): 1992. Census files RESP0792 in PPL–21, series 1294. 1993; July 1, 1993. RES0793. 1994; July 1, 1994. RESD0794. 1995; July 1, 1995. RESD0795. 1996; July 1, 1996. NESTV96 in PPL–57. 1997; July 1, 1997. NESTV97 in PPL–91R. 1998; July 1, 1998. NESTV98. 1999.

Table 2 (page 1 of 2). Persons and families below poverty level, according to selected characteristics, race, and Hispanic origin: United States, selected years 1973–98

[Data are based on household interviews of the civilian noninstitutionalized population]

Selected characteristics, race, and Hispanic origin	1973	1980	1985	1990	1993	1994	1995	1996	1997	1998
All persons				Percent below poverty						
All races.................	11.1	13.0	14.0	13.5	15.1	14.5	13.8	13.7	13.3	12.7
White.....................	8.4	10.2	11.4	10.7	12.2	11.7	11.2	11.2	11.0	10.5
Black.....................	31.4	32.5	31.3	31.9	33.1	30.6	29.3	28.4	26.5	26.1
Asian or Pacific Islander.......	- - -	- - -	- - -	12.2	15.3	14.6	14.6	14.5	14.0	12.5
Hispanic origin	21.9	25.7	29.0	28.1	30.6	30.7	30.3	29.4	27.1	25.6
Mexican.................	- - -	- - -	28.8	28.1	31.6	32.3	31.2	31.0	27.9	27.1
Puerto Rican	- - -	- - -	43.3	40.6	38.4	36.0	38.1	35.7	34.2	30.9
White, non-Hispanic..........	- - -	- - -	- - -	8.8	9.9	9.4	8.5	8.6	8.6	8.2
Related children under 18 years of age in families										
All races.................	14.2	17.9	20.1	19.9	22.0	21.2	20.2	19.8	19.2	18.3
White.....................	9.7	13.4	15.6	15.1	17.0	16.3	15.5	15.5	15.4	14.4
Black.....................	40.6	42.1	43.1	44.2	45.9	43.3	41.5	39.5	36.8	36.4
Asian or Pacific Islander.......	- - -	- - -	- - -	17.0	17.6	17.9	18.6	19.1	19.9	17.5
Hispanic origin	27.8	33.0	39.6	37.7	39.9	41.1	39.3	39.9	36.4	33.6
Mexican.................	- - -	- - -	37.4	35.5	39.5	41.8	39.3	40.7	35.8	34.6
Puerto Rican	- - -	- - -	58.6	56.7	53.8	50.5	53.2	49.4	49.1	43.2
White, non-Hispanic..........	- - -	- - -	- - -	11.6	12.8	11.8	10.6	10.4	10.7	10.0
Related children under 18 years of age in families with female householder and no spouse present										
All races.................	- - -	50.8	53.6	53.4	53.7	52.9	50.3	49.3	49.0	46.1
White.....................	- - -	41.6	45.2	45.9	45.6	45.7	42.5	43.1	44.3	40.0
Black.....................	- - -	64.8	66.9	64.7	65.9	63.2	61.6	58.2	55.3	54.7
Asian or Pacific Islander.......	- - -	- - -	- - -	32.2	32.2	36.8	42.4	48.8	58.3	49.8
Hispanic origin	- - -	65.0	72.4	68.4	66.1	68.3	65.7	67.4	62.8	59.6
Mexican.................	- - -	- - -	64.4	62.4	64.6	69.5	65.9	68.1	62.2	61.5
Puerto Rican	- - -	- - -	85.4	82.7	73.4	73.6	79.6	76.6	71.0	61.6
White, non-Hispanic..........	- - -	- - -	- - -	39.6	39.0	38.0	33.5	34.9	37.2	32.8
All persons				Number below poverty in thousands						
All races.................	22,973	29,272	33,064	33,585	39,265	38,059	36,425	36,529	35,574	34,476
White.....................	15,142	19,699	22,860	22,326	26,226	25,379	24,423	24,650	24,396	23,454
Black.....................	7,388	8,579	8,926	9,837	10,877	10,196	9,872	9,694	9,116	9,091
Asian or Pacific Islander.......	- - -	- - -	- - -	858	1,134	974	1,411	1,454	1,468	1,360
Hispanic origin	2,366	3,491	5,236	6,006	8,126	8,416	8,574	8,697	8,308	8,070
Mexican.................	- - -	- - -	3,220	3,764	5,373	5,781	5,608	5,815	5,509	5,566
Puerto Rican	- - -	- - -	1,011	966	1,061	981	1,183	1,116	1,059	929
White, non-Hispanic..........	- - -	- - -	- - -	16,622	18,882	18,110	16,267	16,462	16,491	15,799
Related children under 18 years of age in families										
All races.................	9,453	11,114	12,483	12,715	14,961	14,610	13,999	13,764	13,422	12,845
White.....................	5,462	6,817	7,838	7,696	9,123	8,826	8,474	8,488	8,441	7,935
Black.....................	3,822	3,906	4,057	4,412	5,030	4,787	4,644	4,411	4,116	4,073
Asian or Pacific Islander.......	- - -	- - -	- - -	356	358	308	532	553	608	542
Hispanic origin	1,364	1,718	2,512	2,750	3,666	3,956	3,938	4,090	3,865	3,670
Mexican.................	- - -	- - -	1,589	1,733	2,520	2,805	2,655	2,853	2,666	2,654
Puerto Rican	- - -	- - -	535	490	537	485	610	545	519	433
White, non-Hispanic..........	- - -	- - -	- - -	5,106	5,819	5,404	4,745	4,656	4,759	4,458

See footnotes at end of table.

Table 2 (page 2 of 2). Persons and families below poverty level, according to selected characteristics, race, and Hispanic origin: United States, selected years 1973–98

[Data are based on household interviews of the civilian noninstitutionalized population]

Selected characteristics, race, and Hispanic origin	1973	1980	1985	1990	1993	1994	1995	1996	1997	1998
Related children under 18 years of age in families with female householder and no spouse present					Number below poverty in thousands					
All races	- - -	5,866	6,716	7,363	8,503	8,427	8,364	7,990	7,928	7,627
White	- - -	2,813	3,372	3,597	4,102	4,099	4,051	4,029	4,186	3,875
Black	- - -	2,944	3,181	3,543	4,104	3,935	3,954	3,619	3,402	3,366
Asian or Pacific Islander.	- - -	- - -	- - -	80	72	59	145	167	200	231
Hispanic origin	- - -	809	1,247	1,314	1,673	1,804	1,872	1,779	1,758	1,739
Mexican.	- - -	- - -	553	615	890	1,054	1,056	948	991	1,092
Puerto Rican	- - -	- - -	449	382	430	394	459	444	392	298
White, non-Hispanic.	- - -	- - -	- - -	2,411	2,636	2,563	2,299	2,419	2,551	2,294

- - - Data not available.

NOTES: The race groups white, black, and Asian include persons of Hispanic and non-Hispanic origin; persons of Hispanic origin may be of any race. Poverty status is based on family income and family size using Bureau of the Census poverty thresholds. See Appendix II. In 1989, 31.2 percent of the American Indian population in the United States, or 585,000 persons, were below the poverty threshold, based on 1989 income data from the 1990 decennial census (U.S. Bureau of the Census, 1990 Census of Population, *Characteristics of American Indians by Tribe and Language*, 1990 CP–3–7). Data for additional years are available (see Appendix III).

SOURCE: U.S. Bureau of the Census. Dalaker J. Poverty in the United States: 1998. Current population reports, series P–60, no 207. Washington: U.S. Government Printing Office. 1999; unpublished data.

Table 3 (page 1 of 2). Crude birth rates, fertility rates, and birth rates by age of mother, according to detailed race and Hispanic origin: United States, selected years 1950–98

[Data are based on the National Vital Statistics System]

Race, Hispanic origin, and year	Crude birth rate[1]	Fertility rate[2]	10–14 years	15–19 years Total	15–17 years	18–19 years	20–24 years	25–29 years	30–34 years	35–39 years	40–44 years	45–54 years[3]
All races				Live births per 1,000 women								
1950	24.1	106.2	1.0	81.6	40.7	132.7	196.6	166.1	103.7	52.9	15.1	1.2
1960	23.7	118.0	0.8	89.1	43.9	166.7	258.1	197.4	112.7	56.2	15.5	0.9
1970	18.4	87.9	1.2	68.3	38.8	114.7	167.8	145.1	73.3	31.7	8.1	0.5
1980	15.9	68.4	1.1	53.0	32.5	82.1	115.1	112.9	61.9	19.8	3.9	0.2
1985	15.8	66.3	1.2	51.0	31.0	79.6	108.3	111.0	69.1	24.0	4.0	0.2
1990	16.7	70.9	1.4	59.9	37.5	88.6	116.5	120.2	80.8	31.7	5.5	0.2
1994	15.2	66.7	1.4	58.9	37.6	91.5	111.1	113.9	81.5	33.7	6.4	0.3
1995	14.8	65.6	1.3	56.8	36.0	89.1	109.8	112.2	82.5	34.3	6.6	0.3
1996	14.7	65.3	1.2	54.4	33.8	86.0	110.4	113.1	83.9	35.3	6.8	0.3
1997	14.5	65.0	1.1	52.3	32.1	83.6	110.4	113.8	85.3	36.1	7.1	0.4
1998	14.6	65.6	1.0	51.1	30.4	82.0	111.2	115.9	87.4	37.4	7.3	0.4
Race of child:[4] White												
1950	23.0	102.3	0.4	70.0	31.3	120.5	190.4	165.1	102.6	51.4	14.5	1.0
1960	22.7	113.2	0.4	79.4	35.5	154.6	252.8	194.9	109.6	54.0	14.7	0.8
1970	17.4	84.1	0.5	57.4	29.2	101.5	163.4	145.9	71.9	30.0	7.5	0.4
1980	14.9	64.7	0.6	44.7	25.2	72.1	109.5	112.4	60.4	18.5	3.4	0.2
Race of mother:[5] White												
1980	15.1	65.6	0.6	45.4	25.5	73.2	111.1	113.8	61.2	18.8	3.5	0.2
1985	15.0	64.1	0.6	43.3	24.4	70.4	104.1	112.3	69.9	23.3	3.7	0.2
1990	15.8	68.3	0.7	50.8	29.5	78.0	109.8	120.7	81.7	31.5	5.2	0.2
1994	14.4	64.9	0.8	51.1	30.7	82.1	106.2	115.5	83.2	33.7	6.2	0.3
1995	14.2	64.4	0.8	50.1	30.0	81.2	106.3	114.8	84.6	34.5	6.4	0.3
1996	14.1	64.3	0.8	48.1	28.4	78.4	107.2	116.1	86.3	35.6	6.7	0.3
1997	13.9	63.9	0.7	46.3	27.1	75.9	106.7	116.6	87.8	36.4	6.9	0.4
1998	14.0	64.6	0.6	45.4	25.9	74.6	107.2	119.1	90.5	37.8	7.2	0.4
Race of child:[4] Black												
1960	31.9	153.5	4.3	156.1	- - -	- - -	295.4	218.6	137.1	73.9	21.9	1.1
1970	25.3	115.4	5.2	140.7	101.4	204.9	202.7	136.3	79.6	41.9	12.5	1.0
1980	22.1	88.1	4.3	100.0	73.6	138.8	146.3	109.1	62.9	24.5	5.8	0.3
Race of mother:[5] Black												
1980	21.3	84.9	4.3	97.8	72.5	135.1	140.0	103.9	59.9	23.5	5.6	0.3
1985	20.4	78.8	4.5	95.4	69.3	132.4	135.0	100.2	57.9	23.9	4.6	0.3
1990	22.4	86.8	4.9	112.8	82.3	152.9	160.2	115.5	68.7	28.1	5.5	0.3
1994	19.5	76.9	4.6	104.5	76.3	148.3	146.0	104.0	65.8	28.9	5.9	0.3
1995	18.2	72.3	4.2	96.1	69.7	137.1	137.1	98.6	64.0	28.7	6.0	0.3
1996	17.8	70.7	3.6	91.4	64.7	132.5	136.8	98.2	63.3	29.1	6.1	0.3
1997	17.7	70.7	3.3	88.2	60.8	130.1	139.0	99.5	64.3	29.7	6.5	0.3
1998	17.7	71.0	2.9	85.4	56.8	126.9	141.9	101.8	64.7	30.5	6.7	0.3
American Indian or Alaska Native mothers[5]												
1980	20.7	82.7	1.9	82.2	51.5	129.5	143.7	106.6	61.8	28.1	8.2	*
1985	19.8	78.6	1.7	79.2	47.7	124.1	139.1	109.6	62.6	27.4	6.0	*
1990	18.9	76.2	1.6	81.1	48.5	129.3	148.7	110.3	61.5	27.5	5.9	*
1994	17.1	70.9	1.9	80.8	51.3	130.3	134.2	104.1	61.2	27.5	5.9	0.4
1995	16.6	69.1	1.8	78.0	47.8	130.7	132.5	98.4	62.2	27.7	6.1	*
1996	16.6	68.7	1.7	73.9	46.4	122.3	133.9	98.5	63.2	28.5	6.3	*
1997	16.6	69.1	1.7	71.8	45.3	117.6	134.9	100.8	64.2	29.3	6.4	0.4
1998	17.1	70.7	1.6	72.1	44.4	118.4	139.3	102.2	66.3	30.2	6.4	*

See footnotes at end of table.

Table 3 (page 2 of 2). Crude birth rates, fertility rates, and birth rates by age of mother, according to detailed race and Hispanic origin: United States, selected years 1950–98

[Data are based on the National Vital Statistics System]

Race, Hispanic origin, and year	Crude birth rate[1]	Fertility rate[2]	10–14 years	15–19 years Total	15–17 years	18–19 years	20–24 years	25–29 years	30–34 years	35–39 years	40–44 years	45–54 years[3]
Asian or Pacific Islander mothers[5]				Live births per 1,000 women								
1980	19.9	73.2	0.3	26.2	12.0	46.2	93.3	127.4	96.0	38.3	8.5	0.7
1985	18.7	68.4	0.4	23.8	12.5	40.8	83.6	123.0	93.6	42.7	8.7	1.2
1990	19.0	69.6	0.7	26.4	16.0	40.2	79.2	126.3	106.5	49.6	10.7	1.1
1994	17.5	66.8	0.7	27.1	16.1	44.1	73.1	118.6	105.2	51.3	11.6	1.0
1995	17.3	66.4	0.7	26.1	15.4	43.4	72.4	113.4	106.9	52.4	12.1	0.8
1996	17.0	65.9	0.6	24.6	14.9	40.4	70.7	111.2	109.2	52.2	12.2	0.8
1997	16.9	66.3	0.5	23.7	14.3	39.3	70.5	113.2	110.3	54.1	11.9	0.9
1998	16.4	64.0	0.4	23.1	13.8	38.3	68.8	110.4	105.1	52.8	12.0	0.9
Hispanic mothers[5,6,7]												
1980	23.5	95.4	1.7	82.2	52.1	126.9	156.4	132.1	83.2	39.9	10.6	0.7
1990	26.7	107.7	2.4	100.3	65.9	147.7	181.0	153.0	98.3	45.3	10.9	0.7
1994	25.5	105.6	2.7	107.7	74.0	158.0	188.2	153.2	95.4	44.3	10.7	0.6
1995	25.2	105.0	2.7	106.7	72.9	157.9	188.5	153.8	95.9	44.9	10.8	0.6
1996	24.8	104.9	2.6	101.8	69.0	151.1	189.5	161.0	98.1	45.1	10.8	0.6
1997	24.2	102.8	2.3	97.4	66.3	144.3	184.2	161.7	97.9	45.0	10.8	0.6
1998	24.3	101.1	2.1	93.6	62.3	140.1	178.4	160.2	98.9	44.9	10.8	0.6
White, non-Hispanic mothers[5,6,7]												
1980	14.2	62.4	0.4	41.2	22.4	67.7	105.5	110.6	59.9	17.7	3.0	0.1
1990	14.4	62.8	0.5	42.5	23.2	66.6	97.5	115.3	79.4	30.0	4.7	0.2
1994	12.8	58.3	0.5	40.4	22.8	67.4	90.9	107.9	80.7	32.1	5.7	0.2
1995	12.6	57.6	0.4	39.3	22.0	66.1	90.0	106.5	82.0	32.9	5.9	0.3
1996	12.4	57.3	0.4	37.6	20.6	63.7	90.1	107.0	83.5	34.0	6.2	0.3
1997	12.2	57.0	0.4	36.0	19.4	61.9	89.8	107.2	85.2	34.9	6.4	0.3
1998	12.3	57.7	0.3	35.2	18.4	60.6	90.7	109.7	88.0	36.4	6.7	0.4
Black, non-Hispanic mothers[5,6,7]												
1980	22.9	90.7	4.6	105.1	77.2	146.5	152.2	111.7	65.2	25.8	5.8	0.3
1990	23.0	89.0	5.0	116.2	84.9	157.5	165.1	118.4	70.2	28.7	5.6	0.3
1994	20.0	79.0	4.7	107.7	78.6	152.9	150.3	107.0	67.5	29.5	6.0	0.3
1995	18.8	74.5	4.3	99.3	72.1	141.9	141.7	102.0	65.9	29.4	6.1	0.3
1996	18.3	72.5	3.8	94.2	66.6	136.6	140.9	100.8	64.9	29.7	6.2	0.3
1997	18.1	72.4	3.4	90.8	62.6	134.0	143.0	101.9	65.8	30.3	6.6	0.3
1998	18.2	73.0	3.0	88.2	58.8	130.9	146.4	104.6	66.6	31.2	6.8	0.3

- - - Data not available.

* Based on fewer than 20 births.

[1] Live births per 1,000 population.

[2] Total number of live births regardless of age of mother per 1,000 women 15–44 years of age.

[3] Prior to 1997 data are for live births to mothers 45–49 years of age per 1,000 women 45–49 years of age. Starting in 1997 data are for live births to mothers 45–54 years of age per 1,000 women 45–49 years of age (see Appendix I, National Vital Statistics System).

[4] Live births are tabulated by race of child.

[5] Live births are tabulated by race and/or Hispanic origin of mother.

[6] Trend data for Hispanics and non-Hispanics are affected by expansion of the reporting area for an Hispanic-origin item on the birth certificate and by immigration. These two factors affect numbers of events, composition of the Hispanic population, and maternal and infant health characteristics. The number of States in the reporting area increased from 22 in 1980, to 23 and the District of Columbia (DC) in 1983–87, 30 and DC in 1988, 47 and DC in 1989, 48 and DC in 1990, 49 and DC in 1991–92, and 50 and DC in 1993 and later years (see Appendix I, National Vital Statistics System).

[7] Rates in 1985 were not calculated because estimates for the Hispanic and non-Hispanic populations were not available.

NOTES: Data are based on births adjusted for underregistration for 1950 and on registered births for all other years. Beginning in 1970, births to persons who were not residents of the 50 States and the District of Columbia are excluded. The race groups, white, black, American Indian or Alaska Native, and Asian or Pacific Islander, include persons of Hispanic and non-Hispanic origin. Conversely, persons of Hispanic origin may be of any race. Data for additional years are available (see Appendix III).

SOURCES: Centers for Disease Control and Prevention, National Center for Health Statistics: Ventura SJ, Martin JA, Curtin SC, Mathews TJ, Park MM. Births: Final data for 1998. National vital statistics reports; vol 48, no 3. Hyattsville, Maryland: 2000; Ventura SJ. Births of Hispanic parentage, 1980 and 1985. Monthly vital statistics report; vol 32 no 6 and vol 36 no 11, suppl. Public Health Service. Hyattsville, Maryland. 1983 and 1988; for age-specific birth rates for 1950–92 see table 1–9 in *Vital statistics of the United States, 1992, vol I, natality,* Washington: Public Health Service, 1995.

Table 4. Women 15–44 years of age who have not had at least 1 live birth, by age: United States, selected years 1960–98

[Data are based on the National Vital Statistics System]

Year[1]	15–19 years	20–24 years	25–29 years	30–34 years	35–39 years	40–44 years
	Percent of women					
1960	91.4	47.5	20.0	14.2	12.0	15.1
1965	92.7	51.4	19.7	11.7	11.4	11.0
1970	93.0	57.0	24.4	11.8	9.4	10.6
1975	92.6	62.5	31.1	15.2	9.6	8.8
1980	93.4	66.2	38.9	19.7	12.5	9.0
1985	93.7	67.7	41.5	24.6	15.4	11.7
1986	93.8	68.0	42.0	25.1	16.1	12.2
1987	93.8	68.2	42.5	25.5	16.9	12.6
1988	93.8	68.4	43.0	25.7	17.7	13.0
1989	93.7	68.4	43.3	25.9	18.2	13.5
1990	93.3	68.3	43.5	25.9	18.5	13.9
1991	93.0	67.9	43.6	26.0	18.7	14.5
1992	92.7	67.3	43.7	26.0	18.8	15.2
1993	92.6	66.7	43.8	26.1	18.8	15.8
1994	92.6	66.1	43.9	26.2	18.7	16.2
1995	92.5	65.5	44.0	26.2	18.6	16.5
1996	92.5	65.0	43.8	26.2	18.5	16.6
1997	92.8	64.9	43.5	26.2	18.4	16.6
1998	93.1	65.1	43.0	26.1	18.3	16.5

[1]As of January 1.

NOTES: Data are based on cohort fertility. See Appendix II, Cohort fertility. Percents are derived from the cumulative childbearing experience of cohorts of women, up to the ages specified. Data on births are adjusted for underregistration and population estimates are corrected for underregistration and misstatement of age. Beginning in 1970, births to persons who were not residents of the 50 States and the District of Columbia are excluded.

SOURCE: Centers for Disease Control and Prevention, National Center for Health Statistics. *Vital statistics of the United States, 1998, Vol 1, natality.*

Table 5. Live births, according to detailed race of mother and Hispanic origin of mother: United States, selected years 1970–98

[Data are based on the National Vital Statistics System]

Race of mother and Hispanic origin of mother	1970	1975	1980	1985	1990	1995	1996	1997	1998
					Total number of live births				
All races	3,731,386	3,144,198	3,612,258	3,760,561	4,158,212	3,899,589	3,891,494	3,880,894	3,941,553
White	3,109,956	2,576,818	2,936,351	3,037,913	3,290,273	3,098,885	3,093,057	3,072,640	3,118,727
Black	561,992	496,829	568,080	581,824	684,336	603,139	594,781	599,913	609,902
American Indian or Alaska Native	22,264	22,690	29,389	34,037	39,051	37,278	37,880	38,572	40,272
Asian or Pacific Islander	- - -	- - -	74,355	104,606	141,635	160,287	165,776	169,769	172,652
Chinese	7,044	7,778	11,671	16,405	22,737	27,380	28,500	28,434	28,058
Japanese	7,744	6,725	7,482	8,035	8,674	8,901	8,902	8,890	8,893
Filipino	8,066	10,359	13,968	20,058	25,770	30,551	31,106	31,501	31,170
Hawaiian and part Hawaiian	- - -	- - -	4,669	4,938	6,099	5,787	5,907	5,687	6,025
Other Asian or Pacific Islander	- - -	- - -	36,565	55,170	78,355	87,668	91,361	95,257	98,506
Hispanic origin (selected States)[1,2]	- - -	- - -	307,163	372,814	595,073	679,768	701,339	709,767	734,661
Mexican	- - -	- - -	215,439	242,976	385,640	469,615	489,666	499,024	516,011
Puerto Rican	- - -	- - -	33,671	35,147	58,807	54,824	54,863	55,450	57,349
Cuban	- - -	- - -	7,163	10,024	11,311	12,473	12,613	12,887	13,226
Central and South American	- - -	- - -	21,268	40,985	83,008	94,996	97,888	97,405	98,226
Other and unknown Hispanic	- - -	- - -	29,622	43,682	56,307	47,860	46,309	45,001	49,849
White, non-Hispanic (selected States)[1]	- - -	- - -	1,245,221	1,394,729	2,626,500	2,382,638	2,358,989	2,333,363	2,361,462
Black, non-Hispanic (selected States)[1]	- - -	- - -	299,646	336,029	661,701	587,781	578,099	581,431	593,127

- - - Data not available.

[1]Trend data for Hispanics and non-Hispanics are affected by expansion of the reporting area for an Hispanic-origin item on the birth certificate and by immigration. These two factors affect numbers of events, composition of the Hispanic population, and maternal and infant health characteristics. The number of States in the reporting area increased from 22 in 1980, to 23 and the District of Columbia (DC) in 1983–87, 30 and DC in 1988, 47 and DC in 1989, 48 and DC in 1990, 49 and DC in 1991–92, and 50 and DC in 1993 and later years (see Appendix I, National Vital Statistics System).
[2]Includes mothers of all races.

NOTES: The race groups, white, black, American Indian or Alaska Native, and Asian or Pacific Islander include persons of Hispanic and non-Hispanic origin. Conversely, persons of Hispanic origin may be of any race. Data for additional years are available (see Appendix III).

SOURCES: Centers for Disease Control and Prevention, National Center for Health Statistics. National Vital Statistics System; Ventura SJ, Martin JA, Curtin SC, Mathews TJ, Park MM. Births: Final data for 1998. National vital statistics reports; vol 48, no 3. Hyattsville, Maryland: 2000; Report of final natality statistics, for each data year 1970–96. Monthly vital statistics report. Hyattsville, Maryland.

Table 6. Prenatal care for live births, according to detailed race of mother and Hispanic origin of mother: United States, selected years 1970–98

[Data are based on the National Vital Statistics System]

Prenatal care, race of mother, and Hispanic origin of mother	1970	1975	1980	1985	1990	1992	1993	1994	1995	1996	1997	1998
Prenatal care began during 1st trimester						Percent of live births[1]						
All races	68.0	72.4	76.3	76.2	75.8	77.7	78.9	80.2	81.3	81.9	82.5	82.8
White.	72.3	75.8	79.2	79.3	79.2	80.8	81.8	82.8	83.6	84.0	84.7	84.8
Black.	44.2	55.5	62.4	61.5	60.6	63.9	66.0	68.3	70.4	71.4	72.3	73.3
American Indian or Alaska Native	38.2	45.4	55.8	57.5	57.9	62.1	63.4	65.2	66.7	67.7	68.1	68.8
Asian or Pacific Islander	---	---	73.7	74.1	75.1	76.6	77.6	79.7	79.9	81.2	82.1	83.1
Chinese	71.8	76.7	82.6	82.0	81.3	83.8	84.6	86.2	85.7	86.8	87.4	88.5
Japanese	78.1	82.7	86.1	84.7	87.0	88.2	87.2	89.2	89.7	89.3	89.3	90.2
Filipino	60.6	70.6	77.3	76.5	77.1	78.7	79.3	81.3	80.9	82.5	83.3	84.2
Hawaiian and part Hawaiian	---	---	68.8	67.7	65.8	69.9	70.6	77.0	75.9	78.5	78.0	78.8
Other Asian or Pacific Islander	---	---	67.4	69.9	71.9	72.8	74.4	76.2	77.0	78.4	79.7	80.9
Hispanic origin (selected States)[2,3]	---	---	60.2	61.2	60.2	64.2	66.6	68.9	70.8	72.2	73.7	74.3
Mexican	---	---	59.6	60.0	57.8	62.1	64.8	67.3	69.1	70.7	72.1	72.8
Puerto Rican.	---	---	55.1	58.3	63.5	67.8	70.0	71.7	74.0	75.0	76.5	76.9
Cuban	---	---	82.7	82.5	84.8	86.8	88.9	90.1	89.2	89.2	90.4	91.8
Central and South American	---	---	58.8	60.6	61.5	66.8	68.7	71.2	73.2	75.0	76.9	78.0
Other and unknown Hispanic	---	---	66.4	65.8	66.4	68.0	70.0	72.1	74.3	74.6	76.0	74.8
White, non-Hispanic (selected States)[2]	---	---	81.2	81.4	83.3	84.9	85.6	86.5	87.1	87.4	87.9	87.9
Black, non-Hispanic (selected States)[2]	---	---	60.7	60.1	60.7	64.0	66.1	68.3	70.4	71.5	72.3	73.3
Prenatal care began during 3d trimester or no prenatal care												
All races	7.9	6.0	5.1	5.7	6.1	5.2	4.8	4.4	4.2	4.0	3.9	3.9
White.	6.3	5.0	4.3	4.8	4.9	4.2	3.9	3.6	3.5	3.3	3.2	3.3
Black.	16.6	10.5	8.9	10.2	11.3	9.9	9.0	8.2	7.6	7.3	7.3	7.0
American Indian or Alaska Native	28.9	22.4	15.2	12.9	12.9	11.0	10.3	9.8	9.5	8.6	8.6	8.5
Asian or Pacific Islander	---	---	6.5	6.5	5.8	4.9	4.6	4.1	4.3	3.9	3.8	3.6
Chinese	6.5	4.4	3.7	4.4	3.4	2.9	2.9	2.7	3.0	2.5	2.4	2.2
Japanese	4.1	2.7	2.1	3.1	2.9	2.4	2.8	1.9	2.3	2.2	2.7	2.1
Filipino	7.2	4.1	4.0	4.8	4.5	4.3	4.0	3.6	4.1	3.3	3.3	3.1
Hawaiian and part Hawaiian	---	---	6.7	7.4	8.7	7.0	6.7	4.7	5.1	5.0	5.4	4.7
Other Asian or Pacific Islander	---	---	9.3	8.2	7.1	5.9	5.4	4.8	5.0	4.6	4.4	4.2
Hispanic origin (selected States)[2,3]	---	---	12.0	12.4	12.0	9.5	8.8	7.6	7.4	6.7	6.2	6.3
Mexican	---	---	11.8	12.9	13.2	10.5	9.7	8.3	8.1	7.2	6.7	6.8
Puerto Rican.	---	---	16.2	15.5	10.6	8.0	7.1	6.5	5.5	5.7	5.4	5.1
Cuban	---	---	3.9	3.7	2.8	2.1	1.8	1.6	2.1	1.6	1.5	1.2
Central and South American	---	---	13.1	12.5	10.9	7.9	7.3	6.5	6.1	5.5	5.0	4.9
Other and unknown Hispanic	---	---	9.2	9.4	8.5	7.5	7.0	6.2	6.0	5.9	5.3	6.0
White, non-Hispanic (selected States)[2]	---	---	3.5	4.0	3.4	2.8	2.7	2.5	2.5	2.4	2.4	2.4
Black, non-Hispanic (selected States)[2]	---	---	9.7	10.9	11.2	9.8	9.0	8.2	7.6	7.3	7.3	7.0

--- Data not available.

[1] Excludes live births for whom trimester when prenatal care began is unknown.

[2] Trend data for Hispanics and non-Hispanics are affected by expansion of the reporting area for an Hispanic-origin item on the birth certificate and by immigration. These two factors affect numbers of events, composition of the Hispanic population, and maternal and infant health characteristics. The number of States in the reporting area increased from 22 in 1980, to 23 and the District of Columbia (DC) in 1983–87, 30 and DC in 1988, 47 and DC in 1989, 48 and DC in 1990, 49 and DC in 1991–92, and 50 and DC in 1993 and later years (see Appendix I, National Vital Statistics System).

[3] Includes mothers of all races.

NOTES: Data for 1970 and 1975 exclude births that occurred in States not reporting prenatal care (see Appendix I). The race groups, white, black, American Indian or Alaska Native, and Asian or Pacific Islander, include persons of Hispanic and non-Hispanic origin. Conversely, persons of Hispanic origin may be of any race. Data for additional years are available (see Appendix III).

SOURCES: Centers for Disease Control and Prevention, National Center for Health Statistics. National Vital Statistics System; Ventura SJ, Martin JA, Curtin SC, Mathews TJ, Park MM. Births: Final data for 1998. National vital statistics reports; vol 48, no 3. Hyattsville, Maryland: 2000; Report of final natality statistics, for each data year 1970–96. Monthly vital statistics report. Hyattsville, Maryland.

Table 7 (page 1 of 2). **Early prenatal care according to race of mother, Hispanic origin of mother, geographic division, and State: United States, average annual 1990–92, 1993–95, and 1996–98**

[Data are based on the National Vital Statistics System]

Geographic division and State	All races			White, non-Hispanic			Black, non-Hispanic		
	1990–92	1993–95	1996–98	1990–92	1993–95	1996–98	1990–92	1993–95	1996–98
	Percent of live births with early prenatal care (beginning in the 1st trimester)								
United States[1]	76.6	80.1	82.4	83.9	86.4	87.7	62.1	68.2	72.4
New England[1]	86.0	88.6	88.1	88.9	91.1	90.6	69.4	76.5	77.8
Maine	85.7	88.8	89.3	85.9	89.2	89.7	79.7	80.2	84.3
New Hampshire[1]	86.3	89.0	89.5	86.5	89.6	89.9	69.2	77.2	77.2
Vermont	83.4	86.1	87.6	83.5	86.4	87.8	*69.2	62.7	*73.6
Massachusetts	85.7	88.8	87.4	89.4	91.7	90.4	69.0	76.7	76.3
Rhode Island	88.0	89.4	89.6	91.0	92.3	92.0	75.1	77.3	80.0
Connecticut	86.3	88.1	88.4	90.8	92.1	91.9	68.8	76.1	79.4
Middle Atlantic	77.1	79.1	81.7	86.4	87.0	88.2	57.0	63.0	68.3
New York	73.7	76.0	80.3	86.0	86.0	87.7	56.1	62.6	69.7
New Jersey	81.6	82.2	81.6	89.4	90.0	89.5	62.8	65.2	64.5
Pennsylvania	79.7	82.0	84.3	85.2	86.5	87.9	54.1	61.7	68.7
East North Central	79.7	82.0	83.4	84.6	86.6	87.5	63.6	66.9	70.1
Ohio	81.8	84.1	85.3	85.0	87.1	87.8	65.5	69.2	72.7
Indiana	77.8	80.2	80.1	80.4	82.5	82.6	59.1	64.8	65.4
Illinois	77.8	80.1	82.2	85.7	88.1	89.3	62.8	65.9	69.5
Michigan	80.0	82.6	84.2	84.9	87.1	88.3	65.5	68.1	71.0
Wisconsin	81.8	83.0	84.3	86.2	87.2	88.0	59.2	63.1	67.5
West North Central	81.5	84.0	85.2	84.6	86.9	88.0	62.9	68.3	72.4
Minnesota	81.3	83.2	84.0	85.0	86.6	87.4	52.0	57.7	65.0
Iowa	85.5	87.1	87.3	86.5	88.2	88.7	70.0	72.0	74.1
Missouri	79.4	83.5	85.9	83.1	86.7	88.4	62.1	68.6	73.4
North Dakota	82.4	83.2	85.0	84.8	84.8	87.1	78.8	83.8	76.8
South Dakota	78.8	81.2	82.2	82.6	84.9	86.0	74.4	74.3	70.5
Nebraska	82.2	83.5	84.1	84.8	86.3	87.0	66.0	68.9	72.0
Kansas	82.1	84.7	85.6	85.0	88.0	89.1	68.8	73.1	76.0
South Atlantic	76.4	81.5	84.3	83.6	87.6	89.5	61.6	69.4	74.3
Delaware	79.3	83.5	83.2	86.3	88.5	88.2	60.4	70.9	73.0
Maryland	84.1	86.6	88.3	90.3	92.1	92.9	71.5	76.0	79.8
District of Columbia	56.1	57.2	67.6	88.4	86.4	89.4	51.3	52.3	62.7
Virginia	80.8	83.2	84.9	86.9	88.6	90.0	66.5	70.9	73.4
West Virginia	74.5	80.4	82.6	75.5	81.0	83.2	51.3	64.1	67.1
North Carolina	77.2	82.0	84.0	84.6	88.4	90.0	61.6	68.7	73.4
South Carolina	69.6	76.0	80.4	79.5	84.4	87.5	54.5	62.6	69.0
Georgia	74.5	81.6	85.8	82.3	87.8	91.0	62.1	72.1	78.6
Florida	75.0	81.3	83.6	81.6	86.7	88.6	59.6	69.3	72.6
East South Central	76.9	80.8	83.0	82.3	85.9	87.9	63.4	67.8	70.7
Kentucky	78.7	82.8	85.6	80.3	84.4	86.8	64.9	68.9	75.9
Tennessee	78.5	81.9	83.7	82.5	85.9	87.7	66.1	69.5	72.0
Alabama	75.3	81.1	82.1	82.8	87.7	88.7	61.2	68.7	69.7
Mississippi	74.4	76.0	79.8	85.1	86.0	89.0	63.1	65.2	69.3
West South Central[1]	70.5	75.7	78.9	79.9	83.6	85.8	60.4	67.9	72.1
Arkansas	71.2	75.2	76.1	76.3	80.0	80.7	55.5	60.6	63.8
Louisiana	75.3	79.0	81.5	85.0	87.2	89.1	62.2	68.3	71.2
Oklahoma[1]	72.5	76.1	78.6	76.6	79.9	81.9	56.1	62.7	68.0
Texas	69.0	74.9	78.6	79.9	84.2	86.8	60.5	69.6	74.8
Mountain	73.6	76.5	78.1	80.8	83.5	84.8	61.2	67.1	71.3
Montana	77.4	81.2	82.5	80.2	83.7	84.9	72.5	79.1	75.9
Idaho	75.0	78.9	78.7	78.0	81.8	81.6	70.7	78.7	72.2
Wyoming	79.6	82.2	81.9	81.7	84.3	83.8	67.8	69.8	69.7
Colorado	78.5	80.2	82.2	83.5	85.4	87.5	65.9	70.1	76.4
New Mexico	59.1	66.7	69.2	69.5	76.8	77.8	51.5	59.6	62.3
Arizona	69.2	71.2	74.7	79.3	81.0	84.4	63.2	67.7	71.5
Utah	84.2	85.2	83.2	86.3	87.5	86.4	68.9	71.4	67.2
Nevada	70.8	74.7	76.1	76.7	81.0	83.3	53.3	63.2	66.8
Pacific	74.3	78.4	81.7	83.4	85.1	86.8	69.9	75.4	79.0
Washington	78.6	82.0	83.2	82.1	85.1	86.0	65.8	73.9	77.0
Oregon	77.1	79.1	80.4	79.4	81.7	83.1	64.6	70.8	78.4
California	73.4	77.7	81.6	84.3	85.6	87.7	70.1	75.4	79.0
Alaska	81.8	83.7	80.9	85.1	86.2	83.4	81.6	85.1	82.3
Hawaii	73.8	80.9	84.3	79.2	85.5	90.1	69.2	82.5	89.5

See footnotes at end of table.

Table 7 (page 2 of 2). Early prenatal care according to race of mother, Hispanic origin of mother, geographic division, and State: United States, average annual 1990–92, 1993–95, and 1996–98

[Data are based on the National Vital Statistics System]

Geographic division and State	Hispanic[2]			American Indian or Alaska Native[3]			Asian or Pacific Islander[3]		
	1990–92	1993–95	1996–98	1990–92	1993–95	1996–98	1990–92	1993–95	1996–98

Percent of live births with early prenatal care (beginning in the 1st trimester)

United States[4]	61.8	68.8	73.4	59.9	65.1	68.2	75.7	79.1	82.2
New England[4]	74.4	78.3	77.4	72.4	76.1	75.8	76.9	82.3	82.2
Maine	80.5	77.5	80.2	71.6	77.2	72.9	75.5	79.7	81.5
New Hampshire[4]	- - -	83.4	77.3	83.9	76.1	86.2	84.1	87.6	84.6
Vermont	69.8	78.2	82.8	*75.7	*66.7	*79.3	74.1	74.5	75.7
Massachusetts	74.0	78.7	75.9	74.0	77.0	71.1	75.0	81.7	81.0
Rhode Island	80.3	82.2	82.6	68.2	77.6	81.5	74.8	78.3	81.5
Connecticut	73.3	76.2	78.2	73.5	73.4	75.2	84.4	85.9	85.9
Middle Atlantic	58.6	63.8	70.7	68.7	71.5	74.2	71.5	74.5	77.8
New York	54.4	61.1	70.5	68.0	68.1	73.2	66.6	71.1	75.0
New Jersey	69.1	69.8	71.0	75.4	79.3	71.8	85.1	83.1	83.2
Pennsylvania	63.4	67.7	71.5	63.5	68.3	78.2	70.8	74.3	78.5
East North Central	66.6	69.7	72.4	65.6	70.3	72.6	74.9	77.7	82.1
Ohio	72.3	75.3	76.8	72.1	77.3	79.4	84.3	85.9	86.0
Indiana	68.2	68.1	65.9	65.5	72.3	68.1	80.5	81.5	81.8
Illinois	65.6	69.1	72.6	66.7	68.9	75.1	78.6	81.0	85.2
Michigan	68.7	71.7	73.2	66.3	74.3	73.9	79.5	82.7	85.6
Wisconsin	66.6	68.6	71.3	63.2	64.7	69.3	48.8	53.4	62.3
West North Central	65.6	66.5	67.8	59.4	64.4	66.9	65.4	69.7	73.2
Minnesota	59.1	60.7	61.7	50.9	57.2	62.1	50.4	56.1	61.2
Iowa	71.1	71.9	71.0	66.8	69.3	69.9	78.8	82.6	82.0
Missouri	76.0	77.2	76.8	68.3	73.4	76.9	81.0	83.4	84.2
North Dakota	73.0	77.9	73.8	61.4	69.4	70.1	76.5	73.6	78.4
South Dakota	75.4	71.7	72.2	59.7	62.2	64.3	73.0	74.4	74.8
Nebraska	62.1	65.3	67.6	62.8	66.6	67.5	73.3	76.3	82.1
Kansas	63.1	63.1	65.9	70.9	75.5	77.7	74.0	78.7	82.5
South Atlantic	69.8	76.0	78.1	66.7	73.6	73.9	77.6	81.3	85.4
Delaware	65.0	68.2	68.7	*66.1	80.9	*76.2	84.4	86.2	84.0
Maryland	75.5	80.6	81.4	79.4	80.9	84.0	86.0	87.4	89.5
District of Columbia	46.6	51.5	64.1	*	*	*	40.7	44.8	73.2
Virginia	64.8	69.4	72.8	75.7	79.4	81.0	77.6	79.5	83.7
West Virginia	61.9	76.2	76.5	*	*64.1	*84.2	73.0	79.9	82.2
North Carolina	66.2	68.2	68.5	68.5	74.5	72.5	79.2	80.1	81.9
South Carolina	59.3	66.0	65.9	61.6	65.9	76.1	73.7	76.8	76.0
Georgia	63.9	72.5	76.0	69.7	78.0	82.9	75.4	81.3	87.3
Florida	71.7	78.6	81.4	55.1	66.8	69.4	78.8	83.3	87.1
East South Central	70.9	71.4	66.7	70.9	73.8	75.7	76.2	80.7	83.4
Kentucky	70.0	76.1	74.0	74.4	78.2	79.4	75.0	81.1	84.6
Tennessee	69.1	69.9	64.5	58.1	69.6	73.8	76.7	81.9	84.0
Alabama	71.3	69.1	62.5	79.7	75.7	80.0	80.2	81.9	83.4
Mississippi	78.0	74.8	77.1	75.0	74.6	72.8	70.5	74.6	80.1
West South Central[4]	58.2	66.3	71.3	60.5	66.8	70.4	77.4	81.9	85.6
Arkansas	58.7	61.0	59.8	59.4	69.5	68.4	74.0	74.7	73.4
Louisiana	76.2	80.3	83.8	75.0	78.3	78.0	74.7	79.6	83.7
Oklahoma[4]	- - -	65.8	68.6	59.4	65.6	69.3	72.5	77.2	81.7
Texas	58.1	66.2	71.4	62.6	69.1	74.1	78.3	82.9	86.6
Mountain	57.4	61.9	65.3	51.6	56.3	60.9	73.1	75.7	78.0
Montana	66.6	72.6	76.7	60.1	63.1	66.4	71.4	76.1	79.7
Idaho	50.1	59.0	61.2	55.6	57.6	59.3	77.7	79.7	78.2
Wyoming	64.2	67.2	71.1	65.4	65.6	65.1	71.7	80.5	84.4
Colorado	63.3	65.2	68.3	58.2	65.7	71.9	71.7	75.5	80.0
New Mexico	54.5	63.2	66.2	46.3	50.9	55.6	61.7	72.7	74.3
Arizona	55.4	59.2	64.1	50.8	56.0	61.0	79.1	78.3	82.4
Utah	69.7	68.0	64.5	54.7	60.7	59.0	70.1	71.7	69.8
Nevada	56.4	61.0	64.0	60.0	63.7	70.3	74.4	76.9	78.5
Pacific	62.5	70.9	76.6	67.3	71.0	72.7	77.0	80.5	83.5
Washington	57.9	66.1	70.8	62.0	69.5	72.1	72.6	77.4	80.5
Oregon	58.0	62.6	66.6	62.2	64.4	66.2	76.3	77.7	80.2
California	62.5	71.1	77.0	65.7	68.2	71.8	78.4	81.1	84.2
Alaska	80.8	82.5	78.1	73.4	76.9	75.7	78.7	81.3	75.2
Hawaii	71.6	78.3	83.0	70.7	81.3	82.9	72.0	79.2	82.3

* Percents preceded by an asterisk are based on fewer than 50 events. Percents not shown are based on fewer than 20 events.
- - - Data not available.
[1]Percents for white and black are substituted for non-Hispanic white and non-Hispanic black for those States and years in which Hispanic origin was not reported on the birth certificate: Oklahoma 1990, and New Hampshire 1990–92.
[2]Persons of Hispanic origin may be of any race.
[3]Includes persons of Hispanic origin.
[4]Percents for Hispanic origin exclude data from States not reporting Hispanic origin on the birth certificate for 1 or more years in 3-year period.

SOURCE: Centers for Disease Control and Prevention, National Center for Health Statistics. National Vital Statistics System.

Table 8. Teenage childbearing, according to detailed race of mother and Hispanic origin of mother: United States, selected years 1970–98

[Data are based on the National Vital Statistics System]

Maternal age, race of mother, and Hispanic origin of mother	1970	1975	1980	1985	1990	1992	1993	1994	1995	1996	1997	1998
Age of mother under 18 years						Percent of live births						
All races	6.3	7.6	5.8	4.7	4.7	4.9	5.1	5.3	5.3	5.1	4.9	4.6
White	4.8	6.0	4.5	3.7	3.6	3.9	4.0	4.2	4.3	4.2	4.1	3.9
Black	14.8	16.3	12.5	10.6	10.1	10.3	10.6	10.8	10.8	10.3	9.7	8.9
American Indian or Alaska Native	7.5	11.2	9.4	7.6	7.2	8.0	8.4	8.7	8.7	8.7	8.6	8.4
Asian or Pacific Islander	- - -	- - -	1.5	1.6	2.1	2.0	2.1	2.2	2.2	2.1	2.0	2.0
Chinese	1.1	0.4	0.3	0.3	0.4	0.3	0.3	0.3	0.3	0.3	0.3	0.3
Japanese	2.0	1.7	1.0	0.9	0.8	0.9	0.9	0.9	0.8	0.9	0.8	0.8
Filipino	3.7	2.4	1.6	1.6	2.0	1.9	2.0	2.2	2.2	2.1	2.1	2.1
Hawaiian and part Hawaiian	- - -	- - -	6.6	5.7	6.5	7.0	7.1	8.0	7.6	6.8	6.7	7.8
Other Asian or Pacific Islander	- - -	- - -	1.2	1.8	2.4	2.3	2.5	2.5	2.5	2.5	2.3	2.3
Hispanic origin (selected States)[1,2]	- - -	- - -	7.4	6.4	6.6	7.1	7.2	7.6	7.6	7.3	7.2	6.9
Mexican	- - -	- - -	7.7	6.9	6.9	7.3	7.5	7.9	8.0	7.7	7.6	7.2
Puerto Rican	- - -	- - -	10.0	8.5	9.1	9.6	10.2	10.8	10.8	10.2	9.5	9.2
Cuban	- - -	- - -	3.8	2.2	2.7	2.5	2.5	3.0	2.8	2.8	2.7	2.9
Central and South American	- - -	- - -	2.4	2.4	3.2	3.6	3.8	4.0	4.1	4.0	3.9	3.6
Other and unknown Hispanic	- - -	- - -	6.5	7.0	8.0	8.9	9.4	9.4	9.0	8.8	8.9	8.8
White, non-Hispanic (selected States)[1]	- - -	- - -	4.0	3.2	3.0	3.1	3.2	3.4	3.4	3.3	3.2	3.0
Black, non-Hispanic (selected States)[1]	- - -	- - -	12.7	10.7	10.2	10.4	10.6	10.9	10.8	10.4	9.8	9.0
Age of mother 18–19 years												
All races	11.3	11.3	9.8	8.0	8.1	7.8	7.8	7.9	7.9	7.9	7.8	7.9
White	10.4	10.3	9.0	7.1	7.3	7.0	7.0	7.1	7.2	·7.2	7.1	7.2
Black	16.6	16.9	14.5	12.9	13.0	12.4	12.1	12.3	12.4	12.5	12.5	12.6
American Indian or Alaska Native	12.8	15.2	14.6	12.4	12.3	11.9	11.9	12.3	12.7	12.3	12.2	12.5
Asian or Pacific Islander	- - -	- - -	3.9	3.4	3.7	3.6	3.6	3.5	3.5	3.2	3.2	3.3
Chinese	3.9	1.7	1.0	0.6	0.8	0.7	0.7	0.7	0.6	0.6	0.6	0.6
Japanese	4.1	3.3	2.3	1.9	2.0	1.7	1.8	1.9	1.7	1.6	1.5	1.6
Filipino	7.1	5.0	4.0	3.7	4.1	3.7	3.8	3.8	4.1	4.0	3.8	4.1
Hawaiian and part Hawaiian	- - -	- - -	13.3	12.3	11.9	11.4	11.3	11.6	11.5	11.6	11.9	11.0
Other Asian or Pacific Islander	- - -	- - -	3.8	3.5	3.9	4.1	4.0	3.9	3.8	3.4	3.3	3.5
Hispanic origin (selected States)[1,2]	- - -	- - -	11.6	10.1	10.2	10.1	10.1	10.2	10.3	10.1	9.8	10.0
Mexican	- - -	- - -	12.0	10.6	10.7	10.7	10.7	10.7	10.8	10.5	10.2	10.3
Puerto Rican	- - -	- - -	13.3	12.4	12.6	11.8	12.1	12.4	12.7	13.0	12.7	12.7
Cuban	- - -	- - -	9.2	4.9	5.0	4.6	4.3	4.3	4.9	4.9	4.7	4.0
Central and South American	- - -	- - -	6.0	5.8	5.9	5.9	6.1	6.4	6.5	6.5	6.5	6.6
Other and unknown Hispanic	- - -	- - -	10.8	10.5	11.1	11.1	11.6	11.4	11.1	11.1	10.9	11.4
White, non-Hispanic (selected States)[1]	- - -	- - -	8.5	6.6	6.6	6.3	6.2	6.3	6.4	6.4	6.3	6.4
Black, non-Hispanic (selected States)[1]	- - -	- - -	14.7	12.9	13.0	12.5	12.2	12.4	12.4	12.6	12.6	12.7

- - - Data not available.

[1]Trend data for Hispanics and non-Hispanics are affected by expansion of the reporting area for an Hispanic-origin item on the birth certificate and by immigration. These two factors affect numbers of events, composition of the Hispanic population, and maternal and infant health characteristics. The number of States in the reporting area increased from 22 in 1980, to 23 and the District of Columbia (DC) in 1983–87, 30 and DC in 1988, 47 and DC in 1989, 48 and DC in 1990, 49 and DC in 1991–92, and 50 and DC in 1993 and later years (see Appendix I, National Vital Statistics System).
[2]Includes mothers of all races.

NOTES: The race groups, white, black, American Indian or Alaska Native, and Asian or Pacific Islander, include persons of Hispanic and non-Hispanic origin. Conversely, persons of Hispanic origin may be of any race. Data for additional years are available (see Appendix III).

SOURCES: Centers for Disease Control and Prevention, National Center for Health Statistics. National Vital Statistics System; Ventura SJ, Martin JA, Curtin SC, Mathews TJ, Park MM. Births: Final data for 1998. National vital statistics reports; vol 48, no 3. Hyattsville, Maryland: 2000; Report of final natality statistics, for each data year 1970–96. Monthly vital statistics report. Hyattsville, Maryland.

Table 9. Nonmarital childbearing according to detailed race of mother, Hispanic origin of mother, and maternal age and birth rates for unmarried women by race of mother and Hispanic origin of mother: United States, selected years 1970–98

[Data are based on the National Vital Statistics System]

Race of mother, Hispanic origin of mother, and maternal age	1970	1975	1980	1985	1990	1992	1993	1994	1995	1996	1997	1998
					Percent of live births to unmarried mothers							
All races	10.7	14.3	18.4	22.0	28.0	30.1	31.0	32.6	32.2	32.4	32.4	32.8
White	5.5	7.1	11.2	14.7	20.4	22.6	23.6	25.4	25.3	25.7	25.8	26.3
Black	37.5	49.5	56.1	61.2	66.5	68.1	68.7	70.4	69.9	69.8	69.2	69.1
American Indian or Alaska Native	22.4	32.7	39.2	46.8	53.6	55.3	55.8	57.0	57.2	58.0	58.7	59.3
Asian or Pacific Islander	- - -	- - -	7.3	9.5	13.2	14.7	15.7	16.2	16.3	16.7	15.6	15.6
Chinese	3.0	1.6	2.7	3.0	5.0	6.1	6.7	7.2	7.9	9.2	6.5	6.4
Japanese	4.6	4.6	5.2	7.9	9.6	9.8	10.0	11.2	10.8	11.4	10.1	9.7
Filipino	9.1	6.9	8.6	11.4	15.9	16.8	17.7	18.5	19.5	19.4	19.5	19.7
Hawaiian and part Hawaiian	- - -	- - -	32.9	37.3	45.0	45.7	47.8	48.6	49.0	49.9	49.1	51.1
Other Asian or Pacific Islander	- - -	- - -	5.4	8.5	12.6	14.9	16.1	16.4	16.2	16.5	15.6	15.2
Hispanic origin (selected States)[1,2]	- - -	- - -	23.6	29.5	36.7	39.1	40.0	43.1	40.8	40.7	40.9	41.6
Mexican	- - -	- - -	20.3	25.7	33.3	36.3	37.0	40.8	38.1	37.9	38.9	39.6
Puerto Rican	- - -	- - -	46.3	51.1	55.9	57.5	59.4	60.2	60.0	60.7	59.4	59.5
Cuban	- - -	- - -	10.0	16.1	18.2	20.2	21.0	22.9	23.8	24.7	24.4	24.8
Central and South American	- - -	- - -	27.1	34.9	41.2	43.9	45.2	45.9	44.1	44.1	41.8	42.0
Other and unknown Hispanic	- - -	- - -	22.4	31.1	37.2	37.6	38.7	43.5	44.0	43.5	43.6	45.3
White, non-Hispanic (selected States)[1]	- - -	- - -	9.6	12.4	16.9	18.5	19.5	20.8	21.2	21.5	21.5	21.9
Black, non-Hispanic (selected States)[1]	- - -	- - -	57.3	62.1	66.7	68.3	68.9	70.7	70.0	70.0	69.4	69.3
					Number of live births, in thousands							
Live births to unmarried mothers	399	448	666	828	1,165	1,225	1,240	1,290	1,254	1,260	1,257	1,294
Maternal age					Percent distribution of live births to unmarried mothers							
Under 20 years	50.1	52.1	40.8	33.8	30.9	29.8	29.7	30.5	30.9	30.4	30.7	30.1
20–24 years	31.8	29.9	35.6	36.3	34.7	35.6	35.4	34.8	34.5	34.2	34.9	35.6
25 years and over	18.1	18.0	23.5	29.9	34.4	34.6	34.9	34.6	34.7	35.3	34.4	34.3
					Live births per 1,000 unmarried women 15–44 years of age[3]							
All races and origins	26.4	24.5	29.4	32.8	43.8	45.2	45.3	46.9	45.1	44.8	44.0	44.3
White[4]	13.9	12.4	18.1	22.5	32.9	35.2	35.9	38.3	37.5	37.6	37.0	37.5
Black[4]	95.5	84.2	81.1	77.0	90.5	86.5	84.0	82.1	75.9	74.4	73.4	73.3
Hispanic origin (selected States)[1,2]	- - -	- - -	- - -	- - -	89.6	95.3	95.2	101.2	95.0	93.2	91.4	90.1
White, non-Hispanic	- - -	- - -	- - -	- - -	- - -	- - -	- - -	28.5	28.2	28.3	27.0	27.4

- - - Data not available.

[1]Trend data for Hispanics and non-Hispanics are affected by expansion of the reporting area for an Hispanic-origin item on the birth certificate and by immigration. These two factors affect numbers of events, composition of the Hispanic population, and maternal and infant health characteristics. The number of States in the reporting area increased from 22 in 1980, to 23 and the District of Columbia (DC) in 1983–87, 30 and DC in 1988, 47 and DC in 1989, 48 and DC in 1990, 49 and DC in 1991–92, and 50 and DC in 1993 and later years (see Appendix I, National Vital Statistics System).

[2]Includes mothers of all races.

[3]Rates computed by relating births to unmarried mothers, regardless of age of mother, to unmarried women 15–44 years of age.

[4]For 1970 and 1975, birth rates are by race of child.

NOTES: National estimates for 1970 and 1975 for unmarried mothers based on births occurring in States reporting marital status of mother (see Appendix I, National Vital Statistics System). The race groups, white, black, American Indian or Alaska Native, and Asian or Pacific Islander, include persons of Hispanic and non-Hispanic origin. Conversely, persons of Hispanic origin may be of any race. In 1995 procedures implemented in California to more accurately identify the marital status of Hispanic mothers account for some of the decline in measures of nonmarital childbearing for women of all races, white women, and Hispanic women between 1994 and 1995. Other reporting changes implemented in California, Nevada, New York City, and Connecticut in 1997 and 1998 have affected trends for all groups. See Appendix I, National Vital Statistics System, Birth certificate items. Data for additional years are available (see Appendix III).

SOURCES: Centers for Disease Control and Prevention, National Center for Health Statistics. National Vital Statistics System; Ventura SJ, Martin JA, Curtin SC, Mathews TJ, Park MM. Births: Final data for 1998. National vital statistics reports; vol 48, no 3. Hyattsville, Maryland: 2000; Ventura SJ. Births to unmarried mothers: United States, 1980–92. Vital Health Stat 21(53). 1995; Report of final natality statistics, for each data year 1993–96. Monthly vital statistics report. Hyattsville, Maryland.

Table 10. Maternal education for live births, according to detailed race of mother and Hispanic origin of mother: United States, selected years 1970–98

[Data are based on the National Vital Statistics System]

Mother's education, race of mother, and Hispanic origin of mother	1970	1975	1980	1985	1990	1992	1993	1994	1995	1996	1997	1998
Less than 12 years of education					Percent of live births[1]							
All races	30.8	28.6	23.7	20.6	23.8	23.6	23.3	22.9	22.6	22.4	22.1	21.9
White	27.1	25.1	20.8	17.8	22.4	22.3	22.0	21.7	21.6	21.6	21.3	21.2
Black	51.2	45.3	36.4	32.6	30.2	30.0	29.8	29.3	28.7	28.2	27.6	26.9
American Indian or Alaska Native	60.5	52.7	44.2	39.0	36.4	35.9	34.8	34.0	33.0	33.0	32.8	32.7
Asian or Pacific Islander	- - -	- - -	21.0	19.4	20.0	19.0	18.1	17.4	16.1	15.0	14.0	12.9
Chinese	23.0	16.5	15.2	15.5	15.8	15.2	14.3	13.7	12.9	12.8	12.3	11.4
Japanese	11.8	9.1	5.0	4.8	3.5	2.4	2.6	2.8	2.6	2.7	2.3	2.4
Filipino	26.4	22.3	16.4	13.9	10.3	9.3	8.8	8.9	8.0	7.4	7.3	6.9
Hawaiian and part Hawaiian	- - -	- - -	20.7	18.7	19.3	18.6	17.3	18.5	17.6	16.9	16.8	18.5
Other Asian or Pacific Islander	- - -	- - -	27.6	24.3	26.8	25.7	24.6	23.3	21.2	19.4	17.8	15.9
Hispanic origin (selected States)[2,3]	- - -	- - -	51.1	44.5	53.9	54.1	53.4	52.7	52.1	51.4	50.3	49.3
Mexican	- - -	- - -	62.8	59.0	61.4	61.3	60.4	59.5	58.6	57.7	56.3	55.2
Puerto Rican	- - -	- - -	55.3	46.6	42.7	41.0	40.3	39.6	38.6	38.1	37.1	35.9
Cuban	- - -	- - -	24.1	21.1	17.8	15.6	14.6	15.0	14.4	14.5	13.7	13.0
Central and South American	- - -	- - -	41.2	37.0	44.2	43.6	43.0	42.0	41.7	40.8	39.6	38.5
Other and unknown Hispanic	- - -	- - -	40.1	36.5	33.3	34.7	33.9	33.9	33.8	33.0	32.8	33.6
White, non-Hispanic (selected States)[2]	- - -	- - -	18.3	15.8	15.2	14.5	14.0	13.5	13.3	13.0	12.9	12.8
Black, non-Hispanic (selected States)[2]	- - -	- - -	37.4	33.5	30.0	29.8	29.6	29.1	28.6	28.0	27.5	26.7
16 years or more of education												
All races	8.6	11.4	14.0	16.7	17.5	18.9	19.5	20.4	21.4	22.1	22.8	23.4
White	9.6	12.7	15.5	18.6	19.3	20.7	21.4	22.2	23.1	23.9	24.6	25.1
Black	2.8	4.3	6.2	7.0	7.2	7.8	8.2	8.7	9.5	10.0	10.5	11.0
American Indian or Alaska Native	2.7	2.2	3.5	3.7	4.4	4.7	5.5	5.7	6.2	6.3	6.8	6.8
Asian or Pacific Islander	- - -	- - -	30.8	30.3	31.0	32.5	33.0	33.9	35.0	36.2	38.0	39.7
Chinese	34.0	37.8	41.5	35.2	40.3	44.0	45.7	46.6	49.0	49.1	51.1	53.8
Japanese	20.7	30.6	36.8	38.1	44.1	46.6	46.3	45.2	46.2	46.8	48.3	49.1
Filipino	28.1	36.6	37.1	35.2	34.5	35.8	36.1	36.6	36.7	38.6	38.6	39.2
Hawaiian and part Hawaiian	- - -	- - -	7.9	6.5	6.8	8.0	8.5	8.9	9.7	11.3	11.0	11.0
Other Asian or Pacific Islander	- - -	- - -	29.2	30.2	27.3	28.0	28.1	29.4	30.5	32.2	34.4	36.7
Hispanic origin (selected States)[2,3]	- - -	- - -	4.2	6.0	5.1	5.4	5.5	5.8	6.1	6.4	6.7	7.0
Mexican	- - -	- - -	2.2	3.0	3.3	3.5	3.5	3.8	4.0	4.2	4.5	4.7
Puerto Rican	- - -	- - -	3.0	4.6	6.5	7.3	7.5	8.1	8.7	8.9	9.2	9.5
Cuban	- - -	- - -	11.6	15.0	20.4	22.5	24.3	24.8	26.5	27.0	27.8	28.6
Central and South American	- - -	- - -	6.1	8.1	8.6	9.2	9.4	9.8	10.3	11.2	11.9	12.5
Other and unknown Hispanic	- - -	- - -	5.5	7.2	8.5	8.5	9.2	9.8	10.5	11.1	11.7	11.5
White, non-Hispanic (selected States)[2]	- - -	- - -	16.4	19.3	22.6	24.4	25.3	26.5	27.7	28.8	29.7	30.4
Black, non-Hispanic (selected States)[2]	- - -	- - -	5.7	6.7	7.3	7.8	8.2	8.7	9.5	10.0	10.6	11.0

- - - Data not available.

[1] Excludes live births for whom education of mother is unknown.

[2] Trend data for Hispanics and non-Hispanics are affected by expansion of the reporting area for an Hispanic-origin item on the birth certificate and by immigration. These two factors affect numbers of events, composition of the Hispanic population, and maternal and infant health characteristics. Data shown only for States with an Hispanic-origin item and education of mother item on their birth certificates. The number of States reporting both items increased from 20 in 1980, to 21 and the District of Columbia (DC) in 1983–87, 26 and DC in 1988, 45 and DC in 1989, 47 and DC in 1990–91, 49 and DC in 1992, and 50 and DC in 1993 and later years (see Appendix I, National Vital Statistics System).

[3] Includes mothers of all races.

NOTES: Excludes births that occurred in States not reporting education (see Appendix I). The race groups, white, black, American Indian or Alaska Native, and Asian or Pacific Islander, include persons of Hispanic and non-Hispanic origin. Conversely, persons of Hispanic origin may be of any race. Maternal education groups shown in this table generally represent the group at highest risk for unfavorable birth outcomes (less than 12 years of education) and the group at lowest risk (16 years or more of education). Data for additional years are available (see Appendix III).

SOURCE: Centers for Disease Control and Prevention, National Center for Health Statistics: National Vital Statistics System.

Table 11. Mothers who smoked cigarettes during pregnancy, according to mother's detailed race, Hispanic origin, age, and educational attainment: Selected States, 1989–98

[Data are based on the National Vital Statistics System]

Characteristic of mother	1989	1990	1992	1993	1994	1995	1996	1997	1998
Race of mother[1]	Percent of mothers who smoked[2]								
All races	19.5	18.4	16.9	15.8	14.6	13.9	13.6	13.2	12.9
White	20.4	19.4	17.9	16.8	15.6	15.0	14.7	14.3	14.0
Black	17.1	15.9	13.8	12.7	11.4	10.6	10.2	9.7	9.5
American Indian or Alaska Native	23.0	22.4	22.5	21.6	21.0	20.9	21.3	20.8	20.2
Asian or Pacific Islander[3]	5.7	5.5	4.8	4.3	3.6	3.4	3.3	3.2	3.1
Chinese	2.7	2.0	1.7	1.1	0.9	0.8	0.7	1.0	0.8
Japanese	8.2	8.0	6.6	6.7	5.4	5.2	4.8	4.7	4.8
Filipino	5.1	5.3	4.8	4.3	3.7	3.4	3.5	3.4	3.3
Hawaiian and part Hawaiian	19.3	21.0	18.5	17.2	16.0	15.9	15.3	15.8	16.8
Other Asian or Pacific Islander	4.2	3.8	3.6	3.2	2.9	2.7	2.7	2.5	2.4
Hispanic origin and race of mother[4]									
Hispanic origin	8.0	6.7	5.8	5.0	4.6	4.3	4.3	4.1	4.0
Mexican	6.3	5.3	4.3	3.7	3.4	3.1	3.1	2.9	2.8
Puerto Rican	14.5	13.6	12.7	11.2	10.9	10.4	11.0	11.0	10.7
Cuban	6.9	6.4	5.9	5.0	4.8	4.1	4.7	4.2	3.7
Central and South American	3.6	3.0	2.6	2.3	1.8	1.8	1.8	1.8	1.5
Other and unknown Hispanic	12.1	10.8	10.1	9.3	8.1	8.2	9.1	8.5	8.0
White, non-Hispanic	21.7	21.0	19.7	18.6	17.7	17.1	16.9	16.5	16.2
Black, non-Hispanic	17.2	15.9	13.8	12.7	11.5	10.6	10.3	9.8	9.6
Age of mother[1]									
Under 15 years	7.7	7.5	6.9	7.0	6.7	7.3	7.7	8.1	7.7
15–19 years	22.2	20.8	18.6	17.5	16.7	16.8	17.2	17.6	17.8
15–17 years	19.0	17.6	15.6	14.8	14.4	14.6	15.4	15.5	15.5
18–19 years	23.9	22.5	20.3	19.1	18.1	18.1	18.3	18.8	19.2
20–24 years	23.5	22.1	20.3	19.2	17.8	17.1	16.8	16.6	16.5
25–29 years	19.0	18.0	16.1	14.8	13.5	12.8	12.3	11.8	11.4
30–34 years	15.7	15.3	14.5	13.4	12.3	11.4	10.9	10.0	9.3
35–39 years	13.6	13.3	13.4	12.8	12.2	12.0	11.7	11.1	10.6
40–54 years[5]	13.2	12.3	11.6	11.0	10.3	10.1	10.1	10.1	10.0
Education of mother[6]	Percent of mothers 20 years of age and over who smoked[2]								
0–8 years	18.9	17.5	15.5	13.9	12.1	11.0	10.3	9.9	9.5
9–11 years	42.2	40.5	37.8	36.1	33.6	32.0	31.1	30.2	29.3
12 years	22.8	21.9	20.7	19.9	18.7	18.3	18.0	17.5	17.1
13–15 years	13.7	12.8	12.1	11.4	10.8	10.6	10.4	9.9	9.6
16 years or more	5.0	4.5	3.9	3.1	2.8	2.7	2.6	2.4	2.2

[1]Includes data for 43 States and the District of Columbia (DC) in 1989, 45 States and DC in 1990, 46 States and DC in 1991–93, and 46 States, DC, and New York City (NYC) in 1994–97. Excludes data for California, Indiana, New York (but includes NYC in 1994–97), and South Dakota (1989–97), Oklahoma (1989–90), and Louisiana and Nebraska (1989), which did not require the reporting of mother's tobacco use during pregnancy on the birth certificate (see Appendix I).
[2]Excludes live births for whom smoking status of mother is unknown.
[3]Maternal tobacco use during pregnancy was not reported on the birth certificates of California and New York, which in 1998 together accounted for 43 percent of the births to Asian or Pacific Islander mothers.
[4]Includes data for 42 States and DC in 1989, 44 States and DC in 1990, 45 States and DC in 1991–92, 46 States and DC in 1993, and 46 States, DC, and NYC in 1994–98. Excludes data for California, Indiana, New York (but includes NYC in 1994–98), and South Dakota (1989–98), New Hampshire (1989–92), Oklahoma (1989–90), and Louisiana and Nebraska (1989), which did not require the reporting of either Hispanic origin of mother or tobacco use during pregnancy on the birth certificate (see Appendix I).
[5]Prior to 1997 data are for live births to mothers 45–49 years of age.
[6]Includes data for 42 States and DC in 1989, 44 States and DC in 1990, 45 States and DC in 1991, 46 States and DC in 1992–93, and 46 States, DC, and NYC in 1994–98. Excludes data for California, Indiana, New York (but includes NYC in 1994–98), and South Dakota (1989–98), Washington (1989–91), Oklahoma (1989–90), and Louisiana and Nebraska (1989), which did not require the reporting of either mother's education or tobacco use during pregnancy on the birth certificate (see Appendix I).

NOTES: The race groups, white, black, American Indian or Alaska Native, and Asian or Pacific Islander, include persons of Hispanic and non-Hispanic origin. Conversely, persons of Hispanic origin may be of any race. Data for additional years are available (see Appendix III).

SOURCES: Centers for Disease Control and Prevention, National Center for Health Statistics. National Vital Statistics System; Ventura SJ, Martin JA, Curtin SC, Mathews TJ, Park MM. Births: Final data for 1998. National vital statistics reports; vol 48, no 3. Hyattsville, Maryland: 2000; Report of final natality statistics, for each data year 1989–96. Monthly vital statistics report. Hyattsville, Maryland.

Table 12. Low-birthweight live births, according to mother's detailed race, Hispanic origin, and smoking status: United States, selected years 1970–98

[Data are based on the National Vital Statistics System]

Birthweight, race of mother, Hispanic origin of mother, and smoking status of mother	1970	1975	1980	1985	1990	1992	1993	1994	1995	1996	1997	1998
Low birthweight (less than 2,500 grams)					Percent of live births[1]							
All races	7.93	7.38	6.84	6.75	6.97	7.08	7.22	7.28	7.32	7.39	7.51	7.57
White	6.85	6.27	5.72	5.65	5.70	5.80	5.98	6.11	6.22	6.34	6.46	6.52
Black	13.90	13.19	12.69	12.65	13.25	13.31	13.34	13.24	13.13	13.01	13.01	13.05
American Indian or Alaska Native	7.97	6.41	6.44	5.86	6.11	6.22	6.42	6.45	6.61	6.49	6.75	6.81
Asian or Pacific Islander	- - -	- - -	6.68	6.16	6.45	6.57	6.55	6.81	6.90	7.07	7.23	7.42
Chinese	6.67	5.29	5.21	4.98	4.69	4.98	4.91	4.76	5.29	5.03	5.06	5.34
Japanese	9.03	7.47	6.60	6.21	6.16	7.00	6.53	6.91	7.26	7.27	6.82	7.50
Filipino	10.02	8.08	7.40	6.95	7.30	7.43	6.99	7.77	7.83	7.92	8.33	8.23
Hawaiian and part Hawaiian	- - -	- - -	7.23	6.49	7.24	6.89	6.76	7.20	6.84	6.77	7.20	7.15
Other Asian or Pacific Islander	- - -	- - -	6.83	6.19	6.65	6.68	6.89	7.06	7.05	7.42	7.54	7.76
Hispanic origin (selected States)[2,3]	- - -	- - -	6.12	6.16	6.06	6.10	6.24	6.25	6.29	6.28	6.42	6.44
Mexican	- - -	- - -	5.62	5.77	5.55	5.61	5.77	5.80	5.81	5.86	5.97	5.97
Puerto Rican	- - -	- - -	8.95	8.69	8.99	9.19	9.23	9.13	9.41	9.24	9.39	9.68
Cuban	- - -	- - -	5.62	6.02	5.67	6.10	6.18	6.27	6.50	6.46	6.78	6.50
Central and South American	- - -	- - -	5.76	5.68	5.84	5.77	5.94	6.02	6.20	6.03	6.26	6.47
Other and unknown Hispanic	- - -	- - -	6.96	6.83	6.87	7.24	7.51	7.54	7.55	7.68	7.93	7.59
White, non-Hispanic (selected States)[2]	- - -	- - -	5.67	5.60	5.61	5.73	5.92	6.06	6.20	6.36	6.47	6.55
Black, non-Hispanic (selected States)[2]	- - -	- - -	12.71	12.61	13.32	13.40	13.43	13.34	13.21	13.12	13.11	13.17
Cigarette smoker[4]	- - -	- - -	- - -	- - -	11.25	11.49	11.84	12.28	12.18	12.13	12.06	12.01
Nonsmoker[4]	- - -	- - -	- - -	- - -	6.14	6.35	6.56	6.71	6.79	6.91	7.07	7.18
Very low birthweight (less than 1,500 grams)												
All races	1.17	1.16	1.15	1.21	1.27	1.29	1.33	1.33	1.35	1.37	1.42	1.45
White	0.95	0.92	0.90	0.94	0.95	0.96	1.01	1.02	1.06	1.09	1.13	1.15
Black	2.40	2.40	2.48	2.71	2.92	2.96	2.96	2.96	2.97	2.99	3.04	3.08
American Indian or Alaska Native	0.98	0.95	0.92	1.01	1.01	0.95	1.05	1.10	1.10	1.21	1.19	1.24
Asian or Pacific Islander	- - -	- - -	0.92	0.85	0.87	0.91	0.86	0.93	0.91	0.99	1.05	1.10
Chinese	0.80	0.52	0.66	0.57	0.51	0.67	0.63	0.58	0.67	0.64	0.74	0.75
Japanese	1.48	0.89	0.94	0.84	0.73	0.85	0.74	0.92	0.87	0.81	0.78	0.84
Filipino	1.08	0.93	0.99	0.86	1.05	1.05	0.95	1.19	1.13	1.20	1.29	1.35
Hawaiian and part Hawaiian	- - -	- - -	1.05	1.03	0.97	1.02	1.14	1.20	0.94	0.97	1.41	1.53
Other Asian or Pacific Islander	- - -	- - -	0.96	0.91	0.92	0.93	0.89	0.93	0.91	1.04	1.07	1.12
Hispanic origin (selected States)[2,3]	- - -	- - -	0.98	1.01	1.03	1.04	1.06	1.08	1.11	1.12	1.13	1.15
Mexican	- - -	- - -	0.92	0.97	0.92	0.94	0.97	0.99	1.01	1.01	1.02	1.02
Puerto Rican	- - -	- - -	1.29	1.30	1.62	1.70	1.66	1.63	1.79	1.70	1.85	1.86
Cuban	- - -	- - -	1.02	1.18	1.20	1.24	1.23	1.31	1.19	1.35	1.36	1.33
Central and South American	- - -	- - -	0.99	1.01	1.05	1.02	1.02	1.06	1.13	1.14	1.17	1.23
Other and unknown Hispanic	- - -	- - -	1.01	0.96	1.09	1.10	1.23	1.29	1.28	1.48	1.35	1.38
White, non-Hispanic (selected States)[2]	- - -	- - -	0.86	0.90	0.93	0.94	1.00	1.01	1.04	1.08	1.12	1.15
Black, non-Hispanic (selected States)[2]	- - -	- - -	2.46	2.66	2.93	2.97	2.99	2.99	2.98	3.02	3.05	3.11
Cigarette smoker[4]	- - -	- - -	- - -	- - -	1.73	1.74	1.77	1.81	1.85	1.85	1.83	1.87
Nonsmoker[4]	- - -	- - -	- - -	- - -	1.18	1.22	1.28	1.30	1.31	1.35	1.40	1.44

- - - Data not available.

[1]Excludes live births with unknown birthweight. Percent based on live births with known birthweight.

[2]Trend data for Hispanics and non-Hispanics are affected by expansion of the reporting area for an Hispanic-origin item on the birth certificate and by immigration. These two factors affect numbers of events, composition of the Hispanic population, and maternal and infant health characteristics. The number of States in the reporting area increased from 22 in 1980, to 23 and the District of Columbia (DC) in 1983–87, 30 and DC in 1988, 47 and DC in 1989, 48 and DC in 1990, 49 and DC in 1991–92, and 50 and DC in 1993 and later years (see Appendix I, National Vital Statistics System).

[3]Includes mothers of all races.

[4]Percent based on live births with known smoking status of mother and known birthweight. Includes data for 43 States and the District of Columbia (DC) in 1989, 45 States and DC in 1990, 46 States and DC in 1991–93, and 46 States, DC, and New York City (NYC) in 1994–98. Excludes data for California, Indiana, New York (but includes NYC in 1994–98), and South Dakota (1989–98), Oklahoma (1989–90), and Louisiana and Nebraska (1989), which did not require the reporting of mother's tobacco use during pregnancy on the birth certificate (see Appendix I).

NOTES: The race groups, white, black, American Indian or Alaska Native, and Asian or Pacific Islander, include persons of Hispanic and non-Hispanic origin. Conversely, persons of Hispanic origin may be of any race. Data for additional years are available (see Appendix III).

SOURCES: Centers for Disease Control and Prevention, National Center for Health Statistics. National Vital Statistics System; Ventura SJ, Martin JA, Curtin SC, Mathews TJ, Park MM. Births: Final data for 1998. National vital statistics reports; vol 48, no-3. Hyattsville, Maryland: 2000; Report of final natality statistics, for each data year 1970–96. Monthly vital statistics report. Hyattsville, Maryland.

Table 13. Low-birthweight live births among mothers 20 years of age and over, by mother's detailed race, Hispanic origin, and educational attainment: United States, 1989–98

[Data are based on the National Vital Statistics System]

Mother's education, race of mother, and Hispanic origin of mother	1989	1990	1992	1993	1994	1995	1996	1997	1998
Less than 12 years of education	Percent of live births weighing less than 2,500 grams[1]								
All races	9.0	8.6	8.4	8.6	8.5	8.4	8.3	8.4	8.4
White	7.3	7.0	6.9	7.1	7.1	7.1	7.1	7.2	7.2
Black	17.0	16.5	16.5	16.4	16.2	16.0	15.5	15.4	15.0
American Indian or Alaska Native	7.3	7.4	7.1	7.6	7.0	8.0	7.7	7.7	8.0
Asian or Pacific Islander	6.6	6.4	6.2	6.4	6.6	6.7	7.1	6.8	7.4
Chinese	5.4	5.2	4.4	4.6	4.6	5.3	5.0	5.1	5.9
Japanese	4.0	10.6	7.0	9.4	7.4	11.0	8.3	2.6	5.0
Filipino	6.9	7.2	6.8	6.2	8.2	7.5	8.0	7.8	7.9
Hawaiian and part Hawaiian	11.0	10.7	9.5	9.1	8.0	9.8	10.1	7.4	8.5
Other Asian or Pacific Islander	6.8	6.4	6.4	6.6	6.8	6.7	7.5	7.1	7.8
Hispanic origin[2,3]	6.0	5.7	5.8	5.8	5.8	5.8	5.8	5.9	5.9
Mexican	5.3	5.2	5.3	5.4	5.4	5.4	5.4	5.6	5.6
Puerto Rican	11.3	10.3	10.4	10.3	10.7	10.5	10.4	10.6	10.7
Cuban	9.4	7.9	7.8	6.5	8.2	9.2	8.0	9.5	7.4
Central and South American	5.8	5.8	5.8	5.8	6.0	6.2	6.0	5.8	6.2
Other and unknown Hispanic	8.2	8.0	7.8	8.1	7.6	7.7	8.0	8.3	7.7
White, non-Hispanic[2]	8.4	8.3	8.3	8.7	8.8	8.9	9.1	9.1	9.1
Black, non-Hispanic[2]	17.6	16.7	16.7	16.7	16.6	16.2	15.8	15.6	15.3
12 years of education									
All races	7.1	7.1	7.2	7.4	7.5	7.6	7.7	7.7	7.9
White	5.7	5.8	5.9	6.1	6.3	6.4	6.6	6.6	6.7
Black	13.4	13.1	13.3	13.4	13.3	13.3	13.2	13.1	13.1
American Indian or Alaska Native	5.6	6.1	6.0	6.1	6.3	6.5	6.0	6.4	6.9
Asian or Pacific Islander	6.4	6.5	6.8	6.6	6.7	7.0	7.0	7.2	7.2
Chinese	5.1	4.9	5.7	4.9	5.3	5.7	4.9	5.2	4.7
Japanese	7.4	6.2	7.4	7.2	7.6	7.4	7.2	7.9	8.0
Filipino	6.8	7.6	7.4	6.5	7.5	7.7	7.8	8.2	8.0
Hawaiian and part Hawaiian	7.0	6.7	7.0	7.1	6.9	6.6	6.5	7.2	6.7
Other Asian or Pacific Islander	6.5	6.7	6.8	7.0	6.8	7.1	7.4	7.3	7.6
Hispanic origin[2,3]	5.9	6.0	6.0	6.2	6.2	6.1	6.2	6.2	6.4
Mexican	5.2	5.5	5.5	5.7	5.8	5.6	5.8	5.7	6.0
Puerto Rican	8.8	8.3	8.3	8.5	8.1	8.7	8.8	8.7	9.4
Cuban	5.3	5.2	6.6	6.6	6.6	6.7	6.0	6.9	6.0
Central and South American	5.7	5.8	5.7	6.1	5.8	5.9	5.9	6.3	6.2
Other and unknown Hispanic	6.1	6.6	7.1	7.4	7.3	7.1	7.5	7.4	7.3
White, non-Hispanic[2]	5.7	5.7	5.9	6.1	6.3	6.5	6.7	6.7	6.8
Black, non-Hispanic[2]	13.6	13.2	13.4	13.5	13.4	13.4	13.3	13.2	13.3
13 years or more of education									
All races	5.5	5.4	5.6	5.8	5.9	6.0	6.2	6.4	6.5
White	4.6	4.6	4.8	5.0	5.1	5.3	5.5	5.7	5.8
Black	11.2	11.1	11.2	11.3	11.5	11.4	11.4	11.4	11.5
American Indian or Alaska Native	5.6	4.7	5.6	5.8	5.9	5.7	6.0	6.2	5.9
Asian or Pacific Islander	6.1	6.0	6.2	6.3	6.6	6.6	6.8	7.0	7.2
Chinese	4.5	4.4	4.7	4.9	4.6	5.1	5.0	4.9	5.3
Japanese	6.6	6.0	6.9	6.3	6.8	7.1	7.2	6.6	7.4
Filipino	7.2	7.0	7.3	6.9	7.5	7.6	7.8	8.1	8.0
Hawaiian and part Hawaiian	6.3	4.7	5.4	5.2	5.9	5.0	5.4	6.6	6.6
Other Asian or Pacific Islander	6.1	6.2	6.2	6.5	6.9	6.7	7.0	7.3	7.5
Hispanic origin[2,3]	5.5	5.5	5.5	5.7	5.8	5.9	6.0	6.2	6.3
Mexican	5.1	5.2	5.1	5.5	5.5	5.6	5.6	5.8	5.8
Puerto Rican	7.4	7.4	7.5	7.4	7.3	7.9	7.8	8.2	8.2
Cuban	4.9	5.0	5.1	5.4	5.7	5.6	6.4	6.0	6.5
Central and South American	5.2	5.6	5.1	5.4	5.5	5.8	5.7	6.1	6.5
Other and unknown Hispanic	5.4	5.2	5.4	5.6	6.5	6.1	6.6	6.7	6.8
White, non-Hispanic[2]	4.6	4.5	4.7	4.9	5.1	5.2	5.4	5.6	5.7
Black, non-Hispanic[2]	11.2	11.1	11.2	11.4	11.5	11.5	11.4	11.5	11.6

[1]Excludes live births with unknown birthweight. Percent based on live births with known birthweight.

[2]Data shown only for States with an Hispanic-origin item and education of mother on their birth certificates. The number of States reporting both items increased from 45, the District of Columbia (DC), and New York City (NYC) in 1989, to 47, DC, and NYC in 1990–91, 49 and DC in 1992, and 50 and DC in 1993 and later years (see Appendix I, National Vital Statistics System).

[3]Includes mothers of all races.

NOTES: Includes data for 48 States, the District of Columbia (DC), and New York City (NYC) in 1989–91 and all 50 States and DC starting in 1992. Excludes data for births to residents of upstate New York and Washington (1989–91), which did not require the reporting of education of mother on the birth certificate (see Appendix I). The race groups, white, black, American Indian or Alaska Native, and Asian or Pacific Islander, include persons of Hispanic and non-Hispanic origin. Conversely, persons of Hispanic origin may be of any race. Data for additional years are available (see Appendix III).

SOURCE: Centers for Disease Control and Prevention, National Center for Health Statistics. National Vital Statistics System.

Table 14 (page 1 of 2). **Low-birthweight live births, according to race of mother, Hispanic origin of mother, geographic division, and State: United States, average annual 1990–92, 1993–95, and 1996–98**

[Data are based on the National Vital Statistics System]

Percent of live births weighing less than 2,500 grams

Geographic division and State	All races			White, non-Hispanic			Black, non-Hispanic		
	1990–92	1993–95	1996–98	1990–92	1993–95	1996–98	1990–92	1993–95	1996–98
United States[1]	7.05	7.27	7.49	5.68	6.06	6.46	13.44	*13.33	13.13
New England[1]	5.99	6.32	6.78	5.17	5.55	6.06	12.21	11.84	11.79
Maine	5.20	5.73	5.88	5.27	5.74	5.95	*	*	*13.27
New Hampshire[1]	5.01	5.20	5.44	4.97	5.04	5.31	*9.30	*10.70	*
Vermont	5.51	5.69	6.32	5.31	5.63	6.22	*	*	*
Massachusetts	5.90	6.29	6.77	5.12	5.53	6.13	11.43	11.48	11.12
Rhode Island	6.15	6.57	7.28	5.50	5.91	6.46	10.55	11.30	11.35
Connecticut	6.79	6.96	7.43	5.21	5.60	6.16	13.73	12.50	12.82
Middle Atlantic	7.44	7.55	7.73	5.50	5.82	6.27	14.03	13.49	13.02
New York	7.69	7.64	7.77	5.45	5.68	6.19	13.74	12.96	12.32
New Jersey	7.18	7.57	7.84	5.29	5.80	6.26	13.70	13.78	13.86
Pennsylvania	7.20	7.39	7.57	5.66	5.99	6.36	14.96	14.43	13.86
East North Central	7.26	7.49	7.64	5.70	6.08	6.47	14.33	14.25	13.73
Ohio	7.32	7.53	7.66	6.04	6.36	6.64	13.91	13.82	13.34
Indiana	6.64	7.10	7.76	5.91	6.42	7.06	12.40	12.73	13.68
Illinois	7.69	7.94	7.96	5.60	5.98	6.44	14.66	14.92	14.22
Michigan	7.61	7.71	7.72	5.67	6.08	6.35	14.91	14.23	13.51
Wisconsin	5.98	6.17	6.40	4.99	5.22	5.58	13.97	13.95	13.21
West North Central	6.06	6.39	6.69	5.32	5.72	6.20	13.02	13.09	12.91
Minnesota	5.19	5.66	5.84	4.51	5.03	5.61	12.71	12.05	11.42
Iowa	5.59	5.86	6.38	5.33	5.60	6.11	12.27	12.33	12.66
Missouri	7.31	7.56	7.68	6.00	6.38	6.65	13.56	13.63	13.48
North Dakota	5.13	5.33	6.15	5.02	5.15	6.17	*9.70	*9.91	*11.69
South Dakota	5.22	5.63	5.73	5.08	5.45	5.72	*	*10.08	*10.36
Nebraska	5.50	6.11	6.60	5.03	5.67	6.32	11.78	12.36	11.58
Kansas	6.30	6.49	6.96	5.74	5.96	6.49	11.89	12.53	13.20
South Atlantic	8.04	8.27	8.45	5.96	6.37	6.75	13.07	13.15	13.09
Delaware	7.70	7.87	8.54	5.66	6.23	6.50	13.77	13.03	14.41
Maryland	8.05	8.49	8.68	5.51	6.08	6.39	13.38	13.52	13.37
District of Columbia	14.93	14.09	13.60	5.74	5.25	6.15	17.45	16.62	16.28
Virginia	7.27	7.50	7.77	5.63	5.91	6.28	12.45	12.59	12.49
West Virginia	7.05	7.52	8.10	6.83	7.29	7.95	12.91	13.59	12.94
North Carolina	8.27	8.66	8.80	6.23	6.75	7.08	13.05	13.59	13.82
South Carolina	8.97	9.26	9.30	6.28	6.75	6.99	13.25	13.49	13.60
Georgia	8.60	8.70	8.62	6.10	6.40	6.58	12.97	12.98	12.83
Florida	7.43	7.65	7.98	5.86	6.26	6.77	12.36	12.33	12.30
East South Central	8.39	8.71	8.98	6.55	6.98	7.42	13.21	13.41	13.48
Kentucky	7.03	7.47	7.94	6.51	6.98	7.49	12.08	12.59	12.73
Tennessee	8.50	8.76	8.89	6.75	7.12	7.46	14.18	14.32	14.07
Alabama	8.53	8.91	9.26	6.28	6.88	7.33	12.83	12.94	13.34
Mississippi	9.72	9.92	10.03	6.63	6.81	7.34	13.08	13.33	13.31
West South Central[1]	7.40	7.50	7.77	5.98	6.27	6.73	13.33	13.10	13.29
Arkansas	8.18	8.20	8.57	6.57	6.89	7.31	13.49	12.80	13.41
Louisiana	9.32	9.55	10.05	6.12	6.43	6.98	13.80	13.86	14.49
Oklahoma[1]	6.62	6.89	7.27	6.02	6.37	6.80	11.93	12.34	12.63
Texas	7.00	7.08	7.30	5.83	6.09	6.54	13.13	12.71	12.51
Mountain	6.83	7.06	7.34	6.41	6.70	7.08	14.20	14.07	13.70
Montana	5.92	6.03	6.56	5.94	5.84	6.28	*	*	*
Idaho	5.65	5.57	6.02	5.61	5.44	5.84	*	*	*
Wyoming	7.23	7.83	8.76	7.05	7.59	8.69	*11.41	*13.98	*15.82
Colorado	8.24	8.46	8.75	7.49	7.90	8.34	16.08	15.46	14.48
New Mexico	7.23	7.39	7.63	6.84	7.39	7.68	12.98	10.43	13.46
Arizona	6.41	6.74	6.80	6.07	6.52	6.63	12.34	13.30	12.88
Utah	5.79	6.04	6.65	5.65	5.89	6.44	12.52	11.25	15.06
Nevada	7.20	7.45	7.57	6.55	6.93	7.28	14.46	14.59	13.78
Pacific	5.76	5.97	6.07	5.01	5.33	5.47	12.52	12.30	11.73
Washington	5.23	5.32	5.63	4.85	4.99	5.25	11.67	10.75	10.32
Oregon	5.03	5.34	5.39	4.77	5.14	5.14	11.36	10.68	10.71
California	5.85	6.08	6.15	5.10	5.48	5.61	12.64	12.46	11.90
Alaska	4.81	5.26	5.78	4.25	4.80	5.30	9.90	10.77	12.00
Hawaii	7.02	7.01	7.34	5.41	5.35	5.35	11.53	11.82	9.79

See footnotes at end of table.

Table 14 (page 2 of 2). Low-birthweight live births, according to race of mother, Hispanic origin of mother, geographic division, and State: United States, average annual 1990–92, 1993–95, and 1996–98

[Data are based on the National Vital Statistics System]

Geographic division and State	Hispanic[2]			American Indian or Alaska Native[3]			Asian or Pacific Islander[3]		
	1990–92	1993–95	1996–98	1990–92	1993–95	1996–98	1990–92	1993–95	1996–98
	Percent of live births weighing less than 2,500 grams								
United States[4]	6.10	6.26	6.38	6.16	6.49	6.69	6.52	6.76	7.24
New England[4]	7.74	8.02	8.28	6.80	7.95	8.17	6.77	6.97	7.19
Maine	*	*7.36	*5.74	*	*	*	*6.33	*7.33	*5.03
New Hampshire[4]	- - -	*5.60	*6.48	*	*	*	*6.82	*7.59	*8.30
Vermont	*	*	*	*	*	*	*	*	*
Massachusetts	7.28	7.76	8.03	*5.76	*6.86	*6.37	6.52	6.46	6.95
Rhode Island	6.76	6.82	7.68	*8.27	*10.21	*10.49	8.21	7.76	8.30
Connecticut	8.79	8.88	8.94	*8.62	*9.07	*10.94	6.98	8.07	7.73
Middle Atlantic	7.92	7.79	7.71	7.73	8.96	8.21	6.62	6.93	7.32
New York	8.08	8.76	7.65	7.09	8.26	7.40	6.53	6.81	7.24
New Jersey	7.17	7 46	7.30	10.36	9.38	12.20	6.71	6.87	7.52
Pennsylvania	8.68	8.99	9.34	*6.75	10.63	7.31	6.86	7.58	7.26
East North Central	6.05	6.16	6.33	6.19	6.70	6.51	6.63	7.04	7.52
Ohio	7.75	7.45	7.38	*6.35	9.81	7.20	6.38	6.51	7.43
Indiana	5.96	6.40	7.00	*9.06	*6.94	*10.98	6.41	5.93	6.50
Illinois	5.85	5.98	6.11	*6.34	8.08	7.70	7.06	7.65	8.02
Michigan	6.05	6.32	6.48	6.39	6.75	6.12	6.12	6.96	7.25
Wisconsin	6.53	6.36	6.56	5.55	5.39	5.71	6.10	6.26	6.81
West North Central	6.13	6.03	6.09	5.82	6.63	6.12	6.26	6.82	7.04
Minnesota	5.78	6.18	6.13	6.11	7.13	6.21	6.08	7.05	6.66
Iowa	6.80	6.08	6.21	*6.31	*5.86	8.48	7.27	7.44	7.63
Missouri	5.92	6.25	6.24	*7.02	*6.64	7.87	6.60	7.19	7.18
North Dakota	*	*6.23	*5.88	5.76	5.87	5.66	*	*8.89	*
South Dakota	*7.21	*6.37	*6.14	5.77	6.44	5.58	*	*	*
Nebraska	6.64	6.30	6.08	4.48	6.11	6.36	6.23	6.38	7.94
Kansas	5.97	5.64	5.95	5.63	8.48	6.40	6.20	5.33	7.49
South Atlantic	6.11	6.22	6.37	7.82	8.42	9.00	6.42	7.05	7.54
Delaware	8.05	6.83	7.76	*	*	*	*6.99	8.68	8.04
Maryland	5.93	6.01	6.29	*	*5.63	*8.48	6.30	7.01	7.15
District of Columbia	6.97	6.78	6.73	*	*	*	7.05	7.31	*8.43
Virginia	5.33	5.70	6.68	*9.43	*7.42	*6.94	5.43	6.51	7.30
West Virginia	*	*9.03	*	*	*	*	*6.31	*7.31	*6.58
North Carolina	5.99	6.01	6.14	8.57	9.11	10.22	6.69	7.45	7.61
South Carolina	5.63	6.28	5.99	*	*8.75	*9.40	6.87	7.10	7.56
Georgia	5.90	6.03	5.36	*	*6.98	*7.21	7.03	6.63	7.51
Florida	6.22	6.32	6.55	6.33	7.35	7.35	6.93	7.53	7.98
East South Central	5.13	5.63	6.53	7.56	7.27	7.73	6.36	6.92	7.60
Kentucky	*4.69	5.96	7.14	*	*	*10.38	5.97	5.27	6.78
Tennessee	4.81	5.85	6.56	*6.62	*7.69	*7.88	7.27	6.84	8.40
Alabama	5.64	4.99	6.51	*	*6.96	*7.60	5.35	7.69	7.94
Mississippi	*5.84	*5.89	5.26	*8.09	*7.52	*6.59	6.37	7.96	6.00
West South Central[4]	6.23	6.43	6.61	5.79	5.71	6.20	6.87	7.04	7.50
Arkansas	4.90	5.93	6.34	*6.36	*7.68	*5.97	7.86	7.81	7.40
Louisiana	5.84	7.35	6.04	7.37	*5.76	8.02	5.86	6.45	8.37
Oklahoma[4]	- - -	6.14	6.13	5.48	5.56	6.07	6.92	6.19	7.02
Texas	6.24	6.43	6.63	7.10	6.00	6.34	6.96	7.16	7.45
Mountain	7.15	7.15	7.22	6.15	6.30	6.72	7.45	8.03	8.57
Montana	8.50	7.76	7.69	5.34	6.07	7.43	*	*8.07	*8.97
Idaho	5.72	6.21	6.95	*6.16	6.53	7.07	*5.82	*6.86	*5.97
Wyoming	8.19	9.96	8.33	8.53	*6.38	7.51	*	*	*
Colorado	8.73	8.55	8.71	9.90	9.14	8.16	9.13	9.36	9.92
New Mexico	7.68	7.62	7.69	6.02	6.16	6.27	7.23	7.46	9.26
Arizona	6.35	6.51	6.52	6.08	6.12	6.57	7.16	7.14	7.54
Utah	7.16	7.27	7.55	5.37	5.75	7.44	6.38	7.01	7.50
Nevada	6.03	5.98	6.26	5.91	7.72	6.23	7.05	8.60	9.17
Pacific	5.24	5.48	5.55	5.80	6.01	6.10	6.41	6.46	6.95
Washington	5.01	5.05	5.53	5.98	5.31	7.09	6.01	5.84	6.12
Oregon	5.36	5.67	5.72	5.87	5.80	5.72	6.30	5.72	6.45
California	5.23	5.48	5.53	6.09	6.88	5.85	6.21	6.32	6.84
Alaska	4.87	5.49	6.48	5.22	5.10	5.73	5.55	6.57	6.43
Hawaii	7.55	6.89	7.08	*7.46	*8.48	*7.37	7.45	7.42	7.95

* Percents preceded by an asterisk are based on fewer than 50 events. Percents not shown are based on fewer than 20 events.
- - - Data not available.
[1]Percents for white and black are substituted for non-Hispanic white and non-Hispanic black for Oklahoma 1990, and New Hampshire 1990–92.
[2]Persons of Hispanic origin may be of any race.
[3]Includes persons of Hispanic origin.
[4]Percents for Hispanic origin exclude data from States not reporting Hispanic origin on the birth certificate for 1 or more years in any 3-year period.

SOURCE: Centers for Disease Control and Prevention, National Center for Health Statistics. National Vital Statistics System.

Table 15 (page 1 of 2). Very low-birthweight live births, according to race of mother, Hispanic origin of mother, geographic division, and State: United States, average annual 1990–92, 1993–95, and 1996–98

[Data are based on the National Vital Statistics System]

Geographic division and State	All races			White, non-Hispanic			Black, non-Hispanic		
	1990–92	1993–95	1996–98	1990–92	1993–95	1996–98	1990–92	1993–95	1996–98
	Percent of live births weighing less than 1,500 grams								
United States[1]	1.29	1.34	1.41	0.94	1.01	1.11	2.96	2.99	3.06
New England[1]	1.11	1.15	1.30	0.89	0.92	1.08	2.90	2.95	3.05
Maine	0.86	1.00	1.05	0.89	1.00	1.06	*	*	*
New Hampshire[1]	0.87	0.83	1.02	0.84	0.81	0.97	*	*	*
Vermont	0.82	0.82	1.08	0.72	0.78	1.04	*	*	*
Massachusetts	1.08	1.15	1.26	0.89	0.94	1.06	2.58	2.79	2.75
Rhode Island	1.16	1.07	1.39	0.95	0.89	1.17	2.79	2.29	2.82
Connecticut	1.36	1.36	1.56	0.92	0.95	1.14	3.40	3.30	3.49
Middle Atlantic	1.43	1.45	1.52	0.93	1.00	1.09	3.25	3.17	3.20
New York	1.46	1.47	1.51	0.87	0.96	1.02	3.14	3.08	3.06
New Jersey	1.41	1.51	1.60	0.97	1.03	1.13	3.11	3.37	3.57
Pennsylvania	1.39	1.37	1.45	0.96	1.03	1.13	3.61	3.17	3.21
East North Central	1.37	1.41	1.46	0.98	1.06	1.15	3.13	3.07	3.08
Ohio	1.34	1.39	1.45	1.03	1.09	1.18	3.00	3.01	2.99
Indiana	1.18	1.28	1.38	0.97	1.11	1.19	2.82	2.68	2.93
Illinois	1.47	1.53	1.55	0.97	1.08	1.18	3.11	3.14	3.14
Michigan	1.50	1.49	1.52	1.01	1.07	1.13	3.38	3.20	3.16
Wisconsin	1.09	1.11	1.21	0.85	0.89	1.00	3.03	2.88	2.93
West North Central	1.06	1.13	1.23	0.87	0.96	1.10	2.80	2.75	2.93
Minnesota	0.93	1.06	1.08	0.75	0.91	1.03	2.60	2.54	2.65
Iowa	0.95	1.01	1.23	0.87	0.94	1.14	2.84	2.72	3.47
Missouri	1.28	1.30	1.35	0.93	1.03	1.06	2.91	2.74	2.93
North Dakota	0.90	0.97	1.11	0.87	0.89	1.10	*	*	*
South Dakota	0.90	0.93	1.06	0.87	0.81	1.00	*	*	*
Nebraska	0.93	1.03	1.27	0.83	0.98	1.22	2.47	2.20	2.88
Kansas	1.12	1.17	1.32	0.98	1.00	1.19	2.67	3.20	3.11
South Atlantic	1.59	1.64	1.72	1.01	1.09	1.19	2.96	3.07	3.14
Delaware	1.60	1.52	1.78	0.99	1.08	1.19	3.47	2.99	3.59
Maryland	1.70	1.80	1.89	0.97	1.09	1.09	3.25	3.35	3.52
District of Columbia	3.55	3.46	3.35	*1.08	*0.73	*1.10	4.25	4.27	4.15
Virginia	1.42	1.48	1.59	0.95	1.02	1.13	2.87	2.93	3.05
West Virginia	1.16	1.25	1.39	1.11	1.21	1.34	2.63	2.15	2.69
North Carolina	1.65	1.78	1.86	1.07	1.22	1.32	3.01	3.26	3.47
South Carolina	1.70	1.79	1.89	1.05	1.16	1.21	2.74	2.87	3.14
Georgia	1.68	1.74	1.75	1.01	1.07	1.15	2.84	3.00	2.98
Florida	1.44	1.45	1.53	1.01	1.04	1.18	2.76	2.81	2.77
East South Central	1.53	1.60	1.74	1.06	1.13	1.28	2.77	2.89	3.07
Kentucky	1.20	1.28	1.46	1.06	1.14	1.33	2.56	2.75	2.86
Tennessee	1.56	1.60	1.67	1.09	1.14	1.25	3.06	3.18	3.22
Alabama	1.63	1.75	1.92	1.06	1.16	1.30	2.73	2.90	3.22
Mississippi	1.76	1.81	1.97	0.97	1.04	1.23	2.60	2.65	2.86
West South Central[1]	1.26	1.34	1.41	0.92	1.03	1.13	2.73	2.83	2.98
Arkansas	1.32	1.49	1.60	0.97	1.20	1.28	2.45	2.48	2.82
Louisiana	1.74	1.89	2.02	0.93	1.07	1.15	2.88	3.04	3.28
Oklahoma[1]	1.08	1.16	1.23	0.95	1.02	1.11	2.26	2.65	2.72
Texas	1.17	1.24	1.30	0.89	0.99	1.10	2.73	2.77	2.84
Mountain	1.01	1.05	1.13	0.93	0.97	1.06	2.68	2.73	2.71
Montana	0.85	0.90	1.06	0.82	0.87	0.97	*	*	*
Idaho	0.85	0.82	0.89	0.86	0.78	0.83	*	*	*
Wyoming	0.83	1.16	1.14	0.78	1.12	1.10	*	*	*
Colorado	1.13	1.19	1.32	0.99	1.06	1.23	2.99	3.04	2.69
New Mexico	0.97	1.05	1.07	0.95	1.14	1.17	*2.71	*1.74	*2.40
Arizona	1.09	1.09	1.13	1.02	1.01	1.07	2.56	2.79	2.79
Utah	0.85	0.89	1.03	0.83	0.85	0.97	*	*	*3.43
Nevada	1.06	1.14	1.18	0.94	1.01	1.07	2.49	2.58	2.67
Pacific	0.99	1.03	1.09	0.83	0.87	0.94	2.70	2.69	2.62
Washington	0.83	0.82	1.02	0.76	0.78	0.93	2.64	2.11	2.52
Oregon	0.83	0.88	0.89	0.78	0.84	0.83	1.89	1.94	*1.79
California	1.02	1.07	1.11	0.85	0.90	0.96	2.72	2.73	2.65
Alaska	0.90	0.94	1.14	0.78	0.84	0.97	*2.23	*2.90	*3.04
Hawaii	1.00	1.01	1.17	0.79	0.83	1.03	3.32	3.40	*2.45

See footnotes at end of table.

Table 15 (page 2 of 2). **Very low-birthweight live births, according to race of mother, Hispanic origin of mother, geographic division, and State: United States, average annual 1990–92, 1993–95, and 1996–98**

[Data are based on the National Vital Statistics System]

Geographic division and State	Hispanic[2]			American Indian or Alaska Native[3]			Asian or Pacific Islander[3]		
	1990–92	1993–95	1996–98	1990–92	1993–95	1996–98	1990–92	1993–95	1996–98
	Percent of live births weighing less than 1,500 grams								
United States[4]	1.03	1.08	1.13	1.01	1.09	1.21	0.88	0.90	1.05
New England[4]	1.46	1.49	1.70	*1.39	*1.28	*1.66	0.99	0.90	1.04
Maine	*	*	*	*	*	*	*	*	*
New Hampshire[4]	- - -	*	*	*	*	*	*	*	*
Vermont	*	*	*	*	*	*	*	*	*
Massachusetts	1.41	1.47	1.65	*	*	*	0.88	0.80	0.90
Rhode Island	1.24	1.18	1.38	*	*	*	*	*	*
Connecticut	1.64	1.64	1.90	*	*	*	*1.28	*1.20	1.35
Middle Atlantic	1.44	1.42	1.43	*1.28	*1.14	*1.45	0.85	0.91	1.01
New York	1.45	1.40	1.39	*1.34	*0.96	*1.23	0.86	0.93	1.01
New Jersey	1.30	1.40	1.41	*	*	*	0.84	0.83	1.03
Pennsylvania	1.68	1.65	1.82	*	*	*	0.85	1.02	1.01
East North Central	1.11	1.19	1.19	1.20	1.31	1.29	0.91	1.00	1.09
Ohio	1.44	1.53	1.51	*	*	*	*0.72	0.98	0.90
Indiana	1.03	1.25	1.39	*	*	*	*	*0.84	*1.00
Illinois	1.10	1.13	1.12	*	*	*	0.99	1.12	1.17
Michigan	1.02	1.19	1.18	*1.29	*1.17	*1.65	*0.96	0.92	0.99
Wisconsin	1.11	1.45	1.43	*1.01	*1.23	*0.88	*0.89	*0.84	1.21
West North Central	1.06	0.98	1.13	1.05	1.36	1.34	0.78	0.87	0.98
Minnesota	*0.84	1.15	1.18	*1.10	*1.32	*1.44	*0.74	0.88	0.97
Iowa	*1.41	*1.18	1.16	*	*	*	*	*	*1.37
Missouri	*1.28	*1.15	1.22	*	*	*	*0.99	*0.81	*0.83
North Dakota	*	*	*	*1.02	*1.08	*1.02	*	*	*
South Dakota	*	*	*	1.07	1.58	1.37	*	*	*
Nebraska	*0.84	*0.87	1.01	*	*	*	*	*	*
Kansas	1.07	0.76	1.12	*	*	*	*	*0.85	*0.94
South Atlantic	1.13	1.09	1.17	1.46	1.72	1.92	0.96	0.97	1.11
Delaware	*	*1.39	*1.12	*	*	*	*	*	*
Maryland	1.06	1.03	1.30	*	*	*	1.03	0.91	1.27
District of Columbia	*1.07	*1.06	*1.23	*	*	*	*1.25	*	*
Virginia	0.97	1.08	1.39	*	*	*	0.73	0.96	1.12
West Virginia	*	*	*	*	*	*	*	*	*
North Carolina	0.96	0.83	0.96	1.78	2.19	2.48	*1.01	*0.92	1.12
South Carolina	*1.28	*1.29	*1.20	*	*	*	*	*	*
Georgia	0.93	1.02	0.96	*	*	*	1.09	1.09	0.99
Florida	1.17	1.13	1.20	*	*	*1.11	1.09	0.94	1.07
East South Central	*0.83	0.97	1.09	*	*1.36	*1.50	0.99	0.91	0.96
Kentucky	*	*	*1.38	*	*	*	*	*	*
Tennessee	*	*0.94	*0.90	*	*	*	*1.34	*0.83	*1.15
Alabama	*	*	*1.23	*	*	*	*	*1.45	*
Mississippi	*	*	*	*	*	*	*	*	*
West South Central[4]	0.96	1.06	1.10	0.85	0.80	1.00	0.86	0.88	0.98
Arkansas	*	*1.27	1.14	*.	*	*	*	*	*
Louisiana	*0.91	*1.15	*1.04	*	*	*	*	*0.83	*1.10
Oklahoma[4]	- - -	0.92	0.94	0.75	0.80	0.90	*	*0.88	*
Texas	0.96	1.06	1.10	*1.17	*0.92	*1.50	0.88	0.86	1.00
Mountain	1.03	1.07	1.12	0.93	0.92	1.07	1.00	1.03	1.15
Montana	*	*	*	*0.89	*0.75	1.36	*	*	*
Idaho	*0.66	0.92	1.13	*	*	*	*	*	*
Wyoming	*	*1.34	*1.22	*	*	*	*	*	*
Colorado	1.13	1.15	1.32	*1.28	0.77	0.81	*1.34	1.19	1.11
New Mexico	0.99	1.04	1.02	0.71	0.77	0.81	*	*	*
Arizona	1.07	1.07	1.09	1.00	0.92	1.07	*1.06	*1.00	*1.00
Utah	0.99	1.10	1.23	*0.97	*1.18	*1.68	*	*0.88	*1.24
Nevada	0.86	0.94	0.95	*	*1.93	*	*	*0.91	1.38
Pacific	0.90	0.97	1.02	0.99	1.08	1.13	0.85	0.86	1.05
Washington	0.82	0.71	0.95	*0.88	1.01	1.30	0.61	0.52	0.94
Oregon	1.12	0.93	1.02	*1.12	*1.09	*	*0.51	*0.97	1.17
California	0.90	0.97	1.02	1.04	1.19	1.06	0.85	0.86	1.02
Alaska	*	*	*1.84	0.99	0.93	1.20	*	*	*
Hawaii	1.17	1.12	0.93	*	*	*	0.97	0.96	1.20

* Percents preceded by an asterisk are based on fewer than 50 events. Percents not shown are based on fewer than 20 events.
- - - Data not available.
[1]Percents for white and black are substituted for non-Hispanic white and non-Hispanic black for Oklahoma 1990, and New Hampshire 1990–92.
[2]Persons of Hispanic origin may be of any race.
[3]Includes persons of Hispanic origin.
[4]Percents for Hispanic origin exclude data from States not reporting Hispanic origin on the birth certificate for 1 or more years in any 3-year period.

SOURCE: Centers for Disease Control and Prevention, National Center for Health Statistics. National Vital Statistics System.

Table 16. Legal abortion ratios, according to selected patient characteristics: United States, selected years 1973–97

[Data are based on reporting by State health departments and by hospitals and other medical facilities]

Characteristic	1973	1975	1980	1985	1990	1991	1992	1993	1994	1995	1996	1997
	Abortions per 100 live births[1]											
Total	19.6	27.2	35.9	35.4	34.5	33.9	33.5	33.4	32.1	31.1	31.4	30.5
Age												
Under 15 years	123.7	119.3	139.7	137.6	84.4	76.7	79.0	74.4	70.4	66.7	72.3	72.9
15–19 years.	53.9	54.2	71.4	68.8	51.5	46.2	44.0	44.0	41.5	39.9	41.5	40.7
20–24 years.	29.4	28.9	39.5	38.6	37.7	37.8	37.6	38.4	36.4	34.9	35.5	34.4
25–29 years.	20.7	19.2	23.7	21.7	22.0	22.1	22.2	22.7	22.2	22.1	22.7	22.3
30–34 years.	28.0	25.0	23.7	19.9	19.1	18.7	18.3	18.0	17.2	16.5	16.5	16.0
35–39 years.	45.1	42.2	41.0	33.6	27.3	26.2	25.6	24.8	23.4	22.4	22.0	20.8
40 years and over	68.4	66.8	80.7	62.3	50.1	46.9	45.4	43.0	41.2	38.7	37.6	35.0
Race												
White[2].	32.6	27.7	33.2	27.7	25.8	24.6	23.6	23.1	21.7	20.4	20.2	19.3
Black[3]	42.0	47.6	54.3	47.2	52.1	50.2	51.8	55.2	53.8	53.4	55.5	54.3
Hispanic origin[4]												
Hispanic	- - -	- - -	- - -	- - -	- - -	30.0	30.7	28.9	27.8	26.5	28.1	26.8
Non-Hispanic.	- - -	- - -	- - -	- - -	- - -	33.2	32.6	30.9	29.0	28.0	28.3	27.2
Marital status												
Married	7.6	9.6	10.5	8.0	8.9	8.9	8.4	8.4	7.9	7.6	7.8	7.3
Unmarried	139.8	161.0	147.6	117.4	87.9	81.5	79.0	78.9	68.9	65.0	65.5	65.7
Previous live births[5]												
0.	43.7	38.4	45.7	45.1	35.8	34.8	32.7	32.4	30.9	28.6	28.7	26.8
1.	23.5	22.0	20.2	21.6	23.0	23.2	22.9	23.1	22.3	22.1	22.3	22.0
2.	36.8	36.8	29.5	29.9	31.7	31.9	31.9	32.2	30.9	30.9	31.1	30.8
3.	46.9	47.7	29.8	18.2	30.2	31.0	30.8	31.5	30.8	31.0	31.5	31.2
4 or more[6].	44.7	43.5	24.3	21.5	27.1	22.6	25.5	23.4	23.3	24.1	24.9	24.7

- - - Data not available.

[1]For calculation of ratios according to each characteristic, abortions with the characteristic unknown have been distributed in proportion to abortions with the characteristic known.

[2]For 1989 and later years, white race includes women of Hispanic ethnicity.

[3]Before 1989 black race includes races other than white.

[4]Includes data for 20–22 States, the District of Columbia, and New York City in 1991–96, and 26 States, the District of Columbia, and New York City in 1997. States with large Hispanic populations that are not included are California, Florida, and Illinois.

[5]For 1973–75 data indicate number of living children.

[6]For 1975 data refer to four previous live births, not four or more. For five or more previous live births, the ratio is 47.3.

NOTES: For each year since 1969 the Centers for Disease Control and Prevention has compiled total abortion data from 50 States, the District of Columbia (DC), and New York City (NYC). The number of States reporting each characteristic varies from year to year. For 1991–97, the number of areas reporting each characteristic was as follows: age, 41–45 States, DC, and NYC; race, 34–38 States, DC, and NYC; marital status, 32–38 States, DC, and NYC; previous live births, 36–39 States, DC, and NYC. Some data for 1996 have been revised and differ from the previous edition of *Health, United States*. Data for additional years are available (see Appendix III).

SOURCES: Centers for Disease Control and Prevention: Abortion Surveillance, 1973, 1975, 1979–80. Public Health Service, DHHS, Atlanta, Ga., May 1975, April 1977, May 1983; CDC Surveillance Summaries. Abortion Surveillance, United States, 1982–83, Vol. 36, No. 1SS, Public Health Service, DHHS, Atlanta, Ga., Feb. 1987; 1984 and 1985, Vol. 38, No. SS–2, Sept. 1989; 1986 and 1987, Vol. 39, No. SS–2, June 1990; 1988, Vol. 40, No. SS–2, July 1991; 1989, Vol. 41, No. SS–5, Sept. 1992; 1990, Vol. 42, No. SS–6, Dec. 1993; 1991, Vol. 44, No. SS–2, May 1995; 1992, Vol. 45, No. SS–3, May 1996; 1993 and 1994, Vol. 46, No. SS–4, Aug. 1997; 1995, Vol. 47, No. SS–2, July 1998; 1996, Vol. 48, No. SS–4, July 1999; 1997, in press, 2000.

Table 17. Legal abortions, according to selected characteristics: United States, selected years 1973–97

[Data are based on reporting by State health departments and by hospitals and other facilities]

Characteristic	1973	1975	1980	1985	1990	1991	1992	1993	1994	1995	1996	1997
				Number of legal abortions reported in thousands								
Centers for Disease Control and Prevention	616	855	1,298	1,329	1,430	1,389	1,359	1,330	1,267	1,211	1,222	1,185
Alan Guttmacher Institute[1]	745	1,034	1,554	1,589	1,609	1,557	1,529	1,500	1,431	1,364	1,366	- - -
						Percent distribution[2]						
Total	100.0	100.0	100.0	100.0	100.0	100.0	100.0	100.0	100.0	100.0	100.0	100.0
Period of gestation[3]												
Under 9 weeks	36.1	44.6	51.7	50.3	51.6	52.3	52.1	52.3	53.7	54.0	54.6	55.5
Under 7 weeks	- - -	- - -	- - -	- - -	- - -	- - -	14.3	14.7	15.7	15.7	16.4	17.7
7 weeks	- - -	- - -	- - -	- - -	- - -	- - -	15.6	16.2	16.5	17.1	17.4	18.1
8 weeks	- - -	- - -	- - -	- - -	- - -	- - -	22.2	21.6	21.6	21.2	20.9	19.6
9–10 weeks	29.4	28.4	26.2	26.6	25.3	25.1	24.2	24.4	23.5	23.1	22.6	21.9
11–12 weeks	17.9	14.9	12.2	12.5	11.7	11.5	12.0	11.6	10.9	10.9	11.0	10.7
13–15 weeks	6.9	5.0	5.1	5.9	6.4	6.1	6.0	6.3	6.3	6.3	6.0	6.2
16–20 weeks	8.0	6.1	3.9	3.9	4.0	3.9	4.2	4.1	4.3	4.3	4.3	4.3
21 weeks and over	1.7	1.0	0.9	0.8	1.0	1.1	1.5	1.3	1.3	1.4	1.5	1.4
Type of procedure												
Curettage	88.4	90.9	95.5	97.5	98.8	98.9	98.9	99.0	99.1	98.9	98.8	97.7
Intrauterine instillation	10.4	6.2	3.1	1.7	0.8	0.7	0.7	0.6	0.5	0.5	0.4	0.4
Other[4]	1.2	2.8	1.4	0.8	0.4	0.4	0.4	0.4	0.4	0.6	0.8	1.9
Location of facility												
In State of residence	74.8	89.2	92.6	92.4	91.8	91.6	92.0	91.4	91.5	91.7	91.9	92.0
Out of State of residence	25.2	10.8	7.4	7.6	8.2	8.4	8.0	8.6	8.5	8.3	8.1	8.0
Previous induced abortions												
0	- - -	81.9	67.6	60.1	57.1	56.1	55.1	54.9	54.8	55.1	54.7	50.8
1	- - -	14.9	23.5	25.7	26.9	27.2	27.4	27.3	27.2	26.9	26.9	29.1
2	- - -	2.5	6.6	9.8	10.1	10.6	11.0	11.0	11.1	10.9	11.2	12.3
3 or more	- - -	0.7	2.3	4.4	5.9	6.1	6.5	6.7	7.0	7.1	7.2	7.8

- - - Data not available.

[1]No survey was conducted in 1983, 1986, 1989, 1990, 1993, or 1994; data for these years are estimated.

[2]Excludes cases for which selected characteristic is unknown.

[3]Percentages for under 7, 7, and 8 weeks may not add to percentage under 9 weeks because some States do not report abortions for detailed gestational age subgroups under 9 weeks.

[4]Includes hysterotomy, hysterectomy, and medical (nonsurgical) procedures.

NOTES: For a discussion of the differences in reported legal abortions between the Centers for Disease Control and Prevention and the Alan Guttmacher Institute, see Appendix I. For each year since 1969 the Centers for Disease Control and Prevention has compiled total abortion data from 50 States, the District of Columbia (DC), and New York City (NYC). The number of States reporting each characteristic varies from year to year. For 1997, the number of areas included in the percentages for each characteristic was as follows: gestational age, 38 States, DC, and NYC; detailed gestational age under 9 weeks, 36 States and NYC; type of procedure, 39 States, DC, and NYC; residence, 43 States, DC, and NYC; previous induced abortions, 37 States and NYC. Data for additional years are available (see Appendix III).

SOURCES: Centers for Disease Control and Prevention: Abortion Surveillance, 1973, 1975, 1979–80. Public Health Service, DHHS, Atlanta, Ga., May 1975, April 1977, May 1983; CDC Surveillance Summaries. Abortion Surveillance, United States, 1982–83, Vol. 36, No. 1SS, Public Health Service, DHHS, Atlanta, Ga., Feb. 1987; 1984 and 1985, Vol. 38, No. SS–2, Sept. 1989; 1986 and 1987, Vol. 39, No. SS–2, June 1990; 1988, Vol. 40, No. SS–2, July 1991; 1989, Vol. 41, No. SS–5, Sept. 1992; 1990, Vol. 42, No. SS–6, Dec. 1993; 1991, Vol. 44, No. SS–2, May 1995; 1992, Vol. 45, No. SS–3, May 1996; 1993 and 1994, Vol. 46, No. SS–4, Aug. 1997; 1995, Vol. 47, No. SS–2, July 1998; 1996, Vol. 48, No. SS–4, July 1999; 1997, in press, 2000; Henshaw, S. K.: Abortion incidence and services in the United States, 1995–1996. Fam. Plann. Perspect. 30(6), Nov.–Dec. 1998.

Table 18 (page 1 of 2). Methods of contraception for women 15–44 years of age, according to race, Hispanic origin, and age: United States, 1982, 1988, and 1995

[Data are based on household interviews of samples of women in the childbearing ages]

Race, Hispanic origin, year, and method of contraception	Age in years				
	15–44	15–19	20–24	25–34	35–44
	Number of women in thousands				
All women:					
1982	54,099	9,521	10,629	19,644	14,305
1988	57,900	9,179	9,413	21,726	17,582
1995	60,201	8,961	9,041	20,758	21,440
White, non-Hispanic:					
1982	41,279	7,010	8,081	14,945	11,243
1988	42,575	6,531	6,630	15,929	13,486
1995	42,522	5,962	6,062	14,565	15,933
Black, non-Hispanic:					
1982	6,825	1,383	1,456	2,392	1,593
1988	7,408	1,362	1,322	2,760	1,965
1995	8,210	1,392	1,328	2,801	2,689
Hispanic:					
1982	4,393	886	811	1,677	1,018
1988	5,557	999	1,003	2,104	1,451
1995	6,702	1,150	1,163	2,450	1,940
All methods	Percent of women using contraception				
All women:					
1982	55.7	24.2	55.8	66.7	61.6
1988	60.3	32.1	59.0	66.3	68.3
1995	64.2	29.8	63.5	71.1	72.3
White, non-Hispanic:					
1982	57.3	23.6	58.7	67.8	63.5
1988	62.9	34.0	62.6	67.7	71.5
1995	66.1	30.5	65.3	72.9	73.6
Black, non-Hispanic:					
1982	51.6	29.8	52.2	63.5	52.0
1988	56.8	35.7	61.8	63.5	58.7
1995	62.1	34.8	67.9	66.8	68.5
Hispanic:					
1982	50.6	*	*36.8	67.2	59.0
1988	50.4	*18.3	40.8	67.4	54.3
1995	59.0	26.1	50.6	69.2	70.8
Female sterilization	Percent of contracepting women				
1982	23.2	0.0	*4.5	22.1	43.5
1988	27.5	*	*4.6	25.0	47.6
1995	27.8	*	4.0	23.8	45.0
Male sterilization					
1982	10.9	*·	*3.6	10.1	19.9
1988	11.7	*	*	10.2	20.8
1995	10.9	–	*	7.8	19.4
Implant[1]					
1982	...	...	...	...	...
1988	...	...	...	...	...
1995	1.3	*	3.7	1.3	*
Injectable[1]					
1982	...	...	...	...	...
1988	...	...	...	...	...
1995	3.0	9.7	6.1	2.8	*0.8
Birth control pill					
1982	28.0	63.9	55.1	25.7	*3.7
1988	30.7	58.8	68.2	32.6	4.3
1995	26.9	43.8	52.1	33.3	8.7
Intrauterine device					
1982	7.1	*	*4.2	9.7	6.9
1988	2.0	0.0	*	2.1	3.1
1995	0.8	–	*	*0.8	*1.1

See footnotes at end of table.

Table 18 (page 2 of 2). Methods of contraception for women 15–44 years of age, according to race, Hispanic origin, and age: United States, 1982, 1988, and 1995

[Data are based on household interviews of samples of women in the childbearing ages]

Race, Hispanic origin, year, and method of contraception	Age in years				
	15–44	15–19	20–24	25–34	35–44
Diaphragm					
1982	8.1	*6.0	10.2	10.3	4.0
1988	5.7	*	*3.7	7.3	6.0
1995	1.9	*	*	1.7	2.8
Condom					
1982	12.0	20.8	10.7	11.4	11.3
1988	14.6	32.8	14.5	13.7	11.2
1995	20.4	36.7	26.4	21.1	14.7

Method of contraception and year	Non-Hispanic		Hispanic
	White	Black	
Female sterilization	Percent of contracepting women		
1982	23.0	21.9	30.0
1988	25.6	37.8	31.7
1995	24.6	40.1	36.6
Male sterilization			
1982	*	13.0	*1.5
1988	14.3	*0.9	*
1995	13.6	*1.7	4.0
Implant[1]			
1982	...	...	...
1988	...	...	...
1995	1.0	*2.3	*2.0
Injectable[1]			
1982	...	...	...
1988	...	...	...
1995	2.4	5.3	4.7
Birth control pill			
1982	30.2	26.8	37.8
1988	29.5	38.1	33.4
1995	28.5	23.8	23.0
Intrauterine device			
1982	19.2	5.8	9.3
1988	1.5	3.2	*5.0
1995	0.7	*	*1.5
Diaphragm			
1982	*	9.2	*3.2
1988	6.6	*2.0	*
1995	2.3	*	*
Condom			
1982	*6.9	13.1	6.3
1988	15.2	10.1	13.6
1995	19.7	20.2	20.5

0.0 Quantity more than zero but less than 0.05.
– Quantity zero.
* Estimates with relative standard error of 20–30 percent are preceded by an asterisk and may have low reliability; those with relative standard error greater than 30 percent are considered unreliable and are not shown.
. . . Data not applicable.
[1]Data collected in 1995 survey only.

NOTES: Method of contraception used in the month of interview. If multiple methods were reported, only the most effective method is shown. Methods are listed in the table in order of effectiveness.

SOURCE: Centers for Disease Control and Prevention, National Center for Health Statistics. National Survey of Family Growth.

Table 19. Breastfeeding by mothers 15–44 years of age by year of baby's birth, according to selected characteristics of mother: United States, average annual 1972–74 to 1993–94

[Data are based on household interviews of samples of women in the childbearing ages]

Selected characteristics of mother	1972–74	1975–77	1978–80	1981–83	1984–86	1987–89	1990–92	1993–94
	Percent of babies breastfed							
Total	30.1	36.7	47.5	58.1	54.5	52.3	54.2	58.1
Race and Hispanic origin[1]								
White, non-Hispanic	32.5	38.9	53.2	64.3	59.7	58.3	59.1	61.2
Black, non-Hispanic	12.5	16.8	19.6	26.0	22.9	21.0	22.9	27.5
Hispanic	33.1	42.9	46.3	52.8	58.9	51.3	58.8	67.4
Education[2]								
No high school diploma or GED[3]	14.0	19.4	27.6	31.4	36.8	30.0	38.6	43.0
High school diploma or GED[3]	25.0	33.6	40.2	54.3	46.7	46.6	46.0	51.2
Some college, no bachelor's degree	35.2	43.5	63.2	66.7	66.1	57.8	60.7	65.9
Bachelor's degree or higher	65.5	66.9	71.3	83.2	75.3	79.2	80.8	80.6
Geographic region								
Northeast	29.9	34.7	49.3	68.2	55.3	49.9	54.0	56.7
Midwest	22.3	30.9	34.4	46.0	50.9	50.4	51.6	49.7
South	30.6	33.1	49.5	57.9	45.3	42.5	43.6	49.7
West	47.1	54.5	66.6	69.9	70.0	69.1	70.5	79.3
Age at baby's birth								
Under 20 years	17.0	22.1	31.4	31.0	30.6	26.2	35.2	45.3
20–24 years	28.7	33.5	44.7	50.8	50.2	46.7	44.7	50.9
25–29 years	38.7	45.9	53.6	62.2	59.8	57.1	56.5	55.9
30–44 years	43.1	47.5	55.2	73.1	65.9	65.3	67.5	71.1
	Percent of breastfed babies who were breastfed 3 months or more[4]							
Total	62.3	66.2	64.7	68.3	63.2	61.5	61.0	56.2
Race and Hispanic origin[1]								
White, non-Hispanic	62.1	66.7	67.6	68.1	62.5	62.3	62.6	56.8
Black, non-Hispanic	47.8	60.7	58.5	61.1	56.8	46.9	56.7	45.4
Hispanic	64.7	62.7	46.3	65.6	66.4	64.3	58.2	55.5
Education[2]								
No high school diploma or GED[3]	54.4	54.7	53.7	50.5	59.8	57.3	55.5	44.5
High school diploma or GED[3]	53.7	62.5	59.4	59.6	58.0	58.3	58.2	49.7
Some college, no bachelor's degree	69.5	77.2	63.8	73.3	63.4	60.7	53.8	60.2
Bachelor's degree or higher	69.2	65.3	79.8	80.9	72.2	68.1	73.8	68.1
Geographic region								
Northeast	64.6	68.2	71.2	75.0	64.8	59.7	72.7	58.7
Midwest	44.4	54.3	53.1	64.4	60.4	58.6	63.1	56.7
South	72.6	74.1	67.6	65.0	60.3	55.2	50.8	50.9
West	69.0	70.6	66.8	69.6	66.9	69.9	60.4	59.0
Age at baby's birth								
Under 20 years	50.0	61.0	48.2	49.1	62.5	56.3	31.9	22.6
20–24 years	57.7	59.4	60.0	63.7	51.9	51.6	54.0	50.6
25–29 years	68.3	71.5	65.1	70.8	65.6	58.3	59.7	63.7
30–44 years	79.4	72.8	81.5	72.8	73.2	73.5	71.8	62.3

[1]Persons of Hispanic origin may be of any race.
[2]For women 22–44 years of age. Education is as of year of interview. See NOTES below.
[3]General equivalency diploma.
[4]For mothers interviewed in the first 3 months of 1995, only babies age 3 months and over are included so they would be eligible for breastfeeding for 3 months or more.

NOTES: Data on breastfeeding during 1972–83 are based on responses to questions in the National Survey of Family Growth (NSFG) Cycle 4, conducted in 1988. Data for 1984–94 are based on the NSFG Cycle 5, conducted in 1995. Data are based on all births to mothers 15–44 years of age at interview, including those births that occurred when the mothers were younger than 15 years of age.

SOURCE: Centers for Disease Control and Prevention, National Center for Health Statistics, Division of Vital Statistics. National Survey of Family Growth, Cycle 4 1988, Cycle 5 1995.

Table 20. Infant, neonatal, and postneonatal mortality rates, according to detailed race of mother and Hispanic origin of mother: United States, selected birth cohorts 1983–97

[Data are based on National Linked Birth/Infant Death Data Sets]

Race of mother and Hispanic origin of mother	Birth cohort								
	1983	1990	1995[1]	1996[1]	1997	1983–85	1986–88	1989–91	1995–97[1]
	Infant[2] deaths per 1,000 live births								
All mothers	10.9	8.9	7.6	7.3	7.2	10.6	9.8	9.0	7.4
White	9.3	7.3	6.3	6.1	6.0	9.0	8.2	7.4	6.1
Black	19.2	16.9	14.6	14.1	13.7	18.7	17.9	17.1	14.1
American Indian or Alaska Native	15.2	13.1	9.0	10.0	8.7	13.9	13.2	12.6	9.2
Asian or Pacific Islander	8.3	6.6	5.3	5.2	5.0	8.3	7.3	6.6	5.1
Chinese	9.5	4.3	3.8	3.2	3.1	7.4	5.8	5.1	3.3
Japanese	*5.6	*5.5	*5.3	*4.2	*5.3	6.0	6.9	5.3	4.9
Filipino	8.4	6.0	5.6	5.8	5.8	8.2	6.9	6.4	5.7
Hawaiian and part Hawaiian	11.2	*8.0	*6.6	*5.6	9.0	11.3	11.1	9.0	7.0
Other Asian or Pacific Islander	8.1	7.4	5.5	5.7	5.0	8.6	7.6	7.0	5.4
Hispanic origin[3],[4]	9.5	7.5	6.3	6.1	6.0	9.2	8.3	7.5	6.1
Mexican	9.1	7.2	6.0	5.8	5.8	8.8	7.9	7.2	5.9
Puerto Rican	12.9	9.9	8.9	8.6	7.9	12.3	11.1	10.4	8.5
Cuban	7.5	7.2	5.3	5.1	5.5	8.0	7.3	6.2	5.3
Central and South American	8.5	6.8	5.5	5.0	5.5	8.2	7.5	6.6	5.3
Other and unknown Hispanic	10.6	8.0	7.4	7.7	6.2	9.8	9.0	8.2	7.1
White, non-Hispanic[4]	9.2	7.2	6.3	6.0	6.0	8.8	8.1	7.3	6.1
Black, non-Hispanic[4]	19.1	16.9	14.7	14.2	13.7	18.5	17.9	17.2	14.2
	Neonatal[2] deaths per 1,000 live births								
All mothers	7.1	5.7	4.9	4.8	4.8	6.9	6.3	5.7	4.8
White	6.1	4.6	4.1	4.0	4.0	5.9	5.2	4.7	4.0
Black	12.5	11.1	9.6	9.4	9.2	12.2	11.7	11.1	9.4
American Indian or Alaska Native	7.5	6.1	3.9	4.7	4.5	6.7	5.9	5.9	4.4
Asian or Pacific Islander	5.2	3.9	3.4	3.3	3.2	5.2	4.5	3.9	3.3
Chinese	5.5	2.3	2.3	1.9	2.1	4.3	3.3	2.7	2.1
Japanese	*3.7	*3.5	*3.3	*2.2	*3.0	3.4	4.4	3.0	2.8
Filipino	5.6	3.5	3.4	4.1	3.6	5.3	4.5	4.0	3.7
Hawaiian and part Hawaiian	*7.0	*4.3	*4.0	*	*6.3	7.4	7.1	4.8	4.5
Other Asian or Pacific Islander	5.0	4.4	3.7	3.7	3.3	5.5	4.7	4.2	3.5
Hispanic origin[3],[4]	6.2	4.8	4.1	4.0	4.0	6.0	5.3	4.8	4.0
Mexican	5.9	4.5	3.9	3.8	3.8	5.7	5.0	4.5	3.8
Puerto Rican	8.7	6.9	6.1	5.6	5.4	8.3	7.2	7.0	5.7
Cuban	*5.0	5.3	*3.6	*3.6	4.0	5.9	5.3	4.6	3.7
Central and South American	5.8	4.4	3.7	3.4	3.9	5.7	4.9	4.4	3.7
Other and unknown Hispanic	6.4	5.0	4.8	5.3	3.7	6.1	5.8	5.2	4.6
White, non-Hispanic[4]	5.9	4.5	4.0	3.9	3.9	5.7	5.1	4.6	4.0
Black, non-Hispanic[4]	12.0	11.0	9.6	9.4	9.2	11.8	11.4	11.1	9.4
	Postneonatal[2] deaths per 1,000 live births								
All mothers	3.8	3.2	2.6	2.5	2.4	3.7	3.5	3.3	2.5
White	3.2	2.7	2.2	2.1	2.1	3.1	3.0	2.7	2.1
Black	6.7	5.9	5.0	4.8	4.5	6.4	6.2	6.0	4.7
American Indian or Alaska Native	7.7	7.0	5.1	5.3	4.2	7.2	7.3	6.7	4.8
Asian or Pacific Islander	3.1	2.7	1.9	1.9	1.8	3.1	2.8	2.6	1.8
Chinese	4.0	*2.0	*1.5	*1.2	*1.0	3.1	2.5	2.4	1.2
Japanese	*	*	*	*	*2.2	2.6	2.5	2.2	2.1
Filipino	*2.8	2.5	2.2	1.8	2.3	2.9	2.4	2.3	2.1
Hawaiian and part Hawaiian	*4.2	*3.8	*	*	*	3.9	4.0	4.1	*2.5
Other Asian or Pacific Islander	3.0	3.0	1.9	2.0	1.7	3.1	2.9	2.8	1.9
Hispanic origin[3],[4]	3.3	2.7	2.1	2.1	2.0	3.2	3.0	2.7	2.1
Mexican	3.2	2.7	2.1	2.1	2.0	3.2	2.9	2.7	2.1
Puerto Rican	4.2	3.0	2.8	3.0	2.5	4.0	3.9	3.4	2.8
Cuban	*2.5	*1.9	*1.7	*	*	2.2	2.0	1.6	1.5
Central and South American	2.6	2.4	1.9	1.6	1.5	2.5	2.6	2.2	1.7
Other and unknown Hispanic	4.2	3.0	2.6	2.5	2.5	3.7	3.2	3.0	2.5
White, non-Hispanic[4]	3.2	2.7	2.2	2.1	2.1	3.1	3.0	2.7	2.2
Black, non-Hispanic[4]	7.0	5.9	5.0	·4.8	4.5	6.7	6.5	6.1	4.8

* Rates preceded by an asterisk are based on fewer than 50 events. Rates not shown are based on fewer than 20 events.

[1]Rates based on a period file using weighted data. Data for 1995–97 not strictly comparable with unweighted birth cohort data for earlier years (see Appendix I, National Vital Statistics System). The 1995–97 weighted mortality rates shown in this table are less than 1 percent to 5 percent higher than unweighted rates for 1995–97.

[2]Infant (under 1 year of age), neonatal (under 28 days), and postneonatal (28–365 days).

[3]Persons of Hispanic origin may be of any race.

[4]Data shown only for States with an Hispanic-origin item on their birth certificates. The number of States reporting the item increased from 23 and the District of Columbia (DC) in 1983–87, to 30 and DC in 1988, 47 and DC in 1989, 48 and DC in 1990, 49 and DC in 1991, and 50 and DC in 1995–97 (see Appendix I).

NOTES: The race groups white, black, American Indian or Alaska Native, and Asian or Pacific Islander include persons of Hispanic and non-Hispanic origin. National linked files do not exist for 1992–94 birth cohorts. Data for additional years are available (see Appendix III).

SOURCE: Centers for Disease Control and Prevention, National Center for Health Statistics. National Vital Statistics System.

Table 21. Infant mortality rates for mothers 20 years of age and over, according to educational attainment, detailed race of mother, and Hispanic origin of mother: United States, selected birth cohorts 1983–97

[Data are based on National Linked Birth/Infant Death Data Sets]

Education of mother, race of mother, and Hispanic origin of mother	1983	1990	1995[1]	1996[1]	1997[1]	1983–85	1986–88	1989–91	1995–97[1]
Less than 12 years of education	\multicolumn{9}{c	}{Infant deaths per 1,000 live births}
All mothers	15.0	10.8	8.9	8.5	8.3	14.6	13.8	11.1	8.6
White	12.5	9.0	7.6	7.1	7.3	12.4	11.4	9.2	7.3
Black	23.4	19.5	17.0	16.6	14.4	21.8	21.1	20.3	16.0
American Indian or Alaska Native	14.5	14.3	12.7	11.3	10.1	15.2	16.8	13.8	11.4
Asian or Pacific Islander[2]	9.7	6.6	5.7	6.4	5.3	9.5	8.2	6.9	5.8
Hispanic origin[3,4]	10.9	7.3	6.0	5.6	5.8	10.6	9.9	7.5	5.8
Mexican	8.7	7.0	5.8	5.4	5.6	9.5	8.3	7.1	5.6
Puerto Rican	15.3	10.1	10.6	9.1	8.8	14.1	12.8	11.7	9.5
Cuban	*14.5	*	*	*	*	*10.5	*9.4	*8.2	*6.7
Central and South American	9.8	7.0	5.1	4.7	6.4	8.6	9.2	6.8	5.4
Other and unknown Hispanic	9.2	9.9	7.3	7.9	*5.6	10.1	10.6	10.0	7.0
White, non-Hispanic[4]	12.8	10.9	9.9	9.5	9.5	12.6	11.8	11.0	9.6
Black, non-Hispanic[4]	24.7	19.7	17.3	16.9	14.7	22.6	21.6	20.6	16.3
12 years of education									
All mothers	10.2	8.8	7.8	7.6	7.5	10.0	9.6	8.9	7.6
White	8.7	7.1	6.4	6.3	6.2	8.5	8.0	7.2	6.3
Black	17.8	16.0	14.7	13.8	13.7	17.7	17.1	16.4	14.1
American Indian or Alaska Native	15.5	13.4	7.9	9.3	8.3	13.4	11.6	12.3	8.5
Asian or Pacific Islander[2]	10.0	7.5	5.5	5.9	5.6	9.3	7.9	7.5	5.6
Hispanic origin[3,4]	8.4	7.0	5.9	5.9	5.6	9.1	8.3	6.8	5.8
Mexican	6.9	6.8	5.7	5.6	5.4	7.8	8.2	6.5	5.6
Puerto Rican	9.5	8.5	6.5	7.7	8.5	10.8	10.1	8.6	7.6
Cuban	*6.9	*8.0	*	*7.2	*5.3	8.6	6.6	7.6	5.4
Central and South American	8.7	6.5	6.1	5.3	5.1	8.7	7.4	6.3	5.5
Other and unknown Hispanic	8.8	7.4	6.5	7.6	5.8	8.8	7.7	7.0	6.6
White, non-Hispanic[4]	8.7	7.1	6.5	6.4	6.3	8.3	7.9	7.3	6.4
Black, non-Hispanic[4]	17.8	16.1	14.8	13.9	13.7	17.9	17.4	16.5	14.2
13 years or more of education									
All mothers	8.1	6.4	5.4	5.3	5.2	7.8	7.2	6.4	5.3
White	7.2	5.4	4.7	4.5	4.5	6.9	6.2	5.5	4.5
Black	15.3	13.7	11.9	11.7	11.4	15.3	14.9	13.7	11.6
American Indian or Alaska Native	12.5	6.8	5.9	7.1	6.9	10.4	8.4	8.1	6.6
Asian or Pacific Islander[2]	6.6	5.1	4.4	4.0	3.9	6.7	5.9	5.1	4.1
Hispanic origin[3,4]	9.0	5.7	5.0	5.1	4.9	7.4	7.0	5.8	5.0
Mexican	*8.3	5.5	5.2	5.1	5.0	7.6	6.4	5.7	5.1
Puerto Rican	10.9	7.3	6.3	6.9	6.0	8.1	6.9	7.8	6.4
Cuban	*	*5.3	*5.3	*3.6	*4.0	5.5	5.9	4.2	4.3
Central and South American	*7.1	5.6	3.7	4.0	4.2	7.2	7.6	5.4	4.0
Other and unknown Hispanic	11.6	5.4	5.2	5.9	4.8	7.9	7.5	5.6	5.3
White, non-Hispanic[4]	7.0	5.4	4.6	4.5	4.4	6.8	6.1	5.4	4.5
Black, non-Hispanic[4]	14.8	13.7	12.0	11.7	11.4	14.7	14.9	13.8	11.7

* Rates preceded by an asterisk are based on fewer than 50 events. Rates not shown are based on fewer than 20 events.

[1] Rates based on a period file using weighted data. Data for 1995–97 not strictly comparable with unweighted birth cohort data for earlier years (see Appendix I, National Vital Statistics System). The 1995–97 weighted mortality rates shown in this table are less than 1 percent to 4 percent higher than unweighted rates for 1995–97.

[2] The States not reporting maternal education on the birth certificate accounted for 49–51 percent of the Asian or Pacific Islander births in the United States in 1983–87, 59 percent in 1988, and 12 percent in 1989–91. Starting in 1992 maternal education was reported by all 50 States and DC.

[3] Persons of Hispanic origin may be of any race.

[4] Data shown only for States with an Hispanic-origin item and education of mother on their birth certificates. The number of States reporting both items increased from 21 and the District of Columbia (DC) in 1983–87, to 26 and DC in 1988, 45 and DC in 1989, 47 and DC in 1990–91, and 50 and DC in 1995–97 (see Appendix I, National Vital Statistics System). The Hispanic-reporting States that did not report maternal education on the birth certificate during 1983–88 together accounted for 28–85 percent of the births in each Hispanic subgroup (except Cuban, 11–16 percent and Puerto Rican, 6–7 percent in 1983–87); and in 1989–91 accounted for 27–39 percent of Central and South American and Puerto Rican births and 2–9 percent of births in other Hispanic subgroups.

NOTES: Data for all mothers and by race based on data for 47 States and the District of Columbia (DC) in 1983–87, 46 States and DC in 1988, 48 States and DC in 1989–91, and 50 and DC in 1995–97. Excludes data for California and Texas (1983–88), Washington (1983–91), and New York (1988–91), which did not require the reporting of maternal education on the birth certificate (see Appendix I). The race groups, white, black, American Indian or Alaska Native, and Asian or Pacific Islander, include persons of Hispanic and non-Hispanic origin. Persons of Hispanic origin may be of any race. National linked files do not exist for 1992–94 birth cohorts. Data for additional years are available (see Appendix III).

SOURCE: Centers for Disease Control and Prevention, National Center for Health Statistics. National Vital Statistics System. National Linked Birth/Infant Death Data Sets.

Table 22. Infant mortality rates according to birthweight: United States, selected birth cohorts 1983–97

[Data are based on National Linked Birth/Infant Death Data Sets]

Birthweight	Birth cohort									
	1983	1985	1987	1988	1989	1990	1991	1995[1]	1996[1]	1997[1]
	Infant deaths per 1,000 live births[2]									
All birthweights	10.9	10.4	9.8	9.6	9.5	8.9	8.6	7.6	7.3	7.2
Less than 2,500 grams.	95.9	93.9	86.5	84.2	83.1	78.1	74.3	65.3	63.6	62.4
Less than 1,500 grams	400.6	387.7	358.0	348.7	343.1	317.6	305.4	270.7	261.5	255.0
Less than 500 grams	890.3	895.9	890.4	878.4	905.6	898.2	889.9	904.9	890.1	885.2
500–999 grams	584.2	559.2	507.9	502.0	480.4	440.1	422.6	351.0	336.9	324.4
1,000–1,499 grams	162.3	145.4	122.2	121.3	118.5	97.9	91.3	69.6	64.7	61.8
1,500–1,999 grams	58.4	54.0	48.8	48.9	46.0	43.8	40.4	33.5	30.6	30.6
2,000–2,499 grams	22.5	20.9	19.5	18.7	17.9	17.8	17.0	13.7	13.6	12.5
2,500 grams or more	4.7	4.3	4.1	4.0	4.0	3.7	3.6	3.0	2.8	2.7
2,500–2,999 grams	8.8	7.9	7.5	7.6	7.4	6.7	6.7	5.5	5.1	5.0
3,000–3,499 grams	4.4	4.3	4.0	3.9	3.8	3.7	3.5	2.9	2.7	2.6
3,500–3,999 grams	3.2	3.0	2.8	2.8	2.8	2.6	2.5	2.0	1.9	1.9
4,000 grams or more.	3.3	3.2	3.0	2.9	2.6	2.4	2.4	2.0	1.8	1.8
4,000–4,499 grams	2.9	2.9	2.6	2.4	2.3	2.2	2.2	1.8	1.7	1.7
4,500–4,999 grams	3.9	3.8	3.4	3.4	3.1	2.5	3.0	2.2	2.1	2.0
5,000 grams or more[3]	14.4	14.7	15.8	20.7	9.6	9.8	8.2	8.5	6.2	4.2

[1]Rates based on a period file using weighted data; not stated birthweight imputed when period of gestation is known and proportionately distributed when period of gestation is unknown. Data for 1995–97 not strictly comparable with unweighted and unimputed birth cohort data for earlier years (see Appendix I, National Vital Statistics System). The 1995, 1996, and 1997 weighted mortality rates with imputed birthweight shown in this table are less than 1 percent to 5 percent higher than unweighted rates with unimputed birthweight for 1995, 1996, and 1997.

[2]For calculation of birthweight-specific infant mortality rates, unknown birthweight has been distributed in proportion to known birthweight separately for live births (denominator) and infant deaths (numerator).

[3]In 1989 a birthweight-gestational age consistency check instituted for the natality file resulted in a decrease in the number of deaths to infants coded with birthweights of 5,000 grams or more and a discontinuity in the mortality trend for infants weighing 5,000 grams or more at birth. Starting with 1989 the rates are believed to be more accurate.

NOTES: National linked files do not exist for 1992–94 birth cohorts. Data for additional years are available (see Appendix III).

SOURCE: Centers for Disease Control and Prevention, National Center for Health Statistics. National Vital Statistics System. National Linked Birth/Infant Death Data Sets.

Table 23. Infant mortality rates, fetal mortality rates, and perinatal mortality rates, according to race: United States, selected years 1950–98

[Data are based on the National Vital Statistics System]

Race and year	Infant[1]	Neonatal[1] Under 28 days	Neonatal[1] Under 7 days	Postneonatal[1]	Fetal mortality rate[2]	Late fetal mortality rate[3]	Perinatal mortality rate[4]
All races		Deaths per 1,000 live births					
1950[5]	29.2	20.5	17.8	8.7	18.4	14.9	32.5
1960[5]	26.0	18.7	16.7	7.3	15.8	12.1	28.6
1970	20.0	15.1	13.6	4.9	14.0	9.5	23.0
1980	12.6	8.5	7.1	4.1	9.1	6.2	13.2
1985	10.6	7.0	5.8	3.7	7.8	4.9	10.7
1990	9.2	5.8	4.8	3.4	7.5	4.3	9.1
1995	7.6	4.9	4.0	2.7	7.0	3.6	7.6
1996	7.3	4.8	3.8	2.5	6.9	3.6	7.4
1997	7.2	4.8	3.8	2.5	6.8	3.5	7.3
1998	7.2	4.8	3.8	2.4	- - -	- - -	- - -
Race of child:[6] White							
1950[5]	26.8	19.4	17.1	7.4	16.6	13.3	30.1
1960[5]	22.9	17.2	15.6	5.7	13.9	10.8	26.2
1970	17.8	13.8	12.5	4.0	12.3	8.6	21.0
1980	11.0	7.5	6.2	3.5	8.1	5.7	11.9
Race of mother:[7] White							
1980	10.9	7.4	6.1	3.5	8.1	5.7	11.8
1985	9.2	6.0	5.0	3.2	6.9	4.5	9.5
1990	7.6	4.8	3.9	2.8	6.4	3.8	7.7
1995	6.3	4.1	3.3	2.2	5.9	3.3	6.5
1996	6.1	4.0	3.2	2.1	5.9	3.3	6.4
1997	6.0	4.0	3.2	2.0	5.8	3.2	6.3
1998	6.0	4.0	3.1	2.0	- - -	- - -	- - -
Race of child:[6] Black							
1950[5]	43.9	27.8	23.0	16.1	32.1	- - -	- - -
1960[5]	44.3	27.8	23.7	16.5	- - -	- - -	- - -
1970	32.6	22.8	20.3	9.9	23.2	- - -	34.5
1980	21.4	14.1	11.9	7.3	14.4	8.9	20.7
Race of mother:[7] Black							
1980	22.2	14.6	12.3	7.6	14.7	9.1	21.3
1985	19.0	12.6	10.8	6.4	12.8	7.2	17.9
1990	18.0	11.6	9.7	6.4	13.3	6.7	16.4
1995	15.1	9.8	8.2	5.3	12.7	5.7	13.8
1996	14.7	9.6	7.8	5.1	12.5	5.5	13.3
1997	14.2	9.4	7.8	4.8	12.5	5.5	13.2
1998	14.3	9.5	7.8	4.8	- - -	- - -	- - -

- - - Data not available.

[1]Infant (under 1 year of age), neonatal (under 28 days), early neonatal (under 7 days), and postneonatal (28 days–11 months).
[2]Number of fetal deaths of 20 weeks or more gestation per 1,000 live births plus fetal deaths.
[3]Number of fetal deaths of 28 weeks or more gestation per 1,000 live births plus late fetal deaths.
[4]Number of late fetal deaths plus infant deaths within 7 days of birth per 1,000 live births plus late fetal deaths.
[5]Includes births and deaths of persons who were not residents of the 50 States and the District of Columbia.
[6]Infant deaths are tabulated by race of decedent; live births and fetal deaths are tabulated by race of child (see Appendix II, Race).
[7]Infant deaths are tabulated by race of decedent; fetal deaths and live births are tabulated by race of mother (see Appendix II, Race).

NOTES: Infant mortality rates in this table are based on infant deaths from the mortality file (numerator) and live births from the natality file (denominator). Inconsistencies in reporting race for the same infant between the birth and death certificate can result in underestimated infant mortality rates for races other than white or black. Infant mortality rates for minority population groups are available from the national linked files of live births and infant deaths and are presented in tables 20–21 and 24–25. Data for additional years are available (see Appendix III).

SOURCES: Centers for Disease Control and Prevention, National Center for Health Statistics. National Vital Statistics System; Vital statistics of the United States, vol II, mortality, part A, for data years 1950–93. Public Health Service. Washington. U.S. Government Printing Office; for 1994–98, data are available on the NCHS Web site at www.cdc.gov/nchs/datawh/statab/unpubd/mortabs.htm; Murphy SL. Deaths: Final data for 1998. National vital statistics reports; vol 48. Hyattsville, Maryland: 2000.

Table 24 (page 1 of 2). Infant mortality rates, according to race, geographic division, and State: United States, average annual 1989–91 and 1995–97

[Data are based on the National Linked Birth/Infant Death Data Sets]

Geographic division and State	All races		White, non-Hispanic		Black, non-Hispanic	
	1989–91	1995–97[1]	1989–91	1995–97[1]	1989–91	1995–97[1]
	Infant[2] deaths per 1,000 live births					
United States	9.0	7.4	7.3	6.1	17.2	14.2
New England[3]	7.3	5.7	6.2	4.8	15.1	11.5
Maine	6.6	5.3	6.2	5.1	*	*
New Hampshire[3]	7.1	4.8	7.2	4.6	*	*
Vermont	6.6	6.3	6.3	6.1	*	
Massachusetts	7.0	5.1	5.9	4.3	14.2	10.6
Rhode Island	8.7	6.5	7.5	5.0	*13.6	*
Connecticut	7.9	6.9	5.9	5.3	17.0	13.6
Middle Atlantic	9.2	7.2	6.6	5.3	18.5	14.3
New York	9.5	7.1	6.3	4.8	18.4	13.5
New Jersey	8.4	6.6	6.1	4.5	17.8	13.8
Pennsylvania	9.2	7.7	7.2	6.2	19.1	16.6
East North Central	9.8	8.2	7.7	6.6	19.1	16.5
Ohio	9.0	8.1	7.7	6.8	16.2	15.3
Indiana	9.4	8.4	8.4	7.5	17.3	15.6
Illinois	10.7	8.8	7.6	6.5	20.5	17.5
Michigan	10.5	8.2	7.7	6.3	20.7	16.3
Wisconsin	8.4	7.0	7.4	5.9	17.0	16.3
West North Central	8.5	7.1	7.4	6.3	17.5	14.7
Minnesota	7.3	6.2	6.4	5.6	18.5	13.4
Iowa	8.2	7.1	7.8	6.7	15.8	*16.5
Missouri	9.7	7.5	8.0	6.2	18.0	14.5
North Dakota	8.0	6.3	7.3	5.8	*	*
South Dakota	9.5	7.4	7.5	6.0	*	
Nebraska	8.1	7.9	7.2	7.3	18.3	*13.5
Kansas	8.5	7.5	7.8	6.7	15.4	17.0
South Atlantic	10.4	8.4	7.6	6.3	17.2	14.2
Delaware	11.2	7.7	8.2	6.2	20.1	12.9
Maryland	9.1	8.7	6.3	5.7	15.0	14.9
District of Columbia	20.3	14.9	*8.2	*	23.9	18.5
Virginia	9.9	7.7	7.4	6.0	18.0	13.6
West Virginia	9.1	8.2	8.8	7.9	*15.7	*17.9
North Carolina	10.7	9.2	8.0	7.0	16.9	15.3
South Carolina	11.8	9.2	8.4	6.3	17.2	14.4
Georgia	11.9	9.1	8.4	6.4	17.9	14.4
Florida	9.4	7.4	7.2	6.1	16.2	12.6
East South Central	10.4	9.1	8.1	7.1	16.5	14.7
Kentucky	8.7	7.3	8.1	7.0	14.4	11.2
Tennessee	10.2	8.7	7.8	6.7	18.2	16.1
Alabama	11.4	9.9	8.6	7.6	16.8	14.6
Mississippi	11.5	10.6	7.9	7.3	15.2	14.5
West South Central[3]	8.4	7.2	7.2	6.5	14.2	12.1
Arkansas	9.8	8.9	8.1	7.7	15.2	13.4
Louisiana[3]	10.2	9.4	7.5	6.7	14.3	13.5
Oklahoma[3]	8.0	8.1	7.3	7.5	12.7	14.3
Texas	7.9	6.4	6.9	6.0	14.1	10.6
Mountain	8.4	6.7	7.9	6.3	16.9	12.5
Montana	9.0	6.9	8.0	6.6	*	*
Idaho	8.9	6.6	8.9	6.4	*	*
Wyoming	8.4	6.8	8.0	6.1	*	*
Colorado	8.7	6.7	8.0	6.1	16.7	13.6
New Mexico	8.4	6.3	8.1	6.2	*17.2	*
Arizona	8.8	7.4	8.2	7.1	17.3	14.1
Utah	7.0	5.8	6.8	5.5	*	*
Nevada	8.6	6.2	7.8	6.3	16.9	10.9
Pacific	7.7	6.0	7.0	5.5	15.4	12.7
Washington	8.0	5.8	7.4	5.4	15.1	12.9
Oregon	8.0	5.8	7.4	5.6	21.3	*11.4
California	7.6	6.0	6.9	5.5	15.4	12.8
Alaska	9.2	7.4	7.2	5.8	*	*
Hawaii	7.0	6.0	5.5	5.2	*13.6	*

See footnotes at end of table.

Table 24 (page 2 of 2). Infant mortality rates, according to race, geographic division, and State: United States, average annual 1989–91 and 1995–97

[Data are based on the National Linked Birth/Infant Death Data Sets]

Geographic division and State	Hispanic[4]		American Indian or Alaska Native[5]		Asian or Pacific Islander[5]	
	1989–91	1995–97[1]	1989–91	1995–97[1]	1989–91	1995–97[1]
	Infant[2] deaths per 1,000 live births					
United States	7.5	6.1	12.6	9.2	6.6	5.1
New England[6]	8.1	7.8	*	*	5.8	4.3
Maine	*	*	*	*	*	*
New Hampshire[6]	- - -	*	*	*	*	*
Vermont	*	*	*	*	*	*
Massachusetts	8.3	6.7	*	*	5.7	*3.7
Rhode Island	*7.2	*9.7	*	*	*	*
Connecticut	7.9	8.8	*	*	*	*
Middle Atlantic	9.1	6.9	*11.6	*	6.4	4.1
New York	9.4	6.6	*15.2	*	6.4	4.1
New Jersey	7.5	7.0	*	*	5.6	4.0
Pennsylvania	10.9	8.9	*	*	7.8	*4.4
East North Central	8.7	7.4	11.6	10.1	6.1	5.3
Ohio	8.0	7.6	*	*	*4.8	*6.2
Indiana	*7.2	8.1	*	*	*	*8.3
Illinois	9.2	7.2	*	*	6.0	5.6
Michigan	7.9	6.7	*10.7	*9.9	*6.1	*3.9
Wisconsin	*7.3	9.6	*11.9	*8.8	*6.7	*3.7
West North Central	9.3	6.8	17.1	13.9	7.4	6.8
Minnesota	*8.4	*6.0	17.3	16.2	*5.1	7.0
Iowa	*11.9	*7.0	*	*	*	*
Missouri	*9.1	*5.3	*	*	*9.1	*
North Dakota	*	*	*13.8	*10.5	*	*
South Dakota	*	*	19.9	15.0	*	*
Nebraska	*8.8	9.2	*18.2	*	*	*
Kansas	8.7	6.9	*	*	*	*
South Atlantic	7.4	5.7	12.7	11.3	6.8	5.6
Delaware	*	*	*	*	*	*
Maryland	7.2	5.7	*	*	7.5	6.8
District of Columbia	*8.8	*	*	*	*	*
Virginia	7.6	6.6	*	*	6.0	4.8
West Virginia	*	*	*	*	*	*
North Carolina	*7.5	6.5	12.2	12.7	*6.3	*5.7
South Carolina	*	*8.1	*	*	*	*
Georgia	9.0	6.7	*	*	*8.2	*5.3
Florida	7.1	5.1	*	*10.6	*6.2	5.5
East South Central	*5.9	6.7	*	*13.7	*7.7	*5.8
Kentucky	*	*	*	*	*	*
Tennessee	*	*6.4	*	*	*	*
Alabama	*	*8.4	*	*	*	*
Mississippi	*	*	*	*	*	*
West South Central[6]	7.0	5.7	8.4	7.6	6.7	5.1
Arkansas	*	*8.6	*	*	*	*
Louisiana[6]	- - -	*	*	*	*	*7.2
Oklahoma[6]	- - -	*5.5	7.8	8.2	*	*
Texas	7.0	5.7	*	*	6.8	5.0
Mountain	7.9	6.7	11.6	8.5	8.1	6.0
Montana	*	*	16.7	*8.6	*	*
Idaho	*7.2	*6.5	*	*	*	*
Wyoming	*	*	*	*	*	*
Colorado	8.5	6.8	*16.5	*	*7.8	*6.6
New Mexico	7.8	6.2	9.8	7.3	*	*
Arizona	8.0	7.4	11.4	8.6	*8.5	*5.3
Utah	*7.0	6.9	*10.0	*	*10.7	*6.9
Nevada	7.0	4.6	*	*	*	*
Pacific	7.1	5.6	14.6	8.0	6.5	5.3
Washington	7.6	4.9	19.6	*7.0	6.2	4.7
Oregon	8.5	6.5	*15.7	*	*8.4	*4.5
California	7.0	5.6	11.0	7.5	6.4	5.1
Alaska	*	*	15.7	10.7	*	*
Hawaii	10.7	*5.8	*	*	7.1	6.2

* Rates preceded by an asterisk are based on fewer than 50 events. Rates not shown are based on fewer than 20 events.   - - - Data not available.
[1]Rates based on period file using weighted data. Data for 1995–97 not strictly comparable with unweighted birth cohort data for earlier years (see Appendix I).
[2]Under 1 year of age.
[3]Rates for white and black are substituted for non-Hispanic white and non-Hispanic black for Louisiana 1989, Oklahoma 1989–90, and New Hampshire 1989–91.
[4]Persons of Hispanic origin may be of any race.   [5]Includes persons of Hispanic origin.
[6]Rates for Hispanic origin exclude data from States not reporting Hispanic origin on the birth certificate for 1 or more years in a 3-year period.

NOTE: National linked files do not exist for 1992–94 birth cohorts.

SOURCE: Centers for Disease Control and Prevention, National Center for Health Statistics. National Vital Statistics System.

Table 25 (page 1 of 2). Neonatal mortality rates, according to race, geographic division, and State: United States, average annual 1989–91 and 1995–97

[Data are based on the National Linked Birth/Infant Death Data Sets]

Geographic division and State	All races		White, non-Hispanic		Black, non-Hispanic	
	1989–91	1995–97[1]	1989–91	1995–97[1]	1989–91	1995–97[1]
	Neonatal[2] deaths per 1,000 live births					
United States	5.7	4.8	4.6	4.0	11.1	9.4
New England[3]	5.1	4.2	4.2	3.5	11.0	8.4
Maine	4.5	3.7	4.2	3.7	*	*
New Hampshire[3]	4.3	3.4	4.4	3.2	*	*
Vermont	4.1	4.2	3.9	4.0	*	*
Massachusetts	4.9	3.8	4.1	3.2	10.4	7.6
Rhode Island	6.4	5.1	5.3	3.8	*9.8	*
Connecticut	5.7	5.1	4.2	4.0	12.5	10.2
Middle Atlantic	6.3	5.0	4.6	3.7	12.3	9.6
New York	6.5	5.0	4.3	3.3	12.6	9.1
New Jersey	5.8	4.6	4.5	3.3	11.4	9.0
Pennsylvania	6.2	5.4	4.9	4.3	12.5	11.4
East North Central	6.3	5.5	4.9	4.4	12.1	10.7
Ohio	5.5	5.4	4.8	4.6	9.8	10.2
Indiana	6.0	5.5	5.2	4.9	11.5	10.3
Illinois	7.0	5.9	5.1	4.6	12.7	11.2
Michigan	6.9	5.4	4.9	4.1	14.0	10.8
Wisconsin	5.1	4.5	4.6	3.8	9.1	10.1
West North Central	5.0	4.5	4.5	4.0	10.2	9.6
Minnesota	4.3	3.8	3.9	3.5	10.7	8.2
Iowa	4.8	4.7	4.5	4.4	*10.5	*11.5
Missouri	6.0	4.8	5.0	3.9	10.6	9.5
North Dakota	5.0	3.8	4.7	3.8	*	*
South Dakota	5.1	4.1	4.5	3.5	*	*
Nebraska	4.5	5.4	4.2	5.1	*9.8	*9.6
Kansas	4.9	4.9	4.6	4.3	8.3	11.6
South Atlantic	6.9	5.7	4.9	4.1	11.7	9.9
Delaware	7.5	5.1	5.8	3.8	12.4	9.7
Maryland	5.9	6.1	3.9	3.7	10.2	10.9
District of Columbia	14.1	10.8	*5.2	*	16.7	13.5
Virginia	6.8	5.4	4.8	4.0	13.0	10.0
West Virginia	5.8	5.5	5.6	5.3	*9.7	*12.5
North Carolina	7.3	6.3	5.3	4.8	11.9	10.6
South Carolina	7.7	6.4	5.4	4.2	11.3	10.3
Georgia	7.9	6.1	5.5	4.1	12.0	10.0
Florida	6.2	4.7	4.7	3.8	10.5	8.2
East South Central	6.6	5.7	5.0	4.3	10.6	9.5
Kentucky	5.0	4.5	4.6	4.2	8.9	7.2
Tennessee	6.5	5.3	4.9	3.9	11.8	10.0
Alabama	7.5	6.5	5.7	4.8	11.1	9.8
Mississippi	7.1	6.6	4.9	4.4	9.5	9.1
West South Central[3]	5.0	4.3	4.2	3.9	8.4	7.4
Arkansas	5.4	5.4	4.5	4.6	8.5	8.1
Louisiana[3]	6.3	6.1	4.8	4.4	8.5	8.6
Oklahoma[3]	4.4	4.8	4.1	4.5	6.3	8.8
Texas	4.7	3.8	4.1	3.5	8.5	6.2
Mountain	4.8	4.2	4.4	3.9	10.1	7.9
Montana	4.6	3.9	4.2	3.7	*	*
Idaho	5.3	4.1	5.2	3.8	*	*
Wyoming	3.9	3.6	3.8	3.1	*	*
Colorado	5.0	4.4	4.7	4.0	10.9	9.3
New Mexico	5.0	3.9	4.8	4.0	*	*
Arizona	5.3	4.8	4.9	4.6	11.0	9.0
Utah	3.7	3.6	3.6	3.4	*	*
Nevada	4.3	3.4	3.8	3.2	*8.3	*5.5
Pacific	4.6	3.8	4.0	3.3	9.2	8.0
Washington	4.3	3.5	3.8	3.3	9.7	8.2
Oregon	4.4	3.3	4.0	3.2	*11.6	*
California	4.6	3.9	4.1	3.4	9.2	8.0
Alaska	4.1	3.9	3.7	3.2	*	*
Hawaii	4.3	3.9	3.5	*3.6	*	*

See footnotes at end of table.

Table 25 (page 2 of 2). Neonatal mortality rates, according to race, geographic division, and State: United States, average annual 1989–91 and 1995–97

[Data are based on the National Linked Birth/Infant Death Data Sets]

Geographic division and State	Hispanic[4]		American Indian or Alaska Native[5]		Asian or Pacific Islander[5]	
	1989–91	1995–97[1]	1989–91	1995–97[1]	1989–91	1995–97[1]
	Neonatal[2] deaths per 1,000 live births					
United States	4.8	4.0	5.9	4.4	3.9	3.3
New England[6]	5.5	5.7	*	*	4.4	3.0
Maine	*	*	*	*	*	*
New Hampshire[6]	- - -	*	*	*	*	*
Vermont	*	*	*	*	*	*
Massachusetts	5.8	5.0	*	*	*3.9	*2.6
Rhode Island	*4.9	*7.6	*	*	*	*
Connecticut	5.3	6.2	*	*	*	*
Middle Atlantic	6.2	4.9	*	*	4.1	2.8
New York	6.4	4.8	*	*	4.1	2.9
New Jersey	5.1	4.7	*	*	*3.4	2.6
Pennsylvania	7.3	6.2	*	*	*5.2	*2.7
East North Central	5.9	4.8	*6.2	*5.8	3.6	3.5
Ohio	*5.4	*5.0	*	*	*	*4.4
Indiana	*4.7	5.7	*	*	*	*
Illinois	6.4	4.5	*	*	3.9	3.8
Michigan	5.2	4.6	*	*	*	*
Wisconsin	*3.9	6.5	*	*	*	*
West North Central	5.3	4.6	6.1	6.3	4.6	4.1
Minnesota	*	*4.4	*4.9	*7.9	*3.2	*3.9
Iowa	*	*	*	*	*	*
Missouri	*	*	*	*	*	*
North Dakota	*	*	*	*	*	*
South Dakota	*	*	*8.2	*7.4	*	*
Nebraska	*	*6.6	*	*	*	*
Kansas	*5.4	*4.3	*	*	*	*
South Atlantic	5.2	3.7	7.4	6.9	4.6	3.6
Delaware	*	*	*	*	*	*
Maryland	*4.7	*3.7	*	*	*4.5	*5.0
District of Columbia	*	*	*	*	*	*
Virginia	*4.8	5.1	*	*	*4.1	*3.5
West Virginia	*	*	*	*	*	*
North Carolina	*5.5	4.6	*7.7	*8.1	*	*4.0
South Carolina	*	*	*	*	*	*
Georgia	*5.7	4.5	*	*	*5.3	*
Florida	5.1	3.2	*	*	*4.4	*3.1
East South Central	*	*4.3	*	*	*	*3.3
Kentucky	*	*	*	*	*	*
Tennessee	*	*	*	*	*	*
Alabama	*	*	*	*	*	*
Mississippi	*	*	*	*	*	*
West South Central[6]	4.2	3.5	4.3	3.5	4.1	3.1
Arkansas	*	*	*	*	*	*
Louisiana[6]	- - -	*	*	*	*	*
Oklahoma[6]	- - -	*3.0	*3.7	3.8	*	*
Texas	4.2	3.5	*	*	4.0	2.9
Mountain	4.7	4.4	5.8	3.8	4.6	4.1
Montana	*	*	*7.6	*	*	*
Idaho	*	*4.8	*	*	*	*
Wyoming	*	*	*	*	*	*
Colorado	4.4	4.4	*	*	*	*4.9
New Mexico	4.9	4.0	4.9	*3.0	*	*
Arizona	5.0	5.0	5.4	3.7	*	*
Utah	*3.6	*4.4	*	*	*	*
Nevada	*4.1	2.9	*	*	*	*
Pacific	4.5	3.7	6.5	3.6	3.7	3.3
Washington	4.9	3.1	*8.5	*	*2.7	*2.9
Oregon	6.5	4.4	*	*	*5.3	*
California	4.4	3.7	6.3	*3.8	3.6	3.2
Alaska	*	*	*5.7	*4.8	*	*
Hawaii	*6.6	*3.7	*	*	4.2	3.9

* Rates preceded by an asterisk are based on fewer than 50 events. Rates not shown are based on fewer than 20 events.   - - - Data not available.

[1]Rates based on period file using weighted data. Data for 1995–97 not strictly comparable with unweighted birth cohort data for earlier years (see Appendix I).

[2]Infants under 28 days of age.

[3]Rates for white and black are substituted for non-Hispanic white and non-Hispanic black for Louisiana 1989, Oklahoma 1989–90, and New Hampshire 1989–91.

[4]Persons of Hispanic origin may be of any race.   [5]Includes persons of Hispanic origin.

[6]Rates for Hispanic origin exclude data from States not reporting Hispanic origin on the birth certificate for 1 or more years in a 3-year period.

NOTE: National linked files do not exist for 1992–94 birth cohorts.

SOURCE: Centers for Disease Control and Prevention, National Center for Health Statistics. National Vital Statistics System.

Table 26. Infant mortality rates and international rankings: Selected countries, selected years, 1960–96

[Data are based on reporting by countries]

| Country[2] | 1960 | 1970 | 1980 | 1990 | 1995 | 1996[3] | International rankings[1] | |
							1960	1996
	Infant[4] deaths per 1,000 live births							
Australia	20.2	17.9	10.7	8.2	5.7	5.8	4	16
Austria	37.5	25.9	14.3	7.8	5.4	5.1	23	11
Belgium	31.2	21.1	12.1	7.9	6.1	5.6	19	13
Bulgaria	45.1	27.3	20.2	14.8	14.8	14.8	29	36
Canada	27.3	18.8	10.4	6.8	6.1	6.1	14	20
Chile	125.1	78.8	33.0	16.0	11.1	11.7	35	33
Costa Rica	74.3	61.5	20.2	15.3	13.2	11.8	32	34
Cuba	37.3	38.7	19.6	10.7	9.4	8.0	22	27
Czech Republic	- - -	- - -	- - -	10.8	7.7	6.0	- - -	18
Czechoslovakia	23.5	22.1	18.4	11.3	- - -	- - -	10	- - -
Denmark	21.5	14.2	8.4	7.5	5.1	5.7	7	14
England and Wales	21.8	18.2	12.0	7.9	6.1	6.1	8	20
Finland	21.0	13.2	7.6	5.6	3.9	4.0	5	3
France	27.4	18.2	10.0	7.3	4.9	4.9	15	9
Germany[5]	35.0	22.5	12.4	7.1	5.3	5.0	21	10
Greece	40.1	29.6	17.9	9.7	8.1	8.1	24	28
Hong Kong	41.5	19.2	11.2	6.2	4.6	4.1	25	6
Hungary	47.6	35.9	23.2	14.8	10.7	10.9	30	31
Ireland	29.3	19.5	11.1	8.2	6.4	5.5	16	12
Israel	31.0	22.0	15.6	9.9	6.9	6.3	18	23
Italy	43.9	29.6	14.6	8.6	6.1	6.0	28	18
Japan	30.4	13.1	7.5	4.6	4.3	3.8	17	1
Kuwait	- - -	39.4	27.7	- - -	10.9	11.5	- - -	32
Netherlands	17.9	12.7	8.6	7.1	5.5	5.7	2	14
New Zealand	22.6	16.7	12.9	8.3	6.7	6.7	9	24
Northern Ireland	27.2	22.9	13.4	7.5	7.1	5.8	13	16
Norway	18.9	12.7	8.1	6.9	4.0	4.0	3	3
Poland	56.1	33.2	21.3	19.4	13.6	12.2	31	35
Portugal	77.5	58.0	24.3	11.0	7.5	6.9	34	25
Puerto Rico	43.3	27.9	18.5	13.4	12.7	10.4	26	30
Romania	75.7	49.4	29.3	26.9	21.2	22.3	33	38
Russia[6]	- - -	- - -	- - -	17.6	18.2	18.2	- - -	37
Scotland	26.4	19.6	12.1	7.7	6.2	6.2	12	22
Singapore	34.8	21.4	11.7	6.7	4.0	3.8	20	1
Slovakia	- - -	- - -	- - -	12.0	11.0	9.9	- - -	29
Spain	43.7	26.5	12.3	7.6	5.5	4.7	27	7
Sweden	16.6	11.0	6.9	6.0	4.1	4.0	1	3
Switzerland	21.1	15.1	9.1	6.8	5.0	4.7	6	7
United States	26.0	20.0	12.6	9.2	7.6	7.3	11	26

- - - Data not available.

[1]Rankings are from lowest to highest infant mortality rates. Some of the variation in infant mortality rates is due to differences among countries in distinguishing between fetal and infant deaths.

[2]Refers to countries, territories, cities, or geographic areas with at least 1 million population and with "complete" counts of live births and infant deaths as indicated in the United Nations Demographic Yearbook.

[3]Rates for Bulgaria, Canada, New Zealand, and Russia are for 1995.

[4]Under 1 year of age.

[5]Rates presented for the years prior to the reunification of Germany were calculated by combining information from the Federal Republic of Germany and the German Democratic Republic.

[6]Excludes infants born alive after less than 28 weeks' gestation, of less than 1,000 grams in weight and 35 centimeters in length, who die within seven days of birth.

SOURCES: United Nations Demographic Yearbook: Historical Supplement 1948–97. First Issue DYB-CD, in press. England and Wales: Office for National Statistics. 1996 Mortality Statistics: Childhood, infant and perinatal. England and Wales. Series DH3, No. 29. London, 1998; Northern Ireland: Registrar General, Northern Ireland. Annual Report (various years). Belfast; Scotland: National Health Service in Scotland. Scottish Stillbirth and Infant Death Report, 1996. Edinburg, 1997; United States and Puerto Rico: Centers for Disease Control and Prevention, National Center for Health Statistics. Vital Statistics of the United States, vol. II, mortality part A (selected years). Washington. Public Health Service.

Table 27 (page 1 of 2). Life expectancy at birth and at 65 years of age, according to sex: Selected countries, 1990 and 1995

[Data are based on reporting by countries]

Country[1]	At birth		At 65 years	
	1990[2]	1995[3]	1990[2]	1995[3]
Male	Life expectancy in years			
Japan	76.2	76.4	16.5	16.5
Sweden	74.8	76.2	15.5	16.0
Israel	74.6	75.3	15.6	15.8
Canada	74.0	75.2	15.5	16.1
Switzerland	74.0	75.1	15.3	16.1
Greece	74.6	75.1	15.8	16.2
Australia	73.3	75.0	14.7	15.6
Norway	73.4	74.9	14.6	15.2
Netherlands	73.9	74.6	14.4	14.7
Italy	73.6	74.4	15.0	15.5
England and Wales	73.2	74.3	14.3	14.7
France	73.4	74.2	16.1	16.6
Spain	73.4	74.2	15.5	16.0
Austria	72.6	73.5	14.7	15.2
Singapore	72.3	73.4	14.4	14.9
Germany	72.0	73.3	14.1	14.7
New Zealand	71.9	73.3	14.3	15.0
Northern Ireland	71.8	73.1	13.2	14.1
Belgium	72.3	73.0	14.0	14.5
Cuba	72.9	73.0	15.9	15.7
Costa Rica	72.1	73.0	14.0	15.2
Finland	71.0	72.8	13.8	14.5
Denmark	72.2	72.8	14.0	14.1
Ireland	72.0	72.5	13.2	13.4
United States	71.8	72.5	15.1	15.6
Scotland	71.2	72.2	13.2	13.8
Chile	69.4	71.6	14.0	14.6
Portugal	70.1	71.2	13.8	14.3
Czech Republic	67.6	69.7	11.7	12.7
Puerto Rico	69.1	69.6	14.9	16.3
Slovakia	68.3	68.2	13.0	12.7
Poland	66.5	67.6	12.5	12.9
Bulgaria	68.2	67.1	12.8	12.6
Romania	66.6	65.5	13.3	12.8
Hungary	65.1	65.3	12.1	12.1
Russian Federation[4]	63.8	58.3	11.9	11.0
Female				
Japan	82.5	82.9	20.6	20.9
France	81.8	82.6	20.7	21.4
Switzerland	81.0	81.9	19.7	20.5
Sweden	80.8	81.6	19.4	19.8
Spain	80.5	81.5	19.2	19.9
Canada	80.8	81.2	19.9	20.1
Australia	79.6	80.9	18.7	19.5
Italy	80.4	80.8	19.0	19.4
Norway	79.9	80.7	18.7	19.3
Netherlands	80.3	80.4	19.2	19.1
Greece	79.8	80.3	18.3	18.5
Finland	79.0	80.3	17.9	18.7
Austria	79.2	80.1	18.2	18.8
Germany	78.6	79.8	17.8	18.6
Belgium	79.1	79.8	18.4	18.9
England and Wales	78.9	79.6	18.2	18.5
Israel	78.1	79.3	17.3	17.8
Singapore	77.5	79.0	17.2	18.1
United States	78.8	78.9	18.9	18.9
New Zealand	78.1	78.9	18.1	18.6

See footnotes at end of table.

Table 27 (page 2 of 2). Life expectancy at birth and at 65 years of age, according to sex: Selected countries, 1990 and 1995

[Data are based on reporting by countries]

Country[1]	At birth		At 65 years	
	1990[2]	1995[3]	1990[2]	1995[3]
Female—Con.	Life expectancy in years			
Puerto Rico	77.2	78.9	17.5	19.4
Portugal	77.3	78.6	17.0	17.7
Northern Ireland	77.5	78.5	17.1	17.7
Ireland	77.7	78.1	17.0	17.0
Denmark	77.9	77.9	18.0	17.6
Chile	76.5	77.9	17.6	17.9
Costa Rica	76.9	77.8	16.8	17.6
Scotland	77.0	77.6	16.9	17.1
Cuba	76.8	76.9	17.8	17.6
Czech Republic	75.5	76.7	15.3	16.2
Poland	75.6	76.4	16.2	16.5
Slovakia	76.5	76.3	16.6	16.3
Bulgaria	74.9	74.9	15.3	15.5
Hungary	73.8	74.6	15.4	15.8
Romania	73.1	73.4	15.2	15.3
Russian Federation[4]	74.3	71.6	15.7	15.0

[1]Refers to countries, territories, cities, or geographic areas.
[2]Data for Slovakia are for 1987. Data for Costa Rica are for 1988. Data for Australia, Belgium, and Puerto Rico are for 1989.
[3]Data for Australia, Bulgaria, Chile, Costa Rica, France, Norway, Spain, and Switzerland are for 1994. Data for Ireland, Italy, and New Zealand are for 1993. Data for Puerto Rico are for 1992.
[4]Data for 1990 from Goskomstat 1997 (Demographic Yearbook of Russia, 1996).

NOTES: Rankings are from highest to lowest life expectancy based on the latest available data for countries or geographic areas with at least 1 million population. This table is based on official mortality data from the countries concerned, as submitted to the United Nations Demographic Yearbook or the World Health Statistics Annual.

SOURCES: World Health Organization: World Health Statistics Annuals. Vols. 1990–1996. Geneva; United Nations: Demographic Yearbook 1991 and 1996. New York; Centers for Disease Control and Prevention, National Center for Health Statistics. Vital statistics of the United States, 1990 and 1995, vol II, mortality, part A. Washington: Public Health Service. 1994 and unpublished.

Table 28. Life expectancy at birth, at 65 years of age, and at 75 years of age, according to race and sex: United States, selected years 1900–98

[Data are based on the National Vital Statistics System]

Specified age and year	All races			White			Black		
	Both sexes	Male	Female	Both sexes	Male	Female	Both sexes	Male	Female
At birth				*Remaining life expectancy in years*					
1900[1,2]	47.3	46.3	48.3	47.6	46.6	48.7	[3]33.0	[3]32.5	[3]33.5
1950[2]	68.2	65.6	71.1	69.1	66.5	72.2	60.7	58.9	62.7
1960[2]	69.7	66.6	73.1	70.6	67.4	74.1	63.2	60.7	65.9
1970	70.8	67.1	74.7	71.7	68.0	75.6	64.1	60.0	68.3
1980	73.7	70.0	77.4	74.4	70.7	78.1	68.1	63.8	72.5
1985	74.7	71.1	78.2	75.3	71.8	78.7	69.3	65.0	73.4
1986	74.7	71.2	78.2	75.4	71.9	78.8	69.1	64.8	73.4
1987	74.9	71.4	78.3	75.6	72.1	78.9	69.1	64.7	73.4
1988	74.9	71.4	78.3	75.6	72.2	78.9	68.9	64.4	73.2
1989	75.1	71.7	78.5	75.9	72.5	79.2	68.8	64.3	73.3
1990	75.4	71.8	78.8	76.1	72.7	79.4	69.1	64.5	73.6
1991	75.5	72.0	78.9	76.3	72.9	79.6	69.3	64.6	73.8
1992	75.8	72.3	79.1	76.5	73.2	79.8	69.6	65.0	73.9
1993	75.5	72.2	78.8	76.3	73.1	79.5	69.2	64.6	73.7
1994	75.7	72.4	79.0	76.5	73.3	79.6	69.5	64.9	73.9
1995	75.8	72.5	78.9	76.5	73.4	79.6	69.6	65.2	73.9
1996	76.1	73.1	79.1	76.8	73.9	79.7	70.2	66.1	74.2
1997	76.5	73.6	79.4	77.1	74.3	79.9	71.1	67.2	74.7
1998	76.7	73.8	79.5	77.3	74.5	80.0	71.3	67.6	74.8
At 65 years									
1900–1902[1,2]	11.9	11.5	12.2	- - -	11.5	12.2	- - -	10.4	11.4
1950[2]	13.9	12.8	15.0	- - -	12.8	15.1	13.9	12.9	14.9
1960[2]	14.3	12.8	15.8	14.4	12.9	15.9	13.9	12.7	15.1
1970	15.2	13.1	17.0	15.2	13.1	17.1	14.2	12.5	15.7
1980	16.4	14.1	18.3	16.5	14.2	18.4	15.1	13.0	16.8
1985	16.7	14.5	18.5	16.8	14.5	18.7	15.2	13.0	16.9
1986	16.8	14.6	18.6	16.9	14.7	18.7	15.2	13.0	17.0
1987	16.9	14.7	18.7	17.0	14.8	18.8	15.2	13.0	17.0
1988	16.9	14.7	18.6	17.0	14.8	18.7	15.1	12.9	16.9
1989	17.1	15.0	18.8	17.2	15.1	18.9	15.2	13.0	16.9
1990	17.2	15.1	18.9	17.3	15.2	19.1	15.4	13.2	17.2
1991	17.4	15.3	19.1	17.5	15.4	19.2	15.5	13.4	17.2
1992	17.5	15.4	19.2	17.6	15.5	19.3	15.7	13.5	17.4
1993	17.3	15.3	18.9	17.4	15.4	19.0	15.5	13.4	17.1
1994	17.4	15.5	19.0	17.5	15.6	19.1	15.7	13.6	17.2
1995	17.4	15.6	18.9	17.6	15.7	19.1	15.6	13.6	17.1
1996	17.5	15.7	19.0	17.6	15.8	19.1	15.8	13.9	17.2
1997	17.7	15.9	19.2	17.8	16.0	19.3	16.1	14.2	17.6
1998	17.8	16.0	19.2	17.8	16.1	19.3	16.1	14.3	17.4
At 75 years									
1980	10.4	8.8	11.5	10.4	8.8	11.5	9.7	8.3	10.7
1985	10.6	9.0	11.7	10.6	9.0	11.7	10.1	8.7	11.1
1986	10.7	9.1	11.7	10.7	9.1	11.8	10.1	8.6	11.1
1987	10.7	9.1	11.8	10.7	9.1	11.8	10.1	8.6	11.1
1988	10.6	9.1	11.7	10.7	9.1	11.7	10.0	8.5	11.0
1989	10.9	9.3	11.9	10.9	9.3	11.9	10.1	8.6	11.0
1990	10.9	9.4	12.0	11.0	9.4	12.0	10.2	8.6	11.2
1991	11.1	9.5	12.1	11.1	9.5	12.1	10.2	8.7	11.2
1992	11.2	9.6	12.2	11.2	9.6	12.2	10.4	8.9	11.4
1993	10.9	9.5	11.9	11.0	9.5	12.0	10.2	8.7	11.1
1994	11.0	9.6	12.0	11.1	9.6	12.0	10.3	8.9	11.2
1995	11.0	9.7	11.9	11.1	9.7	12.0	10.2	8.8	11.1
1996	11.1	9.8	12.0	11.1	9.8	12.0	10.3	9.0	11.2
1997	11.2	9.9	12.1	11.2	9.9	12.1	10.7	9.3	11.5
1998	11.3	10.0	12.2	11.3	10.0	12.2	10.5	9.2	11.3

- - - Data not available.

[1]Death registration area only. The death registration area increased from 10 States and the District of Columbia in 1900 to the coterminous United States in 1933.
[2]Includes deaths of persons who were not residents of the 50 States and the District of Columbia.   [3]Figure is for the all other population.

NOTES: Beginning in 1997 life table methodology was revised to construct complete life tables by single years of age that extend to age 100. (Anderson RN. Method for Constructing Complete Annual U.S. Life Tables. National Center for Health Statistics. Vital Health Stat 2(129). 1999.) Previously abridged life tables were constructed for five-year age groups ending with the age group 85 years and over. Data for additional years are available (see Appendix III).

SOURCES: U.S. Bureau of the Census: U.S. Life Tables 1890, 1901, 1910, and 1901–1910, by Glover JW. Washington. U.S. Government Printing Office, 1921; Centers for Disease Control and Prevention, National Center for Health Statistics: Vital Statistics Rates in the United States, 1940–1960, by Grove RD and Hetzel AM. DHEW Pub. No. (PHS) 1677. Public Health Service. Washington. U.S. Government Printing Office, 1968; Murphy SL. Deaths: Final data for 1998. National vital statistics reports; vol 48. Hyattsville, Maryland: 2000; unpublished data from the Division of Vital Statistics; data for 1960 and earlier years for the black population were computed by the Office of Research and Methodology from data compiled by the Division of Vital Statistics.

Table 29 (page 1 of 2). Age-adjusted death rates, according to detailed race, Hispanic origin, geographic division, and State: United States, average annual 1984–86, 1990–92, and 1996–98

[Data are based on the National Vital Statistics System]

Geographic division and State	All persons			White	Black	American Indian or Alaska Native	Asian or Pacific Islander	Hispanic	White, non-Hispanic
	1984–86	1990–92	1996–98	1996–98	1996–98	1996–98	1996–98	1996–98	1996–98
	Deaths per 100,000 resident population[1]								
United States	547.7	513.4	481.4	458.4	711.8	460.9	274.1	353.5	457.7
New England	514.4	465.0	435.6	430.5	596.6	*	230.9	316.8	426.6
Maine	530.2	479.7	465.2	466.6	*	*	*	*	458.2
New Hampshire	519.8	461.1	443.4	444.9	*	*	204.6	180.4	436.0
Vermont	528.5	476.7	445.0	445.7	*	*	*	*	446.6
Massachusetts	518.7	468.9	429.1	425.9	564.1	*	251.0	315.8	424.0
Rhode Island	517.3	471.8	440.0	433.8	648.8	*	274.7	251.9	428.0
Connecticut	497.3	451.4	433.0	418.0	637.2	*	179.8	352.6	412.5
Middle Atlantic	566.2	527.2	473.2	452.1	654.1	*	233.4	357.4	446.7
New York	573.0	539.2	464.9	448.0	592.6	*	248.2	374.2	434.1
New Jersey	553.6	512.1	462.5	437.1	697.8	*	184.6	281.4	442.4
Pennsylvania	562.5	516.7	490.5	465.4	774.5	*	259.7	471.0	463.2
East North Central	553.0	516.2	488.1	460.0	746.8	*	226.6	300.9	458.8
Ohio	561.6	519.7	497.3	477.5	696.3	*	196.0	381.1	473.3
Indiana	551.2	517.3	502.5	484.7	752.8	*	211.2	246.8	487.0
Illinois	559.5	532.4	493.7	452.0	800.6	*	217.4	290.4	452.2
Michigan	569.6	523.4	487.8	452.4	729.5	*	258.7	346.6	448.7
Wisconsin	488.5	454.4	438.3	425.5	709.9	*	299.3	204.6	427.2
West North Central	497.1	467.4	452.5	436.7	746.5	*	313.6	353.3	434.2
Minnesota	462.6	427.8	403.5	394.4	670.3	820.5	345.6	446.4	390.5
Iowa	472.7	440.4	426.3	422.8	688.7	*	333.3	316.8	422.8
Missouri	549.7	524.8	515.6	490.2	770.9	*	309.6	385.8	490.2
North Dakota	449.6	435.7	416.1	401.7	*	973.9	*	*	390.2
South Dakota	497.2	458.8	441.9	409.0	*	1,119.4	*	*	409.6
Nebraska	484.1	457.0	439.7	428.3	758.3	897.2	274.7	316.4	425.4
Kansas	494.0	463.1	455.5	443.0	720.2	*	273.1	320.6	437.2
South Atlantic	565.0	529.8	504.6	459.5	729.4	*	218.5	322.0	464.9
Delaware	573.9	534.1	511.7	478.3	720.0	*	165.4	356.9	478.0
Maryland	577.6	534.1	506.1	443.2	724.1	*	218.0	#	451.5
District of Columbia	765.8	824.3	732.3	376.5	951.5	*	220.9	#	408.4
Virginia	564.2	520.9	490.1	453.0	698.4	*	225.4	203.0	455.4
West Virginia	593.6	570.2	550.6	547.3	730.9	*	*	186.2	548.6
North Carolina	576.9	546.2	526.7	476.3	744.7	595.3	240.5	182.2	476.8
South Carolina	618.6	584.7	565.9	497.5	776.2	*	260.6	212.2	498.4
Georgia	614.9	578.4	551.2	496.9	742.0	*	275.4	211.9	497.6
Florida	521.2	488.5	466.3	440.7	679.5	*	185.3	350.7	450.5
East South Central	598.3	576.0	566.7	528.6	766.4	*	252.8	296.5	528.7
Kentucky	592.6	560.0	541.7	531.8	717.0	*	245.6	473.6	531.1
Tennessee	583.7	559.9	560.7	526.3	798.5	*	289.6	308.5	526.5
Alabama	604.5	586.2	571.7	525.1	748.3	*	163.5	236.6	525.9
Mississippi	625.3	615.5	608.1	536.5	776.3	*	298.4	178.2	537.0
West South Central	564.6	542.9	514.8	490.3	725.0	*	229.5	399.0	473.7
Arkansas	575.7	560.2	559.8	530.9	780.1	*	352.6	201.4	532.5
Louisiana	623.7	613.0	582.7	512.0	775.3	*	274.8	251.2	517.3
Oklahoma	550.4	533.9	537.8	532.9	700.9	*	330.0	- - -	- - -
Texas	549.4	524.0	487.7	471.5	689.2	*	213.7	407.9	481.0
Mountain	502.4	473.3	453.6	447.3	571.8	617.8	278.7	421.9	443.3
Montana	513.7	479.0	456.1	442.7	*	800.7	*	341.1	440.9
Idaho	488.7	447.9	429.5	428.6	*	556.3	342.3	311.7	429.8
Wyoming	507.5	479.4	463.5	457.8	*	846.5	*	418.4	457.0
Colorado	478.9	451.8	422.4	420.7	550.6	365.0	235.2	420.2	416.2
New Mexico	518.5	489.5	464.1	456.5	420.9	602.0	270.2	466.5	436.2
Arizona	511.9	484.6	470.5	458.8	601.3	684.6	242.9	435.0	452.8
Utah	465.8	418.1	404.1	403.2	591.3	425.1	346.9	374.1	401.5
Nevada	586.6	558.2	537.9	539.8	634.3	391.4	325.3	263.2	553.1

See footnotes at end of table.

Table 29 (page 2 of 2). Age-adjusted death rates, according to detailed race, Hispanic origin, geographic division, and State: United States, average annual 1984–86, 1990–92, and 1996–98

[Data are based on the National Vital Statistics System]

Geographic division and State	All persons			White	Black	American Indian or Alaska Native	Asian or Pacific Islander	Hispanic	White, non-Hispanic
	1984–86	1990–92	1996–98	1996–98	1996–98	1996–98	1996–98	1996–98	1996–98
	Deaths per 100,000 resident population[1]								
Pacific	516.6	482.0	434.9	436.7	657.4	*	302.1	326.4	448.1
Washington	496.9	458.9	429.9	428.4	601.4	555.2	286.8	286.2	428.8
Oregon	510.9	471.5	455.5	454.4	651.9	*	301.4	280.9	455.7
California	523.4	489.6	435.7	437.9	666.8	*	280.8	327.7	454.5
Alaska	561.8	515.1	461.6	425.6	430.0	736.3	308.3	283.5	428.2
Hawaii	418.6	399.1	377.5	355.2	245.1	*	392.1	349.7	358.8

* Data for States with population under 10,000 in the middle year of a 3-year period or fewer than 50 deaths for the 3-year period are considered unreliable and are not shown. Data for American Indians or Alaska Natives in States with more than 10 percent misclassification of American Indian or Alaska Native deaths on death certificates or without information on misclassification are also not shown. (Support Services International, Inc. Methodology for adjusting IHS mortality data for miscoding race-ethnicity of American Indians and Alaska Natives on State death certificates. Report submitted to Indian Health Service. 1996.) Division death rates for American Indians or Alaska Natives are not shown when any State within the division does not meet reliability criteria.
#Estimates of Hispanic death rates in Maryland (79.6 deaths per 1,000 population) and the District of Columbia (DC) (87.5) are substantially lower than for other States and are likely to be underestimates of actual death rates, possibly due to misreporting of Hispanic origin on some death certificates and/or inaccurate Hispanic population estimates for Maryland and DC.
- - - Data not available.
[1] Average annual death rate. Denominators are population estimates for the middle year of each 3-year period, multiplied by 3.

NOTES: Rates are age adjusted to the 1940 U.S. standard million population. See Appendix II, Age adjustment. The race groups, white, black, American Indian or Alaska Native, and Asian or Pacific Islander, include persons of Hispanic and non-Hispanic origin. Conversely, persons of Hispanic origin may be of any race. Bias in death rates results from inconsistent race identification between the death certificate (source of data for numerator of death rates) and data from the Census Bureau (denominator); and from undercounts of some population groups in the census. The net effects of misclassification and under coverage result in death rates estimated to be overstated by 1 percent for the white population and 5 percent for the black population; and death rates estimated to be understated by 21 percent for American Indians, 11 percent for Asians, and 2 percent for Hispanics (Rosenberg HM, Maurer JD, Sorlie PD, Johnson NJ, et al. Quality of death rates by race and Hispanic origin: A summary of current research, 1999. National Center for Health Statistics. Vital Health Stat 2(128). 1999). Data for additional years are available (see Appendix III).

SOURCES: Centers for Disease Control and Prevention, National Center for Health Statistics. Rates computed by the Division of Health and Utilization Analysis from mortality data compiled by the Division of Vital Statistics and from State population estimates prepared by the U.S. Bureau of the Census: 1985 estimate from 0792I intercensal series; 1990 from April 1, 1990 MARS Census File; 1993–94 from vintage 1994 postcensal series; 1995 from vintage 1996 postcensal series; 1996 from vintage 1997 postcensal series; 1997 from vintage 1998 postcensal series.

Table 30 (page 1 of 4). Age-adjusted death rates for selected causes of death, according to sex, detailed race, and Hispanic origin: United States, selected years 1950–98

[Data are based on the National Vital Statistics System]

Sex, race, Hispanic origin, and cause of death	1950[1]	1960[1]	1970	1980	1985	1990	1995	1996	1997	1998
All persons				Deaths per 100,000 resident population						
All causes	841.5	760.9	714.3	585.8	548.9	520.2	503.9	491.6	479.1	471.7
Natural causes	766.6	695.2	636.9	519.7	493.0	465.1	451.7	440.6	429.2	422.6
Diseases of heart	307.2	286.2	253.6	202.0	181.4	152.0	138.3	134.5	130.5	126.6
Ischemic heart disease	- - -	- - -	- - -	149.8	126.1	102.6	89.5	86.7	82.9	79.5
Cerebrovascular diseases	88.8	79.7	66.3	40.8	32.5	27.7	26.7	26.4	25.9	25.1
Malignant neoplasms	125.4	125.8	129.8	132.8	134.4	135.0	129.9	127.9	125.6	123.6
Trachea, bronchus, and lung	11.1	17.7	26.6	34.8	37.6	39.9	38.3	37.9	37.3	37.0
Colorectal	- - -	17.7	16.8	15.5	14.9	13.6	12.7	12.2	12.0	11.8
Prostate[2]	13.4	13.1	13.3	14.4	14.7	16.7	15.4	14.9	13.9	13.2
Breast[3]	22.2	22.3	23.1	22.7	23.3	23.1	21.0	20.2	19.4	18.8
Chronic obstructive pulmonary diseases	4.4	8.2	13.2	15.9	18.8	19.7	20.8	21.0	21.1	21.3
Pneumonia and influenza	26.2	28.0	22.1	12.9	13.5	14.0	12.9	12.8	12.9	13.2
Chronic liver disease and cirrhosis	8.5	10.5	14.7	12.2	9.7	8.6	7.6	7.5	7.4	7.2
Diabetes mellitus	14.3	13.6	14.1	10.1	9.7	11.7	13.3	13.6	13.5	13.6
Human immunodeficiency virus infection	- - -	- - -	- - -	- - -	- - -	9.8	15.6	11.1	5.8	4.6
External causes	73.9	65.7	77.4	66.1	55.9	55.1	52.2	50.9	49.9	49.1
Unintentional injuries	57.5	49.9	53.7	42.3	34.8	32.5	30.5	30.4	30.1	30.1
Motor vehicle-related injuries	23.3	22.5	27.4	22.9	18.8	18.5	16.3	16.2	15.9	15.6
Suicide	11.0	10.6	11.8	11.4	11.5	11.5	11.2	10.8	10.6	10.4
Homicide and legal intervention	5.4	5.2	9.1	10.8	8.3	10.2	9.4	8.5	8.0	7.3
Male										
All causes	1,001.6	949.3	931.6	777.2	723.0	680.2	646.3	623.7	602.8	589.4
Natural causes	892.1	850.7	814.6	675.5	637.9	595.8	567.0	547.2	528.0	516.1
Diseases of heart	383.8	375.5	348.5	280.4	250.1	206.7	184.9	178.8	173.1	166.9
Ischemic heart disease	- - -	- - -	- - -	214.8	179.6	144.0	123.9	119.3	114.2	108.9
Cerebrovascular diseases	91.9	85.4	73.2	44.9	35.5	30.2	28.9	28.5	27.9	26.6
Malignant neoplasms	130.8	143.0	157.4	165.5	166.1	166.3	156.8	153.8	150.4	147.7
Trachea, bronchus, and lung	18.4	32.0	47.5	56.9	58.1	58.5	53.0	51.8	50.5	49.5
Colorectal	- - -	18.6	18.7	18.3	17.9	16.8	15.3	14.8	14.6	14.3
Prostate	13.4	13.1	13.3	14.4	14.7	16.7	15.4	14.9	13.9	13.2
Chronic obstructive pulmonary diseases	6.0	13.7	23.4	26.1	28.1	27.2	26.3	25.9	26.1	25.9
Pneumonia and influenza	30.6	35.0	28.8	17.4	18.4	18.5	16.5	16.2	16.2	16.3
Chronic liver disease and cirrhosis	11.4	14.5	20.2	17.1	13.7	12.2	11.0	10.7	10.5	10.3
Diabetes mellitus	11.4	12.0	13.5	10.2	10.0	12.3	14.4	14.9	14.8	15.2
Human immunodeficiency virus infection	- - -	- - -	- - -	- - -	- - -	17.7	26.2	18.1	9.1	7.2
External causes	109.4	98.5	117.0	101.7	85.2	84.4	79.3	76.5	74.8	73.4
Unintentional injuries	83.7	73.9	80.7	64.0	51.8	47.7	44.1	43.3	42.9	43.0
Motor vehicle-related injuries	36.4	34.5	41.1	34.3	27.3	26.3	22.7	22.3	21.7	21.6
Suicide	17.3	16.6	17.3	18.0	18.8	19.0	18.6	18.0	17.4	17.2
Homicide and legal intervention	8.4	7.9	14.9	17.4	12.8	16.3	14.7	13.3	12.5	11.3
Female										
All causes	688.4	590.6	532.5	432.6	410.3	390.6	385.2	381.0	375.7	372.5
Natural causes	649.2	556.2	492.2	400.1	382.2	363.5	359.1	354.8	349.8	346.8
Diseases of heart	233.9	205.7	175.2	140.3	127.4	108.9	100.4	98.2	95.4	93.3
Ischemic heart disease	- - -	- - -	- - -	98.8	84.2	70.2	61.9	60.4	57.6	55.6
Cerebrovascular diseases	86.0	74.7	60.8	37.6	30.0	25.7	24.8	24.6	24.2	23.6
Malignant neoplasms	120.8	111.2	108.8	109.2	111.7	112.7	110.4	108.8	107.3	105.5
Trachea, bronchus, and lung	3.9	5.7	9.5	17.6	21.8	25.6	26.9	26.9	26.9	27.0
Colorectal	- - -	16.9	15.4	13.4	12.6	11.3	10.6	10.2	10.0	9.9
Breast	22.2	22.3	23.1	22.7	23.3	23.1	21.0	20.2	19.4	18.8
Chronic obstructive pulmonary diseases	2.9	3.5	5.4	8.9	12.5	14.7	17.1	17.6	17.7	18.1
Pneumonia and influenza	22.0	21.8	16.7	9.8	10.1	11.0	10.4	10.4	10.5	11.0
Chronic liver disease and cirrhosis	5.8	6.9	9.8	7.9	6.1	5.3	4.6	4.5	4.5	4.4
Diabetes mellitus	17.1	15.0	14.4	10.0	9.4	11.1	12.4	12.5	12.4	12.3
Human immunodeficiency virus infection	- - -	- - -	- - -	- - -	- - -	2.1	5.2	4.2	2.6	2.2
External causes	39.1	34.4	40.4	32.5	28.1	27.0	26.1	26.2	25.9	25.8
Unintentional injuries	31.7	26.8	28.2	21.8	18.7	17.9	17.5	17.9	17.8	17.8
Motor vehicle-related injuries	10.7	11.0	14.4	11.8	10.5	10.7	10.0	10.2	10.2	9.9
Suicide	4.9	5.0	6.8	5.4	4.9	4.5	4.1	4.0	4.1	4.0
Homicide and legal intervention	2.5	2.6	3.7	4.5	3.9	4.2	4.0	3.6	3.3	3.2

See footnotes at end of table.

Table 30 (page 2 of 4). **Age-adjusted death rates for selected causes of death, according to sex, detailed race, and Hispanic origin: United States, selected years 1950–98**

[Data are based on the National Vital Statistics System]

Sex, race, Hispanic origin, and cause of death	1950[1]	1960[1]	1970	1980	1985	1990	1995	1996	1997	1998
White				Deaths per 100,000 resident population						
All causes	800.4	727.0	679.6	559.4	524.9	492.8	476.9	466.8	456.5	450.4
Natural causes	730.5	665.5	609.2	497.7	471.9	442.0	428.5	419.2	409.7	403.7
Diseases of heart	300.5	281.5	249.1	197.6	176.6	146.9	133.1	129.8	125.9	121.9
Ischemic heart disease	---	---	---	150.6	126.6	102.5	89.0	86.4	82.5	79.2
Cerebrovascular diseases	83.2	74.2	61.8	38.0	30.1	25.5	24.7	24.5	24.0	23.3
Malignant neoplasms	124.7	124.2	127.8	129.6	131.2	131.5	127.0	125.2	122.9	121.0
Trachea, bronchus, and lung	11.2	17.6	26.3	34.2	37.0	39.3	38.0	37.6	37.1	36.8
Colorectal	---	17.9	16.9	15.4	14.7	13.3	12.3	11.8	11.6	11.5
Prostate[2]	13.1	12.4	12.3	13.2	13.4	15.3	14.0	13.5	12.6	12.0
Breast[3]	22.5	22.4	23.4	22.8	23.4	22.9	20.5	19.8	18.9	18.3
Chronic obstructive pulmonary diseases	4.3	8.2	13.4	16.3	19.2	20.1	21.3	21.5	21.7	21.9
Pneumonia and influenza	22.9	24.6	19.8	12.2	12.9	13.4	12.4	12.2	12.4	12.7
Chronic liver disease and cirrhosis	8.6	10.3	13.4	11.0	8.9	8.0	7.4	7.3	7.3	7.1
Diabetes mellitus	13.9	12.8	12.9	9.1	8.6	10.4	11.7	12.0	11.9	12.0
Human immunodeficiency virus infection	---	---	---	---	---	8.0	11.1	7.2	3.3	2.6
External causes	69.9	61.5	70.4	61.9	53.0	50.8	48.4	47.5	46.8	46.7
Unintentional injuries	55.7	47.6	51.0	41.5	34.2	31.8	29.9	29.9	29.6	29.8
Motor vehicle-related injuries	23.1	22.3	26.9	23.4	19.1	18.6	16.4	16.3	15.9	15.7
Suicide	11.6	11.1	12.4	12.1	12.3	12.2	11.9	11.6	11.3	11.2
Homicide and legal intervention	2.6	2.7	4.7	6.9	5.4	5.9	5.5	4.9	4.7	4.4
Black										
All causes	1,236.7	1,073.3	1,044.0	842.5	793.6	789.2	765.7	738.3	705.3	690.9
Natural causes	1,131.0	974.9	910.2	740.2	713.5	701.3	685.8	662.3	632.7	622.2
Diseases of heart	379.6	334.5	307.6	255.7	240.6	213.5	198.8	191.5	185.7	183.3
Ischemic heart disease	---	---	---	150.5	130.9	113.2	103.4	99.4	96.3	92.5
Cerebrovascular diseases	150.9	140.3	114.5	68.5	55.8	48.4	45.0	44.2	42.5	41.4
Malignant neoplasms	129.1	142.3	156.7	172.1	176.6	182.0	171.6	167.8	165.2	161.2
Trachea, bronchus, and lung	8.8	15.8	31.2	43.9	47.6	51.3	47.3	46.1	45.4	44.6
Colorectal	---	15.2	16.6	16.9	17.9	17.9	17.3	16.8	16.8	16.5
Prostate[2]	16.9	22.2	25.4	29.1	31.2	35.3	34.0	33.8	31.4	30.3
Breast[3]	19.3	21.3	21.5	23.3	25.5	27.5	27.5	26.5	26.7	25.3
Chronic obstructive pulmonary diseases	---	---	---	12.5	15.3	16.9	17.6	17.8	17.4	17.7
Pneumonia and influenza	57.0	56.4	40.4	19.2	18.8	19.8	17.8	17.8	17.2	17.4
Chronic liver disease and cirrhosis	7.2	11.7	24.8	21.6	16.3	13.7	9.9	9.2	8.7	8.0
Diabetes mellitus	17.2	22.0	26.5	20.3	20.1	24.8	28.5	28.8	28.9	28.8
Human immunodeficiency virus infection	---	---	---	---	---	25.7	51.8	41.4	24.9	20.6
External causes	105.7	98.4	133.7	101.2	80.1	87.8	79.8	76.0	72.6	68.8
Unintentional injuries	70.9	66.4	74.4	51.2	42.3	39.7	37.4	36.7	36.1	35.7
Motor vehicle-related injuries	24.7	23.4	30.6	19.7	17.4	18.4	16.6	16.7	16.8	16.6
Suicide	4.2	4.7	6.1	6.4	6.4	7.0	6.9	6.6	6.3	5.9
Homicide and legal intervention	30.5	27.4	46.1	40.6	29.2	39.5	33.4	30.6	28.1	25.2
American Indian or Alaska Native										
All causes	---	---	---	564.1	468.2	445.1	468.5	456.7	465.3	458.1
Natural causes	---	---	---	436.5	375.1	360.3	385.4	374.5	381.1	377.3
Diseases of heart	---	---	---	131.2	119.6	107.1	104.5	100.8	102.6	97.1
Ischemic heart disease	---	---	---	87.4	77.3	66.6	65.4	63.8	64.2	57.2
Cerebrovascular diseases	---	---	---	26.6	22.5	19.3	21.6	21.1	19.9	19.6
Malignant neoplasms	---	---	---	70.6	72.0	75.0	80.8	84.9	86.6	83.4
Trachea, bronchus, and lung	---	---	---	13.8	17.5	19.7	22.7	23.8	24.1	25.1
Colorectal	---	---	---	5.6	6.3	6.4	7.6	8.5	9.1	8.2
Prostate[2]	---	---	---	9.6	8.9	7.7	8.8	9.8	8.6	7.4
Breast[3]	---	---	---	8.1	8.0	10.0	10.4	12.7	9.4	10.3
Chronic obstructive pulmonary diseases	---	---	---	7.5	9.8	12.8	13.8	12.6	15.3	15.7
Pneumonia and influenza	---	---	---	19.4	14.9	15.2	14.2	14.0	13.4	14.1
Chronic liver disease and cirrhosis	---	---	---	38.6	23.6	19.8	24.3	20.7	20.6	22.0
Diabetes mellitus	---	---	---	20.0	18.7	20.8	27.3	27.8	30.4	29.6
Human immunodeficiency virus infection	---	---	---	---	---	1.8	7.0	4.2	2.4	2.2
External causes	---	---	---	127.6	93.1	84.8	83.0	82.1	84.3	80.8
Unintentional injuries	---	---	---	95.1	66.2	59.0	56.7	57.6	58.5	55.6
Motor vehicle-related injuries	---	---	---	54.4	36.3	33.2	33.1	34.0	32.3	31.8
Suicide	---	---	---	12.8	12.1	12.4	12.2	13.0	12.9	13.4
Homicide and legal intervention	---	---	---	16.0	12.2	11.1	11.9	10.1	11.0	9.9

See footnotes at end of table.

[Data are based on the National Vital Statistics System]

Sex, race, Hispanic origin, and cause of death	1950[1]	1960[1]	1970	1980	1985	1990	1995	1996	1997	1998
Asian or Pacific Islander				Deaths per 100,000 resident population						
All causes	- - -	- - -	- - -	315.6	305.7	297.6	298.9	277.4	274.8	264.6
Natural causes	- - -	- - -	- - -	280.7	274.4	266.7	269.2	250.3	247.0	240.2
Diseases of heart	- - -	- - -	- - -	93.9	88.6	78.5	78.9	71.7	69.8	67.4
Ischemic heart disease	- - -	- - -	- - -	67.5	58.8	49.7	49.3	44.8	43.5	42.9
Cerebrovascular diseases	- - -	- - -	- - -	29.0	25.5	25.0	25.8	23.9	24.4	22.7
Malignant neoplasms	- - -	- - -	- - -	77.2	80.2	79.8	81.1	76.3	75.4	74.8
Trachea, bronchus, and lung	- - -	- - -	- - -	17.6	16.6	17.7	18.0	16.9	16.9	17.2
Colorectal	- - -	- - -	- - -	9.3	9.6	8.3	8.2	7.7	7.6	7.8
Prostate[2]	- - -	- - -	- - -	4.0	5.9	6.9	7.4	5.8	5.3	4.7
Breast[3]	- - -	- - -	- - -	9.2	9.6	10.0	11.0	8.9	9.2	9.8
Chronic obstructive pulmonary diseases	- - -	- - -	- - -	5.9	8.4	8.7	9.0	8.6	8.6	7.4
Pneumonia and influenza	- - -	- - -	- - -	9.1	9.1	10.4	10.8	9.9	10.1	10.3
Chronic liver disease and cirrhosis	- - -	- - -	- - -	4.5	4.2	3.7	2.7	2.6	2.4	2.4
Diabetes mellitus	- - -	- - -	- - -	6.9	6.1	7.4	9.2	8.8	9.3	8.7
Human immunodeficiency virus infection	- - -	- - -	- - -	- - -	- - -	2.1	3.1	2.2	0.9	0.8
External causes	- - -	- - -	- - -	34.9	31.4	30.9	29.7	27.1	27.7	24.4
Unintentional injuries	- - -	- - -	- - -	21.7	20.1	19.3	17.1	16.1	16.7	14.4
Motor vehicle-related injuries	- - -	- - -	- - -	12.6	12.0	12.5	10.8	9.5	9.7	8.6
Suicide	- - -	- - -	- - -	6.7	6.4	6.0	6.6	6.0	6.2	5.9
Homicide and legal intervention	- - -	- - -	- - -	5.6	4.2	5.2	5.4	4.6	4.3	3.7
Hispanic[4]										
All causes	- - -	- - -	- - -	- - -	397.4	400.2	386.8	365.9	350.3	342.8
Natural causes	- - -	- - -	- - -	- - -	342.7	342.4	334.0	316.9	304.5	298.1
Diseases of heart	- - -	- - -	- - -	- - -	116.0	102.8	92.1	88.6	86.8	84.2
Ischemic heart disease	- - -	- - -	- - -	- - -	77.8	68.0	60.1	58.2	56.8	54.7
Cerebrovascular diseases	- - -	- - -	- - -	- - -	23.8	21.0	20.3	19.5	19.4	19.0
Malignant neoplasms	- - -	- - -	- - -	- - -	75.8	82.4	79.7	77.8	76.4	76.1
Trachea, bronchus, and lung	- - -	- - -	- - -	- - -	13.4	15.9	14.6	14.3	14.2	13.6
Colorectal	- - -	- - -	- - -	- - -	7.5	8.2	7.6	7.3	7.5	7.4
Prostate[2]	- - -	- - -	- - -	- - -	8.5	9.5	10.9	9.9	8.6	9.0
Breast[3]	- - -	- - -	- - -	- - -	11.8	14.1	12.7	12.8	12.6	12.1
Chronic obstructive pulmonary diseases	- - -	- - -	- - -	- - -	8.2	8.7	9.4	8.9	8.7	8.5
Pneumonia and influenza	- - -	- - -	- - -	- - -	12.0	11.5	9.9	9.7	10.0	9.8
Chronic liver disease and cirrhosis	- - -	- - -	- - -	- - -	16.3	14.2	12.9	12.6	12.0	11.7
Diabetes mellitus	- - -	- - -	- - -	- - -	12.8	15.7	19.3	18.8	18.7	18.4
Human immunodeficiency virus infection	- - -	- - -	- - -	- - -	- - -	15.5	23.9	16.3	8.2	6.2
External causes	- - -	- - -	- - -	- - -	54.7	57.8	52.9	49.0	45.8	44.7
Unintentional injuries	- - -	- - -	- - -	- - -	31.8	32.2	29.8	29.0	27.7	28.0
Motor vehicle-related injuries	- - -	- - -	- - -	- - -	16.9	19.3	16.6	16.1	15.2	14.9
Suicide	- - -	- - -	- - -	- - -	6.1	7.3	7.2	6.7	6.1	6.0
Homicide and legal intervention	- - -	- - -	- - -	- - -	15.7	17.7	15.0	12.4	11.1	9.9

See footnotes at end of table.

[Data are based on the National Vital Statistics System]

Sex, race, Hispanic origin, and cause of death	1950[1]	1960[1]	1970	1980	1985	1990	1995	1996	1997	1998
White, non-Hispanic[4]					Deaths per 100,000 resident population					
All causes.................................	---	---	---	---	510.7	493.1	475.2	466.7	458.5	452.7
Natural causes	---	---	---	---	460.7	444.2	428.8	420.7	412.6	406.9
Diseases of heart.........................	---	---	---	---	173.0	148.2	134.1	131.0	127.5	123.6
Ischemic heart disease	---	---	---	---	125.4	103.7	89.8	87.4	83.6	80.3
Cerebrovascular diseases	---	---	---	---	29.2	25.7	24.6	24.4	24.0	23.3
Malignant neoplasms	---	---	---	---	128.3	134.2	129.2	127.6	125.3	123.5
Trachea, bronchus, and lung	---	---	---	---	36.7	40.6	39.2	38.9	38.5	38.3
Colorectal...........................	---	---	---	---	14.4	13.6	12.5	12.1	11.8	11.7
Prostate[2]	---	---	---	---	13.0	15.6	14.1	13.6	12.7	12.1
Breast[3]	---	---	---	---	23.3	23.5	20.9	20.1	19.2	18.7
Chronic obstructive pulmonary diseases	---	---	---	---	19.7	20.7	21.8	22.1	22.4	22.7
Pneumonia and influenza	---	---	---	---	13.2	13.3	12.3	12.2	12.4	12.8
Chronic liver disease and cirrhosis...........	---	---	---	---	8.5	7.5	6.8	6.7	6.7	6.6
Diabetes mellitus	---	---	---	---	8.0	10.1	11.2	11.5	11.3	11.5
Human immunodeficiency virus infection......	---	---	---	---	---	7.0	9.4	6.0	2.6	2.0
External causes...........................	---	---	---	---	50.0	48.9	46.4	46.0	45.9	45.8
Unintentional injuries......................	---	---	---	---	31.9	31.3	29.3	29.3	29.4	29.5
Motor vehicle-related injuries	---	---	---	---	17.8	18.4	16.0	16.0	15.8	15.7
Suicide	---	---	---	---	12.7	12.7	12.2	12.0	11.8	11.8
Homicide and legal intervention	---	---	---	---	4.5	4.2	3.8	3.5	3.5	3.2

- - - Data not available.

[1] Includes deaths of persons who were not residents of the 50 States and the District of Columbia.
[2] Male only.
[3] Female only.
[4] Excludes data from States lacking an Hispanic-origin item on their death certificates. See Appendix I, National Vital Statistics System.

NOTES: Rates are age adjusted to the 1940 U.S. standard million population. See Appendix II, Age adjustment. For data years shown, code numbers for cause of death are based on the current revision of *International Classification of Diseases*. See Appendix II, tables IV, V. Categories for coding human immunodeficiency virus infection deaths were introduced in the United States in 1987. The race groups, white, black, Asian or Pacific Islander, and American Indian or Alaska Native, include persons of Hispanic and non-Hispanic origin. Conversely, persons of Hispanic origin may be of any race. Bias in death rates results from inconsistent race identification between the death certificate (source of data for numerator of death rates) and data from the Census Bureau (denominator); and from undercounts of some population groups in the census. The net effects of misclassification and under coverage result in death rates estimated to be overstated by 1 percent for the white population and 5 percent for the black population; and death rates estimated to be understated by 21 percent for American Indians, 11 percent for Asians, and 2 percent for Hispanics (Rosenberg HM, Maurer JD, Sorlie PD, Johnson NJ, et al. Quality of death rates by race and Hispanic origin: A summary of current research, 1999. National Center for Health Statistics. Vital Health Stat 2(128). 1999). Data for additional years are available (see Appendix III).

SOURCES: Centers for Disease Control and Prevention, National Center for Health Statistics: Grove, RD, Hetzel, AM. *Vital statistics rates in the United States, 1940–1960.* Washington: U.S. Government Printing Office. 1968; *Vital statistics of the United States, vol II, mortality, part A,* for data years 1960–93. Public Health Service. Washington. U.S. Government Printing Office; for 1994–98, data for all persons, white, and black are available on the NCHS Web site at www.cdc.gov/nchs/datawh/statab/unpubd/mortabs.htm; numerator data from National Vital Statistics System, annual mortality files; denominator data from table 1 and unpublished Hispanic population estimates prepared by the Housing and Household Economic Statistics Division, U.S. Bureau of the Census.

[Data are based on the National Vital Statistics System]

Sex, race, Hispanic origin, and cause of death	Crude			Age adjusted[1]				
	1980	1990	1998	1980	1990	1996	1997	1998
All persons	Years lost before age 75 per 100,000 population under 75 years of age							
All causes	10,267.6	8,997.0	7,733.3	9,813.5	8,518.3	7,748.0	7,398.4	7,229.4
Diseases of heart	2,065.3	1,517.6	1,343.2	1,877.5	1,363.0	1,222.6	1,190.2	1,155.5
Ischemic heart disease	1,454.3	942.1	757.5	1,307.4	834.8	704.9	670.2	637.4
Cerebrovascular diseases	332.9	246.2	233.0	302.9	221.1	210.2	207.1	201.2
Malignant neoplasms	1,932.4	1,863.4	1,715.9	1,815.2	1,713.9	1,554.2	1,523.5	1,490.0
Trachea, bronchus, and lung	496.8	516.7	457.8	456.9	466.7	406.2	393.6	385.6
Colorectal	175.8	153.4	142.9	158.5	137.3	123.5	123.3	121.8
Prostate[2]	78.8	89.5	67.6	67.2	76.6	64.6	59.7	57.4
Breast[3]	408.5	416.5	357.5	393.0	381.9	324.3	314.3	301.8
Chronic obstructive pulmonary diseases	164.5	182.5	187.5	141.4	156.9	161.1	158.9	158.1
Pneumonia and influenza	156.4	139.9	122.8	149.1	128.5	114.5	112.6	110.8
Chronic liver disease and cirrhosis	254.1	178.4	159.2	259.1	168.8	145.7	141.7	138.1
Diabetes mellitus	124.6	147.0	174.1	115.1	133.0	153.5	149.9	150.3
Human immunodeficiency virus infection	- - -	391.2	177.2	- - -	366.2	401.9	208.7	163.6
Unintentional injuries	1,688.7	1,221.2	1,051.6	1,688.3	1,263.0	1,136.5	1,115.2	1,103.4
Motor vehicle-related injuries	1,017.6	752.4	596.4	1,010.8	788.8	680.8	661.1	646.3
Suicide	401.6	404.8	365.4	402.8	405.9	387.8	378.0	371.5
Homicide and legal intervention	459.5	452.3	307.1	460.9	466.4	394.7	368.9	337.2
White male								
All causes	12,454.3	10,629.4	8,972.8	11,877.4	10,064.6	8,980.1	8,533.2	8,352.0
Diseases of heart	2,907.1	2,058.7	1,782.0	2,681.9	1,856.8	1,623.5	1,576.7	1,517.1
Ischemic heart disease	2,241.0	1,416.9	1,121.0	2,060.2	1,269.3	1,044.7	990.1	939.5
Cerebrovascular diseases	309.0	222.9	216.5	280.2	198.6	194.4	189.8	185.9
Malignant neoplasms	2,087.1	1,970.9	1,803.9	1,939.8	1,793.9	1,620.7	1,576.4	1,553.6
Trachea, bronchus, and lung	709.2	669.7	560.3	647.9	600.0	501.0	479.8	467.9
Colorectal	194.2	174.7	160.9	176.2	155.7	138.8	137.5	135.9
Prostate	72.6	85.0	61.9	59.1	68.3	56.3	51.5	49.4
Chronic obstructive pulmonary diseases	219.3	208.9	199.9	187.1	177.2	167.5	169.3	166.0
Pneumonia and influenza	156.0	143.3	124.4	147.4	130.5	115.1	116.1	110.3
Chronic liver disease and cirrhosis	306.4	233.5	229.7	307.9	219.1	205.1	200.8	196.9
Diabetes mellitus	114.7	141.0	173.9	107.4	127.5	153.0	143.4	148.6
Human immunodeficiency virus infection	- - -	589.3	164.8	- - -	544.3	448.0	200.7	149.1
Unintentional injuries	2,553.8	1,766.9	1,484.5	2,523.6	1,821.5	1,591.5	1,561.2	1,560.2
Motor vehicle-related injuries	1,579.9	1,085.4	816.9	1,549.8	1,134.9	933.1	897.1	889.3
Suicide	663.0	694.0	630.3	656.4	692.2	665.7	644.7	638.9
Homicide and legal intervention	455.2	384.7	264.4	452.6	391.6	327.7	314.5	287.7
Black male								
All causes	21,081.4	20,744.8	15,998.7	22,338.5	21,250.2	18,994.6	17,373.4	16,626.0
Diseases of heart	3,383.9	2,769.2	2,564.4	4,179.5	3,338.2	2,969.9	2,918.1	2,856.2
Ischemic heart disease	1,805.9	1,249.8	1,088.3	2,283.2	1,561.4	1,326.2	1,308.8	1,241.0
Cerebrovascular diseases	714.1	546.4	495.1	870.2	655.6	583.0	578.8	547.2
Malignant neoplasms	2,495.1	2,444.5	2,137.0	3,070.6	3,021.7	2,576.8	2,517.0	2,438.9
Trachea, bronchus, and lung	853.7	842.5	660.9	1,087.0	1,077.4	849.2	800.4	775.3
Colorectal	176.1	188.6	193.7	215.9	234.0	225.6	229.1	221.1
Prostate	136.9	143.7	124.0	159.1	177.6	160.2	154.6	149.2
Chronic obstructive pulmonary diseases	223.3	241.4	237.5	258.7	278.7	266.7	250.8	260.4
Pneumonia and influenza	467.1	399.2	273.4	492.6	416.8	328.4	291.7	285.6
Chronic liver disease and cirrhosis	610.1	390.5	234.9	791.8	461.4	293.5	265.3	254.3
Diabetes mellitus	199.8	263.0	330.0	245.5	317.8	357.4	380.2	369.3
Human immunodeficiency virus infection	- - -	1,622.4	1,027.0	- - -	1,625.8	2,270.3	1,288.0	1,017.0
Unintentional injuries	2,934.4	2,308.7	1,935.4	2,931.3	2,265.6	1,983.7	1,925.4	1,930.9
Motor vehicle-related injuries	1,289.2	1,163.1	980.2	1,281.2	1,143.1	997.1	987.6	984.1
Suicide	415.7	482.3	406.4	428.1	478.0	465.6	443.1	414.8
Homicide and legal intervention	2,872.4	3,197.7	1,969.7	2,939.9	3,096.6	2,448.4	2,251.2	2,000.0

See footnotes at end of table.

[Data are based on the National Vital Statistics System]

Sex, race, Hispanic origin, and cause of death	Crude			Age adjusted[1]				
	1980	1990	1998	1980	1990	1996	1997	1998
American Indian or Alaska Native male[4]	Years lost before age 75 per 100,000 population under 75 years of age							
All causes	16,368.1	11,879.5	11,173.0	16,915.2	12,125.2	11,607.8	11,907.9	11,701.5
Diseases of heart	1,667.6	1,287.0	1,376.2	2,299.7	1,660.5	1,564.5	1,616.5	1,614.8
Ischemic heart disease	1,024.5	712.6	698.4	1,511.6	985.1	965.7	1,007.5	854.3
Cerebrovascular diseases	190.2	160.3	167.4	256.4	194.1	234.2	196.2	199.1
Malignant neoplasms	661.4	725.2	917.7	912.9	948.4	1,030.9	1,261.7	1,095.3
Trachea, bronchus, and lung	146.5	196.3	263.4	222.7	278.2	347.1	351.5	336.3
Colorectal	44.9	53.1	90.2	64.6	68.9	103.6	135.5	110.3
Prostate	34.2	22.5	30.4	53.1	33.5	58.3	36.4	40.8
Chronic obstructive pulmonary diseases	78.2	100.3	150.1	106.2	128.2	99.1	200.1	178.2
Pneumonia and influenza	343.1	230.2	213.3	370.1	227.5	274.9	249.0	221.2
Chronic liver disease and cirrhosis	943.9	445.9	582.7	1,259.9	530.2	555.6	586.7	638.2
Diabetes mellitus	183.1	191.6	372.8	255.3	256.1	360.0	358.1	449.7
Human immunodeficiency virus infection	- - -	130.2	131.1	- - -	130.3	264.8	139.7	130.9
Unintentional injuries	5,731.6	3,600.0	2,891.3	5,509.9	3,508.2	3,130.9	3,107.1	2,865.9
Motor vehicle-related injuries	3,329.6	2,095.9	1,697.5	3,146.2	2,047.2	1,925.0	1,786.1	1,682.8
Suicide	984.6	968.2	947.8	921.0	945.1	867.0	913.0	941.0
Homicide and legal intervention	1,029.4	778.2	643.5	1,003.6	754.5	677.3	731.5	638.2
Asian or Pacific Islander male[5]								
All causes	6,131.1	5,414.5	4,653.1	6,342.7	5,638.0	5,101.5	4,944.2	4,718.5
Diseases of heart	1,027.0	740.6	775.2	1,237.1	877.9	873.7	855.5	816.0
Ischemic heart disease	697.6	413.4	434.0	863.6	507.1	493.2	485.7	464.0
Cerebrovascular diseases	201.0	176.2	204.7	238.4	208.1	219.3	224.9	215.7
Malignant neoplasms	969.1	965.7	1,011.2	1,160.1	1,132.1	1,031.3	1,062.2	1,061.3
Trachea, bronchus, and lung	230.0	180.4	194.2	293.6	230.6	210.8	225.0	213.9
Colorectal	84.1	85.6	102.1	104.8	103.7	89.1	103.0	106.5
Prostate	10.3	18.6	14.5	12.9	25.0	21.9	16.7	16.9
Chronic obstructive pulmonary diseases	67.1	61.6	66.9	76.8	77.7	88.3	75.7	72.6
Pneumonia and influenza	94.1	72.2	74.9	93.9	79.4	75.5	78.9	77.3
Chronic liver disease and cirrhosis	94.7	84.8	57.1	112.1	95.7	61.8	59.9	57.0
Diabetes mellitus	63.6	60.2	82.2	76.6	74.1	98.5	85.9	89.2
Human immunodeficiency virus infection	- - -	145.8	48.5	- - -	134.5	133.0	54.7	44.5
Unintentional injuries	1,196.8	986.7	667.4	1,143.8	957.1	788.6	755.2	681.9
Motor vehicle-related injuries	732.6	657.3	407.5	699.8	634.9	477.7	425.7	419.1
Suicide	320.0	336.5	324.2	308.9	320.5	324.6	324.1	327.5
Homicide and legal intervention	317.1	347.5	235.2	304.4	330.7	323.8	291.9	240.0
Hispanic male[6]								
All causes	- - -	10,217.2	7,612.8	- - -	10,469.6	8,861.4	8,054.4	7,996.6
Diseases of heart	- - -	897.3	812.8	- - -	1,301.8	1,124.6	1,079.4	1,068.4
Ischemic heart disease	- - -	483.5	421.0	- - -	759.4	631.2	596.6	590.4
Cerebrovascular diseases	- - -	168.7	195.4	- - -	228.9	233.5	228.9	240.4
Malignant neoplasms	- - -	810.1	819.8	- - -	1,131.3	1,042.3	1,041.3	1,059.0
Trachea, bronchus, and lung	- - -	153.1	134.5	- - -	244.1	202.4	189.7	192.0
Colorectal	- - -	64.1	74.0	- - -	98.7	91.8	98.8	103.5
Prostate	- - -	22.0	27.4	- - -	37.8	44.4	35.9	42.5
Chronic obstructive pulmonary diseases	- - -	54.6	62.3	- - -	74.8	72.2	73.2	78.5
Pneumonia and influenza	- - -	139.4	105.4	- - -	152.5	119.0	118.0	116.7
Chronic liver disease and cirrhosis	- - -	340.2	287.3	- - -	454.0	377.9	350.7	354.2
Diabetes mellitus	- - -	107.2	138.7	- - -	160.0	204.0	200.9	194.8
Human immunodeficiency virus infection	- - -	964.3	313.8	- - -	972.6	869.6	434.1	317.3
Unintentional injuries	- - -	2,120.1	1,640.3	- - -	1,972.7	1,632.1	1,551.3	1,613.4
Motor vehicle-related injuries	- - -	1,305.0	893.6	- - -	1,202.0	922.9	872.0	878.7
Suicide	- - -	450.2	361.4	- - -	434.3	413.3	383.7	363.5
Homicide and legal intervention	- - -	1,466.4	800.6	- - -	1,330.1	949.7	841.0	781.4

See footnotes at end of table.

[Data are based on the National Vital Statistics System]

Sex, race, Hispanic origin, and cause of death	Crude			Age adjusted[1]				
	1980	1990	1998	1980	1990	1996	1997	1998
White, non-Hispanic male[6]	Years lost before age 75 per 100,000 population under 75 years of age							
All causes	---	10,530.0	9,039.5	---	9,803.6	8,744.4	8,407.2	8,206.0
Diseases of heart	---	2,175.5	1,910.4	---	1,877.0	1,643.2	1,607.4	1,543.7
Ischemic heart disease	---	1,515.2	1,217.1	---	1,294.4	1,065.8	1,018.1	964.2
Cerebrovascular diseases	---	228.8	216.5	---	195.0	185.9	183.9	176.7
Malignant neoplasms	---	2,102.1	1,937.1	---	1,835.5	1,651.4	1,610.1	1,583.8
Trachea, bronchus, and lung	---	728.5	621.2	---	621.5	519.8	500.9	487.6
Colorectal	---	187.9	172.7	---	159.8	141.5	139.8	137.8
Prostate	---	92.8	66.6	---	70.4	56.8	52.4	49.5
Chronic obstructive pulmonary diseases	---	227.2	219.2	---	183.2	172.0	175.8	170.9
Pneumonia and influenza	---	141.3	125.0	---	125.3	110.9	113.3	107.0
Chronic liver disease and cirrhosis	---	219.1	215.4	---	198.2	183.8	181.6	176.6
Diabetes mellitus	---	144.7	176.9	---	125.9	147.5	137.8	144.2
Human immunodeficiency virus infection	---	531.4	136.7	---	485.9	384.0	164.1	122.0
Unintentional injuries	---	1,689.9	1,432.7	---	1,769.3	1,549.9	1,540.1	1,524.2
Motor vehicle-related injuries	---	1,041.9	791.4	---	1,111.0	914.2	889.4	876.9
Suicide	---	719.4	662.8	---	720.9	692.1	676.5	673.0
Homicide and legal intervention	---	239.2	173.3	---	242.3	200.3	204.4	184.2
White female								
All causes	6,655.6	5,740.0	5,320.2	6,185.7	5,225.3	4,899.9	4,821.5	4,750.6
Diseases of heart	1,142.1	864.1	769.5	915.3	689.3	637.1	626.2	610.0
Ischemic heart disease	758.1	521.1	420.3	584.8	399.6	352.2	332.0	318.5
Cerebrovascular diseases	275.0	200.1	185.6	231.4	165.4	157.3	153.2	149.0
Malignant neoplasms	1,774.6	1,760.8	1,634.2	1,595.5	1,528.7	1,403.1	1,379.3	1,336.8
Trachea, bronchus, and lung	295.3	382.7	380.3	258.1	319.2	304.6	298.7	295.4
Colorectal	165.1	133.2	120.9	137.5	109.5	96.8	97.6	95.6
Breast	418.8	420.7	349.3	390.0	373.0	308.5	298.9	285.5
Chronic obstructive pulmonary diseases	117.4	164.6	182.6	94.8	128.9	142.0	140.1	138.8
Pneumonia and influenza	103.6	92.3	92.8	97.0	81.8	79.8	79.0	80.1
Chronic liver disease and cirrhosis	145.2	95.5	90.9	138.7	84.6	77.1	76.3	74.8
Diabetes mellitus	108.0	121.8	134.7	91.4	101.0	110.9	111.1	108.4
Human immunodeficiency virus infection	---	43.4	30.6	---	41.8	73.2	38.5	29.0
Unintentional injuries	793.0	610.1	576.7	816.8	654.1	634.9	627.6	621.0
Motor vehicle-related injuries	525.0	426.7	368.4	539.1	464.8	434.7	428.0	411.4
Suicide	193.0	166.1	154.4	196.1	165.3	153.6	155.3	152.7
Homicide and legal intervention	132.0	117.2	93.5	136.1	123.5	111.1	101.2	101.6
Black female								
All causes	11,795.1	10,966.0	9,429.8	11,863.1	10,662.7	10,012.6	9,475.2	9,282.7
Diseases of heart	2,020.0	1,665.2	1,563.4	2,189.5	1,756.0	1,636.2	1,534.8	1,541.3
Ischemic heart disease	987.7	711.9	618.9	1,078.5	762.1	682.3	636.6	611.6
Cerebrovascular diseases	600.9	458.3	421.4	656.7	481.2	422.9	419.4	411.2
Malignant neoplasms	1,855.8	1,893.9	1,844.9	2,085.5	2,041.9	1,845.0	1,837.9	1,818.3
Trachea, bronchus, and lung	260.3	328.7	331.8	300.2	364.3	323.1	331.8	330.7
Colorectal	162.6	164.4	160.7	179.2	178.3	160.8	153.2	159.1
Breast	382.8	465.4	468.8	448.6	505.6	484.0	472.7	455.0
Chronic obstructive pulmonary diseases	109.0	149.0	184.6	116.3	157.4	187.4	172.2	182.8
Pneumonia and influenza	252.3	214.2	178.4	245.2	206.1	177.2	177.9	175.2
Chronic liver disease and cirrhosis	323.8	193.2	102.8	378.0	203.4	119.8	113.2	98.8
Diabetes mellitus	248.3	279.1	315.3	271.6	299.0	329.5	318.3	314.3
Human immunodeficiency virus infection	---	427.1	454.5	---	402.5	757.5	492.1	432.1
Unintentional injuries	898.9	767.7	694.3	876.0	748.3	751.9	734.6	690.0
Motor vehicle-related injuries	362.9	381.2	364.4	354.7	376.7	396.9	400.4	368.5
Suicide	88.3	90.0	69.1	91.2	89.0	74.7	74.5	70.0
Homicide and legal intervention	605.3	619.7	395.2	593.1	596.5	470.5	422.2	400.8

See footnotes at end of table.

Table 31 (page 4 of 5). **Years of potential life lost before age 75 for selected causes of death, according to sex, detailed race, and Hispanic origin: United States, selected years 1980–98**

[Data are based on the National Vital Statistics System]

Sex, race, Hispanic origin, and cause of death	Crude			Age adjusted[1]				
	1980	1990	1998	1980	1990	1996	1997	1998
American Indian or Alaska Native female[4]	Years lost before age 75 per 100,000 population under 75 years of age							
All causes	9,077.4	6,086.8	6,606.3	9,126.7	6,192.2	6,797.2	6,563.6	6,765.4
Diseases of heart	714.8	647.0	653.0	870.8	753.2	738.7	754.3	712.2
Ischemic heart disease	323.4	299.7	286.0	442.1	381.1	376.3	365.1	329.8
Cerebrovascular diseases	158.3	167.1	163.4	204.2	191.7	194.6	218.5	183.7
Malignant neoplasms	775.0	860.2	954.8	980.9	1,012.8	1,105.9	1,035.1	1,042.5
Trachea, bronchus, and lung	60.6	138.1	166.5	85.4	176.6	175.2	170.5	190.7
Colorectal	45.8	56.2	80.6	63.9	68.3	85.7	87.0	89.6
Breast	125.9	150.1	167.1	173.5	178.3	210.0	154.7	179.7
Chronic obstructive pulmonary diseases	*	80.1	92.0	*	94.2	110.1	119.1	104.8
Pneumonia and influenza	216.4	152.9	206.5	210.9	154.4	141.1	128.1	203.9
Chronic liver disease and cirrhosis	681.0	381.8	425.5	842.4	415.9	428.0	423.1	435.5
Diabetes mellitus	190.5	186.6	238.3	260.4	233.0	317.8	306.4	270.9
Human immunodeficiency virus infection	- - -	*	*	- - -	*	*	*	*
Unintentional injuries	2,170.7	1,185.9	1,341.1	2,056.6	1,155.4	1,350.9	1,302.8	1,336.6
Motor vehicle-related injuries	1,486.8	778.5	940.8	1,412.6	772.9	924.6	844.2	942.7
Suicide	211.6	153.9	236.0	212.9	152.8	243.1	164.0	241.1
Homicide and legal intervention	342.9	226.8	216.0	345.9	219.8	211.8	223.4	212.1
Asian or Pacific Islander female[5]								
All causes	3,893.8	3,264.7	2,918.4	3,918.3	3,308.2	2,949.8	2,992.2	2,852.1
Diseases of heart	378.1	318.1	307.4	420.4	343.0	318.8	322.5	301.3
Ischemic heart disease	167.1	148.3	137.1	200.5	164.1	139.0	143.8	134.9
Cerebrovascular diseases	192.2	175.3	145.7	215.6	190.0	158.6	168.0	141.6
Malignant neoplasms	870.0	847.0	903.6	949.9	893.7	886.9	863.2	865.3
Trachea, bronchus, and lung	97.3	106.3	124.0	112.1	117.3	103.9	118.6	120.1
Colorectal	79.7	69.7	76.4	89.9	75.7	77.5	72.5	73.0
Breast	175.7	173.1	196.2	190.0	182.0	164.1	170.4	183.0
Chronic obstructive pulmonary diseases	22.1	47.4	38.9	23.2	50.4	52.8	42.2	38.5
Pneumonia and influenza	49.6	59.6	55.0	52.3	60.7	45.8	47.4	54.3
Chronic liver disease and cirrhosis	34.0	30.3	21.9	39.6	32.2	18.8	19.1	20.5
Diabetes mellitus	53.1	44.5	56.4	62.6	50.2	61.4	60.7	56.2
Human immunodeficiency virus infection	- - -	*	*	*	*	18.2	*	*
Unintentional injuries	486.4	419.6	315.5	481.7	424.0	349.5	412.5	332.2
Motor vehicle-related injuries	338.1	325.0	227.0	333.1	328.3	246.4	293.7	239.3
Suicide	159.2	114.7	107.1	151.0	111.3	116.5	118.6	103.8
Homicide and legal intervention	131.0	117.9	83.9	124.8	113.0	97.4	94.8	85.2
Hispanic female[6]								
All causes	- - -	4,753.5	3,957.0	- - -	4,662.3	4,211.1	4,114.5	3,942.8
Diseases of heart	- - -	442.2	396.6	- - -	556.9	458.9	466.2	466.1
Ischemic heart disease	- - -	219.8	188.0	- - -	297.0	241.9	242.3	234.0
Cerebrovascular diseases	- - -	151.9	137.4	- - -	182.8	155.1	155.8	155.7
Malignant neoplasms	- - -	828.7	790.7	- - -	1,014.7	942.3	936.4	911.3
Trachea, bronchus, and lung	- - -	63.3	65.0	- - -	85.4	80.6	87.7	80.1
Colorectal	- - -	54.4	50.8	- - -	70.9	64.8	63.7	61.2
Breast	- - -	201.4	181.0	- - -	254.2	220.2	221.7	210.4
Chronic obstructive pulmonary diseases	- - -	50.6	46.7	- - -	61.6	58.0	58.4	53.3
Pneumonia and influenza	- - -	93.0	68.5	- - -	87.7	74.8	79.3	66.9
Chronic liver disease and cirrhosis	- - -	93.1	71.9	- - -	115.7	95.5	95.2	83.4
Diabetes mellitus	- - -	103.4	126.7	- - -	137.0	164.2	167.9	156.4
Human immunodeficiency virus infection	- - -	152.9	86.8	- - -	146.0	224.2	114.4	87.9
Unintentional injuries	- - -	556.5	496.0	- - -	526.1	520.7	505.9	485.6
Motor vehicle-related injuries	- - -	382.4	330.9	- - -	368.1	355.6	348.6	329.2
Suicide	- - -	89.8	70.0	- - -	88.4	84.8	66.7	72.3
Homicide and legal intervention	- - -	227.5	135.5	- - -	214.0	158.8	142.5	130.9

See footnotes at end of table.

[Data are based on the National Vital Statistics System]

Sex, race, Hispanic origin, and cause of death	Crude			Age adjusted[1]				
	1980	1990	1998	1980	1990	1996	1997	1998.
White, non-Hispanic female[6]	Years lost before age 75 per 100,000 population under 75 years of age							
All causes	- - -	5,788.3	5,449.9	- - -	5,189.9	4,874.5	4,814.2	4,766.9
Diseases of heart	- - -	902.4	816.7	- - -	691.9	643.8	636.7	619.0
Ischemic heart disease	- - -	549.4	450.6	- - -	402.7	356.9	337.8	323.9
Cerebrovascular diseases	- - -	205.5	190.4	- - -	163.4	155.6	151.2	146.1
Malignant neoplasms	- - -	1,861.9	1,742.8	- - -	1,563.0	1,429.5	1,404.2	1,363.6
Trachea, bronchus, and lung	- - -	418.4	424.3	- - -	335.7	321.0	314.8	312.7
Colorectal	- - -	142.6	130.1	- - -	112.6	98.6	99.9	98.1
Breast	- - -	444.4	371.0	- - -	381.3	313.4	303.0	290.4
Chronic obstructive pulmonary diseases	- - -	176.9	201.3	- - -	132.5	147.0	145.2	144.8
Pneumonia and influenza	- - -	90.2	95.2	- - -	78.1	78.0	76.6	79.8
Chronic liver disease and cirrhosis	- - -	95.6	92.6	- - -	82.0	74.9	73.5	73.3
Diabetes mellitus	- - -	123.2	133.8	- - -	98.9	105.7	105.4	103.5
Human immunodeficiency virus infection	- - -	29.1	21.0	- - -	28.2	51.2	27.6	20.0
Unintentional injuries	- - -	607.4	580.7	- - -	661.1	637.3	639.6	635.3
Motor vehicle-related injuries	- - -	425.1	369.1	- - -	470.9	436.7	436.0	420.6
Suicide	- - -	172.6	165.5	- - -	170.9	159.8	165.8	162.4
Homicide and legal intervention	- - -	102.3	85.1	- - -	108.3	99.5	92.0	94.0

- - - Data not available.

* Based on fewer than 20 deaths.

[1]Rates are age adjusted to the 1940 U.S. standard million population. See Appendix II, Age adjustment.

[2]Male only.

[3]Female only.

[4]Interpretation of trends should take into account that population estimates for American Indians increased by 45 percent between 1980 and 1990, partly due to better enumeration techniques in the 1990 decennial census and to the increased tendency for people to identify themselves as American Indian in 1990.

[5]Interpretation of trends should take into account that the Asian population in the United States more than doubled between 1980 and 1990, primarily due to immigration.

[6]Excludes data from States lacking an Hispanic-origin item on their death certificates. See Appendix I, National Vital Statistics System.

NOTES: For data years shown, the code numbers for cause of death are based on the *International Classification of Diseases, Ninth Revision*, described in Appendix II, table V. Categories for coding human immunodeficiency virus infection were introduced in the United States in 1987. Years of potential life lost (YPLL) before age 75 provides a measure of the impact of mortality on the population under 75 years of age. These data are presented as YPLL–75 because the average life expectancy in the United States is over 75 years. YPLL–65 was calculated in *Health, United States, 1995* and earlier editions. See Appendix II, YPLL, for method of calculation. The race groups, white, black, Asian or Pacific Islander, and American Indian or Alaska Native, include persons of Hispanic and non-Hispanic origin. Conversely, persons of Hispanic origin may be of any race. Bias in death rates results from inconsistent race identification between the death certificate (source of data for numerator of death rates) and data from the Census Bureau (denominator); and from undercounts of some population groups in the census. The net effects of misclassification and under coverage result in death rates estimated to be overstated by 1 percent for the white population and 5 percent for the black population; and death rates estimated to be understated by 21 percent for American Indians, 11 percent for Asians, and 2 percent for Hispanics (Rosenberg HM, Maurer JD, Sorlie PD, Johnson NJ, et al. Quality of death rates by race and Hispanic origin: A summary of current research, 1999. National Center for Health Statistics. Vital Health Stat 2(128). 1999). YPLL rates may also be similarly affected. Data for additional years are available (see Appendix III).

SOURCES: Centers for Disease Control and Prevention, National Center for Health Statistics. *Vital statistics of the United States, vol II, mortality, part A*, for data years 1950–93. Public Health Service. Washington. U.S. Government Printing Office; for 1994–98, unpublished data; data computed by the Division of Health and Utilization Analysis from numerator data compiled by the Division of Vital Statistics and denominator data from unrounded national population estimates for race groups from table 1 and unpublished Hispanic population estimates prepared by the Housing and Household Economic Statistics Division, U.S. Bureau of the Census.

Table 32 (page 1 of 4). Leading causes of death and numbers of deaths, according to sex, detailed race, and Hispanic origin: United States, 1980 and 1998

[Data are based on the National Vital Statistics System]

Sex, race, Hispanic origin, and rank order	1980 Cause of death	1980 Deaths	1998 Cause of death	1998 Deaths
All persons				
...	All causes	1,989,841	All causes	2,337,256
1.	Diseases of heart	761,085	Diseases of heart	724,859
2.	Malignant neoplasms	416,509	Malignant neoplasms	541,532
3.	Cerebrovascular diseases	170,225	Cerebrovascular diseases	158,448
4.	Unintentional injuries	105,718	Chronic obstructive pulmonary diseases	112,584
5.	Chronic obstructive pulmonary diseases	56,050	Unintentional injuries	97,835
6.	Pneumonia and influenza	54,619	Pneumonia and influenza	91,871
7.	Diabetes mellitus	34,851	Diabetes mellitus	64,751
8.	Chronic liver disease and cirrhosis	30,583	Suicide	30,575
9.	Atherosclerosis	29,449	Nephritis, nephrotic syndrome, and nephrosis	26,182
10.	Suicide	26,869	Chronic liver disease and cirrhosis	25,192
Male				
...	All causes	1,075,078	All causes	1,157,260
1.	Diseases of heart	405,661	Diseases of heart	353,897
2.	Malignant neoplasms	225,948	Malignant neoplasms	282,065
3.	Unintentional injuries	74,180	Unintentional injuries	63,042
4.	Cerebrovascular diseases	69,973	Cerebrovascular diseases	61,145
5.	Chronic obstructive pulmonary diseases	38,625	Chronic obstructive pulmonary diseases	57,018
6.	Pneumonia and influenza	27,574	Pneumonia and influenza	40,979
7.	Suicide	20,505	Diabetes mellitus	29,584
8.	Chronic liver disease and cirrhosis	19,768	Suicide	24,538
9.	Homicide and legal intervention	19,088	Chronic liver disease and cirrhosis	16,343
10.	Diabetes mellitus	14,325	Homicide and legal intervention	14,023
Female				
...	All causes	914,763	All causes	1,179,996
1.	Diseases of heart	355,424	Diseases of heart	370,962
2.	Malignant neoplasms	190,561	Malignant neoplasms	259,467
3.	Cerebrovascular diseases	100,252	Cerebrovascular diseases	97,303
4.	Unintentional injuries	31,538	Chronic obstructive pulmonary diseases	55,566
5.	Pneumonia and influenza	27,045	Pneumonia and influenza	50,892
6.	Diabetes mellitus	20,526	Diabetes mellitus	35,167
7.	Atherosclerosis	17,848	Unintentional injuries	34,793
8.	Chronic obstructive pulmonary diseases	17,425	Alzheimer's disease	15,671
9.	Chronic liver disease and cirrhosis	10,815	Nephritis, nephrotic syndrome, and nephrosis	13,621
10.	Certain conditions originating in the perinatal period	9,815	Septicemia	13,506
White				
...	All causes	1,738,607	All causes	2,015,984
1.	Diseases of heart	683,347	Diseases of heart	635,549
2.	Malignant neoplasms	368,162	Malignant neoplasms	470,139
3.	Cerebrovascular diseases	148,734	Cerebrovascular diseases	136,855
4.	Unintentional injuries	90,122	Chronic obstructive pulmonary diseases	104,061
5.	Chronic obstructive pulmonary diseases	52,375	Unintentional injuries	82,178
6.	Pneumonia and influenza	48,369	Pneumonia and influenza	81,659
7.	Diabetes mellitus	28,868	Diabetes mellitus	51,706
8.	Atherosclerosis	27,069	Suicide	27,648
9.	Chronic liver disease and cirrhosis	25,240	Chronic liver disease and cirrhosis	21,771
10.	Suicide	24,829	Nephritis, nephrotic syndrome, and nephrosis	21,369
Black				
...	All causes	233,135	All causes	278,440
1.	Diseases of heart	72,956	Diseases of heart	78,294
2.	Malignant neoplasms	45,037	Malignant neoplasms	61,193
3.	Cerebrovascular diseases	20,135	Cerebrovascular diseases	18,237
4.	Unintentional injuries	13,480	Unintentional injuries	12,801
5.	Homicide and legal intervention	10,283	Diabetes mellitus	11,378
6.	Certain conditions originating in the perinatal period	6,961	Homicide and legal intervention	8,420
7.	Pneumonia and influenza	5,648	Pneumonia and influenza	8,326
8.	Diabetes mellitus	5,544	Chronic obstructive pulmonary diseases	7,205
9.	Chronic liver disease and cirrhosis	4,790	Human immunodeficiency virus infection	7,180
10.	Nephritis, nephrotic syndrome, and nephrosis	3,416	Certain conditions originating in the perinatal period	4,841

See footnotes at end of table.

[Data are based on the National Vital Statistics System]

Sex, race, Hispanic origin, and rank order	1980		1998	
	Cause of death	Deaths	Cause of death	Deaths
American Indian or Alaska Native				
...	All causes	6,923	All causes	10,845
1.............	Diseases of heart	1,494	Diseases of heart	2,383
2.............	Unintentional injuries	1,290	Malignant neoplasms	1,834
3.............	Malignant neoplasms	770	Unintentional injuries	1,292
4.............	Chronic liver disease and cirrhosis	410	Diabetes mellitus	645
5.............	Cerebrovascular diseases	322	Cerebrovascular diseases	497
6.............	Pneumonia and influenza	257	Chronic liver disease and cirrhosis	467
7.............	Homicide and legal intervention	219	Pneumonia and influenza	389
8.............	Diabetes mellitus	210	Chronic obstructive pulmonary diseases	369
9.............	Certain conditions originating in the perinatal period	199	Suicide	310
10.............	Suicide	181	Homicide and legal intervention	228
Asian or Pacific Islander				
...	All causes	11,071	All causes	31,987
1.............	Diseases of heart	3,265	Diseases of heart	8,633
2.............	Malignant neoplasms	2,522	Malignant neoplasms	8,366
3.............	Cerebrovascular diseases	1,028	Cerebrovascular diseases	2,859
4.............	Unintentional injuries	810	Unintentional injuries	1,564
5.............	Pneumonia and influenza	342	Pneumonia and influenza	1,497
6.............	Suicide	249	Diabetes mellitus	1,022
7.............	Certain conditions originating in the perinatal period	246	Chronic obstructive pulmonary diseases	949
8.............	Diabetes mellitus	227	Suicide	640
9.............	Homicide and legal intervention	211	Homicide and legal intervention	383
10.............	Chronic obstructive pulmonary diseases	207	Nephritis, nephrotic syndrome, and nephrosis	335
Hispanic				
...	---	---	All causes	98,406
1.............	---		Diseases of heart	24,596
2.............	---		Malignant neoplasms	19,528
3.............	---		Unintentional injuries	8,248
4.............	---		Cerebrovascular diseases	5,587
5.............	---		Diabetes mellitus	4,741
6.............	---		Pneumonia and influenza	3,277
7.............	---		Homicide and legal intervention	2,978
8.............	---		Chronic liver disease and cirrhosis	2,845
9.............	---		Chronic obstructive pulmonary diseases	2,528
10.............	---		Certain conditions originating in the perinatal period	1,987
White male				
...	All causes	933,878	All causes	990,190
1.............	Diseases of heart	364,679	Diseases of heart	309,952
2.............	Malignant neoplasms	198,188	Malignant neoplasms	244,109
3.............	Unintentional injuries	62,963	Unintentional injuries	52,398
4.............	Cerebrovascular diseases	60,095	Chronic obstructive pulmonary diseases	52,172
5.............	Chronic obstructive pulmonary diseases	35,977	Cerebrovascular diseases	51,766
6.............	Pneumonia and influenza	23,810	Pneumonia and influenza	35,795
7.............	Suicide	18,901	Diabetes mellitus	24,249
8.............	Chronic liver disease and cirrhosis	16,407	Suicide	22,174
9.............	Diabetes mellitus	12,125	Chronic liver disease and cirrhosis	14,096
10.............	Atherosclerosis	10,543	Nephritis, nephrotic syndrome, and nephrosis	10,406
Black male				
...	All causes	130,138	All causes	143,417
1.............	Diseases of heart	37,877	Diseases of heart	37,662
2.............	Malignant neoplasms	25,861	Malignant neoplasms	32,523
3.............	Unintentional injuries	9,701	Unintentional injuries	8,788
4.............	Cerebrovascular diseases	9,194	Cerebrovascular diseases	7,765
5.............	Homicide and legal intervention	8,385	Homicide and legal intervention	6,873
6.............	Certain conditions originating in the perinatal period	3,869	Human immunodeficiency virus infection	4,994
7.............	Pneumonia and influenza	3,386	Diabetes mellitus	4,511
8.............	Chronic liver disease and cirrhosis	3,020	Pneumonia and influenza	4,178
9.............	Chronic obstructive pulmonary diseases	2,429	Chronic obstructive pulmonary diseases	4,039
10.............	Diabetes mellitus	2,010	Certain conditions originating in the perinatal period	2,732

See footnotes at end of table.

[Data are based on the National Vital Statistics System]

Sex, race, Hispanic origin, and rank order	1980		1998	
	Cause of death	Deaths	Cause of death	Deaths
American Indian or Alaska Native male				
. . .	All causes	4,193	All causes	5,994
1.	Unintentional injuries	946	Diseases of heart	1,322
2.	Diseases of heart	917	Malignant neoplasms	941
3.	Malignant neoplasms	408	Unintentional injuries	867
4.	Chronic liver disease and cirrhosis	239	Diabetes mellitus	308
5.	Homicide and legal intervention	164	Chronic liver disease and cirrhosis	278
6.	Cerebrovascular diseases	163	Suicide	246
7.	Pneumonia and influenza	148	Chronic obstructive pulmonary diseases	207
8.	Suicide	147	Pneumonia and influenza	197
9.	Certain conditions originating in the perinatal period	107	Cerebrovascular diseases	194
10.	Diabetes mellitus	86	Homicide and legal intervention	170
Asian or Pacific Islander male				
. . .	All causes	6,809	All causes	17,659
1.	Diseases of heart	2,174	Diseases of heart	4,961
2.	Malignant neoplasms	1,485	Malignant neoplasms	4,492
3.	Unintentional injuries	556	Cerebrovascular diseases	1,420
4.	Cerebrovascular diseases	521	Unintentional injuries	989
5.	Pneumonia and influenza	227	Pneumonia and influenza	809
6.	Suicide	159	Chronic obstructive pulmonary diseases	600
7.	Chronic obstructive pulmonary diseases	158	Diabetes mellitus	516
8.	Homicide and legal intervention	151	Suicide	459
9.	Certain conditions originating in the perinatal period	128	Homicide and legal intervention	273
10.	Diabetes mellitus	103	Certain conditions originating in the perinatal period	172
Hispanic male				
. . .	. . .	. . .	All causes	55,821
1.	. . .	. . .	Diseases of heart	12,932
2.	. . .	. . .	Malignant neoplasms	10,465
3.	. . .	. . .	Unintentional injuries	6,229
4.	. . .	. . .	Cerebrovascular diseases	2,646
5.	. . .	. . .	Homicide and legal intervention	2,544
6.	. . .	. . .	Diabetes mellitus	2,203
7.	. . .	. . .	Chronic liver disease and cirrhosis	2,096
8.	. . .	. . .	Pneumonia and influenza	1,657
9.	. . .	. . .	Suicide	1,429
10.	. . .	. . .	Chronic obstructive pulmonary diseases	1,422
White female				
. . .	All causes	804,729	All causes	1,025,794
1.	Diseases of heart	318,668	Diseases of heart	325,597
2.	Malignant neoplasms	169,974	Malignant neoplasms	226,030
3.	Cerebrovascular diseases	88,639	Cerebrovascular diseases	85,089
4.	Unintentional injuries	27,159	Chronic obstructive pulmonary diseases	51,889
5.	Pneumonia and influenza	24,559	Pneumonia and influenza	45,864
6.	Diabetes mellitus	16,743	Unintentional injuries	29,780
7.	Atherosclerosis	16,526	Diabetes mellitus	27,457
8.	Chronic obstructive pulmonary diseases	16,398	Alzheimer's disease	14,723
9.	Chronic liver disease and cirrhosis	8,833	Nephritis, nephrotic syndrome, and nephrosis	10,963
10.	Certain conditions originating in the perinatal period	6,512	Septicemia	10,741
Black female				
. . .	All causes	102,997	All causes	135,023
1.	Diseases of heart	35,079	Diseases of heart	40,632
2.	Malignant neoplasms	19,176	Malignant neoplasms	28,670
3.	Cerebrovascular diseases	10,941	Cerebrovascular diseases	10,472
4.	Unintentional injuries	3,779	Diabetes mellitus	6,867
5.	Diabetes mellitus	3,534	Pneumonia and influenza	4,148
6.	Certain conditions originating in the perinatal period	3,092	Unintentional injuries	4,013
7.	Pneumonia and influenza	2,262	Chronic obstructive pulmonary diseases	3,166
8.	Homicide and legal intervention	1,898	Septicemia	2,564
9.	Chronic liver disease and cirrhosis	1,770	Nephritis, nephrotic syndrome, and nephrosis	2,400
10.	Nephritis, nephrotic syndrome, and nephrosis	1,722	Human immunodeficiency virus infection	2,186

See footnotes at end of table.

Table 32 (page 4 of 4). **Leading causes of death and numbers of deaths, according to sex, detailed race, and Hispanic origin: United States, 1980 and 1998**

[Data are based on the National Vital Statistics System]

Sex, race, Hispanic origin, and rank order	1980		1998	
	Cause of death	Deaths	Cause of death	Deaths
American Indian or Alaska Native female				
. . .	All causes	2,730	All causes	4,851
1.	Diseases of heart	577	Diseases of heart	1,061
2.	Malignant neoplasms	362	Malignant neoplasms	893
3.	Unintentional injuries	344	Unintentional injuries	425
4.	Chronic liver disease and cirrhosis	171	Diabetes mellitus	337
5.	Cerebrovascular diseases	159	Cerebrovascular diseases	303
6.	Diabetes mellitus	124	Pneumonia and influenza	192
7.	Pneumonia and influenza	109	Chronic liver disease and cirrhosis	189
8.	Certain conditions originating in the perinatal period	92	Chronic obstructive pulmonary diseases	162
9.	Nephritis, nephrotic syndrome, and nephrosis	56	Nephritis, nephrotic syndrome, and nephrosis	86
10.	Homicide and legal intervention	55	Septicemia	68
Asian or Pacific Islander female				
. . .	All causes	4,262	All causes	14,328
1.	Diseases of heart	1,091	Malignant neoplasms	3,874
2.	Malignant neoplasms	1,037	Diseases of heart	3,672
3.	Cerebrovascular diseases	507	Cerebrovascular diseases	1,439
4.	Unintentional injuries	254	Pneumonia and influenza	688
5.	Diabetes mellitus	124	Unintentional injuries	575
6.	Certain conditions originating in the perinatal period	118	Diabetes mellitus	506
7.	Pneumonia and influenza	115	Chronic obstructive pulmonary diseases	349
8.	Congenital anomalies	104	Suicide	181
9.	Suicide	90	Nephritis, nephrotic syndrome, and nephrosis	172
10.	Homicide and legal intervention	60	Certain conditions originating in the perinatal period	156
Hispanic female				
. . .	- - -	- - -	All causes	42,585
1.	- - -	- - -	Diseases of heart	11,664
2.	- - -	- - -	Malignant neoplasms	9,063
3.	- - -	- - -	Cerebrovascular diseases	2,941
4.	- - -	- - -	Diabetes mellitus	2,538
5.	- - -	- - -	Unintentional injuries	2,019
6.	- - -	- - -	Pneumonia and influenza	1,620
7.	- - -	- - -	Chronic obstructive pulmonary diseases	1,106
8.	- - -	- - -	Certain conditions originating in the perinatal period	864
9.	- - -	- - -	Chronic liver disease and cirrhosis	749
10.	- - -	- - -	Congenital anomalies	722

. . . Category not applicable.
- - - Data not available.

NOTES: For data years shown, the code numbers for cause of death are based on the *International Classification of Diseases, 9th Revision*, described in Appendix II, table V. Categories for the coding and classification of human immunodeficiency virus infection were introduced in the United States beginning with mortality data for 1987.

SOURCES: Centers for Disease Control and Prevention, National Center for Health Statistics. *Vital statistics of the United States, vol II, mortality, part A*, 1980. Washington: Public Health Service. 1985; Murphy SL. Deaths: Final data for 1998. National vital statistics reports; vol 48. Hyattsville, Maryland: 2000; and data computed by the Division of Health and Utilization Analysis from data compiled by the Division of Vital Statistics.

Table 33 (page 1 of 2). Leading causes of death and numbers of deaths, according to age: United States, 1980 and 1998

[Data are based on the National Vital Statistics System]

Age and rank order	1980		1998	
	Cause of death	Deaths	Cause of death	Deaths
Under 1 year				
. . .	All causes	45,526	All causes	28,371
1.	Congenital anomalies	9,220	Congenital anomalies	6,212
2.	Sudden infant death syndrome	5,510	Disorders relating to short gestation and unspecified low birthweight	4,101
3.	Respiratory distress syndrome	4,989	Sudden infant death syndrome	2,822
4.	Disorders relating to short gestation and unspecified low birthweight	3,648	Newborn affected by maternal complications of pregnancy	1,343
5.	Newborn affected by maternal complications of pregnancy	1,572	Respiratory distress syndrome	1,295
6.	Intrauterine hypoxia and birth asphyxia	1,497	Newborn affected by complications of placenta, cord, and membranes	961
7.	Unintentional injuries	1,166	Infections specific to the perinatal period	815
8.	Birth trauma	1,058	Unintentional injuries	754
9.	Pneumonia and influenza	1,012	Intrauterine hypoxia and birth asphyxia	461
10.	Newborn affected by complications of placenta, cord, and membranes	985	Pneumonia and influenza	441
1–4 years				
. . .	All causes	8,187	All causes	5,251
1.	Unintentional injuries	3,313	Unintentional injuries	1,935
2.	Congenital anomalies	1,026	Congenital anomalies	564
3.	Malignant neoplasms	573	Homicide and legal intervention	399
4.	Diseases of heart	338	Malignant neoplasms	365
5.	Homicide and legal intervention	319	Diseases of heart	214
6.	Pneumonia and influenza	267	Pneumonia and influenza	146
7.	Meningitis	223	Septicemia	89
8.	Meningococcal infection	110	Certain conditions originating in the perinatal period	75
9.	Certain conditions originating in the perinatal period	84	Cerebrovascular diseases	57
10.	Septicemia	71	Benign neoplasms	53
5–14 years				
. . .	All causes	10,689	All causes	7,791
1.	Unintentional injuries	5,224	Unintentional injuries	3,254
2.	Malignant neoplasms	1,497	Malignant neoplasms	1,013
3.	Congenital anomalies	561	Homicide and legal intervention	460
4.	Homicide and legal intervention	415	Congenital anomalies	371
5.	Diseases of heart	330	Diseases of heart	326
6.	Pneumonia and influenza	194	Suicide	324
7.	Suicide	142	Chronic obstructive pulmonary diseases	152
8.	Benign neoplasms	104	Pneumonia and influenza	121
9.	Cerebrovascular diseases	95	Benign neoplasms	84
10.	Chronic obstructive pulmonary diseases	85	Cerebrovascular diseases	82
15–24 years				
. . .	All causes	49,027	All causes	30,627
1.	Unintentional injuries	26,206	Unintentional injuries	13,349
2.	Homicide and legal intervention	6,647	Homicide and legal intervention	5,506
3.	Suicide	5,239	Suicide	4,135
4.	Malignant neoplasms	2,683	Malignant neoplasms	1,699
5.	Diseases of heart	1,223	Diseases of heart	1,057
6.	Congenital anomalies	600	Congenital anomalies	450
7.	Cerebrovascular diseases	418	Chronic obstructive pulmonary diseases	239
8.	Pneumonia and influenza	348	Pneumonia and influenza	215
9.	Chronic obstructive pulmonary diseases	141	Human immunodeficiency virus infection	194
10.	Anemias	133	Cerebrovascular diseases	178

See footnotes at end of table.

Table 33 (page 2 of 2). Leading causes of death and numbers of deaths, according to age: United States, 1980 and 1998

[Data are based on the National Vital Statistics System]

Age and rank order	1980		1998	
	Cause of death	Deaths	Cause of death	Deaths
25–44 years				
. . .	All causes	108,658	All causes	131,382
1.	Unintentional injuries	26,722	Unintentional injuries	27,172
2.	Malignant neoplasms	17,551	Malignant neoplasms	21,407
3.	Diseases of heart	14,513	Diseases of heart	16,800
4.	Homicide and legal intervention	11,136	Suicide	12,202
5.	Suicide	9,855	Human immunodeficiency virus infection	8,658
6.	Chronic liver disease and cirrhosis	4,782	Homicide and legal intervention	8,132
7.	Cerebrovascular diseases	3,154	Chronic liver disease and cirrhosis	3,876
8.	Diabetes mellitus	1,472	Cerebrovascular diseases	3,320
9. . . . . . . :	Pneumonia and influenza	1,467	Diabetes mellitus	2,521
10.	Congenital anomalies	817	Pneumonia and influenza	1,931
45–64 years				
. . .	All causes	425,338	All causes	380,203
1.	Diseases of heart	148,322	Malignant neoplasms	132,771
2.	Malignant neoplasms	135,675	Diseases of heart	100,124
3.	Cerebrovascular diseases	19,909	Unintentional injuries	18,286
4.	Unintentional injuries	18,140	Cerebrovascular diseases	15,362
5.	Chronic liver disease and cirrhosis	16,089	Diabetes mellitus	13,091
6.	Chronic obstructive pulmonary diseases	11,514	Chronic obstructive pulmonary diseases	12,990
7.	Diabetes mellitus	7,977	Chronic liver disease and cirrhosis	11,023
8.	Suicide	7,079	Suicide	8,094
9.	Pneumonia and influenza	5,804	Pneumonia and influenza	6,023
10.	Homicide and legal intervention	4,057	Human immunodeficiency virus infection	4,099
65 years and over				
. . .	All causes	1,341,848	All causes	1,753,220
1.	Diseases of heart	595,406	Diseases of heart	605,673
2.	Malignant neoplasms	258,389	Malignant neoplasms	384,186
3. . . . . , ...	Cerebrovascular diseases	146,417	Cerebrovascular diseases	139,144
4.	Pneumonia and influenza	45,512	Chronic obstructive pulmonary diseases	97,896
5.	Chronic obstructive pulmonary diseases	43,587	Pneumonia and influenza	82,989
6.	Atherosclerosis	28,081	Diabetes mellitus	48,974
7.	Diabetes mellitus	25,216	Unintentional injuries	32,975
8.	Unintentional injuries	24,844	Nephritis, nephrotic syndrome, and nephrosis	22,640
9.	Nephritis, nephrotic syndrome, and nephrosis	12,968	Alzheimer's disease	22,416
10.	Chronic liver disease and cirrhosis	9,519	Septicemia	19,012

. . . Category not applicable.

NOTES: For data years shown, the code numbers for cause of death are based on the *International Classification of Diseases, 9th Revision*, described in Appendix II, table V. Categories for the coding and classification of human immunodeficiency virus infection were introduced in the United States beginning with mortality data for 1987.

SOURCES: Centers for Disease Control and Prevention, National Center for Health Statistics. *Vital statistics of the United States, vol II, mortality, part A*, 1980. Washington: Public Health Service. 1985; Murphy SL. Deaths: Final data for 1998. National vital statistics reports; vol 48. Hyattsville, Maryland: 2000.

Table 34 (page 1 of 2). Age-adjusted death rates, according to race, sex, region, and urbanization: United States, average annual 1984–86, 1989–91, and 1995–97

[Data are based on the National Vital Statistics System]

Sex, region, and urbanization[1]	All races			White			Black		
	1984–86	1989–91	1995–97	1984–86	1989–91	1995–97	1984–86	1989–91	1995–97
Both sexes	Deaths per 100,000 resident population[2]								
All regions:									
Large core metropolitan	575.2	556.5	507.9	536.9	510.8	465.4	810.4	826.5	762.1
Large fringe metropolitan	511.5	474.1	447.1	504.0	464.6	437.8	710.5	691.7	655.9
Medium/small metropolitan	538.2	509.2	489.9	517.7	486.0	468.2	785.2	777.8	731.4
Urban nonmetropolitan	549.8	529.4	509.9	531.1	509.0	492.2	791.6	793.7	729.6
Rural	549.4	534.1	516.7	528.7	511.1	496.5	755.9	758.8	704.6
Northeast:									
Large core metropolitan	592.7	577.4	516.4	552.5	528.1	476.5	799.0	811.6	706.6
Large fringe metropolitan	515.2	472.4	442.6	509.2	464.7	437.5	694.6	670.8	606.0
Medium/small metropolitan	527.4	486.8	461.7	519.0	476.2	451.1	761.4	737.7	703.8
Urban nonmetropolitan	543.3	501.2	476.9	542.8	500.6	477.3	726.4	667.9	580.4
Rural	527.7	497.5	468.5	528.7	497.8	469.5	*	*	*
South:									
Large core metropolitan	587.5	577.7	536.1	522.8	500.5	458.5	834.7	857.8	826.2
Large fringe metropolitan	522.6	491.1	464.3	506.8	472.4	445.5	710.9	695.6	658.6
Medium/small metropolitan	559.4	534.7	517.8	522.6	494.6	481.8	797.5	792.2	742.8
Urban nonmetropolitan	594.4	579.4	563.0	560.0	542.4	532.2	799.9	803.7	743.9
Rural	595.7	583.8	570.1	566.8	553.5	545.7	757.8	759.1	710.2
Midwest:									
Large core metropolitan	600.9	582.4	549.2	544.9	512.1	478.9	824.8	841.3	795.9
Large fringe metropolitan	519.4	478.5	458.8	510.8	467.8	447.5	751.9	727.8	722.8
Medium/small metropolitan	522.1	490.4	473.2	510.0	475.3	457.2	752.8	748.2	733.9
Urban nonmetropolitan	503.8	484.4	465.1	501.5	481.1	462.3	718.3	721.0	623.3
Rural	503.4	488.0	469.7	493.6	475.4	457.9	704.1	782.8	558.1
West:									
Large core metropolitan	527.5	504.0	453.4	523.4	499.9	451.7	757.8	768.1	689.8
Large fringe metropolitan	475.9	445.2	413.9	479.9	448.0	415.4	661.2	661.8	645.7
Medium/small metropolitan	508.5	487.1	463.1	510.1	488.8	465.6	714.5	710.9	608.8
Urban nonmetropolitan	515.3	493.8	467.3	508.7	486.4	462.0	654.1	660.3	477.1
Rural	502.6	468.6	435.0	502.1	465.2	433.5	*	*	*
Male									
All regions:									
Large core metropolitan	757.7	733.5	651.5	707.5	671.9	595.4	1,092.0	1,130.3	1,012.3
Large fringe metropolitan	664.1	607.8	555.7	655.4	595.6	543.8	918.7	899.6	830.0
Medium/small metropolitan	709.8	663.5	621.8	685.5	633.7	593.9	1,029.6	1,035.8	952.8
Urban nonmetropolitan	729.7	695.0	648.9	707.8	669.7	626.6	1,042.4	1,054.4	952.3
Rural	730.3	704.7	660.9	704.7	675.2	635.1	1,005.9	1,016.6	920.0
Northeast:									
Large core metropolitan	784.9	767.6	664.9	730.3	699.5	611.8	1,095.2	1,127.6	946.5
Large fringe metropolitan	671.2	607.9	554.1	663.8	597.8	547.7	910.3	881.3	772.3
Medium/small metropolitan	697.0	635.0	586.0	686.6	621.3	572.9	996.3	982.0	897.8
Urban nonmetropolitan	712.7	652.1	598.9	713.1	652.2	599.9	868.0	808.6	685.9
Rural	696.7	651.2	579.1	699.0	651.3	579.8	*	*	*
South:									
Large core metropolitan	778.7	772.0	694.6	693.6	668.2	593.1	1,124.5	1,179.1	1,105.9
Large fringe metropolitan	683.6	636.4	581.2	664.4	611.9	556.8	926.3	915.0	842.2
Medium/small metropolitan	742.2	702.4	663.3	697.4	649.6	616.4	1,053.6	1,066.2	979.9
Urban nonmetropolitan	800.1	772.2	728.3	760.2	725.6	689.0	1,064.3	1,082.9	983.5
Rural	799.1	778.8	735.5	764.2	740.2	703.6	1,011.1	1,021.8	933.2
Midwest:									
Large core metropolitan	798.5	769.5	710.2	725.8	674.0	616.9	1,107.7	1,147.9	1,064.0
Large fringe metropolitan	674.9	611.2	568.1	664.9	598.2	554.4	957.4	929.9	900.8
Medium/small metropolitan	689.7	638.2	599.7	675.5	619.2	579.4	974.4	979.6	943.6
Urban nonmetropolitan	667.9	635.4	590.5	665.7	632.1	587.7	880.0	874.5	779.0
Rural	666.2	639.7	600.6	653.9	624.4	585.9	891.7	945.5	655.2
West:									
Large core metropolitan	684.5	652.2	573.7	679.9	646.9	570.2	994.0	1,011.4	875.7
Large fringe metropolitan	607.8	561.4	506.2	613.8	565.4	507.6	810.0	812.3	768.1
Medium/small metropolitan	657.4	620.9	574.9	661.6	624.4	577.2	881.1	874.2	727.4
Urban nonmetropolitan	661.0	624.5	574.6	653.2	615.4	567.4	782.9	763.5	532.4
Rural	646.2	596.0	538.0	646.4	590.4	537.1	*	*	*

See footnotes at end of table.

Table 34 (page 2 of 2). **Age-adjusted death rates, according to race, sex, region, and urbanization: United States, average annual 1984–86, 1989–91, and 1995–97**

[Data are based on the National Vital Statistics System]

Sex, region, and urbanization[1]	All races			White			Black		
	1984–86	1989–91	1995–97	1984–86	1989–91	1995–97	1984–86	1989–91	1995–97
Female	Deaths per 100,000 resident population[2]								
All regions:									
Large core metropolitan	432.6	413.5	389.1	403.7	379.9	356.7	599.4	598.2	571.4
Large fringe metropolitan	391.1	367.3	357.3	384.9	360.2	350.1	544.3	526.3	514.9
Medium/small metropolitan	402.6	385.4	380.4	385.3	367.6	363.6	597.9	580.6	559.6
Urban nonmetropolitan	402.6	393.3	391.0	386.4	376.6	376.8	598.1	594.9	556.5
Rural	391.6	385.4	386.3	374.8	367.4	370.4	550.4	551.1	528.3
Northeast:									
Large core metropolitan	446.7	428.3	397.8	417.1	392.6	367.2	589.3	585.4	531.9
Large fringe metropolitan	395.3	367.0	352.3	390.5	361.4	348.2	527.6	507.3	474.8
Medium/small metropolitan	398.9	372.8	361.8	392.3	365.1	353.7	575.4	545.3	543.4
Urban nonmetropolitan	408.0	379.9	373.9	407.2	379.2	374.3	592.0	532.7	460.4
Rural	383.7	366.8	369.9	383.5	367.0	371.2	*	*	*
South:									
Large core metropolitan	436.5	420.2	405.0	386.9	362.9	345.8	617.0	616.0	614.1
Large fringe metropolitan	392.5	372.4	365.7	379.1	358.2	351.2	539.7	523.9	511.9
Medium/small metropolitan	414.5	399.7	397.6	383.1	368.9	369.4	605.6	587.8	564.4
Urban nonmetropolitan	428.4	423.7	424.7	397.2	392.8	399.1	600.1	596.6	563.2
Rural	421.7	417.3	423.9	397.2	392.6	404.2	550.8	549.2	529.9
Midwest:									
Large core metropolitan	451.7	438.3	421.6	410.7	389.0	370.6	610.0	611.5	592.8
Large fringe metropolitan	398.8	375.2	370.9	391.5	366.8	361.8	586.8	565.3	577.0
Medium/small metropolitan	394.0	375.7	372.2	383.8	364.0	360.0	578.4	567.5	565.7
Urban nonmetropolitan	371.5	361.9	359.3	369.1	358.9	356.8	575.5	585.1	482.9
Rural	360.7	355.1	350.4	353.4	345.2	341.6	*	*	493.9
West:									
Large core metropolitan	398.8	377.2	348.1	395.2	373.3	346.3	564.9	565.2	532.3
Large fringe metropolitan	368.9	348.9	334.7	371.5	351.0	336.0	525.6	519.5	528.4
Medium/small metropolitan	380.7	370.5	362.1	381.3	371.3	364.5	551.3	552.7	490.9
Urban nonmetropolitan	384.3	376.0	366.4	379.8	370.8	363.2	521.7	566.7	414.1
Rural	364.6	345.9	332.9	363.6	345.2	330.9	*	*	*

* Data for groups with population under 5,000 in the middle year of a 3-year period are considered unreliable and are not shown.
[1]Urbanization categories for county of residence of decedent are based on a modification of the rural-urban continuum codes, a 1993 classification of counties by the Department of Agriculture. See Appendix II, Urbanization.
[2]Average annual death rate.

NOTES: Rates are age adjusted to the 1940 U.S. standard million population. See Appendix II, Age adjustment. Denominators for rates are population estimates for the middle year of each 3-year period multiplied by 3.

SOURCE: Centers for Disease Control and Prevention, National Center for Health Statistics. Compressed Mortality File. See Appendix I, National Vital Statistics System.

Table 35. Age-adjusted death rates for persons 25–64 years of age for selected causes of death, according to sex and educational attainment: Selected States, 1994–98

[Data are based on the National Vital Statistics System]

Cause of death and year	Both sexes Years of educational attainment[1]			Male Years of educational attainment[1]			Female Years of educational attainment[1]		
	Less than 12	12	13 or more	Less than 12	12	13 or more	Less than 12	12	13 or more
All causes				Deaths per 100,000 population					
1994	571.0	486.1	243.4	762.6	679.2	309.9	379.8	327.6	173.3
1995	581.2	491.7	240.4	770.5	684.9	303.0	391.3	332.4	174.5
1996	556.0	472.4	230.4	733.0	642.6	287.2	379.4	328.9	171.4
1997	531.7	453.6	221.6	690.9	608.0	270.4	370.3	322.3	171.1
1998	538.3	445.6	213.1	698.7	599.5	259.3	377.6	315.9	165.5
Chronic and noncommunicable diseases									
1994	415.8	360.0	183.2	529.8	476.5	216.2	307.2	271.6	147.1
1995	420.4	362.9	181.7	531.6	479.3	212.2	314.2	274.4	147.9
1996	408.6	355.1	178.7	519.3	460.0	209.9	303.8	272.7	145.1
1997	395.9	348.9	177.2	497.3	447.9	207.0	299.1	269.7	145.4
1998	401.8	343.1	171.0	504.9	443.7	199.8	303.9	263.4	140.5
Injury and adverse effects									
1994	98.7	75.3	32.1	153.2	121.6	46.0	40.3	32.6	18.1
1995	99.6	76.3	31.8	153.4	122.8	45.6	41.5	33.1	18.0
1996	94.8	74.9	32.1	143.0	118.6	45.7	42.1	33.6	18.5
1997	95.4	75.4	32.0	142.2	118.7	45.7	42.4	34.4	18.5
1998	96.4	75.4	31.3	143.1	118.2	44.6	44.9	34.7	18.4
Communicable diseases									
1994	56.5	50.8	28.1	79.7	81.2	47.9	32.2	23.3	8.1
1995	61.3	52.5	27.0	85.5	82.9	45.3	35.7	24.8	8.6
1996	52.6	42.4	19.5	70.7	63.9	31.4	33.4	22.6	7.7
1997	40.4	29.2	12.4	51.4	41.4	17.6	28.7	18.2	7.2
1998	40.0	27.1	10.8	50.7	37.7	15.0	28.8	17.8	6.7
HIV infection:									
1994	36.3	36.3	21.0	54.2	62.3	38.9	17.2	12.4	2.9
1995	39.9	37.7	20.1	58.7	63.6	36.9	19.6	13.8	3.4
1996	31.8	27.5	12.7	44.9	44.8	23.1	17.5	11.2	2.4
1997	19.3	14.1	5.7	25.9	22.6	9.9	12.0	6.2	1.6
1998	17.1	11.5	4.1	22.9	17.8	7.2	10.7	5.7	1.1
Other communicable diseases:									
1994	20.2	14.5	7.1	25.5	18.8	8.9	15.0	10.9	5.2
1995	21.4	14.8	6.9	26.8	19.3	8.4	16.0	11.0	5.2
1996	20.8	14.9	6.8	25.8	19.1	8.3	16.0	11.4	5.3
1997	21.1	15.1	6.7	25.4	18.9	7.7	16.8	12.0	5.7
1998	22.9	15.7	6.7	27.9	19.9	7.8	18.1	12.2	5.7

[1]Educational attainment for the numerator is based on the death certificate item "highest grade completed." Educational attainment for the denominator is based on answers to the Current Population Survey question "What is the highest level of school completed or highest degree received?" (Kominski R, Adams A. Educational Attainment in the United States: March 1993 and 1992, U.S. Bureau of the Census, Current Population Reports, P20–476, Washington, DC. 1994.)

NOTES: Rates are age adjusted to the 1940 U.S. standard million population. See Appendix II, Age adjustment. Code numbers for cause of death are based on the *International Classification of Diseases, 9th Revision.* See Appendix II, table V. Based on data from 45 States and the District of Columbia (DC) in 1994–96 and 46 States and DC in 1997–98. See Appendix I. Death records with education not stated are not included in the calculation of age-adjusted death rates shown in this table. Percent not stated averages 3–9 percent of the deaths comprising the age-adjusted death rates for causes of death in this table. Misreporting of education on the death certificate tends to overstate the death rate for high school graduates (12 years of education) because there is a tendency for some people who did not graduate from high school to be reported as high school graduates on the death certificate; by extension, the death rate for the group with less than 12 years of education tends to be understated. Data for the elderly population are not shown because percent with education not stated is somewhat higher for this group and because of possible bias due to misreporting of education on the death certificate. (Sorlie PD, Johnson NJ: Validity of education information on the death certificate, *Epidemiology* 7(4):437–439, 1996.)

SOURCES: Centers for Disease Control and Prevention, National Center for Health Statistics. National Vital Statistics System; denominator data from unpublished population estimates prepared by the Housing and Household Economic Statistics Division, U.S. Bureau of the Census.

Table 36 (page 1 of 4). Death rates for all causes, according to sex, detailed race, Hispanic origin, and age: United States, selected years 1950–98

[Data are based on the National Vital Statistics System]

Sex, race, Hispanic origin, and age	1950[1]	1960[1]	1970	1980	1985	1990	1996	1997	1998	1996–98[2]
All persons				Deaths per 100,000 resident population						
All ages, age adjusted	841.5	760.9	714.3	585.8	548.9	520.2	491.6	479.1	471.7	480.7
All ages, crude	963.8	954.7	945.3	878.3	876.9	863.8	872.5	864.7	864.7	867.3
Under 1 year	3,299.2	2,696.4	2,142.4	1,288.3	1,088.1	971.9	755.7	738.7	751.3	748.5
1–4 years	139.4	109.1	84.5	63.9	51.8	46.8	38.3	35.8	34.6	36.3
5–14 years	60.1	46.6	41.3	30.6	26.5	24.0	21.7	20.8	19.9	20.8
15–24 years	128.1	106.3	127.7	115.4	94.9	99.2	89.6	86.2	82.3	86.0
25–34 years	178.7	146.4	157.4	135.5	124.4	139.2	126.7	115.0	109.6	117.2
35–44 years	358.7	299.4	314.5	227.9	207.7	223.2	221.3	203.2	199.6	207.9
45–54 years	853.9	756.0	730.0	584.0	519.3	473.4	445.9	430.8	423.5	433.1
55–64 years	1,901.0	1,735.1	1,658.8	1,346.3	1,294.2	1,196.9	1,094.1	1,063.6	1,030.7	1,062.2
65–74 years	4,104.3	3,822.1	3,582.7	2,994.9	2,862.8	2,648.6	2,538.4	2,509.8	2,495.1	2,514.5
75–84 years	9,331.1	8,745.2	8,004.4	6,692.6	6,398.7	6,007.2	5,803.1	5,728.2	5,703.2	5,744.1
85 years and over	20,196.9	19,857.5	16,344.9	15,980.3	15,712.4	15,327.4	15,327.2	15,345.2	15,111.7	15,258.4
Male										
All ages, age adjusted	1,001.6	949.3	931.6	777.2	723.0	680.2	623.7	602.8	589.4	605.1
All ages, crude	1,106.1	1,104.5	1,090.3	976.9	948.6	918.4	896.4	880.8	876.4	884.5
Under 1 year	3,728.0	3,059.3	2,410.0	1,428.5	1,219.9	1,082.8	828.0	812.8	818.2	819.7
1–4 years	151.7	119.5	93.2	72.6	58.5	52.4	42.2	39.7	37.6	39.8
5–14 years	70.9	55.7	50.5	36.7	31.8	28.5	25.4	24.0	23.4	24.3
15–24 years	167.9	152.1	188.5	172.3	138.9	147.4	130.6	124.0	119.3	124.6
25–34 years	216.5	187.9	215.3	196.1	179.6	204.3	178.6	160.1	151.7	163.7
35–44 years	428.8	372.8	402.6	299.2	278.9	310.4	298.1	265.7	258.5	274.0
45–54 years	1,067.1	992.2	958.5	767.3	671.6	610.3	573.8	550.5	542.8	555.3
55–64 years	2,395.3	2,309.5	2,282.7	1,815.1	1,711.4	1,553.4	1,388.7	1,336.6	1,296.9	1,339.8
65–74 years	4,931.4	4,914.4	4,873.8	4,105.2	3,856.3	3,491.5	3,233.4	3,191.2	3,143.7	3,189.6
75–84 years	10,426.0	10,178.4	10,010.2	8,816.7	8,501.6	7,888.6	7,249.8	7,116.1	7,019.2	7,126.1
85 years and over	21,636.0	21,186.3	17,821.5	18,801.1	18,614.1	18,056.6	17,547.7	17,461.9	16,763.3	17,242.9
Female										
All ages, age adjusted	688.4	590.6	532.5	432.6	410.3	390.6	381.0	375.7	372.5	376.3
All ages, crude	823.5	809.2	807.8	785.3	809.1	812.0	849.7	849.2	853.5	850.8
Under 1 year	2,854.6	2,321.3	1,863.7	1,141.7	950.6	855.7	680.0	661.1	681.3	674.1
1–4 years	126.7	98.4	75.4	54.7	44.8	41.0	34.3	31.8	31.4	32.5
5–14 years	48.9	37.3	31.8	24.2	21.0	19.3	17.8	17.4	16.2	17.1
15–24 years	89.1	61.3	68.1	57.5	49.6	49.0	46.2	46.3	43.5	45.3
25–34 years	142.7	106.6	101.6	75.9	69.4	74.2	74.7	69.9	68.1	70.9
35–44 years	290.3	229.4	231.1	159.3	138.7	137.9	145.4	141.4	141.5	142.7
45–54 years	641.5	526.7	517.2	412.9	375.2	342.7	323.3	316.1	309.6	316.2
55–64 years	1,404.8	1,196.4	1,098.9	934.3	925.6	878.8	826.7	815.2	788.4	809.7
65–74 years	3,333.2	2,871.8	2,579.7	2,144.7	2,096.9	1,991.2	1,979.0	1,959.0	1,967.7	1,968.6
75–84 years	8,399.6	7,633.1	6,677.6	5,440.1	5,162.1	4,883.1	4,868.3	4,820.5	4,831.9	4,840.0
85 years and over	19,194.7	19,008.4	15,518.0	14,746.9	14,553.9	14,274.3	14,444.7	14,492.3	14,427.4	14,454.6
White male										
All ages, age adjusted	963.1	917.7	893.4	745.3	693.3	644.3	591.4	573.8	562.4	575.7
All ages, crude	1,089.5	1,098.5	1,086.7	983.3	963.6	930.9	918.1	906.3	904.4	909.5
Under 1 year	3,400.5	2,694.1	2,113.2	1,230.3	1,056.5	896.1	683.3	678.1	673.8	678.4
1–4 years	135.5	104.9	83.6	66.1	52.8	45.9	37.1	35.1	32.5	34.9
5–14 years	67.2	52.7	48.0	35.0	30.1	26.4	23.2	22.1	21.2	22.2
15–24 years	152.4	143.7	170.8	167.0	134.2	131.3	113.9	109.0	107.6	110.2
25–34 years	185.3	163.2	176.6	171.3	158.8	176.1	154.8	140.3	133.9	143.2
35–44 years	380.9	332.6	343.5	257.4	243.1	268.2	259.6	235.3	232.7	242.5
45–54 years	984.5	932.2	882.9	698.9	611.7	548.7	515.5	495.8	489.6	500.1
55–64 years	2,304.4	2,225.2	2,202.6	1,728.5	1,625.8	1,467.2	1,305.2	1,252.4	1,215.5	1,256.8
65–74 years	4,864.9	4,848.4	4,810.1	4,035.7	3,770.7	3,397.7	3,158.3	3,122.7	3,082.3	3,121.3
75–84 years	10,526.3	10,299.6	10,098.8	8,829.8	8,486.1	7,844.9	7,205.5	7,086.0	6,988.5	7,091.3
85 years and over	22,116.3	21,750.0	18,551.7	19,097.3	18,980.1	18,268.3	17,870.5	17,767.1	17,048.3	17,546.5

See footnotes at end of table.

[Data are based on the National Vital Statistics System]

Sex, race, Hispanic origin, and age	1950[1]	1960[1]	1970	1980	1985	1990	1996	1997	1998	1996–98[2]
Black male				Deaths per 100,000 resident population						
All ages, age adjusted	1,373.1	1,246.1	1,318.6	1,112.8	1,053.4	1,061.3	967.0	911.9	884.5	920.6
All ages, crude	1,260.3	1,181.7	1,186.6	1,034.1	989.3	1,008.0	939.9	893.9	877.7	903.6
Under 1 year	---	5,306.8	4,298.9	2,586.7	2,219.9	2,112.4	1,748.2	1,671.6	1,717.8	1,712.3
1–4 years	---	208.5	150.5	110.5	90.1	85.8	71.4	67.2	69.2	69.3
5–14 years	95.1	75.1	67.1	47.4	42.3	41.2	38.1	34.8	35.6	36.2
15–24 years	289.7	212.0	320.6	209.1	173.6	252.2	233.0	215.8	194.6	214.3
25–34 years	503.5	402.5	559.5	407.3	351.9	430.8	361.0	308.6	282.0	317.3
35–44 years	878.1	762.0	956.6	689.8	630.2	699.6	629.2	523.7	483.1	544.2
45–54 years	1,905.0	1,624.8	1,777.5	1,479.9	1,292.9	1,261.0	1,190.6	1,114.1	1,082.6	1,127.4
55–64 years	3,773.2	3,316.4	3,256.9	2,873.0	2,779.8	2,618.4	2,395.1	2,320.0	2,269.3	2,327.0
65–74 years	5,310.3	5,798.7	5,803.2	5,131.1	5,172.4	4,946.1	4,431.5	4,298.3	4,186.0	4,304.3
75–84 years	---	8,605.1	9,454.9	9,231.6	9,262.3	9,129.5	8,614.9	8,296.8	8,311.4	8,405.0
85 years and over	---	14,844.8	12,222.3	16,098.8	15,774.2	16,954.9	16,006.3	16,083.5	15,540.9	15,870.3
American Indian or Alaska Native male[3]										
All ages, age adjusted	---	---	---	732.5	602.6	573.1	555.9	584.1	564.9	568.4
All ages, crude	---	---	---	597.1	492.5	476.4	489.8	519.2	513.2	507.5
Under 1 year	---	---	---	1,598.1	1,080.0	1,056.6	874.4	903.0	1,028.1	935.6
1–4 years	---	---	---	82.7	105.3	77.4	72.9	51.6	64.7	63.1
5–14 years	---	---	---	43.7	39.2	33.4	37.8	28.7	29.5	32.0
15–24 years	---	---	---	311.1	214.4	219.8	174.7	180.3	166.4	173.7
25–34 years	---	---	---	360.6	275.0	256.1	260.0	245.4	235.1	246.9
35–44 years	---	---	---	556.8	363.5	365.4	370.0	389.3	373.6	377.6
45–54 years	---	---	---	871.3	687.9	619.9	580.2	673.4	664.2	640.4
55–64 years	---	---	---	1,547.5	1,319.1	1,211.3	1,348.0	1,409.6	1,376.9	1,378.5
65–74 years	---	---	---	2,968.4	2,692.3	2,461.7	2,640.7	2,847.2	2,682.8	2,723.5
75–84 years	---	---	---	5,607.0	5,572.7	5,389.2	4,633.8	4,796.3	4,471.3	4,630.0
85 years and over	---	---	---	12,635.2	8,900.0	11,243.9	7,686.7	7,888.1	8,486.2	8,031.3
Asian or Pacific Islander male[4]										
All ages, age adjusted	---	---	---	416.6	396.9	377.8	355.8	350.3	336.2	347.1
All ages, crude	---	---	---	375.3	344.6	334.3	350.7	351.7	349.8	350.7
Under 1 year	---	---	---	816.5	750.0	605.3	457.6	426.3	397.0	426.3
1–4 years	---	---	---	50.9	43.4	45.0	24.6	25.5	17.6	22.5
5–14 years	---	---	---	23.4	22.5	20.7	17.1	17.3	17.6	17.3
15–24 years	---	---	---	80.8	76.0	76.0	73.2	67.2	59.9	66.7
25–34 years	---	---	---	83.5	77.3	79.6	75.6	71.8	74.4	73.9
35–44 years	---	---	---	128.3	114.4	130.8	125.0	115.7	108.2	116.1
45–54 years	---	---	---	342.3	284.8	287.1	277.0	274.8	276.2	276.0
55–64 years	---	---	---	881.1	869.4	789.1	726.3	750.8	709.3	728.4
65–74 years	---	---	---	2,236.1	2,102.0	2,041.4	1,948.4	1,892.6	1,838.7	1,891.7
75–84 years	---	---	---	5,389.5	5,551.2	5,008.6	4,844.3	4,749.1	4,534.8	4,700.3
85 years and over	---	---	---	13,753.6	12,750.0	12,446.3	11,637.4	11,796.3	11,178.6	11,520.5
Hispanic male[5]										
All ages, age adjusted	---	---	---	---	524.8	531.2	474.8	447.7	442.7	454.6
All ages, crude	---	---	---	---	374.6	411.6	381.3	360.5	366.4	369.3
Under 1 year	---	---	---	---	1,041.8	921.8	686.2	654.3	678.5	672.9
1–4 years	---	---	---	---	53.8	53.8	37.3	34.1	33.1	34.8
5–14 years	---	---	---	---	23.0	26.0	23.5	18.7	20.2	20.8
15–24 years	---	---	---	---	147.5	159.3	140.3	129.1	128.8	132.7
25–34 years	---	---	---	---	202.0	234.0	175.0	154.5	148.4	159.4
35–44 years	---	---	---	---	290.3	341.8	279.7	235.7	226.6	246.6
45–54 years	---	---	---	---	495.4	533.9	493.7	456.1	449.3	465.6
55–64 years	---	---	---	---	1,129.2	1,123.7	1,032.0	957.8	966.3	984.4
65–74 years	---	---	---	---	2,488.9	2,368.2	2,245.4	2,251.7	2,284.9	2,261.2
75–84 years	---	---	---	---	5,724.6	5,369.1	4,966.4	4,750.3	4,564.6	4,749.0
85 years and over	---	---	---	---	11,856.1	12,272.1	10,617.7	10,487.1	9,946.7	10,331.6

See footnotes at end of table.

Table 36 (page 3 of 4). Death rates for all causes, according to sex, detailed race, Hispanic origin, and age: United States, selected years 1950–98

[Data are based on the National Vital Statistics System]

Sex, race, Hispanic origin, and age	1950[1]	1960[1]	1970	1980	1985	1990	1996	1997	1998	1996–98[2]
White, non-Hispanic male[5]					Deaths per 100,000 resident population					
All ages, age adjusted	---	---	---	---	669.7	643.1	589.5	575.3	563.6	576.0
All ages, crude	---	---	---	---	956.3	985.9	982.1	977.3	974.7	978.0
Under 1 year	---	---	---	---	1,002.5	865.4	654.6	662.4	651.5	656.2
1–4 years	---	---	---	---	48.8	43.8	36.2	34.8	31.8	34.3
5–14 years	---	---	---	---	28.9	25.7	22.5	22.4	21.0	22.0
15–24 years	---	---	---	---	125.0	123.4	105.6	102.7	101.2	103.2
25–34 years	---	---	---	---	151.2	165.3	147.2	134.8	128.1	136.9
35–44 years	---	---	---	---	231.8	257.1	252.3	231.4	229.7	237.7
45–54 years	---	---	---	---	587.6	544.5	509.0	494.0	487.2	496.5
55–64 years	---	---	---	---	1,550.8	1,479.7	1,308.7	1,264.7	1,224.0	1,264.8
65–74 years	---	---	---	---	3,648.0	3,434.5	3,181.1	3,154.6	3,112.5	3,149.5
75–84 years	---	---	---	---	8,364.2	7,920.4	7,274.5	7,154.7	7,072.8	7,165.0
85 years and over	---	---	---	---	18,637.2	18,505.4	18,110.1	18,066.9	17,363.4	17,831.7
White female										
All ages, age adjusted	645.0	555.0	501.7	411.1	391.0	369.9	361.9	358.0	355.2	358.3
All ages, crude	803.3	800.9	812.6	806.1	840.1	846.9	896.2	897.8	903.7	899.2
Under 1 year	2,566.8	2,007.7	1,614.6	962.5	799.3	690.0	558.0	546.0	563.6	555.9
1–4 years	112.2	85.2	66.1	49.3	40.0	36.1	28.5	28.0	27.5	28.0
5–14 years	45.1	34.7	29.9	22.9	19.5	17.9	16.4	15.6	15.0	15.7
15–24 years	71.5	54.9	61.6	55.5	48.1	45.9	42.7	43.8	41.2	42.5
25–34 years	112.8	85.0	84.1	65.4	59.4	61.5	62.7	60.0	58.5	60.4
35–44 years	235.8	191.1	193.3	138.2	121.9	117.4	121.6	120.9	122.0	121.5
45–54 years	546.4	458.8	462.9	372.7	341.7	309.3	290.5	285.0	278.3	284.5
55–64 years	1,293.8	1,078.9	1,014.9	876.2	869.1	822.7	779.5	766.3	740.6	761.8
65–74 years	3,242.8	2,779.3	2,470.7	2,066.6	2,027.1	1,923.5	1,919.8	1,900.5	1,912.9	1,911.1
75–84 years	8,481.5	7,696.6	6,698.7	5,401.7	5,111.6	4,839.1	4,826.5	4,786.3	4,792.7	4,801.6
85 years and over	19,679.5	19,477.7	15,980.2	14,979.6	14,745.4	14,400.6	14,642.9	14,681.4	14,620.4	14,647.9
Black female										
All ages, age adjusted	1,106.7	916.9	814.4	631.1	594.8	581.6	561.0	545.5	540.9	549.0
All ages, crude	1,002.0	905.0	829.2	733.3	734.2	747.9	753.5	742.8	746.4	747.5
Under 1 year	---	4,162.2	3,368.8	2,123.7	1,821.4	1,735.5	1,444.0	1,383.9	1,390.1	1,405.8
1–4 years	---	173.3	129.4	84.4	71.1	67.6	63.7	51.0	53.9	56.3
5–14 years	72.8	53.8	43.8	30.5	28.6	27.5	25.9	27.2	23.1	25.4
15–24 years	213.1	107.5	111.9	70.5	59.6	68.7	66.8	62.0	58.0	62.2
25–34 years	393.3	273.2	231.0	150.0	137.6	159.5	153.8	134.6	130.0	139.5
35–44 years	758.1	568.5	533.0	323.9	276.5	298.6	316.4	287.1	284.9	295.9
45–54 years	1,576.4	1,177.0	1,043.9	768.2	667.6	639.4	610.1	590.4	582.0	593.7
55–64 years	3,089.4	2,510.9	1,986.2	1,561.0	1,532.5	1,452.6	1,311.7	1,307.3	1,272.2	1,296.7
65–74 years	4,000.2	4,064.2	3,860.9	3,057.4	2,967.8	2,865.7	2,787.0	2,739.7	2,724.6	2,750.3
75–84 years	---	6,730.0	6,691.5	6,212.1	6,078.0	5,688.3	5,775.9	5,669.3	5,813.8	5,753.2
85 years and over	---	13,052.6	10,706.6	12,367.2	12,703.0	13,309.5	13,398.5	13,701.7	13,580.5	13,561.5
American Indian or Alaska Native female[3]										
All ages, age adjusted	---	---	---	414.1	353.3	335.1	367.7	359.9	363.3	363.5
All ages, crude	---	---	---	380.1	342.5	330.4	396.0	392.6	407.0	398.6
Under 1 year	---	---	---	1,352.6	910.5	688.7	718.2	646.1	825.0	730.0
1–4 years	---	---	---	87.5	54.8	37.8	67.1	66.8	53.5	62.5
5–14 years	---	---	---	33.5	23.0	25.5	23.7	22.2	19.6	21.8
15–24 years	---	---	---	90.3	72.8	69.0	62.5	57.5	64.1	61.4
25–34 years	---	---	---	178.5	121.5	102.3	108.9	116.3	118.3	114.5
35–44 years	---	---	---	286.0	185.6	156.4	196.3	195.6	195.1	195.7
45–54 years	---	---	---	491.4	415.5	380.9	435.4	387.4	388.3	403.1
55–64 years	---	---	---	837.1	851.9	805.9	862.2	866.9	863.6	864.3
65–74 years	---	---	---	1,765.5	1,630.3	1,679.4	1,878.8	1,920.5	1,932.4	1,910.9
75–84 years	---	---	---	3,612.9	3,200.0	3,073.2	3,657.1	3,531.6	3,440.5	3,539.9
85 years and over	---	---	---	8,567.4	7,740.0	8,201.1	6,193.5	5,773.6	6,366.9	6,113.7

See footnotes at end of table.

Table 36 (page 4 of 4). Death rates for all causes, according to sex, detailed race, Hispanic origin, and age: United States, selected years 1950–98

[Data are based on the National Vital Statistics System]

Sex, race, Hispanic origin, and age	1950[1]	1960[1]	1970	1980	1985	1990	1996	1997	1998	1996–98[2]
Asian or Pacific Islander female[4]					Deaths per 100,000 resident population					
All ages, age adjusted	---	---	---	224.6	228.5	228.9	214.4	214.7	207.4	212.0
All ages, crude	---	---	---	222.5	224.9	234.3	257.9	264.3	262.5	261.6
Under 1 year	---	---	---	755.8	622.0	518.2	347.4	343.7	380.2	357.4
1–4 years	---	---	---	35.4	36.8	32.0	25.6	24.7	19.9	23.4
5–14 years	---	---	---	21.5	19.1	13.0	11.4	13.8	12.4	12.6
15–24 years	---	---	---	32.3	30.7	28.8	30.6	33.4	28.8	30.9
25–34 years	---	---	---	45.4	36.5	37.5	35.4	32.4	33.7	33.8
35–44 years	---	---	---	89.7	77.8	69.9	68.7	74.1	61.6	68.0
45–54 years	---	---	---	214.1	184.9	182.7	173.8	166.6	160.5	166.7
55–64 years	---	---	---	440.8	468.0	483.4	417.7	423.4	412.9	417.9
65–74 years	---	---	---	1,027.7	1,130.8	1,089.2	1,090.8	1,117.3	1,083.1	1,096.9
75–84 years	---	---	---	2,833.6	2,873.9	3,127.9	3,118.8	3,052.1	2,917.4	3,023.7
85 years and over	---	---	---	7,923.3	9,808.3	10,254.0	8,599.1	8,414.1	8,618.4	8,544.9
Hispanic female[5]										
All ages, age adjusted	---	---	---	---	286.6	284.9	268.0	263.4	255.5	262.1
All ages, crude	---	---	---	---	251.9	285.4	289.8	288.0	283.6	287.0
Under 1 year	---	---	---	---	793.0	746.6	540.2	572.3	568.7	560.6
1–4 years	---	---	---	---	42.3	42.1	29.6	28.4	27.6	28.5
5–14 years	---	---	---	---	16.0	17.3	16.9	15.6	14.1	15.5
15–24 years	---	---	---	---	36.3	40.6	39.2	38.3	34.0	37.1
25–34 years	---	---	---	---	56.3	62.9	61.1	54.6	51.0	55.5
35–44 years	---	---	---	---	100.0	109.3	108.2	101.1	96.7	101.8
45–54 years	---	---	---	---	251.3	253.3	231.8	228.3	225.8	228.5
55–64 years	---	---	---	---	620.3	607.5	580.9	580.3	543.6	567.6
65–74 years	---	---	---	---	1,449.3	1,453.8	1,400.0	1,381.9	1,384.3	1,388.5
75–84 years	---	---	---	---	3,549.8	3,351.3	3,279.4	3,220.5	3,140.1	3,210.5
85 years and over	---	---	---	---	10,216.9	10,098.7	8,783.9	8,708.6	8,336.0	8,595.7
White, non-Hispanic female[5]										
All ages, age adjusted	---	---	---	---	385.3	372.2	364.1	360.9	359.1	361.3
All ages, crude	---	---	---	---	861.7	903.6	965.0	971.2	982.5	973.0
Under 1 year	---	---	---	---	762.8	655.3	541.1	519.6	544.6	535.0
1–4 years	---	---	---	---	36.6	34.0	27.8	27.3	27.0	27.4
5–14 years	---	---	---	---	19.0	17.6	15.9	15.3	14.9	15.4
15–24 years	---	---	---	---	47.9	46.0	42.4	44.1	41.9	42.8
25–34 years	---	---	---	---	59.0	60.6	61.7	60.0	58.7	60.1
35–44 years	---	---	---	---	122.8	116.8	121.1	121.7	123.7	122.2
45–54 years	---	---	---	---	335.7	312.1	292.0	287.3	280.5	286.5
55–64 years	---	---	---	---	853.3	834.5	787.6	775.7	751.3	771.1
65–74 years	---	---	---	---	1,997.8	1,940.2	1,937.1	1,920.3	1,935.8	1,931.1
75–84 years	---	---	---	---	5,058.5	4,887.3	4,868.1	4,831.1	4,847.8	4,848.8
85 years and over	---	---	---	---	14,561.4	14,533.1	14,826.1	14,864.0	14,839.2	14,843.3

- - - Data not available.

[1]Includes deaths of persons who were not residents of the 50 States and the District of Columbia.

[2]Average annual death rate.

[3]Interpretation of trends should take into account that population estimates for American Indians increased by 45 percent between 1980 and 1990, partly due to better enumeration techniques in the 1990 decennial census and to the increased tendency for people to identify themselves as American Indian in 1990.

[4]Interpretation of trends should take into account that the Asian population in the United States more than doubled between 1980 and 1990, primarily due to immigration.

[5]Excludes data from States lacking an Hispanic-origin item on their death certificates. See Appendix I, National Vital Statistics System.

NOTES: Rates are age adjusted to the 1940 U.S. standard million population. See Appendix II, Age adjustment. The race groups, white, black, Asian or Pacific Islander, and American Indian or Alaska Native, include persons of Hispanic and non-Hispanic origin. Conversely, persons of Hispanic origin may be of any race. Bias in death rates results from inconsistent race identification between the death certificate (source of data for numerator of death rates) and data from the Census Bureau (denominator); and from undercounts of some population groups in the census. The net effects of misclassification and under coverage result in death rates estimated to be overstated by 1 percent for the white population and 5 percent for the black population; and death rates estimated to be understated by 21 percent for American Indians, 11 percent for Asians, and 2 percent for Hispanics (Rosenberg HM, Maurer JD, Sorlie PD, Johnson NJ, et al. Quality of death rates by race and Hispanic origin: A summary of current research, 1999. National Center for Health Statistics. Vital Health Stat 2(128). 1999). Data for additional years are available (see Appendix III).

SOURCES: Centers for Disease Control and Prevention, National Center for Health Statistics. Grove RD and Hetzel AM. *Vital statistics rates in the United States, 1940–60*. Washington: Public Health Service, 1968; *Vital statistics of the United States, vol II, mortality, part A*, for data years 1950–93. Public Health Service. Washington. U.S. Government Printing Office; for 1994–98, data for all persons, white, and black are available on the NCHS Web site at www.cdc.gov/nchs/datawh/statab/unpubd/mortabs.htm; numerator data from National Vital Statistics System, annual mortality files; denominator data from national population estimates for race groups from table 1 and unpublished Hispanic population estimates prepared by the Housing and Household Economic Statistics Division, U.S. Bureau of the Census.

[Data are based on the National Vital Statistics System]

Sex, race, Hispanic origin, and age	1950[1]	1960[1]	1970	1980	1985	1990	1995	1996	1997	1998	1996–98[2]
All persons	Deaths per 100,000 resident population										
All ages, age adjusted	307.2	286.2	253.6	202.0	181.4	152.0	138.3	134.5	130.5	126.6	130.5
All ages, crude	355.5	369.0	362.0	336.0	324.1	289.5	280.7	276.4	271.6	268.2	272.1
Under 1 year	3.5	6.6	13.1	22.8	25.0	20.1	17.1	16.6	16.4	16.1	16.4
1–4 years	1.3	1.3	1.7	2.6	2.2	1.9	1.6	1.4	1.4	1.4	1.4
5–14 years	2.1	1.3	0.8	0.9	1.0	0.9	0.8	0.9	0.8	0.8	0.8
15–24 years	6.8	4.0	3.0	2.9	2.8	2.5	2.9	2.7	3.0	2.8	2.8
25–34 years	19.4	15.6	11.4	8.3	8.3	7.6	8.5	8.3	8.3	8.3	8.3
35–44 years	86.4	74.6	66.7	44.6	38.1	31.4	32.0	30.5	30.1	30.5	30.4
45–54 years	308.6	271.8	238.4	180.2	153.8	120.5	111.0	108.2	104.9	101.4	104.8
55–64 years	808.1	737.9	652.3	494.1	443.0	367.3	322.9	315.2	302.4	286.9	301.2
65–74 years	1,839.8	1,740.5	1,558.2	1,218.6	1,089.8	894.3	799.9	776.2	753.7	735.5	755.2
75–84 years	4,310.1	4,089.4	3,683.8	2,993.1	2,693.1	2,295.7	2,064.7	2,010.2	1,943.6	1,897.3	1,949.5
85 years and over	9,150.6	9,317.8	7,891.3	7,777.1	7,384.1	6,739.9	6,484.1	6,314.5	6,198.9	6,009.6	6,170.4
Male											
All ages, age adjusted	383.8	375.5	348.5	280.4	250.1	206.7	184.9	178.8	173.1	166.9	172.9
All ages, crude	423.4	439.5	422.5	368.6	344.1	297.6	282.7	277.4	272.2	268.0	272.5
Under 1 year	4.0	7.8	15.1	25.5	27.8	21.9	17.5	17.4	18.0	16.2	17.2
1–4 years	1.4	1.4	1.9	2.8	2.2	1.9	1.7	1.4	1.5	1.5	1.5
5–14 years	2.0	1.4	0.9	1.0	0.9	0.9	0.8	0.9	0.9	1.0	0.9
15–24 years	6.8	4.2	3.7	3.7	3.5	3.1	3.6	3.3	3.6	3.5	3.5
25–34 years	22.9	20.1	15.2	11.4	11.6	10.3	11.4	11.0	10.8	10.8	10.9
35–44 years	118.4	112.7	103.2	68.7	58.6	48.1	47.2	44.2	43.7	44.0	44.0
45–54 years	440.5	420.4	376.4	282.6	237.8	183.0	168.6	161.8	157.7	152.2	157.1
55–64 years	1,104.5	1,066.9	987.2	746.8	659.1	537.3	465.4	453.8	434.6	411.1	432.7
65–74 years	2,292.3	2,291.3	2,170.3	1,728.0	1,535.8	1,250.0	1,102.3	1,065.0	1,031.1	997.3	1,031.2
75–84 years	4,825.0	4,742.4	4,534.8	3,834.3	3,496.9	2,968.2	2,615.0	2,529.4	2,443.6	2,377.2	2,448.6
85 years and over	9,659.8	9,788.9	8,426.2	8,752.7	8,251.8	7,418.4	7,039.6	6,834.0	6,658.5	6,330.6	6,598.6
Female											
All ages, age adjusted	233.9	205.7	175.2	140.3	127.4	108.9	100.4	98.2	95.4	93.3	95.6
All ages, crude	288.4	300.6	304.5	305.1	305.2	281.8	278.8	275.5	271.1	268.3	271.6
Under 1 year	2.9	5.4	10.9	20.0	22.0	18.3	16.7	15.7	14.7	16.1	15.5
1–4 years	1.2	1.1	1.6	2.5	2.2	1.9	1.5	1.4	1.2	1.3	1.3
5–14 years	2.2	1.2	0.8	0.9	1.0	0.8	0.7	0.8	0.7	0.7	0.7
15–24 years	6.7	3.7	2.3	2.1	2.1	1.8	2.2	2.0	2.4	2.1	2.2
25–34 years	16.2	11.3	7.7	5.3	5.0	5.0	5.6	5.6	5.8	5.8	5.7
35–44 years	55.1	38.2	32.2	21.4	18.3	15.1	17.1	16.8	16.5	17.3	16.9
45–54 years	177.2	127.5	109.9	84.5	74.4	61.0	56.0	56.9	54.3	52.8	54.6
55–64 years	510.0	429.4	351.6	272.1	252.1	215.7	193.9	189.3	182.1	173.9	181.6
65–74 years	1,419.3	1,261.3	1,082.7	828.6	746.1	616.8	557.8	543.8	529.4	522.6	532.0
75–84 years	3,872.0	3,582.7	3,120.8	2,497.0	2,220.4	1,893.8	1,715.2	1,674.7	1,616.6	1,579.5	1,623.1
85 years and over	8,796.1	9,016.8	7,591.8	7,350.5	7,037.6	6,478.1	6,267.8	6,108.0	6,013.7	5,876.6	5,997.0
White male											
All ages, age adjusted	381.1	375.4	347.6	277.5	246.2	202.0	179.7	174.5	168.7	162.3	168.3
All ages, crude	433.0	454.6	438.3	384.0	360.3	312.7	297.9	293.3	287.7	283.1	288.0
45–54 years	423.6	413.2	365.7	269.8	225.5	170.6	155.7	149.8	145.4	140.2	145.0
55–64 years	1,081.7	1,056.0	979.3	730.6	640.1	516.7	443.0	431.8	411.2	388.1	409.9
65–74 years	2,308.3	2,297.9	2,177.2	1,729.7	1,522.7	1,230.5	1,080.5	1,049.5	1,015.1	981.3	1,015.5
75–84 years	4,907.3	4,839.9	4,617.6	3,883.2	3,527.0	2,983.4	2,616.1	2,536.0	2,453.7	2,381.5	2,455.6
85 years and over	9,950.5	10,135.8	8,818.0	8,958.0	8,481.7	7,558.7	7,165.5	7,014.5	6,829.7	6,478.8	6,764.6
Black male											
All ages, age adjusted	415.5	381.2	375.9	327.3	310.8	275.9	255.9	242.6	236.2	231.8	236.8
All ages, crude	348.4	330.6	330.3	301.0	288.6	256.8	244.2	234.8	230.8	230.5	232.0
45–54 years	624.1	514.0	512.8	433.4	385.2	328.9	317.1	297.7	293.7	282.7	291.1
55–64 years	1,434.0	1,236.8	1,135.4	987.2	935.3	824.0	757.8	740.9	727.8	699.9	722.5
65–74 years	2,140.1	2,281.4	2,237.8	1,847.2	1,839.2	1,632.9	1,482.9	1,381.3	1,335.4	1,312.7	1,342.9
75–84 years	- - -	3,533.6	3,783.4	3,578.8	3,436.6	3,107.1	2,881.4	2,762.0	2,641.6	2,649.3	2,683.3
85 years and over	- - -	6,037.9	5,367.6	6,819.5	6,393.5	6,479.6	5,985.7	5,675.4	5,538.7	5,446.7	5,550.8

See footnotes at end of table.

Table 37 (page 2 of 3). Death rates for diseases of heart, according to sex, detailed race, Hispanic origin, and age: United States, selected years 1950–98

[Data are based on the National Vital Statistics System]

Sex, race, Hispanic origin, and age	1950[1]	1960[1]	1970	1980	1985	1990	1995	1996	1997	1998	1996–98[2]
American Indian or Alaska Native male[3]				Deaths per 100,000 resident population							
All ages, age adjusted	- - -	- - -	- - -	180.9	162.2	144.6	136.7	131.6	136.5	128.7	132.1
All ages, crude	- - -	- - -	- - -	130.6	117.9	108.0	110.4	110.7	116.8	113.2	113.6
45–54 years	- - -	- - -	- - -	238.1	209.1	173.8	151.4	157.5	171.8	151.8	160.3
55–64 years	- - -	- - -	- - -	496.3	438.3	411.0	403.2	404.9	427.2	402.5	411.5
65–74 years	- - -	- - -	- - -	1,009.4	984.6	839.1	918.5	778.0	828.1	793.6	799.9
75–84 years	- - -	- - -	- - -	2,062.2	2,118.2	1,788.8	1,534.9	1,546.5	1,513.8	1,274.0	1,439.0
85 years and over	- - -	- - -	- - -	4,413.7	2,766.7	3,860.3	2,308.7	2,660.1	2,764.2	2,800.9	2,744.2
Asian or Pacific Islander male[4]											
All ages, age adjusted	- - -	- - -	- - -	136.7	123.4	102.6	106.2	98.1	95.9	92.3	95.3
All ages, crude	- - -	- - -	- - -	119.8	103.5	88.7	96.9	97.3	97.4	98.3	97.7
45–54 years	- - -	- - -	- - -	112.0	81.1	70.4	73.4	75.4	72.1	72.9	73.4
55–64 years	- - -	- - -	- - -	306.7	291.2	226.1	214.3	220.7	218.3	210.8	216.4
65–74 years	- - -	- - -	- - -	852.4	753.5	623.5	605.8	581.2	585.1	522.7	562.1
75–84 years	- - -	- - -	- - -	2,010.9	2,025.6	1,642.2	1,680.5	1,534.8	1,432.1	1,493.0	1,485.9
85 years and over	- - -	- - -	- - -	5,923.0	4,937.5	4,617.8	6,372.3	4,338.0	4,392.5	4,110.7	4,272.2
Hispanic male[5]											
All ages, age adjusted	- - -	- - -	- - -	- - -	152.3	136.3	121.9	117.6	113.4	109.3	113.2
All ages, crude	- - -	- - -	- - -	- - -	92.1	91.0	87.5	85.8	83.9	84.9	84.9
45–54 years	- - -	- - -	- - -	- - -	128.1	116.4	103.0	98.7	96.2	96.0	96.9
55–64 years	- - -	- - -	- - -	- - -	398.8	363.0	306.0	310.0	276.9	274.0	286.4
65–74 years	- - -	- - -	- - -,	- - -	972.6	829.9	750.0	725.7	737.2	706.6	723.0
75–84 years	- - -	- - -	- - -	- - -	2,160.8	1,971.3	1,734.5	1,688.6	1,628.7	1,522.0	1,608.2
85 years and over	- - -	- - -	- - -	- - -	4,791.2	4,711.9	4,699.7	4,078.6	3,844.6	3,641.9	3,843.3
White, non-Hispanic male[5]											
All ages, age adjusted	- - -	- - -	- - -	- - -	240.3	204.1	181.2	176.2	171.1	164.6	170.5
All ages, crude	- - -	- - -	- - -	- - -	362.8	336.5	322.0	318.9	315.0	309.8	314.5
45–54 years	- - -	- - -	- - -	- - -	219.9	172.8	157.5	152.1	148.5	142.8	147.7
55–64 years	- - -	- - -	- - -	- - -	610.6	521.3	448.0	435.1	418.1	393.5	415.1
65–74 years	- - -	- - -	- - -	- - -	1,471.3	1,243.4	1,088.3	1,056.4	1,025.1	991.7	1,024.5
75–84 years	- - -	- - -	- - -	- - -	3,514.1	3,007.7	2,635.6	2,559.8	2,477.3	2,411.2	2,481.0
85 years and over	- - -	- - -	- - -	- - -	8,539.3	7,663.4	7,166.3	7,109.2	6,954.2	6,604.4	6,879.3
White female											
All ages, age adjusted	223.6	197.1	167.8	134.6	121.7	103.1	94.9	92.9	90.4	88.1	90.4
All ages, crude	289.4	306.5	313.8	319.2	321.8	298.4	297.4	294.2	289.8	286.8	290.3
45–54 years	141.9	103.4	91.4	71.2	62.5	50.2	45.9	46.9	44.9	43.4	45.0
55–64 years	460.2	383.0	317.7	248.1	227.1	192.4	173.1	167.8	162.5	153.9	161.3
65–74 years	1,400.9	1,229.8	1,044.0	796.7	713.3	583.6	526.3	515.1	500.7	493.8	503.3
75–84 years	3,925.2	3,629.7	3,143.5	2,493.6	2,207.5	1,874.3	1,689.8	1,652.9	1,595.9	1,556.3	1,601.2
85 years and over	9,084.7	9,280.8	7,839.9	7,501.6	7,170.0	6,563.4	6,352.6	6,211.4	6,108.0	5,971.4	6,094.5
Black female											
All ages, age adjusted	349.5	292.6	251.7	201.1	188.3	168.1	156.3	153.4	147.6	146.8	149.2
All ages, crude	289.9	268.5	261.0	249.7	250.3	237.0	231.1	229.0	224.2	224.6	225.9
45–54 years	526.8	360.7	290.9	202.4	176.2	155.3	143.1	144.7	134.8	132.9	137.3
55–64 years	1,210.7	952.3	710.5	530.1	510.7	442.0	384.9	388.4	364.8	361.5	371.4
65–74 years	1,659.4	1,680.5	1,553.2	1,210.3	1,149.9	1,017.5	933.7	890.0	871.6	858.8	873.4
75–84 years	- - -	2,926.9	2,964.1	2,707.2	2,533.4	2,250.9	2,163.1	2,097.7	2,030.5	2,044.8	2,057.4
85 years and over	- - -	5,650.0	5,003.8	5,796.5	5,686.5	5,766.1	5,614.8	5,493.6	5,542.5	5,373.1	5,468.1

See footnotes at end of table.

Table 37 (page 3 of 3). **Death rates for diseases of heart, according to sex, detailed race, Hispanic origin, and age: United States, selected years 1950–98**

[Data are based on the National Vital Statistics System]

Sex, race, Hispanic origin, and age	1950[1]	1960[1]	1970	1980	1985	1990	1995	1996	1997	1998	1996–98[2]
American Indian or Alaska Native female[3]					Deaths per 100,000 resident population						
All ages, age adjusted	---	---	---	88.4	83.7	76.6	77.3	74.9	73.9	70.0	72.9
All ages, crude	---	---	---	80.3	84.3	77.5	87.0	86.7	88.6	89.0	88.1
45–54 years	---	---	---	65.2	59.2	62.0	69.2	61.1	59.7	49.4	56.6
55–64 years	---	---	---	193.5	230.8	197.0	210.2	192.5	172.8	183.3	182.8
65–74 years	---	---	---	577.2	472.7	492.8	503.3	512.8	473.8	440.3	475.1
75–84 years	---	---	---	1,364.3	1,258.8	1,050.3	1,045.6	1,030.0	1,115.2	1,019.8	1,054.7
85 years and over	---	---	---	2,893.3	3,180.0	2,868.7	2,209.8	2,108.8	2,019.5	2,348.9	2,163.9
Asian or Pacific Islander female[4]											
All ages, age adjusted	---	---	---	55.8	59.6	58.3	57.7	50.9	49.3	47.7	49.2
All ages, crude	---	---	---	57.0	60.3	62.0	68.2	66.8	66.9	67.3	67.0
45–54 years	---	---	---	28.6	23.8	17.5	21.6	17.2	18.8	18.4	18.2
55–64 years	---	---	---	92.9	103.0	99.0	93.0	82.3	80.5	70.5	77.6
65–74 years	---	---	---	313.3	341.0	323.9	294.9	282.0	272.8	282.9	279.2
75–84 years	---	---	---	1,053.2	1,056.5	1,130.9	1,063.0	1,009.8	944.0	880.9	941.3
85 years and over	---	---	---	3,211.0	4,208.3	4,161.2	4,717.9	3,394.7	3,326.2	3,385.5	3,368.7
Hispanic female[5]											
All ages, age adjusted	---	---	---	---	86.5	76.0	68.1	64.7	64.7	63.4	64.2
All ages, crude	---	---	---	---	75.0	79.4	78.9	77.0	78.3	77.7	77.7
45–54 years	---	---	---	---	46.6	43.5	32.0	31.3	31.5	31.0	31.3
55–64 years	---	---	---	---	184.8	153.2	137.3	125.1	129.5	122.4	125.6
65–74 years	---	---	---	---	534.0	460.4	402.4	387.6	391.9	399.8	393.3
75–84 years	---	---	---	---	1,456.5	1,259.7	1,150.1	1,152.8	1,102.4	1,071.1	1,107.2
85 years and over	---	---	---	---	4,523.4	4,440.3	4,243.9	3,673.8	3,748.7	3,499.1	3,634.7
White, non-Hispanic female[5]											
All ages, age adjusted	---	---	---	---	120.2	103.7	95.4	93.6	91.3	89.1	91.3
All ages, crude	---	---	---	---	334.2	320.0	321.4	318.9	315.6	313.6	316.0
45–54 years	---	---	---	---	61.3	50.2	46.6	47.5	45.7	44.2	45.7
55–64 years	---	---	---	---	219.6	193.6	173.6	169.0	163.9	155.3	162.6
65–74 years	---	---	---	---	700.4	584.7	529.1	518.0	504.0	496.2	506.1
75–84 years	---	---	---	---	2,201.5	1,890.2	1,697.6	1,663.5	1,609.4	1,571.1	1,614.0
85 years and over	---	---	---	---	7,164.7	6,615.2	6,384.5	6,285.4	6,176.4	6,054.4	6,169.3

- - - Data not available.

[1]Includes deaths of persons who were not residents of the 50 States and the District of Columbia.

[2]Average annual death rate.

[3]Interpretation of trends should take into account that population estimates for American Indians increased by 45 percent between 1980 and 1990, partly due to better enumeration techniques in the 1990 decennial census and to the increased tendency for people to identify themselves as American Indian in 1990.

[4]Interpretation of trends should take into account that the Asian population in the United States more than doubled between 1980 and 1990, primarily due to immigration.

[5]Excludes data from States lacking an Hispanic-origin item on their death certificates. See Appendix I, National Vital Statistics System.

NOTES: Rates are age adjusted to the 1940 U.S. standard million population. See Appendix II, Age adjustment. For data years shown, the code numbers for cause of death are based on the then current *International Classification of Diseases*, which are described in Appendix II, tables IV and V. Age groups were selected to minimize the presentation of unstable age-specific death rates based on small numbers of deaths and for consistency among comparison groups. The race groups, white, black, Asian or Pacific Islander, and American Indian or Alaska Native, include persons of Hispanic and non-Hispanic origin. Conversely, persons of Hispanic origin may be of any race. Bias in death rates results from inconsistent race identification between the death certificate (source of data for numerator of death rates) and data from the Census Bureau (denominator); and from undercounts of some population groups in the census. The net effects of misclassification and under coverage result in death rates estimated to be overstated by 1 percent for the white population and 5 percent for the black population; and death rates estimated to be understated by 21 percent for American Indians, 11 percent for Asians, and 2 percent for Hispanics (Rosenberg HM, Maurer JD, Sorlie PD, Johnson NJ, et al. Quality of death rates by race and Hispanic origin: A summary of current research, 1999. National Center for Health Statistics. Vital Health Stat 2(128). 1999). Data for additional years are available (see Appendix III).

SOURCES: Centers for Disease Control and Prevention, National Center for Health Statistics. *Vital statistics of the United States, vol II, mortality, part A*, for data years 1950–93. Public Health Service. Washington. U.S. Government Printing Office; for 1994–98, data for all persons, white, and black are available on the NCHS Web site at www.cdc.gov/nchs/datawh/statab/unpubd/mortabs.htm; numerator data from National Vital Statistics System, annual mortality files; denominator data from national population estimates for race groups from table 1 and unpublished Hispanic population estimates prepared by the Housing and Household Economic Statistics Division, U.S. Bureau of the Census.

Table 38 (page 1 of 3). Death rates for cerebrovascular diseases, according to sex, detailed race, Hispanic origin, and age: United States, selected years 1950–98

[Data are based on the National Vital Statistics System]

Sex, race, Hispanic origin, and age	1950[1]	1960[1]	1970	1980	1985	1990	1995	1996	1997	1998	1996–98[2]
All persons				Deaths per 100,000 resident population							
All ages, age adjusted	88.8	79.7	66.3	40.8	32.5	27.7	26.7	26.4	25.9	25.1	25.8
All ages, crude	104.0	108.0	101.9	75.1	64.3	57.9	60.1	60.3	59.7	58.6	59.5
Under 1 year	5.1	4.1	5.0	4.4	3.7	3.8	5.8	6.2	7.0	7.8	7.0
1–4 years	0.9	0.8	1.0	0.5	0.3	0.3	0.4	0.3	0.4	0.4	0.4
5–14 years	0.5	0.7	0.7	0.3	0.2	0.2	0.2	0.2	0.2	0.2	0.2
15–24 years	1.6	1.8	1.6	1.0	0.8	0.6	0.5	0.5	0.5	0.5	0.5
25–34 years	4.2	4.7	4.5	2.6	2.2	2.2	1.8	1.8	1.7	1.7	1.7
35–44 years	18.7	14.7	15.6	8.5	7.2	6.5	6.5	6.3	6.3	6.0	6.2
45–54 years	70.4	49.2	41.6	25.2	21.3	18.7	17.6	17.9	16.9	16.5	17.1
55–64 years	194.2	147.3	115.8	65.2	54.8	48.0	46.1	45.3	44.4	42.6	44.0
65–74 years	554.7	469.2	384.1	219.5	172.8	144.4	137.2	135.5	134.8	130.0	133.5
75–84 years	1,499.6	1,491.3	1,254.2	788.6	601.5	499.3	481.4	477.0	462.0	455.4	464.6
85 years and over	2,990.1	3,680.5	3,014.3	2,288.9	1,865.1	1,633.9	1,636.5	1,612.7	1,584.6	1,500.0	1,564.3
Male											
All ages, age adjusted	91.9	85.4	73.2	44.9	35.5	30.2	28.9	28.5	27.9	26.6	27.7
All ages, crude	102.5	104.5	94.5	63.6	52.5	46.8	48.0	48.1	47.8	46.3	47.4
Under 1 year	6.4	5.0	5.8	5.0	4.6	4.4	6.3	6.5	7.6	9.0	7.7
1–4 years	1.1	0.9	1.2	0.4	0.4	0.3	0.4	0.3	0.5	0.3	0.4
5–14 years	0.5	0.7	0.8	0.3	0.2	0.2	0.2	0.2	0.2	0.2	0.2
15–24 years	1.8	1.9	1.8	1.1	0.7	0.7	0.5	0.5	0.6	0.6	0.6
25–34 years	4.2	4.5	4.4	2.6	2.2	2.1	1.9	1.7	1.7	1.7	1.7
35–44 years	17.5	14.6	15.7	8.7	7.4	6.8	7.1	6.7	6.5	6.2	6.5
45–54 years	67.9	52.2	44.4	27.3	23.2	20.5	19.8	20.0	19.2	18.5	19.2
55–64 years	205.2	163.8	138.7	74.7	63.5	54.4	53.4	52.5	51.4	49.5	51.1
65–74 years	589.6	530.7	449.5	259.2	201.4	166.8	155.9	154.7	153.1	145.7	151.2
75–84 years	1,543.6	1,555.9	1,361.6	868.3	661.2	552.7	517.1	508.7	488.7	474.7	490.4
85 years and over	3,048.6	3,643.1	2,895.2	2,199.2	1,730.1	1,533.2	1,537.7	1,512.7	1,500.7	1,347.2	1,450.4
Female											
All ages, age adjusted	86.0	74.7	60.8	37.6	30.0	25.7	24.8	24.6	24.2	23.6	24.1
All ages, crude	105.6	111.4	109.0	86.1	75.5	68.6	71.7	71.9	71.2	70.4	71.2
Under 1 year	3.7	3.2	4.0	3.8	2.7	3.1	5.2	5.9	6.3	6.6	6.3
1–4 years	0.7	0.7	0.7	0.5	0.3	0.3	0.3	0.3	0.3	0.4	0.3
5–14 years	0.4	0.6	0.6	0.3	0.3	0.2	0.2	0.2	0.2	0.2	0.2
15–24 years	1.5	1.6	1.4	0.8	0.8	0.6	0.4	0.4	0.5	0.4	0.4
25–34 years	4.3	4.9	4.7	2.6	2.1	2.2	1.7	1.8	1.7	1.8	1.8
35–44 years	19.9	14.8	15.6	8.4	6.9	6.1	6.0	5.9	6.2	5.7	5.9
45–54 years	72.9	46.3	39.0	23.3	19.4	17.0	15.5	15.9	14.8	14.6	15.1
55–64 years	183.1	131.8	95.3	56.9	47.2	42.2	39.4	38.8	37.9	36.3	37.7
65–74 years	522.1	415.7	333.3	189.0	150.7	126.9	122.2	120.1	120.1	117.2	119.1
75–84 years	1,462.2	1,441.1	1,183.1	741.6	566.3	467.4	458.7	456.5	444.4	442.6	447.8
85 years and over	2,949.4	3,704.4	3,081.0	2,328.2	1,918.9	1,672.7	1,675.0	1,652.4	1,618.4	1,563.3	1,610.4
White male											
All ages, age adjusted	87.0	80.3	68.8	41.9	33.0	27.7	26.5	26.3	25.7	24.5	25.5
All ages, crude	100.5	102.7	93.5	63.3	52.7	47.0	48.6	49.1	48.8	47.3	48.4
45–54 years	53.7	40.9	35.6	21.7	18.1	15.4	14.8	15.2	14.6	14.2	14.7
55–64 years	182.2	139.0	119.9	64.2	54.6	45.8	44.7	43.4	42.3	40.8	42.2
65–74 years	569.7	501.0	420.0	240.4	186.4	153.2	143.5	142.0	141.8	134.9	139.6
75–84 years	1,556.3	1,564.8	1,361.6	854.8	650.0	540.7	503.1	500.1	480.3	464.9	481.4
85 years and over	3,127.1	3,734.8	3,018.1	2,236.9	1,765.6	1,549.8	1,550.0	1,537.7	1,530.6	1,365.9	1,474.8
Black male											
All ages, age adjusted	146.2	141.2	122.5	77.5	62.7	56.1	52.2	50.9	48.6	46.8	48.7
All ages, crude	122.0	122.9	108.8	73.1	59.2	53.1	51.0	50.1	48.3	47.5	48.7
45–54 years	211.9	166.1	136.1	82.1	71.1	68.4	64.1	62.1	59.8	55.7	59.1
55–64 years	522.8	439.9	343.4	189.8	160.7	141.8	134.1	137.5	135.5	129.2	134.0
65–74 years	783.6	899.2	780.1	472.8	379.7	327.2	291.5	292.2	274.3	255.8	274.0
75–84 years	- - -	1,475.2	1,445.7	1,067.6	814.4	723.7	700.2	653.0	600.5	621.3	624.7
85 years and over	- - -	2,700.0	1,963.1	1,873.2	1,429.0	1,430.5	1,393.9	1,329.5	1,281.6	1,243.1	1,283.7

See footnotes at end of table.

Table 38 (page 2 of 3). Death rates for cerebrovascular diseases, according to sex, detailed race, Hispanic origin, and age: United States, selected years 1950–98

[Data are based on the National Vital Statistics System]

Sex, race, Hispanic origin, and age	1950[1]	1960[1]	1970	1980	1985	1990	1995	1996	1997	1998	1996–98[2]
American Indian or Alaska Native male[3]				Deaths per 100,000 resident population							
All ages, age adjusted	- - -	- - -	- - -	30.7	24.9	20.5	23.5	21.4	20.1	18.5	20.0
All ages, crude	- - -	- - -	- - -	23.2	18.5	16.0	20.1	18.7	18.5	16.6	17.9
45–54 years	- - -	- - -	- - -	*	*	*	28.4	19.9	*	17.6	17.4
55–64 years	- - -	- - -	- - -	72.0	*	39.8	45.7	42.9	49.4	53.5	48.7
65–74 years	- - -	- - -	- - -	170.5	200.0	120.3	153.1	139.1	112.5	109.8	120.3
75–84 years	- - -	- - -	- - -	535.1	372.7	325.9	290.1	319.4	324.0	257.8	299.0
85 years and over	- - -	- - -	- - -	1,384.7	733.3	949.8	748.8	550.4	707.9	450.2	569.6
Asian or Pacific Islander male[4]											
All ages, age adjusted	- - -	- - -	- - -	32.3	28.0	26.9	31.2	26.9	28.3	26.5	27.2
All ages, crude	- - -	- - -	- - -	28.7	24.0	23.4	28.6	27.0	28.8	28.1	28.0
45–54 years	- - -	- - -	- - -	17.0	13.9	15.6	17.3	19.5	18.3	16.9	18.2
55–64 years	- - -	- - -	- - -	59.9	48.8	51.8	62.1	55.6	58.0	56.0	56.5
65–74 years	- - -	- - -	- - -	197.9	155.6	167.9	162.3	161.4	160.9	160.9	161.1
75–84 years	- - -	- - -	- - -	619.5	583.7	485.7	571.8	430.0	524.0	456.5	470.4
85 years and over	- - -	- - -	- - -	1,399.0	1,387.5	1,196.6	1,808.5	1,348.7	1,219.4	1,149.6	1,233.4
Hispanic male[5]											
All ages, age adjusted	- - -	- - -	- - -	- - -	27.7	22.7	23.1	22.3	22.1	21.8	22.0
All ages, crude	- - -	- - -	- - -	- - -	17.2	15.6	17.1	16.8	16.7	17.4	16.9
45–54 years	- - -	- - -	- - -	- - -	23.6	20.0	20.5	23.1	20.4	22.3	21.9
55–64 years	- - -	- - -	- - -	- - -	63.9	49.4	46.1	50.7	52.7	53.0	52.2
65–74 years	- - -	- - -	- - -	- - -	163.5	126.4	132.2	114.8	134.9	124.0	124.7
75–84 years	- - -	- - -	- - -	- - -	396.7	356.6	349.9	348.6	304.2	296.0	314.8
85 years and over	- - -	- - -	- - -	- - -	1,152.1	866.3	996.3	866.3	787.8	795.7	814.9
White, non-Hispanic male[5]											
All ages, age adjusted	- - -	- - -	- - -	- - -	31.6	27.9	26.3	26.1	25.6	24.3	25.4
All ages, crude	- - -	- - -	- - -	- - -	52.2	50.7	52.3	53.0	53.1	51.3	52.5
45–54 years	- - -	- - -	- - -	- - -	16.0	14.9	14.1	14.2	13.9	13.2	13.8
55–64 years	- - -	- - -	- - -	- - -	50.5	45.2	43.9	42.0	41.1	39.4	40.8
65–74 years	- - -	- - -	- - -	- - -	178.5	154.8	143.1	142.0	141.1	134.7	139.3
75–84 years	- - -	- - -	- - -	- - -	637.0	548.8	507.4	505.1	486.0	471.1	487.0
85 years and over	- - -	- - -	- - -	- - -	1,735.1	1,583.6	1,552.4	1,560.6	1,562.9	1,391.9	1,501.7
White female											
All ages, age adjusted	79.7	68.7	56.2	35.2	27.9	23.8	23.1	22.9	22.5	22.0	22.5
All ages, crude	103.3	110.1	109.8	88.8	78.4	71.8	76.0	76.3	75.7	75.0	75.7
45–54 years	55.0	33.8	30.5	18.7	15.5	13.5	12.7	12.8	11.6	11.3	11.9
55–64 years	156.9	103.0	78.1	48.7	40.0	35.8	33.6	33.3	31.8	31.3	32.1
65–74 years	498.1	383.3	303.2	172.8	137.9	116.3	112.6	110.2	111.4	108.6	110.1
75–84 years	1,471.3	1,444.7	1,176.8	730.3	552.9	457.6	449.5	446.7	437.5	434.2	439.4
85 years and over	3,017.9	3,795.7	3,167.6	2,367.8	1,944.9	1,691.4	1,690.0	1,679.3	1,645.8	1,589.6	1,637.3
Black female											
All ages, age adjusted	155.6	139.5	107.9	61.7	50.6	42.7	39.6	39.2	37.9	37.2	38.1
All ages, crude	128.3	127.7	112.2	77.9	68.6	60.7	60.4	59.7	58.0	57.9	58.5
45–54 years	248.9	166.2	119.4	61.9	50.8	44.1	36.4	38.6	38.6	39.9	39.1
55–64 years	567.7	452.0	272.4	138.7	113.6	97.0	85.5	82.9	84.0	76.5	81.1
65–74 years	754.4	830.5	673.5	362.2	285.6	236.8	221.2	216.4	204.8	197.3	206.1
75–84 years	- - -	1,413.1	1,338.3	918.6	753.8	596.0	583.2	586.5	540.0	560.0	562.0
85 years and over	- - -	2,578.9	2,210.5	1,896.3	1,657.1	1,496.5	1,568.8	1,443.6	1,433.1	1,398.4	1,424.5

See footnotes at end of table.

Table 38 (page 3 of 3). Death rates for cerebrovascular diseases, according to sex, detailed race, Hispanic origin, and age: United States, selected years 1950–98

[Data are based on the National Vital Statistics System]

Sex, race, Hispanic origin, and age	1950[1]	1960[1]	1970	1980	1985	1990	1995	1996	1997	1998	1996–98[2]
American Indian or Alaska Native female[3]					Deaths per 100,000 resident population						
All ages, age adjusted	- - -	- - -	- - -	23.3	20.6	18.5	19.9	20.6	19.9	20.2	20.2
All ages, crude	- - -	- - -	- - -	22.1	21.8	19.3	23.8	25.5	24.3	25.4	25.1
45–54 years	- - -	- - -	- - -	*	*	*	*	24.6	*	18.8	19.0
55–64 years	- - -	- - -	- - -	*	40.4	40.7	43.5	29.7	49.4	47.5	42.4
65–74 years	- - -	- - -	- - -	128.3	121.2	100.5	112.3	127.7	109.0	126.4	121.0
75–84 years	- - -	- - -	- - -	404.2	317.6	282.0	321.7	354.9	319.7	324.6	332.7
85 years and over	- - -	- - -	- - -	1,123.6	1,000.0	776.2	697.3	700.0	570.0	618.1	627.3
Asian or Pacific Islander female[4]											
All ages, age adjusted	- - -	- - -	- - -	25.9	23.6	23.4	21.6	21.5	21.4	19.6	20.8
All ages, crude	- - -	- - -	- - -	26.5	23.3	24.3	24.9	27.5	27.8	26.4	27.2
45–54 years	- - -	- - -	- - -	20.3	15.1	19.7	16.2	16.2	14.2	11.4	13.8
55–64 years	- - -	- - -	- - -	44.5	49.0	42.5	39.1	36.3	40.7	31.0	35.9
65–74 years	- - -	- - -	- - -	136.1	130.8	124.0	103.3	111.2	109.3	113.4	111.3
75–84 years	- - -	- - -	- - -	449.6	387.0	396.6	405.2	409.2	409.8	388.8	402.0
85 years and over	- - -	- - -	- - -	1,545.2	1,383.3	1,395.0	1,432.5	1,243.3	1,097.8	1,006.4	1,108.7
Hispanic female[5]											
All ages, age adjusted	- - -	- - -	- - -	- - -	20.6	19.5	18.1	17.1	17.0	16.6	16.9
All ages, crude	- - -	- - -	- - -	- - -	18.3	20.2	20.1	19.6	19.6	19.6	19.6
45–54 years	- - -	- - -	- - -	- - -	15.8	15.2	15.1	15.3	12.7	14.2	14.0
55–64 years	- - -	- - -	- - -	- - -	35.8	38.8	35.7	35.2	32.4	30.1	32.5
65–74 years	- - -	- - -	- - -	- - -	108.6	102.9	98.2	90.3	96.8	93.0	93.4
75–84 years	- - -	- - -	- - -	- - -	339.8	309.5	287.4	284.3	286.3	279.1	283.1
85 years and over	- - -	- - -	- - -	- - -	1,191.5	1,060.4	932.4	837.8	774.5	756.1	787.2
White, non-Hispanic female[5]											
All ages, age adjusted	- - -	- - -	- - -	- - -	27.2	23.9	23.1	23.0	22.6	22.1	22.6
All ages, crude	- - -	- - -	- - -	- - -	81.0	77.4	82.2	82.9	82.6	82.1	82.5
45–54 years	- - -	- - -	- - -	- - -	14.3	13.2	12.4	12.4	11.3	10.9	11.5
55–64 years	- - -	- - -	- - -	- - -	37.8	35.7	33.0	32.7	31.5	31.1	31.7
65–74 years	- - -	- - -	- - -	- - -	133.5	117.1	112.4	110.7	111.5	108.9	110.4
75–84 years	- - -	- - -	- - -	- - -	551.6	463.1	452.9	450.4	442.0	439.5	443.9
85 years and over	- - -	- - -	- - -	- - -	1,926.2	1,720.4	1,704.8	1,707.4	1,675.3	1,621.5	1,667.0

- - - Data not available.

* Based on fewer than 20 deaths.

[1]Includes deaths of persons who were not residents of the 50 States and the District of Columbia.

[2]Average annual death rate.

[3]Interpretation of trends should take into account that population estimates for American Indians increased by 45 percent between 1980 and 1990, partly due to better enumeration techniques in the 1990 decennial census and to the increased tendency for people to identify themselves as American Indian in 1990.

[4]Interpretation of trends should take into account that the Asian population in the United States more than doubled between 1980 and 1990, primarily due to immigration.

[5]Excludes data from States lacking an Hispanic-origin item on their death certificates. See Appendix I, National Vital Statistics System.

NOTES: Rates are age adjusted to the 1940 U.S. standard million population. See Appendix II, Age adjustment. For data years shown, the code numbers for cause of death are based on the then current *International Classification of Diseases*, which are described in Appendix II, tables IV and V. Age groups were selected to minimize the presentation of unstable age-specific death rates based on small numbers of deaths and for consistency among comparison groups. The race groups, white, black, Asian or Pacific Islander, and American Indian or Alaska Native, include persons of Hispanic and non-Hispanic origin. Conversely, persons of Hispanic origin may be of any race. Bias in death rates results from inconsistent race identification between the death certificate (source of data for numerator of death rates) and data from the Census Bureau (denominator); and from undercounts of some population groups in the census. The net effects of misclassification and under coverage result in death rates estimated to be overstated by 1 percent for the white population and 5 percent for the black population; and death rates estimated to be understated by 21 percent for American Indians, 11 percent for Asians, and 2 percent for Hispanics (Rosenberg HM, Maurer JD, Sorlie PD, Johnson NJ, et al. Quality of death rates by race and Hispanic origin: A summary of current research, 1999. National Center for Health Statistics. Vital Health Stat 2(128). 1999). Data for additional years are available (see Appendix III).

SOURCES: Centers for Disease Control and Prevention, National Center for Health Statistics. Grove RD and Hetzel AM. *Vital statistics rates in the United States, 1940–60*. Washington: Public Health Service, 1968; *Vital statistics of the United States, vol II, mortality, part A*, for data years 1950–93. Public Health Service. Washington. U.S. Government Printing Office; for 1994–98, data for all persons, white, and black are available on the NCHS Web site at www.cdc.gov/nchs/datawh/statab/unpubd/mortabs.htm; numerator data from National Vital Statistics System, annual mortality files; denominator data from national population estimates for race groups from table 1 and unpublished Hispanic population estimates prepared by the Housing and Household Economic Statistics Division, U.S. Bureau of the Census.

Table 39 (page 1 of 4). **Death rates for malignant neoplasms, according to sex, detailed race, Hispanic origin, and age: United States, selected years 1950–98**

[Data are based on the National Vital Statistics System]

Sex, race, Hispanic origin, and age	1950[1]	1960[1]	1970	1980	1985	1990	1995	1996	1997	1998	1996–98[2]
All persons				Deaths per 100,000 resident population							
All ages, age adjusted	125.4	125.8	129.8	132.8	134.4	135.0	129.9	127.9	125.6	123.6	125.6
All ages, crude	139.8	149.2	162.8	183.9	194.0	203.2	204.9	203.4	201.6	200.3	201.8
Under 1 year	8.7	7.2	4.7	3.2	3.1	2.3	1.8	2.3	2.4	2.1	2.3
1–4 years	11.7	10.9	7.5	4.5	3.8	3.5	3.1	2.7	2.9	2.4	2.7
5–14 years	6.7	6.8	6.0	4.3	3.5	3.1	2.7	2.7	2.7	2.6	2.6
15–24 years	8.6	8.3	8.3	6.3	5.4	4.9	4.6	4.5	4.5	4.6	4.5
25–34 years	20.0	19.5	16.5	13.7	13.2	12.6	11.9	12.0	11.6	11.3	11.7
35–44 years	62.7	59.7	59.5	48.6	45.9	43.3	40.3	39.3	38.9	38.2	38.8
45–54 years	175.1	177.0	182.5	180.0	170.1	158.9	142.2	137.9	135.1	132.3	135.0
55–64 years	390.7	396.8	423.0	436.1	454.6	449.6	416.0	406.5	395.7	383.8	395.1
65–74 years	698.8	713.9	751.2	817.9	845.5	872.3	868.2	861.6	847.3	841.3	850.1
75–84 years	1,153.3	1,127.4	1,169.2	1,232.3	1,271.8	1,348.5	1,364.8	1,351.5	1,335.2	1,326.3	1,337.5
85 years and over	1,451.0	1,450.0	1,320.7	1,594.6	1,615.4	1,752.9	1,823.8	1,798.3	1,805.0	1,749.4	1,783.6
Male											
All ages, age adjusted	130.8	143.0	157.4	165.5	166.1	166.3	156.8	153.8	150.4	147.7	150.6
All ages, crude	142.9	162.5	182.1	205.3	213.4	221.3	219.5	217.2	214.6	213.6	215.1
Under 1 year	9.7	7.7	4.4	3.7	3.0	2.4	1.8	2.2	2.3	2.2	2.3
1–4 years	12.5	12.4	8.3	5.2	4.3	3.7	3.6	3.1	3.1	2.4	2.9
5–14 years	7.4	7.6	6.7	4.9	3.9	3.5	3.0	3.0	2.8	2.9	2.9
15–24 years	9.7	10.2	10.4	7.8	6.4	5.7	5.5	5.1	5.2	5.4	5.3
25–34 years	17.7	18.8	16.3	13.4	13.2	12.6	11.7	11.5	11.5	10.9	11.3
35–44 years	45.6	48.9	53.0	44.0	42.4	38.5	36.5	35.6	34.5	34.4	34.8
45–54 years	156.2	170.8	183.5	188.7	175.2	162.5	143.7	140.7	138.0	136.5	138.3
55–64 years	413.1	459.9	511.8	520.8	536.9	532.9	480.5	469.1	453.4	441.1	454.2
65–74 years	791.5	890.5	1,006.8	1,093.2	1,105.2	1,122.2	1,089.9	1,080.9	1,058.4	1,045.5	1,061.6
75–84 years	1,332.6	1,389.4	1,588.3	1,790.5	1,839.7	1,914.4	1,842.3	1,802.7	1,770.2	1,745.6	1,772.3
85 years and over	1,668.3	1,741.2	1,720.8	2,369.5	2,451.8	2,739.9	2,837.3	2,733.1	2,712.5	2,562.6	2,666.2
Female											
All ages, age adjusted	120.8	111.2	108.8	109.2	111.7	112.7	110.4	108.8	107.3	105.5	107.2
All ages, crude	136.8	136.4	144.4	163.6	175.7	186.0	191.0	190.2	189.2	187.7	189.0
Under 1 year	7.6	6.8	5.0	2.7	3.2	2.2	1.8	2.4	2.5	1.9	2.3
1–4 years	10.8	9.3	6.7	3.7	3.4	3.2	2.6	2.3	2.6	2.4	2.5
5–14 years	6.0	6.0	5.2	3.6	3.1	2.8	2.4	2.4	2.5	2.3	2.4
15–24 years	7.6	6.5	6.2	4.8	4.3	4.1	3.6	3.8	3.7	3.7	3.8
25–34 years	22.2	20.1	16.7	14.0	13.2	12.6	12.2	12.6	11.7	11.7	12.0
35–44 years	79.3	70.0	65.6	53.1	49.2	48.1	44.0	42.9	43.1	42.1	42.7
45–54 years	194.0	183.0	181.5	171.8	165.3	155.5	140.7	135.2	132.3	128.2	131.8
55–64 years	368.2	337.7	343.2	361.7	381.8	375.2	357.5	349.6	343.2	331.6	341.3
65–74 years	612.3	560.2	557.9	607.1	645.3	677.4	690.7	685.2	676.8	675.2	679.1
75–84 years	1,000.7	924.1	891.9	903.1	937.8	1,010.3	1,061.5	1,060.0	1,050.6	1,048.6	1,053.0
85 years and over	1,299.7	1,263.9	1,096.7	1,255.7	1,281.4	1,372.1	1,429.1	1,426.8	1,439.2	1,412.5	1,426.0
White male											
All ages, age adjusted	130.9	141.6	154.3	160.5	160.4	160.3	151.8	149.2	145.9	143.6	146.2
All ages, crude	147.2	166.1	185.1	208.7	218.1	227.7	228.1	225.8	223.3	223.0	224.0
25–34 years	17.7	18.8	16.2	13.6	13.1	12.3	11.3	11.3	11.2	10.7	11.1
35–44 years	44.5	46.3	50.1	41.1	39.8	35.8	34.2	33.5	32.3	32.6	32.8
45–54 years	150.8	164.1	172.0	175.4	162.0	149.9	134.3	131.8	129.0	126.5	129.1
55–64 years	409.4	450.9	498.1	497.4	512.0	508.2	460.0	448.9	432.4	422.4	434.3
65–74 years	798.7	887.3	997.0	1,070.7	1,076.5	1,090.7	1,064.6	1,057.3	1,038.7	1,030.1	1,042.1
75–84 years	1,367.6	1,413.7	1,592.7	1,779.7	1,817.1	1,883.2	1,810.9	1,771.0	1,746.1	1,722.4	1,746.0
85 years and over	1,732.7	1,791.4	1,772.2	2,375.6	2,449.1	2,715.1	2,805.2	2,723.9	2,695.5	2,554.3	2,654.7
Black male											
All ages, age adjusted	126.1	158.5	198.0	229.9	239.9	248.1	226.8	221.9	214.8	208.1	214.9
All ages, crude	106.6	136.7	171.6	205.5	214.9	221.9	209.1	207.3	203.0	199.0	203.1
25–34 years	18.0	18.4	18.8	14.1	14.9	15.7	15.2	14.0	14.5	12.9	13.8
35–44 years	55.7	72.9	81.3	73.8	69.9	64.3	57.5	55.0	54.3	50.0	53.0
45–54 years	211.7	244.7	311.2	333.0	315.9	302.6	250.7	242.7	235.3	241.0	239.7
55–64 years	490.8	579.7	689.2	812.5	851.3	859.2	755.3	741.2	723.3	697.4	720.3
65–74 years	636.4	938.5	1,168.9	1,417.2	1,532.8	1,613.9	1,509.6	1,473.2	1,412.4	1,344.7	1,409.6
75–84 years	- - -	1,053.3	1,624.8	2,029.6	2,229.6	2,478.3	2,426.8	2,421.8	2,298.4	2,284.5	2,333.6
85 years and over	- - -	1,155.2	1,387.0	2,393.9	2,629.0	3,238.3	3,338.2	3,209.7	3,306.2	3,050.5	3,186.3

See footnotes at end of table.

Table 39 (page 2 of 4). Death rates for malignant neoplasms, according to sex, detailed race, Hispanic origin, and age: United States, selected years 1950–98

[Data are based on the National Vital Statistics System]

Sex, race, Hispanic origin, and age	1950[1]	1960[1]	1970	1980	1985	1990	1995	1996	1997	1998	1996–98[2]
American Indian or Alaska Native male[3]				Deaths per 100,000 resident population							
All ages, age adjusted	---	---	---	82.1	87.1	83.5	94.0	94.0	104.0	95.7	97.9
All ages, crude	---	---	---	58.1	62.8	61.4	74.2	75.9	84.7	80.6	80.4
25–34 years	---	---	---	*	*	*	*	*	*	*	6.6
35–44 years	---	---	---	*	28.8	22.8	16.0	18.4	25.0	26.8	23.5
45–54 years	---	---	---	86.9	89.4	86.9	88.0	76.0	109.3	90.6	92.2
55–64 years	---	---	---	213.4	276.6	246.2	300.3	325.5	336.2	286.7	315.7
65–74 years	---	---	---	613.0	584.6	530.6	670.4	680.1	761.6	711.3	717.7
75–84 years	---	---	---	936.4	963.6	1,038.4	1,111.9	1,036.6	1,041.1	1,070.7	1,050.2
85 years and over	---	---	---	1,471.2	1,133.3	1,654.4	1,081.5	1,284.2	1,011.3	1,067.0	1,116.1
Asian or Pacific Islander male[4]											
All ages, age adjusted	---	---	---	96.4	101.0	99.6	98.3	93.8	91.7	91.1	92.2
All ages, crude	---	---	---	81.9	82.6	82.7	87.1	87.1	87.0	89.0	87.7
25–34 years	---	---	---	6.3	10.0	9.2	8.8	7.8	9.4	9.4	8.9
35–44 years	---	---	---	29.4	25.7	27.7	27.4	27.4	26.1	26.0	26.5
45–54 years	---	---	---	108.2	98.0	92.6	86.6	85.7	89.0	91.5	88.9
55–64 years	---	---	---	298.5	315.0	274.6	255.4	247.5	261.6	246.5	251.8
65–74 years	---	---	---	581.2	631.3	687.2	640.6	663.6	596.2	630.8	629.9
75–84 years	---	---	---	1,147.6	1,251.2	1,229.7	1,278.9	1,199.8	1,160.3	1,095.3	1,148.8
85 years and over	---	---	---	1,798.7	1,800.0	1,837.0	2,712.8	1,668.4	1,674.0	1,556.0	1,628.9
Hispanic male[5]											
All ages, age adjusted	---	---	---	---	92.1	99.8	98.6	93.1	91.4	92.6	92.3
All ages, crude	---	---	---	---	56.1	65.5	68.9	65.8	65.4	68.7	66.7
25–34 years	---	---	---	---	9.7	8.0	9.2	8.0	8.8	8.5	8.4
35–44 years	---	---	---	---	23.0	22.5	25.4	22.0	22.5	21.8	22.1
45–54 years	---	---	---	---	83.4	96.6	85.8	81.6	87.3	87.7	85.6
55–64 years	---	---	---	---	259.0	294.0	276.8	262.2	256.0	258.7	258.9
65–74 years	---	---	---	---	599.1	655.5	667.1	647.9	627.2	666.2	647.3
75–84 years	---	---	---	---	1,216.6	1,233.4	1,272.1	1,178.3	1,123.5	1,087.5	1,127.2
85 years and over	---	---	---	---	1,700.7	2,019.4	1,858.7	1,637.8	1,658.8	1,551.0	1,613.2
White, non-Hispanic male[5]											
All ages, age adjusted	---	---	---	---	156.0	163.3	154.0	151.7	148.6	146.2	148.8
All ages, crude	---	---	---	---	217.4	246.2	247.1	246.2	244.7	243.9	245.0
25–34 years	---	---	---	---	13.5	12.8	11.4	11.8	11.5	10.9	11.4
35–44 years	---	---	---	---	39.1	36.8	34.7	34.4	33.1	33.7	33.7
45–54 years	---	---	---	---	159.9	153.9	137.0	134.9	131.9	129.1	131.9
55–64 years	---	---	---	---	496.4	520.6	469.9	458.6	443.3	432.2	444.4
65–74 years	---	---	---	---	1,044.2	1,109.0	1,081.1	1,073.6	1,057.8	1,047.5	1,059.7
75–84 years	---	---	---	---	1,766.1	1,906.6	1,825.6	1,791.6	1,765.7	1,745.8	1,767.2
85 years and over	---	---	---	---	2,327.6	2,744.4	2,814.6	2,764.3	2,738.3	2,599.8	2,697.5
White female											
All ages, age adjusted	119.4	109.5	107.6	107.7	110.5	111.2	108.9	107.6	106.0	104.1	105.9
All ages, crude	139.9	139.8	149.4	170.3	184.4	196.1	202.4	201.8	200.4	199.1	200.4
25–34 years	20.9	18.8	16.3	13.5	12.7	11.9	11.5	12.1	11.2	11.2	11.5
35–44 years	74.5	66.6	62.4	50.9	47.3	46.2	42.0	40.5	40.6	39.3	40.1
45–54 years	185.8	175.7	177.3	166.4	161.6	150.9	136.1	131.0	128.4	123.3	127.5
55–64 years	362.5	329.0	338.6	355.5	376.3	368.5	352.6	347.3	339.6	326.5	337.6
65–74 years	616.5	562.1	554.7	605.2	644.9	675.1	689.6	684.6	674.6	675.7	678.4
75–84 years	1,026.6	939.3	903.5	905.4	938.2	1,011.8	1,060.2	1,059.9	1,049.7	1,051.1	1,053.5
85 years and over	1,348.3	1,304.9	1,126.6	1,266.8	1,285.4	1,372.3	1,428.2	1,430.1	1,435.8	1,415.1	1,426.8

See footnotes at end of table.

Table 39 (page 3 of 4). Death rates for malignant neoplasms, according to sex, detailed race, Hispanic origin, and age: United States, selected years 1950–98

[Data are based on the National Vital Statistics System]

Sex, race, Hispanic origin, and age	1950[1]	1960[1]	1970	1980	1985	1990	1995	1996	1997	1998	1996–98[2]
Black female					Deaths per 100,000 resident population						
All ages, age adjusted	131.9	127.8	123.5	129.7	131.8	137.2	134.1	130.7	131.2	128.9	130.3
All ages, crude	111.8	113.8	117.3	136.5	145.2	156.1	159.1	157.9	160.5	158.5	159.0
25–34 years	34.3	31.0	20.9	18.3	17.2	18.7	16.8	16.4	16.2	15.6	16.1
35–44 years	119.8	102.4	94.6	73.5	69.0	67.4	62.2	62.8	62.9	64.1	63.2
45–54 years	277.0	254.8	228.6	230.2	212.4	209.9	192.7	182.8	180.6	180.9	181.4
55–64 years	484.6	442.7	404.8	450.4	474.9	482.4	443.6	422.2	426.4	419.9	422.8
65–74 years	477.3	541.6	615.8	662.4	704.2	773.2	799.6	790.6	789.7	770.2	783.5
75–84 years	- - -	696.3	763.3	923.9	986.3	1,059.9	1,154.1	1,150.9	1,166.5	1,138.3	1,151.9
85 years and over	- - -	728.9	791.5	1,159.9	1,284.2	1,431.3	1,490.3	1,507.2	1,602.3	1,513.5	1,540.8
American Indian or Alaska Native female[3]											
All ages, age adjusted	- - -	- - -	- - -	62.1	60.5	69.6	70.7	78.6	72.8	74.3	75.1
All ages, crude	- - -	- - -	- - -	50.4	52.5	62.1	69.9	77.1	71.8	74.9	74.6
25–34 years	- - -	- - -	- - -	*	*	*	11.1	*	11.0	*	9.0
35–44 years	- - -	- - -	- - -	36.9	23.4	31.0	33.5	38.5	36.8	33.4	36.2
45–54 years	- - -	- - -	- - -	96.9	90.1	104.5	85.2	111.2	88.3	94.9	97.9
55–64 years	- - -	- - -	- - -	198.4	192.3	213.2	223.2	249.2	245.5	255.8	250.3
65–74 years	- - -	- - -	- - -	350.8	378.8	438.9	427.7	487.3	467.5	481.1	478.6
75–84 years	- - -	- - -	- - -	446.4	505.9	554.3	723.9	721.4	613.4	599.9	643.2
85 years and over	- - -	- - -	- - -	786.5	700.0	843.7	736.6	638.0	561.9	649.0	616.3
Asian or Pacific Islander female[4]											
All ages, age adjusted	- - -	- - -	- - -	59.8	62.8	63.6	68.4	63.2	63.0	62.4	62.8
All ages, crude	- - -	- - -	- - -	54.1	57.5	60.5	71.5	69.7	71.1	71.0	70.6
25–34 years	- - -	- - -	- - -	9.5	9.9	7.3	10.6	9.6	7.0	9.3	8.6
35–44 years	- - -	- - -	- - -	38.7	33.1	29.8	28.6	29.9	31.5	27.7	29.7
45–54 years	- - -	- - -	- - -	99.8	91.3	93.9	98.0	88.7	81.1	83.3	84.3
55–64 years	- - -	- - -	- - -	174.7	195.5	196.2	211.4	179.6	176.7	186.8	181.2
65–74 years	- - -	- - -	- - -	301.9	330.8	346.2	351.2	347.8	376.4	362.7	362.5
75–84 years	- - -	- - -	- - -	522.1	589.1	641.4	722.6	703.6	662.1	639.9	666.7
85 years and over	- - -	- - -	- - -	800.0	908.3	971.7	1,307.7	917.8	1,014.0	908.8	946.4
Hispanic female[5]											
All ages, age adjusted	- - -	- - -	- - -	- - -	64.1	70.0	66.1	66.7	65.4	63.8	65.3
All ages, crude	- - -	- - -	- - -	- - -	49.8	60.7	60.5	62.1	61.4	60.4	61.3
25–34 years	- - -	- - -	- - -	- - -	9.7	9.7	9.2	10.3	10.3	9.6	10.1
35–44 years	- - -	- - -	- - -	- - -	30.9	34.8	31.2	30.0	30.5	29.8	30.1
45–54 years	- - -	- - -	- - -	- - -	90.1	100.5	89.7	85.3	84.7	86.7	85.6
55–64 years	- - -	- - -	- - -	- - -	199.4	205.4	197.6	202.4	201.6	189.9	197.7
65–74 years	- - -	- - -	- - -	- - -	356.3	404.8	382.3	405.3	388.2	390.4	394.4
75–84 years	- - -	- - -	- - -	- - -	599.7	663.0	659.6	637.8	622.4	588.5	615.3
85 years and over	- - -	- - -	- - -	- - -	906.1	1,022.7	938.2	913.9	888.6	835.2	876.9

See footnotes at end of table.

Table 39 (page 4 of 4). Death rates for malignant neoplasms, according to sex, detailed race, Hispanic origin, and age: United States, selected years 1950–98

[Data are based on the National Vital Statistics System]

Sex, race, Hispanic origin, and age	1950[1]	1960[1]	1970	1980	1985	1990	1995	1996	1997	1998	1996–98[2]
White, non-Hispanic female[5]					Deaths per 100,000 resident population						
All ages, age adjusted	- - -	- - -	- - -	- - -	108.9	113.6	111.1	109.8	108.1	106.3	108.0
All ages, crude	- - -	- - -	- - -	- - -	187.1	210.6	218.4	218.3	217.3	216.9	217.5
25–34 years	- - -	- - -	- - -	- - -	12.2	11.9	11.7	12.2	11.2	11.3	11.6
35–44 years	- - -	- - -	- - -	- - -	47.2	47.0	42.7	41.2	41.4	40.1	40.9
45–54 years	- - -	- - -	- - -	- - -	158.8	154.9	139.3	133.9	131.2	125.7	130.2
55–64 years	- - -	- - -	- - -	- - -	372.7	379.5	362.7	356.6	348.5	335.7	346.7
65–74 years	- - -	- - -	- - -	- - -	638.3	688.5	703.1	697.9	688.7	691.2	692.6
75–84 years	- - -	- - -	- - -	- - -	917.7	1,027.2	1,070.5	1,075.3	1,063.9	1,068.3	1,069.1
85 years and over	- - -	- - -	- - -	- - -	1,241.6	1,385.7	1,438.4	1,448.8	1,452.5	1,435.7	1,445.5

- - - Data not available.

* Based on fewer than 20 deaths.

[1]Includes deaths of persons who were not residents of the 50 States and the District of Columbia.

[2]Average annual death rate.

[3]Interpretation of trends should take into account that population estimates for American Indians increased by 45 percent between 1980 and 1990, partly due to better enumeration techniques in the 1990 decennial census and to the increased tendency for people to identify themselves as American Indian in 1990.

[4]Interpretation of trends should take into account that the Asian population in the United States more than doubled between 1980 and 1990, primarily due to immigration.

[5]Excludes data from States lacking an Hispanic-origin item on their death certificates. See Appendix I, National Vital Statistics System.

NOTES: Rates are age adjusted to the 1940 U.S. standard million population. See Appendix II, Age adjustment. For data years shown, the code numbers for cause of death are based on the then current *International Classification of Diseases*, which are described in Appendix II, tables IV and V. Age groups were selected to minimize the presentation of unstable age-specific death rates based on small numbers of deaths and for consistency among comparison groups. The race groups, white, black, Asian or Pacific Islander, and American Indian or Alaska Native, include persons of Hispanic and non-Hispanic origin. Conversely, persons of Hispanic origin may be of any race. Bias in death rates results from inconsistent race identification between the death certificate (source of data for numerator of death rates) and data from the Census Bureau (denominator); and from undercounts of some population groups in the census. The net effects of misclassification and under coverage result in death rates estimated to be overstated by 1 percent for the white population and 5 percent for the black population; and death rates estimated to be understated by 21 percent for American Indians, 11 percent for Asians, and 2 percent for Hispanics (Rosenberg HM, Maurer JD, Sorlie PD, Johnson NJ, et al. Quality of death rates by race and Hispanic origin: A summary of current research, 1999. National Center for Health Statistics. Vital Health Stat 2(128). 1999). Data for additional years are available (see Appendix III).

SOURCES: Centers for Disease Control and Prevention, National Center for Health Statistics. Grove RD and Hetzel AM. *Vital statistics rates in the United States, 1940–60*. Washington: Public Health Service, 1968; *Vital statistics of the United States, vol II, mortality, part A*, for data years 1950–93. Public Health Service. Washington. U.S. Government Printing Office; for 1994–98, data for all persons, white, and black are available on the NCHS Web site at www.cdc.gov/nchs/datawh/statab/unpubd/mortabs.htm; numerator data from National Vital Statistics System, annual mortality files; denominator data from national population estimates for race groups from table 1 and unpublished Hispanic population estimates prepared by the Housing and Household Economic Statistics Division, U.S. Bureau of the Census.

Table 40 (page 1 of 3). **Death rates for malignant neoplasms of trachea, bronchus, and lung, according to sex, detailed race, Hispanic origin, and age: United States, selected years 1950–98**

[Data are based on the National Vital Statistics System]

Sex, race, Hispanic origin, and age	1950	1960	1970	1980	1985	1990	1995	1996	1997	1998	1996–98[1]
All persons					Deaths per 100,000 resident population						
All ages, age adjusted	11.1	17.7	26.6	34.8	37.6	39.9	38.3	37.9	37.3	37.0	37.4
All ages, crude	12.1	20.3	32.1	45.8	51.5	56.8	57.5	57.3	57.3	57.2	57.3
Under 25 years	0.1	0.0	0.1	0.0	0.0	0.0	0.0	0.0	0.0	0.0	0.0
25–34 years	0.8	1.0	0.9	0.6	0.6	0.7	0.7	0.7	0.6	0.6	0.6
35–44 years	4.5	6.8	11.0	9.2	7.8	6.8	6.0	6.2	6.2	6.1	6.2
45–54 years	20.4	29.6	43.4	54.1	50.9	46.8	38.0	36.8	34.6	33.3	34.9
55–64 years	48.7	75.3	109.1	138.2	153.8	160.6	142.9	138.7	134.3	131.4	134.7
65–74 years	59.7	108.1	164.5	233.3	261.2	288.4	297.1	296.1	295.7	296.7	296.2
75–84 years	55.8	91.5	163.2	240.5	282.0	333.3	361.4	364.4	368.5	367.7	366.9
85 years and over	42.3	65.6	101.7	176.0	195.2	242.5	284.0	280.9	297.6	289.9	289.6
Male											
All ages, age adjusted	18.4	32.0	47.5	56.9	58.1	58.5	53.0	51.8	50.5	49.5	50.6
All ages, crude	19.9	35.4	53.4	68.6	72.5	75.1	71.6	70.6	69.7	69.3	69.8
Under 25 years	0.0	0.0	0.1	0.1	*	0.0	0.1	*	*	0.0	0.0
25–34 years	1.1	1.4	1.3	0.8	0.7	0.9	0.8	0.7	0.6	0.6	0.6
35–44 years	7.1	10.5	16.1	11.9	10.0	8.5	7.1	7.3	7.1	7.0	7.1
45–54 years	35.0	50.6	76.0	76.0	67.5	59.7	47.0	45.8	42.7	40.8	43.1
55–64 years	83.8	139.3	189.7	213.6	223.5	222.9	187.4	181.4	173.7	168.4	174.4
65–74 years	98.7	204.3	320.8	403.9	416.2	430.4	417.0	409.3	404.0	401.7	405.0
75–84 years	82.6	167.1	330.8	488.8	537.6	572.9	552.1	547.2	543.0	534.7	541.5
85 years and over	62.5	107.7	194.0	368.1	433.2	513.2	543.8	520.7	543.8	512.4	525.4
Female											
All ages, age adjusted	3.9	5.7	9.5	17.6	21.8	25.6	26.9	26.9	26.9	27.0	26.9
All ages, crude	4.5	4.7	11.9	24.3	31.7	39.4	44.1	44.6	45.4	45.7	45.2
Under 25 years	0.1	0.0	0.0	*	*	*	*	*	*	*	0.0
25–34 years	0.5	5.4	0.5	0.5	0.6	0.5	0.6	0.6	0.5	0.6	0.6
35–44 years	1.9	3.2	6.1	6.5	5.6	5.2	5.0	5.1	5.4	5.3	5.3
45–54 years	5.8	9.2	21.0	33.7	35.2	34.5	29.4	28.2	26.9	26.0	27.0
55–64 years	13.6	15.4	36.8	72.0	92.1	105.0	102.6	99.9	98.5	97.6	98.7
65–74 years	23.3	24.4	43.1	102.7	141.8	177.6	201.1	204.9	208.2	211.3	208.1
75–84 years	32.9	32.8	52.4	94.1	131.7	190.1	240.3	246.4	254.3	257.2	252.7
85 years and over	28.2	38.8	50.0	91.9	100.2	138.1	182.8	185.6	198.4	197.8	194.1
White male											
All ages, age adjusted	18.8	31.9	46.9	55.5	56.4	56.6	51.6	50.5	49.4	48.4	49.4
All ages, crude	20.8	36.4	37.5	70.2	74.5	77.8	74.9	73.9	73.1	72.7	73.2
45–54 years	35.1	49.2	63.3	70.9	62.7	55.2	43.7	42.7	39.6	37.5	39.9
55–64 years	85.4	139.2	186.8	205.6	214.2	213.7	180.4	174.4	167.4	162.5	168.0
65–74 years	101.5	207.5	325.0	401.0	409.5	422.1	411.3	404.9	400.4	399.2	401.5
75–84 years	85.5	170.4	336.7	493.5	540.3	572.2	548.8	543.7	540.1	531.7	538.4
85 years and over	67.4	109.4	199.6	374.1	440.0	516.3	542.4	524.5	549.1	516.6	529.8
Black male											
All ages, age adjusted	14.3	33.0	56.6	77.2	82.6	86.2	75.8	73.5	70.6	68.5	70.8
All ages, crude	12.1	28.1	47.7	66.6	71.2	73.7	67.0	65.8	64.1	63.0	64.3
45–54 years	34.4	68.4	115.4	133.8	122.5	114.9	87.6	85.3	79.4	78.8	81.1
55–64 years	68.3	146.8	234.3	321.1	351.5	358.6	295.3	287.0	270.1	263.2	273.2
65–74 years	54.2	168.3	300.5	472.3	539.6	585.4	547.9	520.8	507.9	487.5	505.3
75–84 years	- - -	107.3	271.6	472.9	556.4	645.4	660.8	660.8	660.1	647.5	656.0
85 years and over	- - -	82.8	137.0	311.3	382.3	499.5	573.2	544.7	553.8	533.1	543.7
American Indian or Alaska Native male[2]											
All ages, age adjusted	- - -	- - -	- - -	21.1	26.7	28.1	31.2	33.5	33.8	34.4	33.9
All ages, crude	- - -	- - -	- - -	14.2	18.4	20.0	23.9	25.6	26.5	27.8	26.7
45–54 years	- - -	- - -	- - -	*	*	26.6	26.5	24.4	32.1	30.2	29.0
55–64 years	- - -	- - -	- - -	72.0	85.1	97.8	106.1	139.7	124.9	109.9	124.5
65–74 years	- - -	- - -	- - -	202.8	223.1	194.3	256.0	267.9	268.4	294.5	277.1
75–84 years	- - -	- - -	- - -	*	263.6	356.2	338.4	308.2	339.9	376.7	343.0
85 years and over	- - -	- - -	- - -	*	*	*	*	*	*	*	201.4

See footnotes at end of table.

[Data are based on the National Vital Statistics System]

Sex, race, Hispanic origin, and age	1950	1960	1970	1980	1985	1990	1995	1996	1997	1998	1996–98[1]
Asian or Pacific Islander male[3]					Deaths per 100,000 resident population						
All ages, age adjusted	---	---	---	26.7	25.8	25.7	24.8	24.8	24.2	24.7	24.6
All ages, crude	---	---	---	22.1	20.4	20.7	21.5	22.4	22.4	23.5	22.8
45–54 years	---	---	---	33.3	21.7	18.8	19.6	15.4	17.4	17.3	16.7
55–64 years	---	---	---	94.4	98.1	74.4	67.1	69.8	72.8	66.6	69.7
65–74 years	---	---	---	174.3	180.8	215.8	191.9	206.9	194.5	215.3	205.7
75–84 years	---	---	---	301.3	295.3	307.5	324.9	341.1	300.4	318.4	319.5
85 years and over	---	---	---	*	350.0	421.3	572.2	343.0	367.1	332.9	347.1
Hispanic male[4]											
All ages, age adjusted	---	---	---	---	22.4	25.7	23.3	22.0	21.3	21.0	21.4
All ages, crude	---	---	---	---	12.9	16.2	15.6	14.8	14.6	15.0	14.8
45–54 years	---	---	---	---	16.7	21.5	17.7	18.3	17.3	15.7	17.1
55–64 years	---	---	---	---	68.6	80.7	68.7	66.3	58.9	58.9	61.3
65–74 years	---	---	---	---	169.9	195.5	183.5	175.7	176.1	173.4	175.0
75–84 years	---	---	---	---	292.1	313.4	303.5	277.9	274.0	271.4	274.2
85 years and over	---	---	---	---	393.8	420.7	352.5	278.9	332.9	264.1	291.3
White, non-Hispanic male[4]											
All ages, age adjusted	---	---	---	---	54.9	58.2	52.9	52.0	51.0	50.1	51.0
All ages, crude	---	---	---	---	74.5	84.7	81.8	81.4	81.2	80.8	81.1
45–54 years	---	---	---	---	62.6	57.8	45.4	44.4	41.4	39.3	41.6
55–64 years	---	---	---	---	209.8	221.0	186.8	180.7	175.0	169.6	175.0
65–74 years	---	---	---	---	398.4	431.4	420.3	414.9	412.1	411.6	412.8
75–84 years	---	---	---	---	518.2	580.4	554.9	552.1	549.5	542.6	548.0
85 years and over	---	---	---	---	413.8	520.9	543.4	533.1	557.7	528.7	539.7
White female											
All ages, age adjusted	4.0	4.7	9.5	17.6	22.1	25.9	27.4	27.4	27.4	27.4	27.4
All ages, crude	4.7	5.9	12.3	25.6	33.9	42.4	48.0	48.6	49.3	49.7	49.2
45–54 years	5.7	5.0	20.9	33.0	35.4	34.6	29.5	28.4	26.8	25.8	27.0
55–64 years	13.7	8.8	37.2	71.9	92.4	105.7	104.7	102.9	100.9	99.7	101.1
65–74 years	23.7	13.8	42.9	104.6	145.5	181.3	205.0	210.0	213.2	216.6	213.3
75–84 years	34.0	20.0	52.6	95.2	134.8	194.6	246.1	251.5	259.7	263.1	258.1
85 years and over	29.3	25.4	50.6	92.4	99.3	138.3	184.0	188.2	200.5	200.3	196.5
Black female											
All ages, age adjusted	3.4	4.8	10.2	18.5	21.8	26.4	26.9	26.6	27.3	27.5	27.2
All ages, crude	2.8	4.3	9.4	18.3	22.5	28.1	30.2	30.5	31.9	32.2	31.5
45–54 years	7.5	11.3	23.9	43.4	39.1	41.3	34.9	33.0	33.6	33.4	33.4
55–64 years	12.9	17.9	33.5	79.9	103.5	117.9	106.5	99.3	101.8	102.6	101.3
65–74 years	14.0	18.1	46.1	88.0	117.2	164.3	195.3	196.1	200.5	202.5	199.7
75–84 years	---	31.3	49.1	79.4	101.2	148.1	188.6	209.3	220.1	222.4	217.4
85 years and over	---	34.2	44.8	85.8	114.3	134.9	163.7	162.1	184.2	176.6	174.4
American Indian or Alaska Native female[2]											
All ages, age adjusted	---	---	---	7.5	10.1	13.4	15.9	15.8	16.1	17.6	16.5
All ages, crude	---	---	---	6.0	8.2	11.2	15.0	15.2	15.2	16.9	15.8
45–54 years	---	---	---	*	*	22.9	*	*	*	18.0	15.5
55–64 years	---	---	---	*	38.5	53.7	47.8	62.3	65.8	62.0	63.4
65–74 years	---	---	---	*	93.9	78.5	131.8	102.1	130.0	157.0	130.1
75–84 years	---	---	---	*	*	111.8	185.0	192.9	141.3	130.6	154.0
85 years and over	---	---	---	*	*	*	*	*	*	*	84.9

See footnotes at end of table.

[Data are based on the National Vital Statistics System]

Sex, race, Hispanic origin, and age	1950	1960	1970	1980	1985	1990	1995	1996	1997	1998	1996–98[1]
Asian or Pacific Islander female[3]				Deaths per 100,000 resident population							
All ages, age adjusted	---	---	---	9.5	8.9	11.1	12.8	10.8	11.3	11.5	11.2
All ages, crude	---	---	---	8.4	7.9	10.5	13.4	12.0	12.9	13.2	12.7
45–54 years	---	---	---	13.5	12.5	11.3	12.1	11.1	9.8	9.9	10.2
55–64 years	---	---	---	24.6	26.0	38.3	39.1	29.8	32.3	35.9	32.7
65–74 years	---	---	---	62.4	60.7	71.6	86.1	76.1	79.7	82.0	79.4
75–84 years	---	---	---	117.7	97.8	137.9	162.9	149.5	147.3	138.6	144.8
85 years and over	---	---	---	*	*	172.9	281.9	179.0	170.5	176.3	175.2
Hispanic female[4]											
All ages, age adjusted	---	---	---	---	6.4	8.5	7.9	8.3	8.7	7.9	8.3
All ages, crude	---	---	---	---	4.9	7.2	7.3	7.8	8.1	7.5	7.8
45–54 years	---	---	---	---	6.8	8.7	7.1	6.1	7.1	7.3	6.8
55–64 years	---	---	---	---	17.4	25.1	24.8	25.9	27.7	23.9	25.8
65–74 years	---	---	---	---	49.1	66.8	56.8	65.8	67.2	59.5	64.1
75–84 years	---	---	---	---	73.6	94.3	103.6	98.8	101.3	95.0	98.3
85 years and over	---	---	---	---	110.7	118.2	117.0	124.8	116.0	105.5	114.8
White, non-Hispanic female[4]											
All ages, age adjusted	---	---	---	---	22.6	26.9	28.5	28.6	28.6	28.8	28.6
All ages, crude	---	---	---	---	35.6	46.2	52.6	53.5	54.4	55.2	54.4
45–54 years	---	---	---	---	36.6	36.6	31.3	30.1	28.4	27.4	28.6
55–64 years	---	---	---	---	93.4	111.3	110.5	108.4	106.3	105.6	106.7
65–74 years	---	---	---	---	149.4	186.4	212.0	217.5	221.3	226.1	221.6
75–84 years	---	---	---	---	138.1	199.1	250.5	257.2	265.6	270.0	264.4
85 years and over	---	---	---	---	100.9	139.0	185.1	190.6	203.3	203.9	199.4

0.0 Quantity more than zero but less than 0.05.
* Based on fewer than 20 deaths.
- - - Data not available.
[1]Average annual death rate.
[2]Interpretation of trends should take into account that population estimates for American Indians increased by 45 percent between 1980 and 1990, partly due to better enumeration techniques in the 1990 decennial census and to the increased tendency for people to identify themselves as American Indian in 1990.
[3]Interpretation of trends should take into account that the Asian population in the United States more than doubled between 1980 and 1990, primarily due to immigration.
[4]Excludes data from States lacking an Hispanic-origin item on their death certificates. See Appendix I, National Vital Statistics System.

NOTES: Rates are age adjusted to the 1940 U.S. standard million population. See Appendix II, Age adjustment. For data years shown, the code numbers for cause of death are based on the then current *International Classification of Diseases* (ICD), which are described in Appendix II, tables IV and V. Starting with *Health, United States, 2000* this table presents trends for malignant neoplasms of trachea, bronchus, and lung, ICD 162, replacing malignant neoplasms of the respiratory system, ICD 160–165, shown in previous editions. Age groups were selected to minimize the presentation of unstable age-specific death rates based on small numbers of deaths and for consistency among comparison groups. The race groups, white, black, Asian or Pacific Islander, and American Indian or Alaska Native, include persons of Hispanic and non-Hispanic origin. Conversely, persons of Hispanic origin may be of any race. Bias in death rates results from inconsistent race identification between the death certificate (source of data for numerator of death rates) and data from the Census Bureau (denominator); and from undercounts of some population groups in the census. The net effects of misclassification and under coverage result in death rates estimated to be overstated by 1 percent for the white population and 5 percent for the black population; and death rates estimated to be understated by 21 percent for American Indians, 11 percent for Asians, and 2 percent for Hispanics (Rosenberg HM, Maurer JD, Sorlie PD, Johnson NJ, et al. Quality of death rates by race and Hispanic origin: A summary of current research, 1999. National Center for Health Statistics. Vital Health Stat 2(128). 1999). Data for additional years are available (see Appendix III).

SOURCES: Centers for Disease Control and Prevention, National Center for Health Statistics. Grove RD and Hetzel AM. *Vital statistics rates in the United States, 1940–60.* Washington: Public Health Service, 1968; *Vital statistics of the United States, vol II, mortality, part A,* for data years 1950–93. Public Health Service. Washington. U.S. Government Printing Office; for 1994–98, data for all persons, white, and black are available on the NCHS Web site at www.cdc.gov/nchs/datawh/statab/unpubd/mortabs.htm; numerator data from National Vital Statistics System, annual mortality files; denominator data from national population estimates for race groups from table 1 and unpublished Hispanic population estimates prepared by the Housing and Household Economic Statistics Division, U.S. Bureau of the Census.

Table 41 (page 1 of 2). Death rates for malignant neoplasm of breast for females, according to detailed race, Hispanic origin, and age: United States, selected years 1950–98

[Data are based on the National Vital Statistics System]

Race, Hispanic origin, and age	1950[1]	1960[1]	1970	1980	1985	1990	1995	1996	1997	1998	1996–98[2]
All persons				Deaths per 100,000 resident population							
All ages, age adjusted	22.2	22.3	23.1	22.7	23.3	23.1	21.0	20.2	19.4	18.8	19.5
All ages, crude	24.7	26.1	28.4	30.6	32.8	34.0	32.6	31.8	30.7	30.2	30.9
Under 25 years	*	*	*	*	0.0	*	*	0.0	*	*	0.0
25–34 years	3.8	3.8	3.9	3.3	3.0	2.9	2.7	2.7	2.6	2.6	2.6
35–44 years	20.8	20.2	20.4	17.9	17.5	17.8	15.0	14.2	14.0	13.4	13.9
45–54 years	46.9	51.4	52.6	48.1	47.1	45.4	41.4	38.8	37.8	35.8	37.5
55–64 years	70.4	70.8	77.6	80.5	84.2	78.6	69.8	67.4	64.4	62.2	64.6
65–74 years	94.0	90.0	93.8	101.1	107.8	111.7	103.3	99.1	94.1	93.3	95.5
75–84 years	139.8	129.9	127.4	126.4	136.2	146.3	142.0	139.8	132.2	131.4	134.4
85 years and over	195.5	191.9	157.1	169.3	178.5	196.8	203.7	204.9	198.5	194.7	199.3
White											
All ages, age adjusted	22.5	22.4	23.4	22.8	23.4	22.9	20.5	19.8	18.9	18.3	19.0
All ages, crude	25.7	27.2	29.9	32.3	34.7	35.9	34.1	33.3	31.9	31.5	32.2
35–44 years	20.8	19.7	20.2	17.3	16.8	17.1	14.1	12.9	12.9	12.2	12.6
45–54 years	47.1	51.2	53.0	48.1	46.8	44.3	39.2	36.9	36.1	33.8	35.6
55–64 years	70.9	71.8	79.3	81.3	84.7	78.5	68.7	67.2	62.8	60.7	63.5
65–74 years	96.3	91.6	95.9	103.7	109.9	113.3	103.9	99.8	93.6	94.1	95.9
75–84 years	143.6	132.8	129.6	128.4	138.8	148.2	143.0	140.6	132.3	132.2	135.0
85 years and over	204.2	199.7	161.9	171.7	180.9	198.0	205.9	207.1	199.9	196.4	201.0
Black											
All ages, age adjusted	19.3	21.3	21.5	23.3	25.5	27.5	27.5	26.5	26.7	25.3	26.2
All ages, crude	16.4	18.7	19.7	22.9	25.9	29.0	30.2	29.9	30.4	29.2	29.8
35–44 years	21.0	24.8	24.4	24.1	26.1	25.8	23.1	24.6	23.1	23.0	23.6
45–54 years	46.5	54.4	52.0	52.7	55.5	60.5	62.6	59.1	56.4	55.7	57.0
55–64 years	64.3	63.2	64.7	79.9	90.4	93.1	88.8	82.9	88.1	82.1	84.4
65–74 years	67.0	72.3	77.3	84.3	100.7	112.2	117.3	109.9	117.7	104.9	110.8
75–84 years	---	87.5	101.8	114.1	117.6	140.5	151.6	152.9	154.0	146.5	151.1
85 years and over	---	92.1	112.1	149.9	159.4	201.5	198.6	206.9	211.2	206.6	208.2
American Indian or Alaska Native[3]											
All ages, age adjusted	---	---	---	8.1	8.0	10.0	10.4	12.7	9.4	10.3	10.8
All ages, crude	---	---	---	6.1	6.9	8.6	9.8	12.1	9.0	10.1	10.4
35–44 years	---	---	---	*	*	*	*	*	*	*	7.9
45–54 years	---	---	---	*	*	23.9	24.0	28.0	19.6	21.2	22.8
55–64 years	---	---	---	*	*	*	39.1	43.9	32.9	38.2	38.3
65–74 years	---	---	---	*	*	*	45.4	66.0	48.2	42.8	52.2
75–84 years	---	---	---	*	*	*	*	*	*	*	59.1
85 years and over	---	---	---	*	*	*	*	*	*	*	68.5
Asian or Pacific Islander[4]											
All ages, age adjusted	---	---	---	9.2	9.6	10.0	11.0	8.9	9.2	9.8	9.3
All ages, crude	---	---	---	8.2	8.6	9.3	11.1	9.6	9.9	10.6	10.0
35–44 years	---	---	---	10.4	7.2	8.4	8.3	8.8	8.2	7.8	8.3
45–54 years	---	---	---	23.4	21.9	26.4	30.2	22.0	23.2	22.9	22.7
55–64 years	---	---	---	35.7	39.5	33.8	39.4	23.0	33.1	40.0	32.3
65–74 years	---	---	---	*	32.5	38.5	37.4	40.2	34.1	35.0	36.4
75–84 years	---	---	---	*	50.0	48.0	44.9	51.0	40.6	42.3	44.4
85 years and over	---	---	---	*	*	*	*	*	68.8	54.3	59.4
Hispanic[5]											
All ages, age adjusted	---	---	---	---	11.8	14.1	12.7	12.8	12.6	12.1	12.5
All ages, crude	---	---	---	---	8.8	11.5	10.9	11.4	11.2	10.7	11.1
35–44 years	---	---	---	---	10.4	11.7	9.7	11.0	9.9	9.8	10.2
45–54 years	---	---	---	---	26.4	32.8	27.7	27.4	26.7	25.3	26.4
55–64 years	---	---	---	---	43.5	45.8	43.8	39.7	45.4	43.1	42.8
65–74 years	---	---	---	---	40.9	64.8	55.7	56.5	52.9	54.7	54.7
75–84 years	---	---	---	---	64.5	67.2	75.5	85.6	71.6	63.6	73.2
85 years and over	---	---	---	---	85.7	102.8	105.4	104.5	101.9	85.9	96.8

See footnotes at end of table.

Table 41 (page 2 of 2). Death rates for malignant neoplasm of breast for females, according to detailed race, Hispanic origin, and age: United States, selected years 1950–98

[Data are based on the National Vital Statistics System]

Race, Hispanic origin, and age	1950[1]	1960[1]	1970	1980	1985	1990	1995	1996	1997	1998	1996–98[2]
White, non-Hispanic[5]					Deaths per 100,000 resident population						
All ages, age adjusted	- - -	- - -	- - -	- - -	23.3	23.5	20.9	20.1	19.2	18.7	19.3
All ages, crude	- - -	- - -	- - -	- - -	35.6	38.5	36.8	35.9	34.4	34.2	34.8
35–44 years	- - -	- - -	- - -	- - -	16.9	17.5	14.4	12.9	13.1	12.4	12.8
45–54 years	- - -	- - -	- - -	- - -	46.8	45.2	39.9	37.5	36.7	34.4	36.1
55–64 years	- - -	- - -	- - -	- - -	85.1	80.6	70.2	69.0	63.8	61.7	64.8
65–74 years	- - -	- - -	- - -	- - -	108.6	115.7	106.2	102.0	95.7	96.3	98.0
75–84 years	- - -	- - -	- - -	- - -	139.4	151.4	145.2	142.6	134.4	135.0	137.3
85 years and over	- - -	- - -	- - -	- - -	175.6	201.5	208.3	211.7	203.3	200.6	205.1

* Based on fewer than 20 deaths.

0.0 Quantity more than zero but less than 0.05.

- - - Data not available.

[1]Includes deaths of persons who were not residents of the 50 States and the District of Columbia.

[2]Average annual death rate.

[3]Interpretation of trends should take into account that population estimates for American Indians increased by 45 percent between 1980 and 1990, partly due to better enumeration techniques in the 1990 decennial census and to the increased tendency for people to identify themselves as American Indian in 1990.

[4]Interpretation of trends should take into account that the Asian population in the United States more than doubled between 1980 and 1990, primarily due to immigration.

[5]Excludes data from States lacking an Hispanic-origin item on their death certificates. See Appendix I, National Vital Statistics System.

NOTES: Rates are age adjusted to the 1940 U.S. standard million population. See Appendix II, Age adjustment. For data years shown, the code numbers for cause of death are based on the then current *International Classification of Diseases*, which are described in Appendix II, tables IV and V. Age groups were selected to minimize the presentation of unstable age-specific death rates based on small numbers of deaths and for consistency among comparison groups. The race groups, white, black, Asian or Pacific Islander, and American Indian or Alaska Native, include persons of Hispanic and non-Hispanic origin. Conversely, persons of Hispanic origin may be of any race. Bias in death rates results from inconsistent race identification between the death certificate (source of data for numerator of death rates) and data from the Census Bureau (denominator); and from undercounts of some population groups in the census. The net effects of misclassification and under coverage result in death rates estimated to be overstated by 1 percent for the white population and 5 percent for the black population; and death rates estimated to be understated by 21 percent for American Indians, 11 percent for Asians, and 2 percent for Hispanics (Rosenberg HM, Maurer JD, Sorlie PD, Johnson NJ, et al. Quality of death rates by race and Hispanic origin: A summary of current research, 1999. National Center for Health Statistics. Vital Health Stat 2(128). 1999). Data for additional years are available (see Appendix III).

SOURCES: Centers for Disease Control and Prevention, National Center for Health Statistics. *Vital statistics of the United States, vol II, mortality, part A*, for data years 1950–93. Public Health Service. Washington. U.S. Government Printing Office; for 1994–98, data for all persons, white, and black are available on the NCHS Web site at www.cdc.gov/nchs/datawh/statab/unpubd/mortabs.htm; numerator data from National Vital Statistics System, annual mortality files; denominator data from national population estimates for race groups from table 1 and unpublished Hispanic population estimates prepared by the Housing and Household Economic Statistics Division, U.S. Bureau of the Census.

Table 42 (page 1 of 3). Death rates for chronic obstructive pulmonary diseases, according to sex, detailed race, Hispanic origin, and age: United States, selected years 1980–98

[Data are based on the National Vital Statistics System]

Sex, race, Hispanic origin, and age	1980	1985	1990	1992	1993	1994	1995	1996	1997	1998	1996–98[1]
All persons				Deaths per 100,000 resident population							
All ages, age adjusted	15.9	18.8	19.7	19.9	21.4	21.0	20.8	21.0	21.1	21.3	21.1
All ages, crude	24.7	31.4	34.9	36.0	39.2	39.0	39.2	40.0	40.7	41.7	40.8
Under 1 year	1.6	1.4	1.4	1.1	1.4	1.4	1.1	1.0	1.3	1.0	1.1
1–4 years	0.4	0.3	0.4	0.4	0.3	0.3	0.2	0.3	0.3	0.3	0.3
5–14 years	0.2	0.3	0.3	0.3	0.4	0.3	0.4	0.4	0.3	0.4	0.4
15–24 years	0.3	0.5	0.5	0.5	0.6	0.6	0.7	0.7	0.5	0.6	0.6
25–34 years	0.5	0.6	0.7	0.7	0.7	0.9	0.9	0.9	0.9	0.8	0.9
35–44 years	1.6	1.6	1.6	1.8	1.8	1.8	2.0	2.0	2.0	2.0	2.0
45–54 years	9.8	10.2	9.1	8.3	8.7	9.0	8.9	8.7	8.4	8.2	8.4
55–64 years	42.7	47.9	48.9	48.3	51.0	49.2	47.3	47.0	46.3	44.8	46.0
65–74 years	129.1	149.2	152.5	155.5	167.8	163.8	160.6	161.6	165.3	169.1	165.3
75–84 years	224.4	289.5	321.1	326.5	357.3	351.9	351.8	358.3	359.6	365.8	361.3
85 years and over	274.0	365.4	433.3	460.9	493.9	509.7	527.8	540.9	561.9	569.3	557.7
Male											
All ages, age adjusted	26.1	28.1	27.2	26.4	27.8	26.9	26.3	25.9	26.1	25.9	26.0
All ages, crude	35.1	40.3	40.8	40.5	43.2	42.3	42.0	42.0	42.7	43.2	42.6
Under 1 year	1.9	2.0	1.6	1.7	1.5	1.7	1.4	1.3	1.6	1.2	1.4
1–4 years	0.5	*	0.5	0.4	0.4	0.3	0.2	0.4	0.3	0.4	0.4
5–14 years	0.2	0.3	0.4	0.3	0.4	0.4	0.5	0.5	0.4	0.4	0.4
15–24 years	0.4	0.4	0.5	0.6	0.7	0.8	0.7	0.7	0.7	0.8	0.7
25–34 years	0.6	0.6	0.7	0.7	0.6	0.9	0.9	0.8	1.0	0.9	0.9
35–44 years	1.7	1.6	1.7	1.8	1.8	1.8	1.7	1.9	1.9	1.9	1.9
45–54 years	12.1	11.3	9.4	8.7	9.5	9.3	9.0	8.9	8.8	8.2	8.6
55–64 years	59.9	60.8	58.6	56.3	58.1	55.9	52.9	52.2	50.5	49.6	50.7
65–74 years	210.0	218.9	204.0	199.7	208.4	202.0	196.9	192.6	201.3	201.2	198.3
75–84 years	437.4	505.2	500.0	478.6	512.1	490.4	482.5	478.8	469.6	471.5	473.2
85 years and over	583.4	758.1	815.1	830.9	883.1	874.9	896.2	878.6	902.8	869.8	883.5
Female											
All ages, age adjusted	8.9	12.5	14.7	15.5	17.1	17.1	17.1	17.6	17.7	18.1	17.8
All ages, crude	15.0	23.0	29.2	31.8	35.4	35.9	36.4	38.0	38.8	40.2	39.0
Under 1 year	1.3	*	1.2	*	1.2	1.1	*	*	*	*	0.8
1–4 years	*	*	*	0.4	*	*	*	*	*	*	0.2
5–14 years	0.3	0.4	0.3	0.3	0.3	0.2	0.2	0.4	0.3	0.3	0.3
15–24 years	0.3	0.5	0.5	0.5	0.4	0.5	0.6	0.6	0.4	0.5	0.5
25–34 years	0.5	0.6	0.7	0.6	0.8	0.9	0.9	0.9	0.8	0.8	0.9
35–44 years	1.5	1.5	1.5	1.7	1.8	1.7	2.2	2.1	2.1	2.0	2.1
45–54 years	7.7	9.2	8.8	7.9	8.0	8.7	8.8	8.4	8.1	8.2	8.2
55–64 years	27.6	36.6	40.3	41.0	44.6	43.1	42.2	42.4	42.6	40.5	41.8
65–74 years	67.1	95.5	112.3	120.7	135.6	133.4	131.5	136.7	136.1	143.0	138.6
75–84 years	98.7	162.7	214.2	233.4	261.5	265.2	268.8	280.4	287.6	295.8	288.0
85 years and over	138.7	208.6	286.0	317.6	344.6	368.8	384.3	406.7	424.5	444.7	425.7
White male											
All ages, age adjusted	26.7	28.7	27.4	26.8	28.2	27.3	26.6	26.3	26.5	26.4	26.4
All ages, crude	37.9	43.7	44.3	44.4	47.3	46.4	46.1	46.1	47.0	47.7	46.9
35–44 years	1.2	1.3	1.3	1.5	1.3	1.4	1.4	1.5	1.5	1.5	1.5
45–54 years	11.4	10.5	8.6	8.3	9.0	8.7	8.3	8.5	8.3	7.6	8.1
55–64 years	60.0	60.6	58.7	56.6	58.5	56.7	53.2	52.3	51.0	50.0	51.1
65–74 years	218.4	225.2	208.1	204.6	213.3	206.9	201.6	198.4	207.5	208.5	204.8
75–84 years	459.8	525.5	513.5	494.1	525.2	504.2	496.3	491.1	481.4	485.5	486.0
85 years and over	611.2	798.1	847.0	862.5	917.6	907.7	924.0	917.5	940.1	904.8	920.4
Black male											
All ages, age adjusted	20.9	24.8	26.5	24.8	26.6	25.7	25.4	24.8	24.5	24.3	24.5
All ages, crude	19.3	23.4	25.2	23.8	25.7	24.9	24.9	24.7	24.6	24.7	24.7
35–44 years	5.8	5.3	5.3	4.7	5.4	4.9	4.3	5.2	4.8	5.0	5.0
45–54 years	19.7	19.5	18.8	15.1	16.9	16.6	17.3	15.4	14.9	15.1	15.1
55–64 years	66.6	69.6	67.4	64.8	65.9	61.0	62.0	63.2	56.6	56.6	58.7
65–74 years	142.0	178.2	184.5	175.1	184.9	181.7	175.1	161.6	170.7	164.2	165.5
75–84 years	229.8	321.8	390.9	354.5	407.1	374.1	366.5	380.7	374.9	372.1	375.8
85 years and over	271.6	374.2	498.0	559.8	560.6	561.7	613.6	579.5	586.5	570.9	578.8

See footnotes at end of table.

Table 42 (page 2 of 3). Death rates for chronic obstructive pulmonary diseases, according to sex, detailed race, Hispanic origin, and age: United States, selected years 1980–98

[Data are based on the National Vital Statistics System]

Sex, race, Hispanic origin, and age	1980	1985	1990	1992	1993	1994	1995	1996	1997	1998	1996–98[1]
American Indian or Alaska Native male[2]					Deaths per 100,000 resident population						
All ages, age adjusted	11.2	14.1	18.5	14.7	17.3	16.5	16.4	13.7	20.3	19.7	18.0
All ages, crude	8.4	10.5	13.8	11.3	13.4	13.4	13.4	11.9	17.9	17.7	15.9
35–44 years	*	*	*	*	*	*	*	*	*	*	
45–54 years	*	*	*	*	*	*	*	*	*	*	9.6
55–64 years	*	46.8	*	39.8	42.4	33.3	39.2	*	54.0	47.5	43.0
65–74 years	*	*	135.7	102.9	138.9	130.4	129.3	115.9	127.8	139.8	128.0
75–84 years	*	272.7	363.8	276.8	313.9	301.8	253.8	229.7	339.9	317.3	297.3
85 years and over	*	*	*	*	*	*	*	421.9	488.8	500.2	471.8
Asian or Pacific Islander male[3]											
All ages, age adjusted	9.8	12.0	13.1	11.6	13.5	12.8	13.5	13.0	12.7	11.0	12.2
All ages, crude	8.7	10.1	11.3	10.3	11.9	11.5	12.3	12.7	12.9	11.9	12.5
35–44 years	*	*	*	*	*	*	*	*	*	*	1.0
45–54 years	*	*	*	*	*	*	*	*	*	*	2.7
55–64 years	*	24.4	22.1	19.6	19.8	15.7	16.4	19.2	16.6	17.1	17.6
65–74 years	70.6	72.7	91.4	94.6	94.1	85.5	91.7	89.9	86.2	74.7	83.4
75–84 years	155.7	246.5	258.6	206.1	278.2	264.2	263.6	294.8	276.3	216.4	260.2
85 years and over	472.4	462.5	615.2	483.8	645.7	660.6	847.8	421.7	568.2	553.5	517.8
Hispanic male[4]											
All ages, age adjusted	---	11.8	12.2	11.3	12.4	12.4	12.7	11.4	11.5	11.4	11.5
All ages, crude	---	7.2	8.4	8.1	9.0	9.0	9.4	8.7	9.0	9.3	9.0
35–44 years	---	*	*	2.1	1.3	1.3	1.1	1.1	1.5	1.3	1.3
45–54 years	---	5.9	4.1	4.5	3.1	4.6	3.9	4.0	3.5	3.7	3.7
55–64 years	---	21.5	17.2	16.5	21.1	18.2	18.8	18.8	17.6	17.7	18.0
65–74 years	---	67.5	81.0	76.7	77.1	80.3	78.8	68.4	77.2	73.4	73.1
75–84 years	---	261.8	252.4	223.9	244.4	253.5	273.8	240.3	220.2	231.7	230.5
85 years and over	---	462.5	613.9	483.5	666.5	616.2	634.5	579.5	634.3	541.7	583.9
White, non-Hispanic male[4]											
All ages, age adjusted	---	29.1	28.2	27.2	28.5	27.8	27.1	26.9	27.3	27.2	27.1
All ages, crude	---	45.3	48.5	48.2	51.5	50.7	50.4	50.9	52.2	52.9	52.0
35–44 years	---	1.3	1.4	1.4	1.3	1.4	1.4	1.5	1.5	1.5	1.5
45–54 years	---	10.7	9.0	8.3	9.2	8.9	8.7	8.7	8.6	7.9	8.4
55–64 years	---	61.6	61.3	58.5	60.1	58.8	55.2	54.1	53.3	52.3	53.2
65–74 years	---	229.9	213.4	208.4	217.6	211.5	206.5	204.0	214.2	215.9	211.4
75–84 years	---	528.7	523.7	498.2	529.8	510.3	501.9	499.5	491.0	495.8	495.4
85 years and over	---	782.4	860.6	873.1	909.1	908.6	924.5	928.0	951.1	920.4	933.0
White female											
All ages, age adjusted	9.2	12.9	15.2	16.1	17.8	17.8	17.8	18.3	18.5	18.9	18.6
All ages, crude	16.4	25.5	32.8	35.8	40.0	40.6	41.2	43.0	44.1	45.7	44.3
35–44 years	1.3	1.3	1.2	1.3	1.4	1.3	1.7	1.7	1.7	1.6	1.7
45–54 years	7.6	9.1	8.3	7.5	7.6	8.3	8.4	8.0	7.8	7.7	7.8
55–64 years	28.7	37.8	41.9	43.2	47.0	45.2	44.3	44.6	44.8	42.7	44.0
65–74 years	71.0	101.1	118.8	127.7	143.8	141.8	139.8	145.3	145.3	153.0	147.8
75–84 years	104.0	171.0	226.3	246.9	276.1	280.1	282.8	296.4	304.2	312.9	304.6
85 years and over	144.2	217.6	298.4	330.7	361.2	384.9	402.0	423.6	445.0	466.6	445.5
Black female											
All ages, age adjusted	6.3	8.8	10.7	11.2	12.2	12.4	12.5	13.1	12.7	13.3	13.0
All ages, crude	6.8	10.0	12.6	13.7	14.9	15.4	15.8	17.0	16.5	17.5	17.0
35–44 years	3.4	2.8	3.8	4.3	5.3	5.1	5.4	5.0	5.0	5.3	5.1
45–54 years	9.3	11.2	14.0	13.3	12.6	13.5	12.9	13.2	12.2	14.2	13.2
55–64 years	20.8	30.6	33.4	32.1	35.2	35.8	34.7	34.8	35.8	33.8	34.8
65–74 years	32.7	48.3	64.7	73.5	78.3	79.2	78.3	84.3	81.4	84.8	83.5
75–84 years	41.1	76.6	96.0	105.6	120.2	122.1	136.6	137.6	136.9	148.9	141.2
85 years and over	63.2	94.0	133.0	169.0	163.5	195.0	191.4	236.5	220.9	231.1	229.5

See footnotes at end of table.

Table 42 (page 3 of 3). Death rates for chronic obstructive pulmonary diseases, according to sex, detailed race, Hispanic origin, and age: United States, selected years 1980–98

[Data are based on the National Vital Statistics System]

Sex, race, Hispanic origin, and age	1980	1985	1990	1992	1993	1994	1995	1996	1997	1998	1996–98[1]
American Indian or Alaska Native female[2]				Deaths per 100,000 resident population							
All ages, age adjusted	4.5	6.5	8.9	9.3	13.3	11.1	12.0	11.8	11.4	12.6	11.9
All ages, crude	3.8	5.9	8.7	9.3	12.9	11.5	12.5	13.4	12.2	13.6	13.1
35–44 years	*	*	*	*	*	*	*	*	*	*	*
45–54 years	*	*	*	*	*	*	*	*	*	*	7.3
55–64 years	*	*	*	*	38.1	34.0	40.6	32.6	35.7	31.6	33.3
65–74 years	*	*	56.4	62.3	114.6	73.8	77.8	78.7	88.1	118.2	95.3
75–84 years	*	*	116.7	128.9	172.2	189.7	168.9	192.9	137.5	165.8	165.1
85 years and over	*	*	*	*	*	*	*	265.8	171.0	162.3	197.2
Asian or Pacific Islander female[3]											
All ages, age adjusted	2.5	5.4	5.2	4.5	5.0	5.3	5.8	5.3	5.6	4.7	5.2
All ages, crude	2.6	5.1	5.2	4.9	5.4	5.8	6.5	6.5	7.2	6.4	6.7
35–44 years	*	*	*	*	*	*	*	*	*	*	1.1
45–54 years	*	*	*	*	*	*	3.6	*	*	*	2.3
55–64 years	*	13.5	15.2	9.2	7.8	9.4	10.0	11.1	9.2	6.7	8.9
65–74 years	*	35.0	26.5	29.6	31.0	29.4	29.8	32.7	32.2	28.5	31.1
75–84 years	*	76.1	80.6	79.7	102.4	105.5	120.1	81.1	117.7	92.4	97.3
85 years and over	*	208.3	232.5	190.7	191.8	238.0	272.6	240.9	242.3	252.3	245.5
Hispanic female[4]											
All ages, age adjusted	---	5.7	6.4	5.9	6.9	6.7	7.1	7.2	6.7	6.3	6.7
All ages, crude	---	4.8	6.3	6.3	7.3	7.3	7.9	8.3	7.8	7.4	7.8
35–44 years	---	*	*	1.3	1.2	1.3	1.5	1.3	1.1	1.9	1.5
45–54 years	---	*	4.9	4.2	3.6	4.1	4.6	4.1	4.4	3.2	3.9
55–64 years	---	13.8	14.4	10.8	12.2	12.1	12.5	13.0	11.7	11.6	12.1
65–74 years	---	35.0	36.6	34.5	44.8	41.2	41.4	40.9	38.6	38.3	39.3
75–84 years	---	99.1	101.1	109.2	123.0	114.5	116.7	134.1	119.3	116.6	123.0
85 years and over	---	175.0	269.0	250.2	290.5	308.4	367.2	342.8	322.6	261.1	306.4
White, non-Hispanic female[4]											
All ages, age adjusted	---	13.6	15.7	16.4	18.2	18.3	18.3	18.9	19.1	19.6	19.2
All ages, crude	---	27.7	35.7	38.7	43.3	44.4	45.0	47.2	48.6	50.7	48.8
35–44 years	---	1.2	1.2	1.3	1.4	1.3	1.7	1.7	1.8	1.5	1.7
45–54 years	---	9.6	8.5	7.5	7.7	8.5	8.6	8.2	8.1	8.0	8.1
55–64 years	---	39.8	43.7	44.8	49.0	47.3	46.6	46.8	47.3	45.1	46.4
65–74 years	---	107.6	122.8	130.8	147.0	146.2	144.0	150.4	151.2	160.0	153.8
75–84 years	---	179.4	231.9	250.1	280.1	285.6	288.4	302.5	310.9	320.9	311.5
85 years and over	---	221.4	302.1	330.9	358.7	383.6	401.2	426.8	447.9	473.7	450.0

* Based on fewer than 20 deaths.

- - - Data not available.

[1]Average annual death rate.

[2]Interpretation of trends should take into account that population estimates for American Indians increased by 45 percent between 1980 and 1990, partly due to better enumeration techniques in the 1990 decennial census and to the increased tendency for people to identify themselves as American Indian in 1990.

[3]Interpretation of trends should take into account that the Asian population in the United States more than doubled between 1980 and 1990, primarily due to immigration.

[4]Excludes data from States lacking an Hispanic-origin item on their death certificates. See Appendix I, National Vital Statistics System.

NOTES: Rates are age adjusted to the 1940 U.S. standard million population. See Appendix II, Age adjustment. For data years shown, the code numbers for cause of death are based on the then current *International Classification of Diseases*, which are described in Appendix II, tables IV and V. Age groups were selected to minimize the presentation of unstable age-specific death rates based on small numbers of deaths and for consistency among comparison groups. The race groups, white, black, Asian or Pacific Islander, and American Indian or Alaska Native, include persons of Hispanic and non-Hispanic origin. Conversely, persons of Hispanic origin may be of any race. Bias in death rates results from inconsistent race identification between the death certificate (source of data for numerator of death rates) and data from the Census Bureau (denominator); and from undercounts of some population groups in the census. The net effects of misclassification and under coverage result in death rates estimated to be overstated by 1 percent for the white population and 5 percent for the black population; and death rates estimated to be understated by 21 percent for American Indians, 11 percent for Asians, and 2 percent for Hispanics (Rosenberg HM, Maurer JD, Sorlie PD, Johnson NJ, et al. Quality of death rates by race and Hispanic origin: A summary of current research, 1999. National Center for Health Statistics. Vital Health Stat 2(128). 1999). Data for additional years are available (see Appendix III).

SOURCES: Centers for Disease Control and Prevention, National Center for Health Statistics. *Vital statistics of the United States, vol II, mortality, part A*, for data years 1980–93. Public Health Service. Washington. U.S. Government Printing Office; for 1994–98, data for all persons, white, and black are available on the NCHS Web site at www.cdc.gov/nchs/datawh/statab/unpubd/mortabs.htm; numerator data from National Vital Statistics System, annual mortality files; denominator data from national population estimates for race groups from table 1 and unpublished Hispanic population estimates prepared by the Housing and Household Economic Statistics Division, U.S. Bureau of the Census.

Table 43 (page 1 of 2). Death rates for human immunodeficiency virus (HIV) infection, according to sex, detailed race, Hispanic origin, and age: United States, selected years 1987–98

[Data are based on the National Vital Statistics System]

Sex, race, Hispanic origin, and age	1987	1989	1990	1992	1993	1994	1995	1996	1997	1998	1996–98[1]
All persons					Deaths per 100,000 resident population						
All ages, age adjusted	5.5	8.7	9.8	12.6	13.8	15.4	15.6	11.1	5.8	4.6	7.2
All ages, crude	5.6	8.9	10.1	13.2	14.5	16.2	16.4	11.7	6.2	5.0	7.6
Under 1 year	2.3	3.1	2.7	2.5	2.2	2.5	1.5	1.1	*	*	0.6
1–4 years	0.7	0.8	0.8	1.0	1.3	1.3	1.3	0.9	0.4	0.2	0.5
5–14 years	0.1	0.2	0.2	0.3	0.4	0.5	0.5	0.5	0.3	0.1	0.3
15–24 years	1.3	1.6	1.5	1.6	1.7	1.8	1.7	1.1	0.8	0.5	0.8
25–34 years	11.7	17.9	19.7	24.6	27.0	29.3	29.1	19.9	10.1	7.5	12.6
35–44 years	14.0	23.5	27.4	35.6	39.1	44.1	44.4	31.4	16.1	12.9	20.1
45–54 years	8.0	13.3	15.2	20.3	22.6	25.6	26.3	19.3	10.4	9.0	12.8
55–64 years	3.5	5.4	6.2	8.5	8.8	10.4	11.0	8.4	4.9	4.3	5.8
65–74 years	1.3	1.8	2.0	2.8	2.9	3.1	3.6	2.7	1.8	1.6	2.1
75–84 years	0.8	0.7	0.7	0.8	0.8	0.9	0.7	0.8	0.6	0.5	0.6
85 years and over	*	*	*	*	*	*	*	*	*	*	0.3
Male											
All ages, age adjusted	10.0	15.8	17.7	22.3	24.1	26.4	26.2	18.1	9.1	7.2	11.5
All ages, crude	10.2	16.4	18.5	23.6	25.5	28.0	28.0	19.5	9.8	7.8	12.3
Under 1 year	2.2	2.7	2.4	2.3	2.1	2.1	1.7	1.1	*	*	0.7
1–4 years	0.7	0.7	0.8	1.1	1.3	1.2	1.2	0.9	0.3	*	0.5
5–14 years	0.2	0.2	0.3	0.4	0.4	0.5	0.5	0.5	0.3	0.1	0.3
15–24 years	2.2	2.6	2.2	2.3	2.3	2.3	2.1	1.3	0.8	0.5	0.9
25–34 years	20.7	31.5	34.5	42.2	46.0	48.5	47.1	31.4	15.1	10.7	19.2
35–44 years	26.3	43.6	50.2	63.5	68.5	76.2	75.9	51.8	25.5	20.1	32.3
45–54 years	15.5	25.6	29.1	38.1	41.7	46.3	46.9	33.6	17.4	15.2	21.8
55–64 years	6.8	10.5	12.0	15.9	16.5	19.1	19.9	14.9	8.5	7.3	10.2
65–74 years	2.4	3.3	3.7	5.3	5.4	5.8	6.4	5.1	3.4	2.9	3.8
75–84 years	1.2	1.2	1.1	1.6	1.4	1.4	1.3	1.5	1.0	0.9	1.1
85 years and over	*	*	*	*	*	*	*	*	*	*	*
Female											
All ages, age adjusted	1.1	1.8	2.1	3.2	3.8	4.8	5.2	4.2	2.6	2.2	3.0
All ages, crude	1.1	1.8	2.2	3.2	3.9	4.9	5.3	4.3	2.7	2.3	3.1
Under 1 year	2.5	3.5	3.0	2.7	2.4	2.9	1.2	*	*	*	0.6
1–4 years	0.7	0.8	0.8	1.0	1.3	1.3	1.5	1.0	0.4	*	0.5
5–14 years	*	0.1	0.2	0.2	0.4	0.5	0.5	0.4	0.2	0.2	0.3
15–24 years	0.3	0.6	0.7	0.9	1.1	1.3	1.4	1.0	0.7	0.6	0.8
25–34 years	2.8	4.4	4.9	6.9	8.0	10.1	11.1	8.5	5.1	4.4	6.0
35–44 years	2.1	3.9	5.2	8.2	10.2	12.5	13.4	11.3	6.8	5.8	7.9
45–54 years	0.8	1.6	1.9	3.4	4.4	5.8	6.7	5.7	3.8	3.1	4.2
55–64 years	0.5	0.8	1.1	1.9	1.9	2.6	2.9	2.5	1.6	1.6	1.9
65–74 years	0.5	0.7	0.8	0.9	1.0	1.0	1.4	0.8	0.5	0.6	0.6
75–84 years	0.5	0.4	0.4	0.4	0.4	0.6	0.3	0.3	0.4	0.3	0.3
85 years and over	*	*	*	*	*	*	*	*	*	*	*
All ages, age adjusted											
White male	8.4	13.2	15.0	18.1	19.0	20.1	19.6	12.5	5.6	4.3	7.5
Black male	25.4	40.3	44.2	61.8	70.0	81.7	84.3	66.4	38.5	31.2	45.1
American Indian or Alaska Native male	*	2.9	3.3	4.9	8.3	9.3	11.3	6.9	3.6	3.8	4.8
Asian or Pacific Islander male	2.2	3.6	4.0	4.3	5.1	6.6	5.8	4.1	1.6	1.3	2.3
Hispanic male[2]	17.8	27.0	27.2	33.0	33.6	39.3	39.0	26.0	13.1	9.8	16.1
White, non-Hispanic male[2]	6.4	12.2	13.4	15.9	16.7	17.7	17.1	10.7	4.6	3.5	6.2
White female	0.6	0.9	1.1	1.6	1.9	2.3	2.5	1.8	1.0	0.8	1.2
Black female	4.7	8.1	9.9	14.3	17.3	21.8	24.0	20.2	13.3	11.7	15.0
American Indian or Alaska Native female	*	*	*	*	*	*	2.7	*	*	*	1.1
Asian or Pacific Islander female	*	*	*	0.5	0.7	0.7	0.6	0.5	*	*	0.3
Hispanic female[2]	2.1	4.0	3.7	5.6	6.5	7.7	8.5	6.2	3.3	2.6	4.0
White, non-Hispanic female[2]	0.2	0.6	0.7	1.0	1.2	1.6	1.8	1.3	0.7	0.5	0.8

See footnotes at end of table.

Table 43 (page 2 of 2). Death rates for human immunodeficiency virus (HIV) infection, according to sex, detailed race, Hispanic origin, and age: United States, selected years 1987–98

[Data are based on the National Vital Statistics System]

Sex, race, Hispanic origin, and age	1987	1989	1990	1992	1993	1994	1995	1996	1997	1998	1996–98[1]
Age 25–44 years					Deaths per 100,000 resident population						
All persons	12.7	20.5	23.2	29.9	32.9	36.7	36.9	25.9	13.2	10.4	16.5
White male	19.2	30.8	35.0	42.8	45.5	48.4	46.9	29.6	13.2	9.9	17.6
Black male	60.2	94.1	102.0	137.4	155.3	178.0	182.0	139.1	76.7	59.4	91.5
American Indian or Alaska Native male	*	7.4	7.7	13.4	20.9	23.6	31.3	18.4	10.7	8.7	12.6
Asian or Pacific Islander male. . .	4.1	7.5	8.1	9.4	10.8	13.8	12.6	8.1	3.6	2.6	4.7
Hispanic male[2]	36.8	58.2	59.3	68.9	71.0	78.0	78.9	50.5	24.9	18.9	31.3
White, non-Hispanic male[2]	14.3	28.2	31.6	38.1	40.2	43.4	41.5	25.8	11.0	8.2	15.0
White female.	1.2	1.9	2.3	3.6	4.4	5.5	6.0	4.4	2.4	1.8	2.9
Black female	11.6	20.1	23.6	34.4	40.4	49.8	54.5	46.6	29.3	26.1	33.9
American Indian or Alaska Native female	*	*	*	*	*	*	*	*	*	*	2.5
Asian or Pacific Islander female .	*	*	*	*	1.2	1.5	1.2	*	*	*	0.7
Hispanic female[2]	4.9	9.3	8.9	12.5	14.2	17.3	18.0	12.8	6.7	5.0	8.1
White, non-Hispanic female[2]	0.3	1.3	1.5	2.3	2.9	3.9	4.2	3.1	1.7	1.3	2.0
Age 45–64 years											
All persons	5.8	9.7	11.1	15.2	16.8	19.3	20.1	15.0	8.3	7.2	10.1
White male	9.9	16.4	18.6	23.4	24.7	26.4	26.3	17.4	8.0	6.8	10.6
Black male	27.3	46.1	53.0	86.4	101.2	127.1	136.6	114.1	71.8	63.5	82.5
American Indian or Alaska Native male.	*	*	*	*	*	*	*	*	*	*	4.4
Asian or Pacific Islander male. . .	*	6.1	6.5	7.1	9.2	10.6	9.5	8.2	2.4	2.5	4.3
Hispanic male[2]	25.8	37.0	37.9	52.5	52.2	69.2	67.1	48.8	24.7	18.5	30.1
White, non-Hispanic male[2]	8.0	15.3	16.9	20.3	21.5	22.6	22.6	14.3	6.4	5.5	8.6
White female.	0.5	0.7	0.9	1.5	1.8	2.1	2.4	1.9	1.1	0.9	1.3
Black female	2.6	5.6	7.5	12.9	16.5	24.1	27.2	24.4	17.6	15.5	19.1
American Indian or Alaska Native female	*	*	*	*	*	*	*	*	*	*	*
Asian or Pacific Islander female .	*	*	*	*	*	*	*	*	*	*	*
Hispanic female[2]	*	3.5	3.1	6.8	8.2	9.9	12.4	9.7	5.3	4.9	6.5
White, non-Hispanic female[2]	0.3	0.5	0.7	1.0	1.1	1.4	1.5	1.2	0.7	0.5	0.8

* Based on fewer than 20 deaths.

[1] Average annual death rate.

[2] Data shown only for States with an Hispanic-origin item on their death certificates. See Appendix I, National Vital Statistics System.

NOTES: Rates are age adjusted to the 1940 U.S. standard million population. See Appendix II, Age adjustment. Categories for the coding and classification of human immunodeficiency virus infection were introduced in the United States beginning with mortality data for 1987. Age groups were selected to minimize the presentation of unstable age-specific death rates based on small numbers of deaths and for consistency among comparison groups. The race groups, white, black, Asian or Pacific Islander, and American Indian or Alaska Native, include persons of Hispanic and non-Hispanic origin. Conversely, persons of Hispanic origin may be of any race. Bias in death rates results from inconsistent race identification between the death certificate (source of data for numerator of death rates) and data from the Census Bureau (denominator); and from undercounts of some population groups in the census. The net effects of misclassification and under coverage result in death rates estimated to be overstated by 1 percent for the white population and 5 percent for the black population; and death rates estimated to be understated by 21 percent for American Indians, 11 percent for Asians, and 2 percent for Hispanics (Rosenberg HM, Maurer JD, Sorlie PD, Johnson NJ, et al. Quality of death rates by race and Hispanic origin: A summary of current research, 1999. National Center for Health Statistics. Vital Health Stat 2(128). 1999). Data for additional years are available (see Appendix III).

SOURCES: Centers for Disease Control and Prevention, National Center for Health Statistics. Vital statistics of the United States, vol II, mortality, part A, for data years 1987–93. Public Health Service. Washington. U.S. Government Printing Office; for 1994–98, data for all persons, white, and black are available on the NCHS Web site at www.cdc.gov/nchs/datawh/statab/unpubd/mortabs.htm; numerator data from National Vital Statistics System, annual mortality files; denominator data from national population estimates for race groups from table 1 and unpublished Hispanic population estimates prepared by the Housing and Household Economic Statistics Division, U.S. Bureau of the Census.

Table 44. Maternal mortality for complications of pregnancy, childbirth, and the puerperium, according to race, Hispanic origin, and age: United States, selected years 1950–98

[Data are based on the National Vital Statistics System]

Race, Hispanic origin, and age	1950[1]	1960[1]	1970	1980	1985	1990	1995	1996	1997	1998
	Number of deaths									
All persons...............	2,960	1,579	803	334	295	343	277	294	327	281
White.................	1,873	936	445	193	156	177	129	159	179	158
Black.................	1,041	624	342	127	124	153	133	121	125	104
American Indian or Alaska Native.....	- - -	- - -	- - -	3	7	4	1	6	2	2
Asian or Pacific Islander	- - -	- - -	- - -	11	8	9	14	8	21	17
Hispanic[2].................	- - -	- - -	- - -	- - -	29	47	43	39	57	42
White, non-Hispanic[2].............	- - -	- - -	- - -	- - -	60	125	84	114	121	116
All persons	Deaths per 100,000 live births									
All ages, age adjusted.............	73.7	32.1	21.5	9.4	7.6	7.6	6.3	6.4	7.6	6.1
All ages, crude	83.3	37.1	21.5	9.2	7.8	8.2	7.1	7.6	8.4	7.1
Under 20 years.................	70.7	22.7	18.9	7.6	6.9	7.5	3.9	*	5.7	*
20–24 years.................	47.6	20.7	13.0	5.8	5.4	6.1	5.7	5.0	6.6	5.0
25–29 years.................	63.5	29.8	17.0	7.7	6.4	6.0	6.0	6.6	7.9	6.7
30–34 years.................	107.7	50.3	31.6	13.6	8.9	9.5	7.3	7.6	8.3	7.5
35 years and over[3]	222.0	104.3	81.9	36.3	25.0	20.7	15.9	19.0	16.1	14.5
White										
All ages, age adjusted.............	53.1	22.4	14.4	6.7	4.9	5.1	3.6	4.1	5.2	4.2
All ages, crude	61.1	26.0	14.3	6.6	5.1	5.4	4.2	5.1	5.8	5.1
Under 20 years.................	44.9	14.8	13.8	5.8	5.8	*	*	*	4.2	3.1
20–24 years.................	35.7	15.3	8.4	4.2	3.3	3.9	3.5	*	4.2	3.1
25–29 years.................	45.0	20.3	11.1	5.4	4.6	4.8	4.0	4.0	5.4	4.9
30–34 years.................	75.9	34.3	18.7	9.3	5.1	5.0	4.0	5.0	5.4	4.9
35 years and over[3]	174.1	73.9	59.3	25.5	17.5	12.6	9.1	14.9	11.5	11.0
Black										
All ages, age adjusted.............	- - -	92.0	65.5	24.9	22.1	21.7	20.9	19.9	20.1	16.1
All ages, crude	- - -	103.6	60.9	22.4	21.3	22.4	22.1	20.3	20.8	17.1
Under 20 years.................	- - -	54.8	32.3	13.1	*	*	*	*	*	*
20–24 years.................	- - -	56.9	41.9	13.9	14.6	14.7	15.3	15.1	15.3	12.7
25–29 years.................	- - -	92.8	65.2	22.4	19.4	14.9	21.0	25.5	24.3	17.2
30–34 years.................	- - -	150.6	117.8*	44.0	38.0	44.2	31.2	28.6	32.9	27.7
35 years and over[3]	- - -	299.5	207.5	100.6	77.2	79.7	61.4	49.9	40.4	37.2
Hispanic[2,4]										
All ages, age adjusted.............	- - -	- - -	- - -	- - -	7.1	7.4	5.4	4.8	7.6	5.2
All ages, crude	- - -	- - -	- - -	- - -	7.8	7.9	6.3	5.6	8.0	5.7
White, non-Hispanic[2]										
All ages, age adjusted.............	- - -	- - -	- - -	- - -	4.0	4.4	3.3	3.9	4.4	4.0
All ages, crude	- - -	- - -	- - -	- - -	4.3	4.8	3.5	4.8	5.2	4.9

- - - Data not available.
* Based on fewer than 20 deaths.
[1]Includes deaths of persons who were not residents of the 50 States and the District of Columbia.
[2]Hispanic and White, non-Hispanic data exclude data from States lacking an Hispanic-origin item on their death and birth certificates. See Appendix I, National Vital Statistics System.
[3]Rates computed by relating deaths of women 35 years and over to live births to women 35–49 years.
[4]Age-specific maternal mortality rates are not calculated because rates based on fewer than 20 deaths are unreliable.

NOTES: Rates are age adjusted to the 1940 U.S. standard million population. See Appendix II, Age adjustment. For data years shown, the code numbers for cause of death are based on the then current International Classification of Diseases, described in Appendix II, tables IV and V. The race groups, white, black, Asian or Pacific Islander, and American Indian or Alaska Native, include persons of Hispanic and non-Hispanic origin. Conversely, persons of Hispanic origin may be of any race. For 1950 and 1960, rates are based on live births by race of child; for all other years, rates are based on live births by race of mother. See Appendix I, National Vital Statistics System. Rates are not calculated for American Indian or Alaska Native and Asian or Pacific Islander mothers because rates based on fewer than 20 deaths are unreliable. Data for additional years are available (see Appendix III).

SOURCES: Centers for Disease Control and Prevention, National Center for Health Statistics: Vital statistics of the United States, vol I, natality and vol II, mortality, part A, for data years 1950–93. Public Health Service. Washington. U.S. Government Printing Office; for 1994–98, unpublished data.

Table 45 (page 1 of 4). Death rates for motor vehicle-related injuries, according to sex, detailed race, Hispanic origin, and age: United States, selected years 1950–98

[Data are based on the National Vital Statistics System]

Sex, race, Hispanic origin, and age	1950[1]	1960[1]	1970	1980	1985	1990	1995	1996	1997	1998	1996–98[2]
All persons					Deaths per 100,000 resident population						
All ages, age adjusted	23.3	22.5	27.4	22.9	18.8	18.5	16.3	16.2	15.9	15.6	15.9
All ages, crude	23.1	21.3	26.9	23.5	19.3	18.8	16.5	16.5	16.2	16.1	16.3
Under 1 year	8.4	8.1	9.8	7.0	4.9	4.9	4.7	5.7	4.3	4.3	4.8
1–14 years	9.8	8.6	10.5	8.2	7.0	6.0	5.3	5.2	5.1	4.8	5.0
1–4 years	11.5	10.0	11.5	9.2	7.2	6.3	5.2	5.3	5.0	5.0	5.1
5–14 years	8.8	7.9	10.2	7.9	6.9	5.9	5.4	5.2	5.1	4.8	5.0
15–24 years	34.4	38.0	47.2	44.8	35.7	34.1	29.5	29.2	27.9	26.9	28.0
25–34 years	24.6	24.3	30.9	29.1	23.0	23.6	19.8	19.1	18.9	18.4	18.8
35–44 years	20.3	19.3	24.9	20.9	17.2	16.9	15.4	15.6	15.2	15.6	15.5
45–64 years	25.2	23.0	26.5	18.0	15.4	15.7	14.2	14.4	14.7	14.7	14.6
45–54 years	22.2	21.4	25.5	18.6	15.2	15.6	13.9	14.1	14.3	14.4	14.3
55–64 years	29.0	25.1	27.9	17.4	15.6	15.9	14.6	15.0	15.3	15.1	15.1
65 years and over	43.1	34.7	36.2	22.5	21.7	23.1	22.7	23.0	23.6	23.7	23.4
65–74 years	39.1	31.4	32.8	19.2	17.9	18.6	17.6	18.3	18.2	18.5	18.4
75–84 years	52.7	41.8	43.5	28.1	27.4	29.1	28.6	28.3	29.0	28.9	28.7
85 years and over	45.1	37.9	34.2	27.6	26.5	31.2	31.4	30.1	32.7	31.5	31.4
Male											
All ages, age adjusted	36.4	34.5	41.1	34.3	27.3	26.3	22.7	22.3	21.7	21.6	21.9
All ages, crude	35.4	31.8	39.7	35.3	28.0	26.7	22.7	22.4	22.0	22.0	22.1
Under 1 year	9.1	8.6	9.3	7.3	5.0	5.0	4.9	5.7	4.3	4.6	4.8
1–14 years	12.3	10.7	13.0	10.0	8.5	7.0	6.2	5.9	5.7	5.6	5.7
1–4 years	13.0	11.5	12.9	10.2	8.3	6.9	5.6	5.7	5.3	5.4	5.5
5–14 years	11.9	10.4	13.1	9.9	8.6	7.0	6.4	6.0	5.8	5.7	5.8
15–24 years	56.7	61.2	73.2	68.4	52.7	49.5	41.4	40.7	38.1	37.3	38.7
25–34 years	40.8	40.1	49.4	46.3	35.9	35.7	29.1	27.5	27.5	27.0	27.4
35–44 years	32.5	29.9	37.7	31.7	25.2	24.7	21.9	21.8	21.2	21.7	21.6
45–64 years	37.7	33.3	38.9	26.5	22.0	21.9	19.7	19.8	20.0	20.4	20.1
45–54 years	33.6	31.6	37.2	27.6	21.9	22.0	19.6	19.6	19.9	20.3	20.0
55–64 years	43.1	35.6	40.9	25.4	22.1	21.7	19.8	20.1	20.2	20.5	20.3
65 years and over	66.6	52.1	54.4	33.9	30.4	32.1	30.8	31.4	31.9	32.1	31.8
65–74 years	59.1	45.8	47.3	27.3	23.0	24.2	22.3	23.9	23.6	23.5	23.7
75–84 years	85.0	66.0	68.2	44.3	41.3	41.2	39.7	38.7	39.7	39.7	39.4
85 years and over	78.1	62.7	63.1	56.1	55.3	64.5	61.9	59.0	60.4	61.2	60.3
Female											
All ages, age adjusted	10.7	11.0	14.4	11.8	10.5	10.7	10.0	10.2	10.2	9.9	10.1
All ages, crude	10.9	11.0	14.7	12.3	11.0	11.3	10.6	10.7	10.2	9.9	10.7
Under 1 year	7.6	7.5	10.4	6.7	4.7	4.9	4.4	5.8	4.4	4.0	4.7
1–14 years	7.2	6.3	7.9	6.3	5.4	4.9	4.5	4.4	4.4	4.0	4.3
1–4 years	10.0	8.4	10.0	8.1	6.0	5.6	4.8	4.8	4.7	4.6	4.7
5–14 years	5.7	5.4	7.2	5.7	5.1	4.7	4.3	4.2	4.3	3.8	4.1
15–24 years	12.6	15.1	21.6	20.8	18.2	17.9	17.1	17.1	17.1	16.1	16.7
25–34 years	9.3	9.2	13.0	12.2	10.1	11.5	10.4	10.7	10.4	9.9	10.3
35–44 years	8.5	9.1	12.9	10.4	9.4	9.2	9.0	9.4	9.2	9.7	9.4
45–64 years	12.6	13.1	15.3	10.3	9.5	10.1	9.1	9.4	9.6	9.3	9.5
45–54 years	10.9	11.6	14.5	10.2	9.0	9.6	8.5	8.8	8.9	8.8	8.8
55–64 years	14.9	15.2	16.2	10.5	9.9	10.8	9.9	10.3	10.8	10.1	10.4
65 years and over	21.9	20.3	23.1	15.0	15.8	17.2	17.2	17.2	17.8	17.8	17.6
65–74 years	20.6	19.0	21.6	13.0	14.0	14.1	13.8	13.9	13.8	14.5	14.1
75–84 years	25.2	23.0	27.2	18.5	19.2	21.9	21.5	21.5	22.0	21.8	21.8
85 years and over	22.1	22.0	18.0	15.2	15.0	18.3	19.6	18.6	21.5	19.2	19.8
White male											
All ages, age adjusted	35.9	34.0	40.1	34.8	27.6	26.3	22.6	22.2	21.6	21.5	21.8
All ages, crude	35.1	31.5	39.1	35.9	28.3	26.7	22.6	22.4	21.9	21.9	22.1
Under 1 year	9.1	8.8	9.1	7.0	4.6	4.8	4.3	5.2	3.7	4.6	4.5
1–14 years	12.4	10.6	12.5	9.8	8.3	6.6	5.9	5.7	5.4	5.1	5.4
15–24 years	58.3	62.7	75.2	73.8	56.5	52.5	43.2	42.2	39.8	39.4	40.5
25–34 years	39.1	38.6	47.0	46.6	35.8	35.4	28.8	27.0	26.8	26.3	26.7
35–44 years	30.9	28.4	35.2	30.7	24.3	23.7	21.1	21.4	20.7	21.2	21.1
45–64 years	36.2	31.7	36.5	25.2	20.8	20.6	18.9	19.2	19.2	19.6	19.3
65 years and over	67.1	52.1	54.2	32.7	29.9	31.4	30.2	31.1	31.8	31.9	31.6

See footnotes at end of table.

[Data are based on the National Vital Statistics System]

Sex, race, Hispanic origin, and age	1950[1]	1960[1]	1970	1980	1985	1990	1995	1996	1997	1998	1996–98[2]
Black male			Deaths per 100,000 resident population								
All ages, age adjusted	39.8	38.2	50.1	32.9	28.0	28.9	25.3	24.9	24.9	25.0	25.0
All ages, crude	37.2	33.1	44.3	31.1	27.1	28.1	24.6	24.3	24.2	24.5	24.3
Under 1 year	---	---	10.6	7.8	*	*	8.3	7.6	7.8	*	6.9
1–14 years	---	11.2	16.3	11.4	9.7	8.9	7.8	7.6	7.6	8.5	7.9
15–24 years	41.6	46.4	58.1	34.9	32.0	36.1	34.3	35.2	32.7	30.3	32.7
25–34 years	57.4	51.0	70.4	44.9	37.7	39.5	32.9	32.5	33.2	34.5	33.4
35–44 years	45.9	43.6	59.5	41.2	34.7	33.5	28.9	26.6	27.0	26.9	26.8
45–64 years	54.6	47.8	61.7	39.5	32.9	33.3	26.9	26.8	28.9	29.0	28.3
65 years and over	52.6	48.2	53.4	42.4	35.2	36.3	36.3	35.6	32.3	36.0	34.6
American Indian or Alaska Native male[3]											
All ages, age adjusted	---	---	---	77.4	52.3	49.0	45.4	45.4	‡43.3	41.0	43.2
All ages, crude	---	---	---	74.6	51.7	47.6	43.8	44.2	42.2	39.9	42.1
1–14 years	---	---	---	15.1	16.2	11.6	8.5	13.5	8.2	10.1	10.6
15–24 years	---	---	---	126.1	77.3	75.2	76.6	69.6	67.6	60.4	65.8
25–34 years	---	---	---	107.0	84.0	78.2	73.1	70.5	64.3	55.9	63.6
35–44 years	---	---	---	82.8	55.8	57.0	50.4	48.8	54.7	51.3	51.6
45–64 years	---	---	---	77.4	52.2	45.9	42.5	39.8	37.8	44.5	40.7
65 years and over	---	---	---	97.0	*	43.0	*	43.5	50.1	36.2	43.2
Asian or Pacific Islander male[4]											
All ages, age adjusted	---	---	---	17.1	16.2	15.8	13.6	11.9	11.7	10.9	11.5
All ages, crude	---	---	---	17.1	16.0	15.8	13.1	11.5	11.4	10.8	11.2
1–14 years	---	---	---	8.2	5.2	6.3	4.3	2.9	2.7	3.2	3.0
15–24 years	---	---	---	27.2	28.1	25.7	20.6	22.4	15.7	16.3	18.1
25–34 years	---	---	---	18.8	18.4	17.0	13.2	13.3	15.7	12.5	13.9
35–44 years	---	---	---	13.1	12.0	12.2	10.4	9.9	8.5	9.3	9.3
45–64 years	---	---	---	13.7	13.4	15.1	15.0	9.7	12.1	12.3	11.4
65 years and over	---	---	---	37.3	37.3	33.6	34.4	23.9	31.0	22.9	25.9
Hispanic male[5]											
All ages, age adjusted	---	---	---	---	25.3	29.1	24.5	23.2	21.4	21.7	22.1
All ages, crude	---	---	---	---	25.6	29.2	23.5	22.3	20.8	20.8	21.3
1–14 years	---	---	---	---	7.7	7.2	5.8	5.6	5.1	5.4	5.3
15–24 years	---	---	---	---	44.9	48.2	42.4	37.5	35.3	36.0	36.3
25–34 years	---	---	---	---	31.2	41.0	31.6	28.0	27.4	27.4	27.6
35–44 years	---	---	---	---	26.3	28.0	23.8	23.9	22.9	21.5	22.7
45–64 years	---	---	---	---	25.9	28.9	23.0	23.8	21.3	21.5	22.2
65 years and over	---	---	---	---	22.9	35.3	35.1	35.2	28.6	31.3	31.7
White, non-Hispanic male[5]											
All ages, age adjusted	---	---	---	---	25.3	25.7	21.9	21.7	21.3	21.2	21.4
All ages, crude	---	---	---	---	25.9	26.0	22.0	21.9	21.7	21.7	21.8
1–14 years	---	---	---	---	7.8	6.4	5.8	5.5	5.4	5.0	5.3
15–24 years	---	---	---	---	53.3	52.3	42.3	42.0	40.1	39.4	40.5
25–34 years	---	---	---	---	33.2	34.0	27.5	26.1	26.2	25.5	25.9
35–44 years	---	---	---	---	21.6	23.1	20.3	20.5	20.0	20.8	20.4
45–64 years	---	---	---	---	18.0	19.8	18.2	18.4	18.8	19.2	18.8
65 years and over	---	---	---	---	27.6	31.1	29.6	30.5	31.7	31.8	31.3
White female											
All ages, age adjusted	10.6	11.1	14.4	12.3	10.8	11.0	10.3	10.4	10.3	10.0	10.3
All ages, crude	10.9	11.2	14.8	12.8	11.4	11.6	10.8	11.0	10.9	10.7	10.9
Under 1 year	7.8	7.5	10.2	7.1	3.9	4.7	4.5	5.7	4.3	3.3	4.4
1–14 years	7.2	6.2	7.5	6.2	5.4	4.8	4.3	4.3	4.1	3.9	4.1
15–24 years	12.6	15.6	22.7	23.0	20.0	19.5	18.4	18.1	18.4	17.3	18.0
25–34 years	9.0	9.0	12.7	12.2	10.1	11.6	10.4	10.8	10.3	10.0	10.4
35–44 years	8.1	8.9	12.3	10.6	9.4	9.2	9.0	9.3	9.0	9.6	9.3
45–64 years	12.7	13.1	15.1	10.4	9.5	9.9	8.9	9.3	9.4	9.1	9.3
65 years and over	22.2	20.8	23.7	15.3	16.2	17.4	17.7	17.4	17.9	18.1	17.8

See footnotes at end of table.

Table 45 (page 3 of 4). Death rates for motor vehicle-related injuries, according to sex, detailed race, Hispanic origin, and age: United States, selected years 1950–98

[Data are based on the National Vital Statistics System]

Sex, race, Hispanic origin, and age	1950[1]	1960[1]	1970	1980	1985	1990	1995	1996	1997	1998	1996–98[2]
Black female					Deaths per 100,000 resident population						
All ages, age adjusted	10.3	10.0	13.8	8.4	8.2	9.3	8.9	9.4	9.8	9.2	9.5
All ages, crude	10.2	9.7	13.4	8.3	8.3	9.4	9.0	9.5	9.9	9.3	9.6
Under 1 year	---	8.1	11.9	*	8.1	7.0	*	7.8	*	9.4	7.6
1–14 years	---	6.9	10.2	6.3	5.1	5.3	5.1	4.8	5.6	4.8	5.1
15–24 years	11.5	9.9	13.4	8.0	9.1	9.9	10.7	13.3	11.3	10.3	11.6
25–34 years	10.7	9.8	13.3	10.6	9.3	11.1	10.5	10.9	11.2	8.9	10.4
35–44 years	11.1	11.0	16.1	8.3	9.1	9.4	9.8	9.6	10.2	11.1	10.3
45–64 years	11.8	12.7	16.7	9.2	9.0	10.7	9.4	8.9	11.0	10.6	10.2
65 years and over	14.3	13.2	15.7	9.5	11.2	13.5	11.5	13.1	14.2	13.8	13.7
American Indian or Alaska Native female[3]											
All ages, age adjusted	---	---	---	32.5	20.9	17.8	21.0	22.6	21.3	22.8	22.2
All ages, crude	---	---	---	32.0	20.6	17.3	20.4	21.8	20.9	22.3	21.7
1–14 years	---	---	---	15.0	9.2	8.1	9.1	9.7	10.0	9.4	9.7
15–24 years	---	---	---	42.3	29.5	31.4	32.7	27.1	24.5	30.4	27.4
25–34 years	---	---	---	52.5	30.2	18.8	36.7	31.9	27.6	33.4	31.0
35–44 years	---	---	---	38.1	27.0	18.2	19.4	23.0	21.5	21.7	22.1
45–64 years	---	---	---	32.6	19.5	17.6	17.1	27.1	22.5	24.1	24.5
65 years and over	---	---	---	*	*	*	*	*	35.7	27.7	28.3
Asian or Pacific Islander female[4]											
All ages, age adjusted	---	---	---	8.4	8.0	9.2	8.2	7.2	8.0	6.6	7.2
All ages, crude	---	---	---	8.2	7.9	9.0	8.0	7.4	8.0	6.6	7.3
1–14 years	---	---	---	7.4	5.0	3.6	3.0	2.3	3.2	2.4	2.6
15–24 years	---	---	---	7.4	7.4	11.4	12.4	8.3	11.5	9.4	9.8
25–34 years	---	---	---	7.3	8.4	7.3	5.1	5.6	6.1	6.1	5.9
35–44 years	---	---	---	8.6	7.0	7.5	6.2	7.5	6.9	4.6	6.3
45–64 years	---	---	---	8.5	8.6	11.8	10.8	8.9	8.6	7.5	8.3
65 years and over	---	---	---	18.6	20.5	24.3	19.7	21.3	20.7	16.7	19.5
Hispanic female[5]											
All ages, age adjusted	---	---	---	---	8.3	9.2	8.5	8.7	8.5	8.1	8.4
All ages, crude	---	---	---	---	7.9	8.9	8.3	8.5	8.3	7.8	8.2
1–14 years	---	---	---	---	4.8	4.8	4.4	4.7	3.9	3.8	4.1
15–24 years	---	---	---	---	10.1	11.6	12.8	11.8	13.1	11.4	12.1
25–34 years	---	---	---	---	7.5	9.4	7.7	9.0	8.3	8.5	8.6
35–44 years	---	---	---	---	8.8	8.0	8.1	7.7	8.1	7.4	7.7
45–64 years	---	---	---	---	9.4	11.4	9.2	9.7	9.0	9.6	9.4
65 years and over	---	---	---	---	14.8	14.9	13.9	13.9	14.1	11.2	13.0

See footnotes at end of table.

Table 45 (page 4 of 4). Death rates for motor vehicle-related injuries, according to sex, detailed race, Hispanic origin, and age: United States, selected years 1950–98

[Data are based on the National Vital Statistics System]

Sex, race, Hispanic origin, and age	1950[1]	1960[1]	1970	1980	⌐5	1990	1995	1996	1997	1998	1996–98[2]
White, non-Hispanic female[5]					Deaths per 100,000 resident population						
All ages, age adjusted	- - -	- - -	- - -	- - -	10.4	11.1	10.3	10.4	10.4	10.2	10.3
All ages, crude	- - -	- - -	- - -	- - -	10.9	11.7	10.9	11.0	11.1	11.0	11.1
1–14 years	- - -	- - -	- - -	- - -	4.9	4.7	4.2	4.2	4.1	3.8	4.0
15–24 years	- - -	- - -	- - -	- - -	20.2	20.4	19.0	18.8	19.2	18.3	18.7
25–34 years	- - -	- - -	- - -	- - -	9.8	11.7	10.6	10.8	10.4	10.1	10.4
35–44 years	- - -	- - -	- - -	- - -	8.6	9.3	8.9	9.3	9.0	9.8	9.3
45–64 years	- - -	- - -	- - -	- - -	8.6	9.7	8.7	9.0	9.4	9.0	9.1
65 years and over	- - -	- - -	- - -	- - -	15.3	17.5	17.7	17.4	18.0	18.4	17.9

- - - Data not available.
* Based on fewer than 20 deaths.
[1]Includes deaths of persons who were not residents of the 50 States and the District of Columbia.
[2]Average annual death rate.
[3]Interpretation of trends should take into account that population estimates for American Indians increased by 45 percent between 1980 and 1990, partly due to better enumeration techniques in the 1990 decennial census and to the increased tendency for people to identify themselves as American Indian in 1990.
[4]Interpretation of trends should take into account that the Asian population in the United States more than doubled between 1980 and 1990, primarily due to immigration.
[5]Excludes data from States lacking an Hispanic-origin item on their death certificates. See Appendix I, National Vital Statistics System.

NOTES: Rates are age adjusted to the 1940 U.S. standard million population. See Appendix II, Age adjustment. For data years shown, the code numbers for cause of death are based on the then current *International Classification of Diseases*, which are described in Appendix II, tables IV and V. Age groups were selected to minimize the presentation of unstable age-specific death rates based on small numbers of deaths and for consistency among comparison groups. The race groups, white, black, Asian or Pacific Islander, and American Indian or Alaska Native, include persons of Hispanic and non-Hispanic origin. Conversely, persons of Hispanic origin may be of any race. Bias in death rates results from inconsistent race identification between the death certificate (source of data for numerator of death rates) and data from the Census Bureau (denominator); and from undercounts of some population groups in the census. The net effects of misclassification and under coverage result in death rates estimated to be overstated by 1 percent for the white population and 5 percent for the black population; and death rates estimated to be understated by 21 percent for American Indians, 11 percent for Asians, and 2 percent for Hispanics (Rosenberg HM, Maurer JD, Sorlie PD, Johnson NJ, et al. Quality of death rates by race and Hispanic origin: A summary of current research, 1999. National Center for Health Statistics. Vital Health Stat 2(128). 1999). Data for additional years are available (see Appendix III).

SOURCES: Centers for Disease Control and Prevention, National Center for Health Statistics. Grove RD and Hetzel AM. *Vital statistics rates in the United States, 1940–60*. Washington: Public Health Service, 1968; *Vital statistics of the United States, vol II, mortality, part A*, for data years 1950–93. Public Health Service. Washington. U.S. Government Printing Office; for 1994–98, data for all persons, white, and black are available on the NCHS Web site at www.cdc.gov/nchs/datawh/statab/unpubd/mortabs.htm; numerator data from National Vital Statistics System, annual mortality files; denominator data from national population estimates for race groups from table 1 and unpublished Hispanic population estimates prepared by the Housing and Household Economic Statistics Division, U.S. Bureau of the Census.

Table 46 (page 1 of 3). Death rates for homicide and legal intervention, according to sex, detailed race, Hispanic origin, and age: United States, selected years 1950–98

[Data are based on the National Vital Statistics System]

Sex, race, Hispanic origin, and age	1950[1]	1960[1]	1970	1980	1985	1990	1995	1996	1997	1998	1996–98[2]
All persons					Deaths per 100,000 resident population						
All ages, age adjusted	5.4	5.2	9.1	10.8	8.3	10.2	9.4	8.5	8.0	7.3	7.9
All ages, crude	5.3	4.7	8.3	10.7	8.4	10.0	8.7	7.9	7.4	6.8	7.4
Under 1 year	4.4	4.8	4.3	5.9	5.4	8.4	8.1	8.8	8.3	8.5	8.6
1–14 years	0.6	0.6	1.1	1.5	1.6	1.8	1.9	1.7	1.5	1.6	1.6
1–4 years	0.6	0.7	1.9	2.5	2.5	2.6	2.9	2.7	2.4	2.6	2.6
5–14 years	0.5	0.5	0.9	1.2	1.2	1.5	1.5	1.3	1.2	1.2	1.2
15–24 years	6.3	5.9	11.7	15.6	11.9	19.9	20.3	18.1	16.8	14.8	16.5
25–44 years	9.3	8.9	15.2	17.6	13.3	14.9	12.3	11.1	10.5	9.8	10.5
25–34 years	9.9	9.7	16.6	19.6	14.8	17.7	15.1	13.4	12.8	11.8	12.7
35–44 years	8.8	8.1	13.7	15.1	11.3	11.8	9.7	9.0	8.4	8.0	8.4
45–64 years	5.2	5.3	8.8	9.1	7.0	6.4	5.5	5.2	4.9	4.4	4.8
45–54 years	6.1	6.2	10.1	11.1	8.1	7.6	6.2	5.9	5.6	5.0	5.5
55–64 years	4.0	4.2	7.1	7.0	5.7	5.0	4.5	4.1	3.9	3.4	3.8
65 years and over	3.0	2.7	4.6	5.6	4.3	4.0	3.2	3.0	3.0	2.6	2.9
65–74 years	3.2	2.8	5.0	5.7	4.3	3.8	3.3	3.0	2.9	2.5	2.8
75–84 years	2.6	2.4	4.0	5.2	4.3	4.3	3.1	2.9	2.9	2.7	2.8
85 years and over	2.3	2.4	4.2	5.3	4.2	4.6	3.3	3.0	3.8	2.5	3.1
Male											
All ages, age adjusted	8.4	7.9	14.9	17.4	12.8	16.3	14.7	13.3	12.5	11.3	12.4
All ages, crude	8.1	7.1	13.4	17.3	13.0	16.2	13.8	12.5	11.8	10.6	11.6
Under 1 year	4.5	4.7	4.5	6.3	5.6	8.8	8.9	8.7	9.4	8.9	9.0
1–14 years	0.6	0.6	1.2	1.6	1.8	2.0	2.3	1.9	1.8	1.7	1.8
1–4 years	0.5	0.7	1.9	2.7	2.5	2.7	3.1	2.7	2.7	2.9	2.7
5–14 years	0.6	0.5	1.0	1.2	1.4	1.7	1.9	1.6	1.5	1.3	1.4
15–24 years	9.6	9.1	19.0	24.5	18.6	32.9	33.9	30.4	28.2	24.8	27.8
25–44 years	14.7	13.6	25.0	29.4	21.0	24.0	19.1	17.3	16.3	15.0	16.2
25–34 years	15.5	14.9	27.6	32.5	23.3	28.3	23.7	21.4	20.5	18.8	20.3
35–44 years	13.8	12.3	22.2	24.9	17.9	19.0	14.6	13.5	12.5	11.8	12.6
45–64 years	8.4	8.3	14.9	15.4	11.1	10.3	8.6	8.0	7.6	6.8	7.4
45–54 years	9.9	9.6	17.0	18.6	12.9	12.1	9.6	8.9	8.5	7.8	8.4
55–64 years	6.5	6.6	12.2	11.9	9.2	8.1	7.2	6.6	6.1	5.3	6.0
65 years and over	4.9	4.3	7.8	8.9	6.2	5.8	4.3	4.1	4.3	3.6	4.0
65–74 years	5.3	4.6	8.6	9.3	6.5	5.8	4.6	4.3	4.3	3.7	4.1
75–84 years	4.0	3.7	6.0	8.1	5.8	5.7	3.7	3.8	3.8	3.5	3.7
85 years and over	2.5	3.6	7.4	7.5	5.0	6.8	4.2	3.7	5.9	3.3	4.3
Female											
All ages, age adjusted	2.5	2.6	3.7	4.5	3.9	4.2	4.0	3.6	3.3	3.2	3.4
All ages, crude	2.4	2.4	3.4	4.5	4.0	4.2	3.8	3.5	3.2	3.1	3.3
Under 1 year	4.2	4.9	4.1	5.6	5.2	8.0	7.2	8.9	7.3	8.1	8.1
1–14 years	0.6	0.5	1.0	1.4	1.4	1.6	1.5	1.6	1.2	1.4	1.4
1–4 years	0.7	0.7	1.9	2.2	2.4	2.4	2.6	2.7	2.2	2.4	2.4
5–14 years	0.5	0.4	0.7	1.1	1.0	1.2	1.0	1.1	0.9	1.1	1.0
15–24 years	3.1	2.8	4.6	6.6	5.1	6.3	6.0	5.1	4.7	4.3	4.7
25–44 years	4.2	4.3	5.9	6.4	5.7	6.0	5.7	5.0	4.6	4.6	4.7
25–34 years	4.5	4.6	6.0	7.0	6.4	7.2	6.5	5.5	5.1	4.9	5.2
35–44 years	3.8	4.1	5.7	5.7	4.9	4.8	4.9	4.5	4.3	4.3	4.4
45–64 years	1.9	2.5	3.1	3.4	3.2	2.8	2.6	2.5	2.4	2.1	2.3
45–54 years	2.3	2.9	3.7	4.1	3.7	3.2	3.0	3.0	2.7	2.4	2.7
55–64 years	1.4	2.0	2.5	2.8	2.7	2.3	2.1	1.9	2.0	1.6	1.8
65 years and over	1.4	1.3	2.3	3.3	3.0	2.8	2.4	2.1	2.2	1.9	2.1
65–74 years	1.3	1.3	2.2	3.0	2.6	2.2	2.2	1.9	1.9	1.6	1.8
75–84 years	1.4	1.3	2.7	3.5	3.4	3.4	2.7	2.4	2.2	2.1	2.2
85 years and over	2.1	1.6	2.5	4.3	3.8	3.8	2.9	2.7	3.0	2.2	2.6
White male											
All ages, age adjusted	3.9	3.9	7.3	10.9	8.1	8.9	8.2	7.3	7.0	6.4	6.9
All ages, crude	3.9	3.6	6.8	10.9	8.2	9.0	7.8	7.0	6.7	6.1	6.6
Under 1 year	4.3	3.8	2.9	4.3	3.8	6.4	7.1	6.5	7.8	6.7	7.0
1–14 years	0.4	0.5	0.7	1.2	1.3	1.3	1.5	1.4	1.3	1.1	1.2
15–24 years	3.7	4.4	7.9	15.5	11.0	15.4	16.5	14.0	13.2	12.2	13.1
25–44 years	5.9	5.9	12.0	17.4	12.9	13.3	11.0	9.9	9.5	8.7	9.4
25–34 years	5.4	6.2	13.0	18.9	14.0	15.1	12.9	11.5	11.4	10.2	11.0
35–44 years	6.4	5.5	11.0	15.5	11.5	11.4	9.2	8.4	7.8	7.5	7.9
45–64 years	5.0	4.7	8.4	9.9	7.5	7.0	5.8	5.5	5.3	4.7	5.2
65 years and over	3.9	3.2	5.5	6.7	4.5	4.1	3.0	3.2	3.4	2.8	3.1

See footnotes at end of table.

Table 46 (page 2 of 3). Death rates for homicide and legal intervention, according to sex, detailed race, Hispanic origin, and age: United States, selected years 1950–98

[Data are based on the National Vital Statistics System]

Sex, race, Hispanic origin, and age	1950[1]	1960[1]	1970	1980	1985	1990	1995	1996	1997	1998	1996–98[2]
Black male					Deaths per 100,000 resident population						
All ages, age adjusted	51.1	44.9	82.1	71.9	50.2	68.7	57.6	52.6	48.3	43.1	48.0
All ages, crude	47.3	36.6	67.6	66.6	49.0	69.2	56.3	51.5	47.1	42.1	46.8
Under 1 year	- - -	10.3	14.3	18.6	16.7	21.4	19.4	23.1	18.1	21.8	21.0
1–14 years	- - -	1.5	4.4	4.1	4.2	5.8	6.1	4.8	4.7	4.9	4.8
15–24 years	58.9	46.4	102.5	84.3	65.9	138.3	132.0	123.1	113.3	96.5	110.8
25–44 years	97.8	84.9	143.3	130.1	87.5	106.2	77.9	71.0	65.0	59.0	65.0
25–34 years	110.5	92.0	158.5	145.1	95.6	125.4	98.3	89.5	82.9	75.0	82.5
35–44 years	83.7	77.5	126.2	110.3	74.9	82.3	56.2	52.0	47.1	43.4	47.5
45–64 years	47.6	45.4	83.0	70.8	46.3	41.7	34.6	30.5	27.4	25.8	27.9
65 years and over	16.7	17.9	33.7	31.1	26.2	25.9	19.9	15.6	14.4	11.9	14.0
American Indian or Alaska Native male[3]											
All ages, age adjusted	- - -	- - -	- - -	23.9	20.0	17.5	18.0	15.7	16.7	14.9	15.8
All ages, crude	- - -	- - -	- - -	23.4	19.0	17.3	17.8	15.3	16.4	14.6	15.4
15–24 years	- - -	- - -	- - -	36.0	27.1	27.7	32.2	26.6	27.7	22.8	25.7
25–44 years	- - -	- - -	- - -	39.7	30.2	26.0	28.4	23.6	23.9	21.5	23.0
45–64 years	- - -	- - -	- - -	22.1	21.2	15.5	13.2	12.7	13.3	15.5	13.9
Asian or Pacific Islander male[4]											
All ages, age adjusted	- - -	- - -	- - -	8.5	5.8	7.7	8.3	7.3	6.6	5.5	6.5
All ages, crude	- - -	- - -	- - -	8.3	6.0	7.9	8.0	7.2	6.5	5.4	6.4
15–24 years	- - -	- - -	- - -	9.3	8.6	14.9	19.4	15.6	13.4	9.6	12.9
25–44 years	- - -	- - -	- - -	11.3	8.9	9.7	8.1	8.4	7.6	6.9	7.6
45–64 years	- - -	- - -	- - -	10.4	5.4	7.0	8.4	7.6	6.5	4.7	6.2
Hispanic male[5]											
All ages, age adjusted	- - -	- - -	- - -	- - -	26.7	29.8	25.1	20.4	18.2	16.6	18.4
All ages, crude	- - -	- - -	- - -	- - -	27.6	31.5	25.2	20.9	18.6	16.7	18.7
Under 1 year	- - -	- - -	- - -	- - -	*	8.7	5.9	6.4	8.2	8.7	7.8
1–14 years	- - -	- - -	- - -	- - -	1.5	3.1	3.3	2.5	1.8	1.7	2.0
15–24 years	- - -	- - -	- - -	- - -	42.9	56.2	63.5	48.9	42.7	41.1	44.2
25–44 years	- - -	- - -	- - -	- - -	47.3	47.2	31.7	26.4	24.1	21.4	24.0
25–34 years	- - -	- - -	- - -	- - -	51.4	51.9	37.1	31.2	28.8	27.0	29.0
35–44 years	- - -	- - -	- - -	- - -	40.1	39.8	24.2	20.2	18.3	15.0	17.8
45–64 years	- - -	- - -	- - -	- - -	19.9	20.9	14.8	13.9	11.6	9.0	11.4
65 years and over	- - -	- - -	- - -	- - -	9.3	9.4	5.5	4.0	6.4	4.9	5.1
White, non-Hispanic male[5]											
All ages, age adjusted	- - -	- - -	- - -	- - -	6.2	5.8	5.1	4.7	4.8	4.4	4.6
All ages, crude	- - -	- - -	- - -	- - -	6.4	6.0	5.1	4.7	4.8	4.4	4.6
Under 1 year	- - -	- - -	- - -	- - -	4.6	5.4	6.7	6.4	7.4	6.1	6.7
1–14 years	- - -	- - -	- - -	- - -	1.2	0.9	1.1	1.1	1.1	1.0	1.1
15–24 years	- - -	- - -	- - -	- - -	7.7	7.7	7.3	6.4	6.5	5.8	6.3
25–44 years	- - -	- - -	- - -	- - -	9.5	9.0	7.6	6.9	6.9	6.4	6.7
25–34 years	- - -	- - -	- - -	- - -	9.6	9.6	8.2	7.3	7.6	6.6	7.2
35–44 years	- - -	- - -	- - -	- - -	9.3	8.3	7.1	6.6	6.3	6.4	6.4
45–64 years	- - -	- - -	- - -	- - -	6.4	5.8	4.8	4.6	4.7	4.2	4.5
65 years and over	- - -	- - -	- - -	- - -	4.4	3.7	2.7	3.1	3.1	2.7	3.0
White female											
All ages, age adjusted	1.4	1.5	2.2	3.2	2.9	2.8	2.8	2.5	2.3	2.2	2.3
All ages, crude	1.4	1.4	2.1	3.2	2.9	2.8	2.7	2.5	2.3	2.2	2.3
Under 1 year	3.9	3.5	2.9	4.3	4.3	5.1	5.0	6.8	4.6	5.9	5.8
1–14 years	0.4	0.4	0.7	1.1	1.1	1.0	1.1	1.1	0.9	1.1	1.0
15–24 years	1.3	1.5	2.7	4.7	3.6	4.0	4.0	3.3	3.2	2.8	3.1
25–44 years	2.0	2.1	3.3	4.2	4.1	3.8	3.8	3.3	3.1	3.2	3.2
45–64 years	1.5	1.7	2.1	2.6	2.6	2.3	2.2	2.1	1.9	1.7	1.9
65 years and over	1.2	1.2	1.9	2.9	2.6	2.2	2.0	1.8	1.9	1.7	1.8

See footnotes at end of table.

[Data are based on the National Vital Statistics System]

Sex, race, Hispanic origin, and age	1950[1]	1960[1]	1970	1980	1985	1990	1995	1996	1997	1998	1996–98[2]
Black female					Deaths per 100,000 resident population						
All ages, age adjusted	11.7	11.8	15.0	13.7	10.9	13.0	11.0	10.2	9.3	8.6	9.4
All ages, crude	11.5	10.4	13.3	13.5	11.1	13.5	11.1	10.2	9.3	8.6	9.3
Under 1 year	- - -	13.8	10.7	12.8	10.7	22.8	19.2	21.1	21.6	22.1	21.6
1–14 years	- - -	1.2	3.1	3.3	3.3	4.7	3.6	3.9	3.0	3.4	3.5
15–24 years	16.5	11.9	17.7	18.4	14.2	18.9	16.8	14.7	13.3	12.6	13.5
25–44 years	22.5	22.8	25.4	22.3	17.8	20.9	17.4	15.8	14.3	13.0	14.3
45–64 years	6.8	10.3	13.4	10.8	7.9	6.5	5.9	6.0	6.1	5.0	5.7
65 years and over	3.6	3.0	7.4	8.0	7.8	9.5	6.9	5.2	4.6	4.0	4.6
American Indian or Alaska Native female[3]											
All ages, age adjusted	- - -	- - -	- - -	8.3	4.8	4.9	5.6	4.5	5.2	4.9	4.9
All ages, crude	- - -	- - -	- - -	7.7	4.5	4.9	5.6	4.4	5.3	4.9	4.9
15–24 years	- - -	- - -	- - -	*	*	*	*	*	*	*	4.5
25–44 years	- - -	- - -	- - -	13.7	*	6.9	9.1	*	7.3	10.2	7.3
45–64 years	- - -	- - -	- - -	*	*	*	*	*	*	*	4.8
Asian or Pacific Islander female[4]											
All ages, age adjusted	- - -	- - -	- - -	3.0	2.7	2.7	2.6	2.1	2.2	2.0	2.1
All ages, crude	- - -	- - -	- - -	3.1	2.8	2.8	2.7	2.1	2.2	2.0	2.1
15–24 years	- - -	- - -	- - -	*	*	*	3.7	3.7	2.8	*	2.9
25–44 years	- - -	- - -	- - -	4.6	2.9	3.8	3.8	2.1	2.3	2.3	2.3
45–64 years	- - -	- - -	- - -	*	*	*	2.3	*	2.5	2.2	2.1
Hispanic female[5]											
All ages, age adjusted	- - -	- - -	- - -	- - -	4.2	4.6	4.4	3.4	3.1	2.9	3.2
All ages, crude	- - -	- - -	- - -	- - -	4.3	4.7	4.3	3.5	3.1	2.9	3.2
Under 1 year	- - -	- - -	- - -	- - -	*	*	*	7.7	*	*	6.0
1–14 years	- - -	- - -	- - -	- - -	1.5	1.9	1.8	1.5	1.2	1.2	1.3
15–24 years	- - -	- - -	- - -	- - -	5.7	8.1	6.9	5.1	4.8	4.2	4.7
25–44 years	- - -	- - -	- - -	- - -	6.8	6.1	5.8	4.8	4.5	4.3	4.5
45–64 years	- - -	- - -	- - -	- - -	3.2	3.3	3.4	2.7	2.5	2.0	2.4
65 years and over	- - -	- - -	- - -	- - -	*	*	2.3	*	*	*	1.4
White, non-Hispanic female[5]											
All ages, age adjusted	- - -	- - -	- - -	- - -	2.8	2.5	2.4	2.2	2.1	2.1	2.2
All ages, crude	- - -	- - -	- - -	- - -	2.9	2.6	2.4	2.3	2.1	2.1	2.2
Under 1 year	- - -	- - -	- - -	- - -	4.1	4.4	4.4	6.0	3.9	5.8	5.2
1–14 years	- - -	- - -	- - -	- - -	1.0	0.8	0.9	1.0	0.8	1.0	0.9
15–24 years	- - -	- - -	- - -	- - -	3.5	3.3	3.4	2.7	2.8	2.5	2.7
25–44 years	- - -	- - -	- - -	- - -	3.9	3.5	3.3	3.1	2.9	3.0	3.0
45–64 years	- - -	- - -	- - -	- - -	2.6	2.2	1.9	2.0	1.8	1.7	1.8
65 years and over	- - -	- - -	- - -	- - -	3.0	2.2	2.0	1.9	2.0	1.6	1.8

- - - Data not available.

* Based on fewer than 20 deaths.

[1]Includes deaths of persons who were not residents of the 50 States and the District of Columbia.

[2]Average annual death rate.

[3]Interpretation of trends should take into account that population estimates for American Indians increased by 45 percent between 1980 and 1990, partly due to better enumeration techniques in the 1990 decennial census and to the increased tendency for people to identify themselves as American Indian in 1990.

[4]Interpretation of trends should take into account that the Asian population in the United States more than doubled between 1980 and 1990, primarily due to immigration.

[5]Excludes data from States lacking an Hispanic-origin item on their death certificates. See Appendix I, National Vital Statistics System.

NOTES: Rates are age adjusted to the 1940 U.S. standard million population. See Appendix II, Age adjustment. For data years shown, the code numbers for cause of death are based on the then current International Classification of Diseases, which are described in Appendix II, tables IV and V. Age groups were selected to minimize the presentation of unstable age-specific death rates based on small numbers of deaths and for consistency among comparison groups. The race groups, white, black, Asian or Pacific Islander, and American Indian or Alaska Native, include persons of Hispanic and non-Hispanic origin. Conversely, persons of Hispanic origin may be of any race. Bias in death rates results from inconsistent race identification between the death certificate (source of data for numerator of death rates) and data from the Census Bureau (denominator); and from undercounts of some population groups in the census. The net effects of misclassification and under coverage result in death rates estimated to be overstated by 1 percent for the white population and 5 percent for the black population; and death rates estimated to be understated by 21 percent for American Indians, 11 percent for Asians, and 2 percent for Hispanics (Rosenberg HM, Maurer JD, Sorlie PD, Johnson NJ, et al. Quality of death rates by race and Hispanic origin: A summary of current research, 1999. National Center for Health Statistics. Vital Health Stat 2(128). 1999). Data for additional years are available (see Appendix III).

SOURCES: Centers for Disease Control and Prevention, National Center for Health Statistics. Grove RD and Hetzel AM. Vital statistics rates in the United States, 1940–60. Washington: Public Health Service, 1968; Vital statistics of the United States, vol II, mortality, part A, for data years 1950–93. Public Health Service. Washington. U.S. Government Printing Office; for 1994–98, data for all persons, white, and black are available on the NCHS Web site at www.cdc.gov/nchs/datawh/statab/unpubd/mortabs.htm; numerator data from National Vital Statistics System, annual mortality files; denominator data from national population estimates for race groups from table 1 and unpublished Hispanic population estimates prepared by the Housing and Household Economic Statistics Division, U.S. Bureau of the Census.

[Data are based on the National Vital Statistics System]

Sex, race, Hispanic origin, and age	1950[1]	1960[1]	1970	1980	1985	1990	1995	1996	1997	1998	1996–98[2]
All persons				Deaths per 100,000 resident population							
All ages, age adjusted	11.0	10.6	11.8	11.4	11.5	11.5	11.2	10.8	10.6	10.4	10.6
All ages, crude	11.4	10.6	11.6	11.9	12.4	12.4	11.9	11.6	11.4	11.3	11.5
Under 1 year	...	...	...	...	...	...	...	...	...	...	...
1–4 years	...	...	...	...	...	...	...	...	...	...	...
5–14 years	0.2	0.3	0.3	0.4	0.8	0.8	0.9	0.8	0.8	0.8	0.8
15–24 years	4.5	5.2	8.8	12.3	12.8	13.2	13.3	12.0	11.4	11.1	11.5
25–44 years	11.6	12.2	15.4	15.6	15.0	15.2	15.3	15.0	14.8	14.6	14.8
25–34 years	9.1	10.0	14.1	16.0	15.3	15.2	15.4	14.5	14.3	13.8	14.2
35–44 years	14.3	14.2	16.9	15.4	14.6	15.3	15.2	15.5	15.3	15.4	15.4
45–64 years	23.5	22.0	20.6	15.9	16.3	15.3	14.1	14.4	14.2	14.1	14.3
45–54 years	20.9	20.7	20.0	15.9	15.7	14.8	14.6	14.9	14.7	14.8	14.8
55–64 years	27.0	23.7	21.4	15.9	16.8	16.0	13.3	13.7	13.5	13.1	13.4
65 years and over	30.0	24.5	20.8	17.6	20.4	20.5	18.1	17.3	16.8	16.9	17.0
65–74 years	29.3	23.0	20.8	16.9	18.7	17.9	15.8	15.0	14.4	14.1	14.5
75–84 years	31.1	27.9	21.2	19.1	23.9	24.9	20.7	20.0	19.3	19.7	19.7
85 years and over	28.8	26.0	19.0	19.2	19.4	22.2	21.6	20.2	20.8	21.0	20.7
Male											
All ages, age adjusted	17.3	16.6	17.3	18.0	18.8	19.0	18.6	18.0	17.4	17.2	17.5
All ages, crude	17.8	16.5	16.8	18.6	20.0	20.4	19.8	19.3	18.7	18.6	18.8
Under 1 year	...	...	...	...	...	...	...	...	...	...	...
1–4 years	...	...	...	...	...	...	...	...	...	...	...
5–14 years	0.3	0.4	0.5	0.6	1.2	1.1	1.3	1.1	1.2	1.2	1.2
15–24 years	6.5	8.2	13.5	20.2	21.0	22.0	22.5	20.0	18.9	18.5	19.2
25–44 years	17.2	17.9	20.9	24.0	23.7	24.4	24.9	24.3	23.8	23.5	23.8
25–34 years	13.4	14.7	19.8	25.0	24.7	24.8	25.6	24.0	23.6	22.9	23.5
35–44 years	21.3	21.0	22.1	22.5	22.3	23.9	24.1	24.6	23.9	24.0	24.1
45–64 years	37.1	34.4	30.0	23.7	25.3	24.3	22.5	23.0	22.5	22.4	22.6
45–54 years	32.0	31.6	27.9	22.9	23.6	23.2	22.8	23.3	22.5	23.1	22.9
55–64 years	43.6	38.1	32.7	24.5	27.1	25.7	22.0	22.7	22.4	21.3	22.1
65 years and over	52.8	44.0	38.4	35.0	40.9	41.6	36.3	35.2	33.9	34.1	34.4
65–74 years	50.5	39.6	36.0	30.4	33.9	32.2	28.7	27.7	26.4	26.2	26.8
75–84 years	58.3	52.5	42.8	42.3	53.1	56.1	44.8	43.4	40.9	42.0	42.1
85 years and over	58.3	57.4	42.4	50.6	56.2	65.9	63.1	59.9	60.3	57.8	59.3
Female											
All ages, age adjusted	4.9	5.0	6.8	5.4	4.9	4.5	4.1	4.0	4.1	4.0	4.1
All ages, crude	5.1	4.9	6.6	5.5	5.2	4.8	4.4	4.4	4.4	4.4	4.4
Under 1 year	...	...	...	...	...	...	...	...	...	...	...
1–4 years	...	...	...	...	...	...	...	...	...	...	...
5–14 years	0.1	0.1	0.2	0.2	0.4	0.4	0.4	0.4	0.4	0.4	0.4
15–24 years	2.6	2.2	4.2	4.3	4.3	3.9	3.7	3.6	3.5	3.3	3.5
25–44 years	6.2	6.6	10.2	7.7	6.5	6.2	5.8	5.8	6.0	6.0	5.9
25–34 years	4.9	5.5	8.6	7.1	5.9	5.6	5.2	5.0	5.0	4.9	5.0
35–44 years	7.5	7.7	11.9	8.5	7.1	6.8	6.5	6.6	6.8	6.9	6.8
45–64 years	9.9	10.2	12.0	8.9	8.0	7.1	6.1	6.4	6.5	6.4	6.4
45–54 years	9.9	10.2	12.6	9.4	8.3	6.9	6.7	7.0	7.3	7.0	7.1
55–64 years	9.9	10.2	11.4	8.4	7.8	7.3	5.3	5.5	5.4	5.5	5.5
65 years and over	9.4	8.4	8.1	6.1	6.6	6.4	5.5	4.8	4.9	4.7	4.8
65–74 years	10.1	8.4	9.0	6.5	6.9	6.7	5.4	4.8	4.7	4.3	4.6
75–84 years	8.1	8.9	7.0	5.5	6.7	6.3	5.5	5.0	5.2	4.9	5.0
85 years and over	8.2	6.0	5.9	5.5	4.7	5.4	5.5	4.4	4.9	5.8	5.0
White male											
All ages, age adjusted	18.1	17.5	18.2	18.9	19.9	20.1	19.7	19.1	18.4	18.3	18.6
All ages, crude	19.0	17.6	18.0	19.9	21.6	22.0	21.4	20.9	20.2	20.3	20.5
15–24 years	6.6	8.6	13.9	21.4	22.3	23.2	23.5	20.9	19.5	19.3	19.9
25–44 years	17.9	18.5	21.5	24.6	24.8	25.4	26.3	25.7	25.3	25.2	25.4
45–64 years	39.3	36.5	31.9	25.0	27.0	26.0	24.2	24.9	24.2	24.2	24.4
65 years and over	55.8	46.7	41.1	37.2	43.7	44.2	38.7	37.8	36.1	36.6	36.8
65–74 years	53.2	42.0	38.7	32.5	35.8	34.2	30.3	29.6	28.0	27.9	28.5
75–84 years	61.9	55.7	45.5	45.5	57.0	60.2	47.5	46.1	43.4	44.7	44.7
85 years and over	61.9	61.3	45.8	52.8	60.9	70.3	68.2	65.4	65.0	62.7	64.3

See footnotes at end of table.

Table 47 (page 2 of 3). Death rates for suicide, according to sex, detailed race, Hispanic origin, and age: United States, selected years 1950–98

[Data are based on the National Vital Statistics System]

Sex, race, Hispanic origin, and age	1950[1]	1960[1]	1970	1980	1985	1990	1995	1996	1997	1998	1996–98[2]
Black male					Deaths per 100,000 resident population						
All ages, age adjusted	7.0	7.8	9.9	11.1	11.5	12.4	12.4	11.8	11.2	10.5	11.2
All ages, crude	6.3	6.4	8.0	10.3	11.0	12.0	11.9	11.4	10.9	10.2	10.8
15–24 years	4.9	4.1	10.5	12.3	13.3	15.1	18.0	16.7	16.0	15.0	15.9
25–44 years	9.8	12.6	16.1	19.2	17.8	19.6	18.6	17.8	17.0	15.2	16.7
45–64 years	12.7	13.0	12.4	11.8	12.9	13.1	11.8	11.8	10.5	11.1	11.1
65 years and over	9.0	9.9	8.7	11.4	15.8	14.9	14.3	12.6	13.6	11.6	12.6
65–74 years	10.0	11.3	8.7	11.1	16.7	14.7	13.5	12.7	12.9	11.4	12.4
75–84 years	- - -	6.6	8.9	10.5	15.6	14.4	16.6	12.5	14.1	12.5	13.0
85 years and over	- - -	6.9	*	*	*	*	*	*	*	*	13.1
American Indian or Alaska Native male[3]											
All ages, age adjusted	- - -	- - -	- - -	20.8	19.9	21.0	20.1	20.0	21.3	21.4	20.9
All ages, crude	- - -	- - -	- - -	20.9	20.3	20.9	19.6	19.9	20.9	21.1	20.6
15–24 years	- - -	- - -	- - -	45.3	42.0	49.1	34.2	32.1	38.4	41.8	37.5
25–44 years	- - -	- - -	- - -	31.2	30.2	27.8	31.8	34.8	32.6	33.3	33.5
45–64 years	- - -	- - -	- - -	*	*	*	15.0	11.5	15.5	11.3	12.8
65 years and over	- - -	- - -	- - -	*	*	*	*	*	*	*	14.0
Asian or Pacific Islander male[4]											
All ages, age adjusted	- - -	- - -	- - -	9.0	8.5	8.8	9.7	8.6	9.4	9.1	9.1
All ages, crude	- - -	- - -	- - -	8.8	8.4	8.7	9.4	8.6	9.2	9.1	9.0
15–24 years	- - -	- - -	- - -	10.8	14.2	13.5	16.0	11.9	12.2	10.9	11.7
25–44 years	- - -	- - -	- - -	11.0	9.3	10.6	11.5	11.5	10.6	11.9	11.3
45–64 years	- - -	- - -	- - -	13.0	10.4	9.7	9.1	8.6	12.3	10.2	10.4
65 years and over	- - -	- - -	- - -	18.6	16.7	16.8	20.3	16.0	21.0	21.0	19.4
Hispanic male[5]											
All ages, age adjusted	- - -	- - -	- - -	- - -	10.4	12.4	12.3	11.1	10.4	10.1	10.5
All ages, crude	- - -	- - -	- - -	- - -	9.8	11.4	11.5	10.6	9.8	9.4	9.9
15–24 years	- - -	- - -	- - -	- - -	13.8	14.7	18.3	15.5	14.4	13.4	14.4
25–44 years	- - -	- - -	- - -	- - -	14.8	16.2	15.5	14.6	13.9	13.0	13.8
45–64 years	- - -	- - -	- - -	- - -	12.3	16.1	14.2	13.3	11.6	11.5	12.1
65 years and over	- - -	- - -	- - -	- - -	14.7	23.4	19.9	17.7	17.7	20.0	18.5
White, non-Hispanic male[5]											
All ages, age adjusted	- - -	- - -	- - -	- - -	20.3	20.8	20.2	19.7	19.3	19.2	19.4
All ages, crude	- - -	- - -	- - -	- - -	22.3	23.1	22.3	22.0	21.5	21.6	21.7
15–24 years	- - -	- - -	- - -	- - -	22.6	24.4	23.8	21.4	20.2	20.2	20.6
25–44 years	- - -	- - -	- - -	- - -	25.1	26.4	27.3	27.1	26.8	26.7	26.9
45–64 years	- - -	- - -	- - -	- - -	27.3	26.8	24.8	25.6	25.1	25.1	25.2
65 years and over	- - -	- - -	- - -	- - -	46.4	45.4	39.2	38.6	36.8	37.3	37.5
White female											
All ages, age adjusted	5.3	5.3	7.2	5.7	5.3	4.8	4.4	4.4	4.4	4.4	4.4
All ages, crude	5.5	5.3	7.1	5.9	5.6	5.3	4.8	4.8	4.9	4.8	4.8
15–24 years	2.7	2.3	4.2	4.6	4.7	4.2	3.9	3.8	3.7	3.5	3.6
25–44 years	6.6	7.0	11.0	8.1	7.0	6.6	6.3	6.4	6.6	6.6	6.5
45–64 years	10.6	10.9	13.0	9.6	8.7	7.7	6.7	7.0	7.2	7.1	7.1
65 years and over	9.9	8.8	8.5	6.4	6.9	6.8	5.7	5.0	5.1	5.0	5.0

See footnotes at end of table.

Table 47 (page 3 of 3). Death rates for suicide, according to sex, detailed race, Hispanic origin, and age: United States, selected years 1950–98

[Data are based on the National Vital Statistics System]

Sex, race, Hispanic origin, and age	1950[1]	1960[1]	1970	1980	1985	1990	1995	1996	1997	1998	1996–98[2]
Black female					Deaths per 100,000 resident population						
All ages, age adjusted	1.7	1.9	2.9	2.4	2.1	2.4	2.0	2.0	1.9	1.8	1.9
All ages, crude	1.5	1.6	2.6	2.2	2.1	2.3	2.0	2.0	1.9	1.8	1.9
15–24 years	1.8	*	3.8	2.3	2.0	2.3	2.2	2.3	2.4	2.2	2.3
25–44 years	2.3	3.0	4.8	4.3	3.2	3.8	3.4	2.9	2.7	2.7	2.8
45–64 years	2.7	3.1	2.9	2.5	2.8	2.9	2.0	2.3	2.4	2.2	2.3
65 years and over	2.0	1.9	2.6	*	2.7	1.9	2.2	2.1	1.6	1.2	1.6
American Indian or Alaska Native female[3]											
All ages, age adjusted	- - -	- - -	- - -	5.0	4.4	3.8	4.4	5.9	4.4	5.6	5.3
All ages, crude	- - -	- - -	- - -	4.7	4.4	3.7	4.2	5.6	4.2	5.4	5.1
15–24 years	- - -	- - -	- - -	*	*	*	*	10.2	*	*	8.3
25–44 years	- - -	- - -	- - -	10.7	*	*	7.1	9.0	6.4	8.0	7.8
45–64 years	- - -	- - -	- - -	*	*	*	*	*	*	*	5.6
65 years and over	- - -	- - -	- - -	*	*	*	*	*	*	*	*
Asian or Pacific Islander female[4]											
All ages, age adjusted	- - -	- - -	- - -	4.7	4.4	3.4	3.7	3.6	3.4	3.1	3.3
All ages, crude	- - -	- - -	- - -	4.7	4.3	3.4	3.8	3.7	3.6	3.3	3.5
15–24 years	- - -	- - -	- - -	*	5.8	3.9	5.2	3.0	4.7	2.7	3.5
25–44 years	- - -	- - -	- - -	5.4	4.2	3.8	3.8	4.5	3.7	4.0	4.1
45–64 years	- - -	- - -	- - -	7.9	5.4	5.0	4.9	5.2	4.4	4.3	4.6
65 years and over	- - -	- - -	- - -	*	13.6	8.5	9.0	8.4	8.9	7.2	8.1
Hispanic female[5]											
All ages, age adjusted	- - -	- - -	- - -	- - -	1.8	2.3	2.0	2.2	1.7	1.9	1.9
All ages, crude	- - -	- - -	- - -	- - -	1.6	2.2	1.9	2.1	1.6	1.8	1.8
15–24 years	- - -	- - -	- - -	- - -	2.1	3.1	2.6	3.3	2.4	2.8	2.8
25–44 years	- - -	- - -	- - -	- - -	2.1	3.1	2.7	2.8	2.2	2.2	2.4
45–64 years	- - -	- - -	- - -	- - -	3.2	2.5	2.7	2.6	2.3	2.7	2.5
65 years and over	- - -	- - -	- - -	- - -	*	*	*	2.5	*	2.5	2.3
White, non-Hispanic female[5]											
All ages, age adjusted	- - -	- - -	- - -	- - -	5.7	5.0	4.6	4.5	4.7	4.6	4.7
All ages, crude	- - -	- - -	- - -	- - -	6.2	5.6	5.1	5.0	5.3	5.2	5.2
15–24 years	- - -	- - -	- - -	- - -	4.7	4.3	4.0	3.8	3.9	3.6	3.8
25–44 years	- - -	- - -	- - -	- - -	7.7	7.0	6.7	6.7	7.2	7.2	7.0
45–64 years	- - -	- - -	- - -	- - -	9.2	8.0	7.0	7.3	7.6	7.4	7.4
65 years and over	- - -	- - -	- - -	- - -	7.5	7.0	5.8	5.1	5.2	5.2	5.2

. . . Category not applicable.
- - - Data not available.
* Based on fewer than 20 deaths.
[1]Includes deaths of persons who were not residents of the 50 States and the District of Columbia.
[2]Average annual death rate.
[3]Interpretation of trends should take into account that population estimates for American Indians increased by 45 percent between 1980 and 1990, partly due to better enumeration techniques in the 1990 decennial census and to the increased tendency for people to identify themselves as American Indian in 1990.
[4]Interpretation of trends should take into account that the Asian population in the United States more than doubled between 1980 and 1990, primarily due to immigration.
[5]Excludes data from States lacking an Hispanic-origin item on their death certificates. See Appendix I, National Vital Statistics System.

NOTES: Rates are age adjusted to the 1940 U.S. standard million population. See Appendix II, Age adjustment. For data years shown, the code numbers for cause of death are based on the then current *International Classification of Diseases*, which are described in Appendix II, tables IV and V. Age groups chosen to show data for American Indians, Asians, Hispanics, and non-Hispanic whites were selected to minimize the presentation of unstable age-specific death rates based on small numbers of deaths and for consistency among comparison groups. The race groups, white, black, Asian or Pacific Islander, and American Indian or Alaska Native, include persons of Hispanic and non-Hispanic origin. Conversely, persons of Hispanic origin may be of any race. Bias in death rates results from inconsistent race identification between the death certificate (source of data for numerator of death rates) and data from the Census Bureau (denominator); and from undercounts of some population groups in the census. The net effects of misclassification and under coverage result in death rates estimated to be overstated by 1 percent for the white population and 5 percent for the black population; and death rates estimated to be understated by 21 percent for American Indians, 11 percent for Asians, and 2 percent for Hispanics (Rosenberg HM, Maurer JD, Sorlie PD, Johnson NJ, et al. Quality of death rates by race and Hispanic origin: A summary of current research, 1999. National Center for Health Statistics. Vital Health Stat 2(128). 1999). Data for additional years are available (see Appendix III).

SOURCES: Centers for Disease Control and Prevention, National Center for Health Statistics. Grove RD and Hetzel AM. *Vital statistics rates in the United States, 1940–60.* Washington: Public Health Service, 1968; *Vital statistics of the United States, vol II, mortality, part A,* for data years 1950–93. Public Health Service. Washington. U.S. Government Printing Office; for 1994–98, data for all persons, white, and black are available on the NCHS Web site at www.cdc.gov/nchs/datawh/statab/unpubd/mortabs.htm; numerator data from National Vital Statistics System, annual mortality files; denominator data from national population estimates for race groups from table 1 and unpublished Hispanic population estimates prepared by the Housing and Household Economic Statistics Division, U.S. Bureau of the Census.

Table 48 (page 1 of 3). Death rates for firearm-related injuries, according to sex, detailed race, Hispanic origin, and age: United States, selected years 1970–98

[Data are based on the National Vital Statistics System]

Sex, race, Hispanic origin, and age	1970	1980	1985	1990	1994	1995	1996	1997	1998	1996–98[1]
All persons				Deaths per 100,000 resident population						
All ages, age adjusted	14.0	14.8	12.8	14.6	15.1	13.9	12.9	12.2	11.3	12.1
All ages, crude	13.0	14.9	13.3	14.9	14.8	13.7	12.8	12.1	11.4	12.1
Under 1 year	*	*	*	*	*	*	*	*	*	0.2
1–14 years	1.6	1.4	1.4	1.5	1.6	1.6	1.3	1.1	1.1	1.2
1–4 years	1.0	0.7	0.7	0.6	0.6	0.6	0.5	0.5	0.5	0.5
5–14 years	1.7	1.6	1.8	1.9	2.0	2.0	1.6	1.4	1.4	1.4
15–24 years	15.5	20.6	17.2	25.8	30.8	27.2	24.2	22.3	19.9	22.1
25–44 years	20.9	22.5	17.9	19.3	18.8	17.2	16.1	15.4	14.4	15.3
25–34 years	22.2	24.3	19.3	21.8	21.9	20.1	18.3	17.8	16.3	17.5
35–44 years	19.6	20.0	16.0	16.3	15.6	14.4	14.0	13.2	12.8	13.3
45–64 years	17.6	15.2	14.3	13.6	12.2	11.8	11.9	11.3	10.7	11.3
45–54 years	18.1	16.4	14.7	13.9	12.8	12.1	12.3	11.5	10.9	11.6
55–64 years	17.0	13.9	13.9	13.3	11.4	11.4	11.2	11.0	10.4	10.8
65 years and over	13.8	13.5	15.6	16.0	14.3	14.2	13.9	13.2	13.1	13.4
65–74 years	14.5	13.8	15.1	14.4	12.6	12.9	12.6	11.9	11.3	11.9
75–84 years	13.4	13.4	17.7	19.4	16.9	16.4	15.9	14.9	15.5	15.4
85 years and over	10.2	11.6	12.2	14.7	15.1	14.6	14.5	14.3	14.3	14.4
Male										
All ages, age adjusted	23.8	25.3	21.9	25.4	26.2	24.1	22.4	21.1	19.6	21.0
All ages, crude	22.2	25.7	22.8	26.2	26.0	23.9	22.5	21.2	19.8	21.2
Under 1 year	*	*	*	*	*	*	*	*	*	*
1–14 years	2.3	2.0	2.1	2.2	2.3	2.3	1.8	1.7	1.5	1.7
1–4 years	1.2	0.9	0.8	0.7	0.7	0.8	0.5	0.5	0.6	0.6
5–14 years	2.7	2.5	2.7	2.9	3.0	2.9	2.4	2.1	1.9	2.1
15–24 years	26.4	34.8	29.1	44.7	54.0	47.6	42.2	38.9	34.7	38.6
25–44 years	34.1	38.1	29.7	32.6	31.7	28.9	27.0	25.8	24.2	25.7
25–34 years	36.5	41.4	32.1	37.0	37.4	34.3	31.4	30.5	28.0	30.0
35–44 years	31.6	33.2	26.6	27.4	26.0	23.7	22.9	21.5	20.9	21.8
45–64 years	31.0	25.9	24.5	23.4	21.0	20.2	20.4	19.4	18.4	19.4
45–54 years	30.7	27.3	24.4	23.2	21.3	20.4	20.5	19.3	18.3	19.4
55–64 years	31.3	24.5	24.6	23.7	20.5	20.0	20.2	19.7	18.4	19.4
65 years and over	29.7	29.7	34.2	35.3	31.2	30.9	30.2	28.5	28.5	29.1
65–74 years	29.5	27.8	30.0	28.2	24.6	25.3	24.8	23.1	22.2	23.4
75–84 years	31.0	33.0	42.7	46.9	39.9	37.7	36.4	34.1	35.1	35.2
85 years and over	26.2	34.9	38.2	49.3	49.7	47.4	46.7	45.8	44.9	45.8
Female										
All ages, age adjusted	4.8	4.8	4.2	4.3	4.2	4.0	3.6	3.4	3.3	3.4
All ages, crude	4.4	4.7	4.2	4.3	4.1	3.9	3.6	3.4	3.3	3.4
Under 1 year	*	*	*	*	*	*	*	*	*	*
1–14 years	0.8	0.7	0.7	0.8	0.9	0.8	0.7	0.6	0.7	0.7
1–4 years	0.9	0.5	0.5	0.5	0.5	0.5	0.4	0.5	0.4	0.4
5–14 years	0.8	0.7	0.8	1.0	1.0	0.9	0.8	0.7	0.8	0.8
15–24 years	4.8	6.1	5.0	6.0	6.5	6.0	5.1	4.8	4.5	4.8
25–44 years	8.3	7.4	6.2	6.1	6.0	5.6	5.2	5.0	4.7	5.0
25–34 years	8.4	7.5	6.6	6.7	6.5	5.9	5.2	5.1	4.7	5.0
35–44 years	8.2	7.2	5.8	5.4	5.5	5.3	5.1	4.9	4.7	4.9
45–64 years	5.4	5.4	5.0	4.5	4.1	4.0	3.9	3.7	3.6	3.7
45–54 years	6.4	6.2	5.6	4.9	4.6	4.3	4.4	4.1	3.9	4.1
55–64 years	4.2	4.6	4.5	4.0	3.3	3.5	3.1	3.0	3.1	3.1
65 years and over	2.4	2.5	3.2	3.1	2.7	2.8	2.6	2.5	2.3	2.5
65–74 years	2.8	3.1	3.6	3.6	3.0	3.0	2.8	2.9	2.4	2.7
75–84 years	1.7	1.7	3.0	2.9	2.5	2.8	2.6	2.3	2.5	2.5
85 years and over	*	1.3	1.8	1.3	1.8	1.8	1.7	1.7	1.6	1.6
White male										
All ages, age adjusted	18.2	21.1	19.4	20.5	20.4	19.3	18.0	17.1	16.2	17.1
All ages, crude	17.6	21.8	20.7	21.8	21.1	20.1	19.0	18.1	17.4	18.1
1–14 years	1.8	1.9	2.1	1.9	1.8	1.9	1.5	1.4	1.3	1.4
15–24 years	16.9	28.4	24.1	29.5	34.2	31.4	26.9	24.8	23.1	24.9
25–44 years	24.2	29.5	25.0	25.7	24.9	23.6	22.0	21.2	20.3	21.2
25–34 years	24.3	31.1	26.3	27.8	27.6	26.1	23.6	23.1	21.2	22.7
35–44 years	24.1	27.1	23.3	23.3	22.3	21.2	20.6	19.5	19.5	19.9
45–64 years	27.4	23.3	23.6	22.8	20.6	19.7	20.2	19.4	18.5	19.3
65 years and over	29.9	30.1	35.4	36.8	32.5	32.3	31.8	30.0	30.3	30.7

See footnotes at end of table.

[Data are based on the National Vital Statistics System]

Sex, race, Hispanic origin, and age	1970	1980	1985	1990	1994	1995	1996	1997	1998	1996–98[1]
Black male				Deaths per 100,000 resident population						
All ages, age adjusted	73.4	61.8	42.2	61.5	65.1	55.6	52.0	47.4	41.6	47.0
All ages, crude	60.6	57.7	41.3	61.9	63.8	54.0	50.6	46.1	40.3	45.6
1–14 years	5.3	3.0	2.7	4.4	5.2	4.6	3.6	3.1	2.4	3.0
15–24 years	97.3	77.9	61.3	138.0	169.6	140.2	131.6	119.9	101.8	117.6
25–44 years	126.2	114.1	71.8	90.3	84.5	71.2	67.0	61.8	55.3	61.3
25–34 years	145.6	128.4	79.8	108.6	109.0	94.4	88.6	84.0	75.3	82.7
35–44 years	104.2	92.3	59.2	66.1	57.7	46.6	44.7	39.5	35.9	40.0
45–64 years	71.1	55.6	36.9	34.5	29.1	29.1	27.0	23.3	22.1	24.1
65 years and over	30.6	29.7	26.3	23.9	23.2	21.4	19.1	17.8	14.2	17.0
American Indian or Alaska Native male[2]										
All ages, age adjusted	- - -	26.5	24.9	20.8	24.6	23.4	19.4	20.7	19.7	19.9
All ages, crude	- - -	27.5	24.4	20.5	24.1	22.9	19.1	20.1	19.3	19.5
15–24 years	- - -	55.3	39.8	49.1	54.6	45.5	40.0	39.4	43.3	40.9
25–44 years	- - -	43.9	40.3	25.4	33.8	34.1	26.7	29.3	25.6	27.2
45–64 years	- - -	*	21.2	*	13.6	15.6	13.8	13.9	13.4	13.7
65 years and over	- - -	*	*	*	*	*	*	*	*	13.5
Asian or Pacific Islander male[3]										
All ages, age adjusted	- - -	8.1	7.1	9.2	10.9	10.8	8.7	9.0	7.2	8.3
All ages, crude	- - -	8.2	7.3	9.4	10.8	10.4	8.6	8.7	7.0	8.1
15–24 years	- - -	10.8	12.6	21.0	26.9	27.1	19.6	19.7	13.9	17.7
25–44 years	- - -	12.8	9.8	10.9	13.0	11.3	10.0	9.6	8.7	9.4
45–64 years	- - -	10.4	6.7	8.1	7.4	8.6	7.7	8.7	6.1	7.5
65 years and over	- - -	*	*	*	*	*	*	7.7	8.0	7.0
Hispanic male[4]										
All ages, age adjusted	- - -	- - -	25.3	28.9	29.9	28.0	22.5	19.9	18.3	20.2
All ages, crude	- - -	- - -	26.0	29.9	30.0	27.6	22.6	19.9	18.1	20.2
1–14 years	- - -	- - -	1.4	2.6	2.3	2.9	1.9	1.4	1.3	1.5
15–24 years	- - -	- - -	42.0	55.5	72.0	70.7	54.4	47.9	44.9	49.0
25–44 years	- - -	- - -	43.2	42.7	38.8	33.5	27.5	24.5	22.6	24.9
25–34 years	- - -	- - -	47.3	47.3	45.5	39.9	32.8	29.3	28.6	30.2
35–44 years	- - -	- - -	35.9	35.4	29.5	24.9	20.8	18.7	15.6	18.3
45–64 years	- - -	- - -	19.2	21.4	19.2	17.2	16.2	13.7	10.7	13.4
65 years and over	- - -	- - -	12.4	19.1	14.7	15.6	11.7	12.3	14.2	12.8
White, non-Hispanic male[4]										
All ages, age adjusted	- - -	- - -	18.4	18.7	18.1	17.2	16.4	15.9	15.2	15.8
All ages, crude	- - -	- - -	19.9	20.4	19.5	18.6	18.0	17.5	17.0	17.5
1–14 years	- - -	- - -	2.0	1.6	1.6	1.6	1.4	1.4	1.3	1.4
15–24 years	- - -	- - -	22.0	24.1	26.3	23.3	20.4	19.4	18.1	19.3
25–44 years	- - -	- - -	23.0	23.3	22.4	21.6	20.6	20.3	19.6	20.2
25–34 years	- - -	- - -	23.7	24.7	23.9	22.9	21.2	21.4	19.3	20.7
35–44 years	- - -	- - -	22.0	21.6	20.9	20.4	20.1	19.4	19.8	19.7
45–64 years	- - -	- - -	23.0	22.7	20.5	19.7	20.2	19.8	19.0	19.6
65 years and over	- - -	- - -	37.3	37.4	33.2	32.7	32.6	30.8	31.1	31.5
White female										
All ages, age adjusted	4.0	4.2	3.9	3.7	3.6	3.5	3.1	3.1	3.0	3.1
All ages, crude	3.7	4.1	4.0	3.8	3.6	3.5	3.2	3.2	3.0	3.2
15–24 years	3.4	5.1	4.4	4.8	4.9	4.6	3.8	3.8	3.4	3.7
25–44 years	6.9	6.2	5.6	5.3	5.2	5.0	4.6	4.7	4.4	4.5
45–64 years	5.0	5.1	5.0	4.5	4.1	4.0	3.9	3.8	3.7	3.8
65 years and over	2.2	2.5	3.2	3.1	2.7	2.9	2.6	2.6	2.4	2.5

See footnotes at end of table.

Table 48 (page 3 of 3). Death rates for firearm-related injuries, according to sex, detailed race, Hispanic origin, and age: United States, selected years 1970–98

[Data are based on the National Vital Statistics System]

Sex, race, Hispanic origin, and age	1970	1980	1985	1990	1994	1995	1996	1997	1998	1996–98[1]
Black female				Deaths per 100,000 resident population						
All ages, age adjusted	11.4	9.1	6.6	7.8	8.0	6.8	6.5	5.6	5.2	5.7
All ages, crude	10.0	8.8	6.5	7.8	7.8	6.6	6.4	5.4	5.0	5.6
15–24 years	15.2	12.3	8.3	13.3	15.5	13.5	12.0	10.6	10.2	10.9
25–44 years	19.4	16.1	11.4	12.4	11.9	10.0	9.8	8.0	7.5	8.4
45–64 years	10.2	8.2	5.8	4.8	4.6	4.1	4.1	3.4	3.2	3.5
65 years and over	4.3	3.1	3.7	3.1	2.9	2.6	3.0	2.2	1.8	2.3
American Indian or Alaska Native female[2]										
All ages, age adjusted	- - -	6.1	4.3	3.6	4.5	4.5	3.8	3.2	4.3	3.8
All ages, crude	- - -	5.8	4.1	3.4	4.4	4.4	3.7	3.0	4.2	3.6
15–24 years	- - -	*	*	*	*	*	*	*	*	5.3
25–44 years	- - -	10.2	*	*	7.5	7.7	5.9	*	6.9	5.4
45–64 years	- - -	*	*	*	*	*	*	*	*	4.4
65 years and over	- - -	*	*	*	*	*	*	*	*	*
Asian or Pacific Islander female[3]										
All ages, age adjusted	- - -	2.0	1.7	2.0	2.1	2.2	1.7	1.8	1.8	1.8
All ages, crude	- - -	2.1	1.7	2.1	2.1	2.2	1.7	1.7	1.8	1.7
15–24 years	- - -	*	*	*	4.0	4.2	3.7	3.2	*	3.1
25–44 years	- - -	3.2	2.2	2.7	2.6	2.9	2.1	1.9	2.2	2.1
45–64 years	- - -	*	*	*	*	*	*	*	2.1	1.9
65 years and over	- - -	*	*	*	*	*	*	*	*	*
Hispanic female[4]										
All ages, age adjusted	- - -	- - -	3.2	3.6	3.5	3.5	2.8	2.4	2.3	2.5
All ages, crude	- - -	- - -	3.2	3.6	3.4	3.4	2.7	2.3	2.2	2.4
15–24 years	- - -	- - -	5.1	6.9	6.9	6.6	5.0	4.5	4.0	4.5
25–44 years	- - -	- - -	5.5	5.1	5.0	4.9	4.1	3.3	3.0	3.5
45–64 years	- - -	- - -	2.2	2.4	2.4	2.4	2.3	2.2	1.6	2.0
65 years and over	- - -	- - -	*	*	*	*	*	*	*	1.0
White, non-Hispanic female[4]										
All ages, age adjusted	- - -	- - -	3.9	3.6	3.5	3.4	3.1	3.2	3.0	3.1
All ages, crude	- - -	- - -	4.1	3.7	3.6	3.5	3.2	3.3	3.1	3.2
15–24 years	- - -	- - -	4.5	4.3	4.5	4.1	3.5	3.6	3.3	3.4
25–44 years	- - -	- - -	5.6	5.1	5.1	4.8	4.5	4.8	4.5	4.6
45–64 years	- - -	- - -	5.1	4.6	4.1	4.1	4.0	3.9	3.8	3.9
65 years and over	- - -	- - -	3.4	3.2	2.7	2.9	2.7	2.7	2.5	2.6

* Based on fewer than 20 deaths.

- - - Data not available.

[1] Average annual death rate.

[2] Interpretation of trends should take into account that population estimates for American Indians increased by 45 percent between 1980 and 1990, partly due to better enumeration techniques in the 1990 decennial census and to the increased tendency for people to identify themselves as American Indian in 1990.

[3] Interpretation of trends should take into account that the Asian population in the United States more than doubled between 1980 and 1990, primarily due to immigration.

[4] Excludes data from States lacking an Hispanic-origin item on their death certificates. See Appendix I, National Vital Statistics System.

NOTES: Rates are age adjusted to the 1940 U.S. standard million population. See Appendix II, Age adjustment. For data years shown, the code numbers for cause of death are based on the then current *International Classification of Diseases*, which are described in Appendix II, tables IV and V. Age groups chosen to show data for American Indians, Asians, Hispanics, and non-Hispanic whites were selected to minimize the presentation of unstable age-specific death rates based on small numbers of deaths and for consistency among comparison groups. The race groups, white, black, Asian or Pacific Islander, and American Indian or Alaska Native, include persons of Hispanic and non-Hispanic origin. Conversely, persons of Hispanic origin may be of any race. Bias in death rates results from inconsistent race identification between the death certificate (source of data for numerator of death rates) and data from the Census Bureau (denominator); and from undercounts of some population groups in the census. The net effects of misclassification and under coverage result in death rates estimated to be overstated by 1 percent for the white population and 5 percent for the black population; and death rates estimated to be understated by 21 percent for American Indians, 11 percent for Asians, and 2 percent for Hispanics (Rosenberg HM, Maurer JD, Sorlie PD, Johnson NJ, et al. Quality of death rates by race and Hispanic origin: A summary of current research, 1999. National Center for Health Statistics. Vital Health Stat 2(128). 1999). Data for additional years are available (see Appendix III).

SOURCES: Centers for Disease Control and Prevention, National Center for Health Statistics. *Vital statistics of the United States, vol II, mortality, part A,* for data years 1950–93. Public Health Service. Washington. U.S. Government Printing Office; for 1994–98, data for all persons, white, and black are available on the NCHS Web site at www.cdc.gov/nchs/datawh/statab/unpubd/mortabs.htm; numerator data from National Vital Statistics System, annual mortality files; denominator data from national population estimates for race groups from table 1 and unpublished Hispanic population estimates prepared by the Housing and Household Economic Statistics Division, U.S. Bureau of the Census.

Table 49. Deaths from selected occupational diseases for males, according to age: United States, selected years 1970–98

[Data are based on the National Vital Statistics System]

Age and cause of death	1970	1975	1980	1985	1990	1991	1992	1993	1994	1995	1996	1997	1998
25 years and over						Number of deaths[1]							
Malignant neoplasm of peritoneum and pleura (mesothelioma)	602	591	552	571	629	607	618	551	511	546	574	557	563
Coalworkers' pneumoconiosis	1,155	973	977	947	727	692	631	564	491	531	533	483	415
Asbestosis	25	43	96	130	282	247	270	308	325	342	345	387	439
Silicosis	351	243	202	138	146	150	110	123	113	110	95	93	90
25–64 years													
Malignant neoplasm of peritoneum and pleura (mesothelioma)	308	280	241	210	199	190	193	164	161	163	146	154	156
Coalworkers' pneumoconiosis	294	188	136	89	49	48	32	34	21	40	20	25	19
Asbestosis	17	22	30	29	50	35	34	32	35	32	33	33	36
Silicosis	90	64	49	30	35	29	25	25	25	15	19	19	14
65 years and over													
Malignant neoplasm of peritoneum and pleura (mesothelioma)	294	311	311	361	430	417	425	387	350	383	428	403	407
Coalworkers' pneumoconiosis	861	785	841	858	678	644	599	530	470	491	513	458	396
Asbestosis	8	21	66	101	232	212	236	276	290	310	312	354	403
Silicosis	261	179	153	108	111	121	85	98	88	95	76	74	76

[1]This table classifies deaths according to underlying cause. Additional deaths for which occupational diseases are classified as nonunderlying causes can be identified from multiple cause of death data from the National Vital Statistics System. The numbers of such deaths are shown below for males 25 years of age and over.

Nonunderlying cause of death	1980	1985	1990	1991	1992	1993	1994	1995	1996	1997	1998
Malignant neoplasm of peritoneum and pleura (mesothelioma)	135	102	105	96	87	84	103	83	74	81	82
Coalworkers' pneumoconiosis	1,587	1,652	1,248	1,227	1,130	1,052	974	876	874	800	678
Asbestosis	228	382	619	660	653	661	701	796	778	741	738
Silicosis	232	187	152	155	130	145	109	122	111	96	84

NOTES: Selection of occupational diseases based on definitions in D. Rutstein et al.: Sentinel health events (occupational): A basis for physician recognition and public health surveillance, *Am. J. Public Health* 73(9):1054–1062, Sept. 1983. For data years shown, the code numbers for cause of death are based on the then current *International Classification of Diseases*, which are described in Appendix II, tables IV and V. Data for additional years are available (see Appendix III).

SOURCE: Centers for Disease Control and Prevention, National Center for Health Statistics. National Vital Statistics System.

Table 50. Occupational injury deaths by industry: United States, 1992–98

[Data are compiled from various Federal, State, and local administrative sources]

Industry[1]	1992	1993	1994	1995	1996	1997	1998[2]
	Deaths per 100,000 employed workers[3]						
Total work force	5.2	5.2	5.3	4.9	4.8	4.8	4.5
Private sector	5.5	5.6	5.7	5.1	5.1	5.0	4.8
Agriculture, forestry, and fishing.	24.0	26.7	23.9	22.3	22.4	23.5	23.3
Mining.	27.1	26.0	26.9	25.0	27.0	25.0	23.6
Construction	14.1	13.8	14.8	14.7	14.0	14.1	14.5
Manufacturing	3.8	3.9	3.9	3.5	3.5	3.6	3.3
Transportation and public utilities.	13.4	13.0	13.4	12.6	13.4	13.3	11.8
Wholesale trade.	5.3	5.5	5.8	5.1	5.5	4.9	4.5
Retail trade	3.8	3.9	3.8	3.3	3.2	3.1	2.6
Finance, insurance, and							
real estate.	1.6	1.5	1.4	1.6	1.5	1.2	1.1
Services	2.5	2.4	2.6	2.2	2.2	2.0	2.0
Government[4]	3.7	3.4	3.4	3.9	3.1	3.2	3.0
	Number of deaths						
Total work force	6,217	6,331	6,632	6,275	6,202	6,238	6,026
Private sector	5,497	5,643	5,959	5,495	5,597	5,616	5,428
Agriculture, forestry, and fishing.	808	864	852	800	806	833	831
Mining.	181	174	180	156	153	158	146
Construction	919	932	1,028	1,055	1,047	1,107	1,171
Manufacturing	765	767	789	709	725	744	694
Transportation and public utilities.	895	894	949	901	970	1,008	909
Wholesale trade.	253	252	271	256	270	241	228
Retail trade	734	795	808	687	681	670	569
Finance, insurance, and							
real estate.	122	118	113	125	116	97	92
Services	757	774	853	749	776	727	757
Not classified.	63	73	116	57	53	31	31
Government[4]	720	688	673	780	605	622	598

[1]Classified according to the Standard Industrial Classification Manual, 1987 (see Appendix II, table VII).
[2]Preliminary data.
[3]Excludes deaths to workers under the age of 16 years. Employment data in denominators are annual average estimates of employed civilians 16 years of age and over from the Current Population Survey (CPS) plus resident military figures from the Bureau of the Census.
[4]Includes fatalities to workers employed by governmental organizations regardless of industry.

NOTES: Fatalities and rates are based on revised data and may differ from originally published data from the Census of Fatal Occupational Injuries (CFOI). See Appendix I. CFOI began collecting fatality data in 1992. For data for prior years, see CDC. Fatal Occupational Injuries—United States, 1980–1994. MMWR 1998;47(15):297–302, which reports trend data from the National Traumatic Occupational Fatalities (NTOF) surveillance system. NTOF was established at the National Institute of Occupational Safety and Health (NIOSH) in 1980 to monitor occupational injury deaths through death certificates.

SOURCE: Department of Labor, Bureau of Labor Statistics. Census of Fatal Occupational Injuries (CFOI).

Table 51. Occupational injuries with lost workdays in the private sector, according to industry: United States, selected years 1980–98

[Data are based on employer records from a sample of business establishments]

Industry	1980	1985	1990	1991	1992	1993	1994	1995	1996	1997	1998
	Number of injuries with lost workdays in thousands										
Total private sector[1]	2,491.0	2,484.7	2,987.3	2,794.0	2,776.1	2,772.5	2,848.3	2,767.6	2,646.3	2,682.6	2,612.0
Agriculture, fishing, and forestry[1]	39.3	45.2	57.2	54.3	52.3	51.2	48.5	51.7	49.0	53.8	53.8
Mining	66.2	43.9	35.6	31.4	25.6	24.2	24.0	22.8	19.5	22.6	16.9
Construction	242.6	272.8	296.3	239.9	226.8	226.5	241.7	217.9	216.8	227.4	217.0
Manufacturing	1,009.5	825.1	975.0	886.0	833.7	819.5	859.4	838.1	782.9	785.4	782.6
Transportation, communication, and public utilities	263.0	243.5	293.3	283.5	266.1	284.1	301.5	289.2	293.0	281.3	261.3
Wholesale trade	191.1	188.4	211.5	204.1	205.3	205.3	214.0	214.7	203.9	200.7	211.1
Retail trade	330.2	399.9	483.9	457.0	476.7	480.4	477.7	459.6	433.9	456.9	434.7
Finance, insurance, and real estate	38.1	45.5	63.7	62.2	64.4	61.7	58.8	52.2	49.5	47.6	39.6
Services	311.1	420.6	570.8	575.6	625.1	619.6	622.8	621.4	597.8	606.9	594.9
	Injuries with lost workdays per 100 full-time equivalents[2]										
Total private sector[1]	3.9	3.6	3.9	3.7	3.6	3.5	3.5	3.4	3.1	3.1	2.9
Agriculture, fishing, and forestry[1]	5.6	5.6	5.7	5.2	5.2	4.8	4.6	4.2	3.8	4.0	3.8
Mining	6.4	4.7	4.9	4.4	4.0	3.8	3.8	3.8	3.2	3.7	2.7
Construction	6.5	6.8	6.6	6.0	5.7	5.4	5.4	4.8	4.4	4.4	4.0
Manufacturing	5.2	4.4	5.3	5.0	4.7	4.6	4.7	4.6	4.3	4.2	4.2
Transportation, communication, and public utilities	5.4	4.9	5.4	5.3	4.9	5.2	5.3	5.0	5.0	4.7	4.2
Wholesale trade	3.8	3.5	3.6	3.6	3.6	3.6	3.6	3.5	3.3	3.1	3.2
Retail trade	2.9	3.1	3.4	3.3	3.3	3.2	3.2	2.9	2.7	2.8	2.6
Finance, insurance, and real estate	0.8	0.9	1.1	1.0	1.1	1.0	0.9	0.9	0.8	0.8	0.6
Services	2.3	2.5	2.7	2.8	2.9	2.7	2.7	2.7	2.5	2.4	2.3

[1]Excludes farms with fewer than 11 employees.

[2]Incidence rate calculated as (N/EH) x 200,000, where N = total number of injuries with lost workdays in a calendar year, EH = total hours worked by all full-time and part-time employees in a calendar year, and 200,000 = base for 100 full-time equivalent employees working 40 hours per week, 50 weeks per year.

NOTES: Industry is coded based on various editions of the *Standard Industrial Classification Manual* as follows: data for 1980–87 are based on the 1972 edition, 1977 supplement; and data for 1988–98 are based on the 1987 edition (see Appendix II, Industry). Data for additional years are available (see Appendix III).

SOURCE: U.S. Department of Labor, Bureau of Labor Statistics. Workplace injuries and illnesses, 1980–98 editions. 1982–99.

Table 52. Selected notifiable disease rates, according to disease: United States, selected years 1950–98

[Data are based on reporting by State health departments]

Disease	1950	1960	1970	1980	1985	1990	1995	1996	1997	1998
	Cases per 100,000 population									
Diphtheria	3.83	0.51	0.21	0.00	0.00	0.00	–	0.01	0.01	0.00
Haemophilus influenzae, invasive	- - -	- - -	- - -	- - -	- - -	- - -	0.45	0.45	0.44	0.44
Hepatitis A	- - -	- - -	27.87	12.84	10.03	12.64	12.13	11.70	11.22	8.59
Hepatitis B	- - -	- - -	4.08	8.39	11.50	8.48	4.19	4.01	3.90	3.80
Lyme disease	- - -	- - -	- - -	- - -	- - -	- - -	4.49	6.21	4.79	6.39
Meningococcal disease	- - -	- - -	1.23	1.25	1.04	0.99	1.25	1.30	1.24	1.01
Mumps	- - -	- - -	55.55	3.86	1.30	2.17	0.35	0.29	0.27	0.25
Pertussis (whooping cough)	79.82	8.23	2.08	0.76	1.50	1.84	1.97	2.94	2.46	2.74
Poliomyelitis, total	22.02	1.77	0.02	0.00	0.00	0.00	0.00	0.01	0.01	0.00
Paralytic[1]	- - -	1.40	0.02	0.00	0.00	0.00	0.00	0.01	0.01	0.00
Rocky Mountain spotted fever	- - -	- - -	0.19	0.52	0.30	0.26	0.23	0.32	0.16	0.14
Rubella (German measles)	- - -	- - -	27.75	1.72	0.26	0.45	0.05	0.10	0.07	0.13
Rubeola (measles)	211.01	245.42	23.23	5.96	1.18	11.17	0.12	0.20	0.06	0.04
Salmonellosis, excluding typhoid fever	- - -	3.85	10.84	14.88	27.37	19.54	17.66	17.15	15.66	16.17
Shigellosis	15.45	6.94	6.79	8.41	7.14	10.89	12.32	9.80	8.64	8.74
Tuberculosis[2]	- - -	30.83	18.28	12.25	9.30	10.33	8.70	8.04	7.42	6.79
Sexually transmitted diseases:[3]										
Syphilis[4]	146.02	68.78	45.26	30.51	28.39	54.52	26.39	20.07	17.43	14.19
Primary and secondary	16.73	9.06	10.89	12.06	11.40	20.34	6.30	4.29	3.20	2.61
Early latent	39.71	10.11	8.08	9.00	9.11	22.27	10.15	7.61	6.21	4.71
Late and late latent[5]	70.22	45.91	24.94	9.30	7.74	10.35	9.25	7.68	7.62	6.56
Congenital[6]	8.97	2.48	0.97	0.12	0.11	1.53	0.70	0.49	0.40	0.30
Chlamydia[7]	- - -	- - -	- - -	- - -	17.42	160.83	190.42	192.87	206.95	236.57
Gonorrhea[8]	192.50	145.40	297.22	445.10	382.98	277.45	149.44	123.24	122.02	132.88
Chancroid	3.34	0.94	0.70	0.30	0.87	1.69	0.23	0.15	0.09	0.07
	Number of cases									
Diphtheria	5,796	918	435	3	3	4	–	2	4	1
Haemophilus influenzae, invasive	- - -	- - -	- - -	- - -	- - -	- - -	1,180	1,170	1,162	1,194
Hepatitis A	- - -	- - -	56,797	29,087	23,210	31,441	31,582	31,032	30,021	23,229
Hepatitis B	- - -	- - -	8,310	19,015	26,611	21,102	10,805	10,637	10,416	10,258
Lyme disease	- - -	- - -	- - -	- - -	- - -	- - -	11,700	16,455	12,801	16,801
Meningococcal disease	- - -	- - -	2,505	2,840	2,479	2,451	3,243	3,437	3,308	2,725
Mumps	- - -	- - -	104,953	8,576	2,982	5,292	906	751	683	666
Pertussis (whooping cough)	120,718	14,809	4,249	1,730	3,589	4,570	5,137	7,796	6,564	7,405
Poliomyelitis, total	33,300	3,190	33	9	8	6	7	5	5	1
Paralytic[1]	- - -	2,525	31	9	8	6	7	5	5	1
Rocky Mountain spotted fever	- - -	- - -	380	1,163	714	651	590	831	409	365
Rubella (German measles)	- - -	- - -	56,552	3,904	630	1,125	128	238	181	364
Rubeola (measles)	319,124	441,703	47,351	13,506	2,822	27,786	309	508	138	100
Salmonellosis, excluding typhoid fever	- - -	6,929	22,096	33,715	65,347	48,603	45,970	45,471	41,901	43,694
Shigellosis	23,367	12,487	13,845	19,041	17,057	27,077	32,080	25,978	23,117	23,626
Tuberculosis[2]	- - -	55,494	37,137	27,749	22,201	25,701	22,860	21,337	19,851	18,361
Sexually transmitted diseases:[3]										
Syphilis[4]	217,558	122,538	91,382	68,832	67,563	135,043	69,345	53,226	46,642	37,977
Primary and secondary	23,939	16,145	21,982	27,204	27,131	50,578	16,543	11,388	8,556	6,993
Early latent	59,256	18,017	16,311	20,297	21,689	55,397	26,657	20,187	16,631	12,613
Late and late latent[5]	113,569	81,798	50,348	20,979	18,414	25,750	24,295	20,356	20,385	17,570
Congenital[6]	13,377	4,416	1,953	277	329	3,865	1,850	1,295	1,070	801
Chlamydia[7]	- - -	- - -	- - -	- - -	25,848	323,663	478,577	490,615	531,529	607,602
Gonorrhea[8]	286,746	258,933	600,072	1,004,029	911,419	690,042	392,651	326,805	326,564	355,642
Chancroid	4,977	1,680	1,416	788	2,067	4,212	607	386	246	189

0.00 Rate greater than zero but less than 0.005.

– Quantity zero.

- - - Data not available.

[1]Data beginning in 1986 may be updated due to retrospective case evaluations or late reports.

[2]Case reporting for tuberculosis began in 1953. Data prior to 1975 are not comparable with subsequent years' data because of changes in reporting criteria effective in 1975.

[3]Newly reported civilian cases prior to 1991; includes military cases beginning in 1991 and adjustments to the number of cases through June 15, 1999, for states submitting hardcopy reports and through July 19, 1999, for states reporting electronically. For 1950, data for Alaska and Hawaii not included.

[4]Includes stage of syphilis not stated.

[5]Includes cases of unknown duration.

[6]Data reported for 1989 and later years reflect change in case definition introduced in 1988. Through 1994, all cases of congenitally acquired syphilis; as of 1995, congenital syphilis less than 1 year of age.

[7]Chlamydia was non-notifiable in 1994 and earlier years (see Appendix I). For 1998, cases for New York based exclusively on those reported by New York City.

[8]Data for 1994 do not include cases from Georgia.

NOTES: The total resident population was used to calculate all rates except sexually transmitted diseases, for which the civilian resident population was used prior to 1991. For sexually transmitted diseases, 1997 population estimates were used to calculate 1998 rates. Population data from those States where diseases were not notifiable or not available were excluded from rate calculation. See Appendix I for information on underreporting of notifiable diseases. Some numbers for 1990–97 have been revised and differ from the previous edition of *Health, United States*. Data for additional years are available (see Appendix III).

SOURCES: Centers for Disease Control and Prevention. Summary of notifiable diseases, United States, 1998. Morbidity and mortality weekly report; 47(53). Atlanta, Georgia: Public Health Service. 1999; National Center for HIV, STD, and TB Prevention, Division of STD Prevention. Sexually transmitted disease surveillance, 1998. Atlanta, Georgia: Public Health Service. Centers for Disease Control and Prevention, 1999.

Table 53. Acquired immunodeficiency syndrome (AIDS) cases, according to age at diagnosis, sex, detailed race, and Hispanic origin: United States, selected years 1985–99

[Data are based on reporting by State health departments]

Age at diagnosis, sex, race, and Hispanic origin	All years[1]	All years[1]	1985	1990	1994	1995	1996	1997	1998	January–June 1999	12 months ending June 30, 1999
	Percent distribution[2]	Number, by year of report									Cases per 100,000 population[3]
All races	. . .	687,863	8,164	41,502	76,982	70,715	66,247	58,016	46,247	23,238	16.9
Male											
All males, 13 years and over	100.0	570,211	7,511	36,249	62,725	56,957	52,461	45,111	35,404	17,781	32.8
White, non-Hispanic	49.9	284,410	4,754	20,856	29,451	26,141	23,130	17,465	13,955	6,629	17.0
Black, non-Hispanic	33.7	191,919	1,710	10,261	22,417	20,915	20,054	18,736	14,654	7,681	125.7
Hispanic[4]	15.3	86,988	990	4,758	10,071	9,157	8,559	8,233	6,213	3,212	55.2
American Indian or Alaska Native[5] . .	0.3	1,670	8	81	206	199	167	168	116	72	18.4
Asian or Pacific Islander[5]	0.8	4,475	49	263	527	491	479	380	324	131	7.6
13–19 years	0.4	2,036	28	107	227	226	202	182	140	57	0.8
20–29 years	16.2	92,540	1,504	6,938	9,678	8,408	7,062	5,771	4,298	2,093	22.9
30–39 years	45.6	259,917	3,589	16,698	28,898	25,793	23,808	20,117	15,292	7,597	67.7
40–49 years	26.9	153,154	1,634	8,844	17,183	16,249	15,441	13,554	10,947	5,573	54.0
50–59 years	8.1	46,314	597	2,651	5,049	4,716	4,424	4,112	3,528	1,829	26.3
60 years and over	2.8	16,250	159	1,011	1,690	1,565	1,524	1,375	1,199	632	6.2
Female											
All females, 13 years and over	100.0	109,459	523	4,529	13,287	13,012	13,134	12,459	10,475	5,328	9.2
White, non-Hispanic	23.2	25,383	142	1,224	3,074	3,052	2,846	2,462	2,011	989	2.4
Black, non-Hispanic	59.5	65,131	279	2,544	7,843	7,610	8,077	7,817	6,728	3,431	49.5
Hispanic[4]	16.3	17,868	99	730	2,275	2,233	2,064	2,037	1,607	851	14.6
American Indian or Alaska Native[5] . .	0.3	335	2	8	41	37	45	36	31	21	4.5
Asian or Pacific Islander[5]	0.5	583	1	19	50	72	78	63	57	23	1.2
13–19 years	1.2	1,368	4	66	174	158	174	176	143	80	1.1
20–29 years	21.8	23,850	178	1,115	2,933	2,676	2,670	2,417	1,928	1,002	10.8
30–39 years	45.3	49,539	232	2,076	5,996	5,954	5,887	5,463	4,446	2,224	20.4
40–49 years	22.4	24,487	45	780	3,075	3,071	3,249	3,236	2,876	1,413	13.7
50–59 years	6.2	6,762	26	272	766	819	828	816	793	452	5.8
60 years and over	3.2	3,453	38	220	343	334	326	351	289	157	1.2
Children											
All children, under 13 years	100.0	8,193	130	724	970	746	652	446	368	129	0.6
White, non-Hispanic	18.3	1,499	26	158	140	117	96	63	58	16	0.1
Black, non-Hispanic	61.1	5,007	86	389	634	484	429	290	235	79	2.7
Hispanic[4]	19.5	1,598	18	168	180	135	123	86	72	32	0.8
American Indian or Alaska Native[5] . .	0.4	29	–	5	3	2	3	2	–	1	0.2
Asian or Pacific Islander[5]	0.6	46	–	4	11	5	1	3	2	–	0.0
Under 1 year	39.4	3,224	63	317	351	270	219	132	96	49	2.4
1–12 years	60.6	4,969	67	407	619	476	433	314	272	80	0.5

. . . Category not applicable.
– Quantity zero.
0.0 Quantity more than zero but less than 0.05.
[1] Includes cases prior to 1985 and through June 30, 1999.
[2] Percents may not sum to 100 percent due to rounding.
[3] Computed using official postcensus resident population estimates for 1998 from the U.S. Bureau of the Census.
[4] Persons of Hispanic origin may be of any race.
[5] Excludes persons of Hispanic origin.

NOTES: The AIDS case reporting definitions were expanded in 1985, 1987, and 1993. See Appendix II, AIDS. Excludes data for U.S. dependencies and possessions and independent nations in free association with the United States. Data for all years have been updated through June 30, 1999, to include temporally delayed case reports and may differ from previous editions of *Health, United States*. Similar data as of December 31, 1999, are available in the Centers for Disease Control and Prevention, HIV/AIDS Surveillance Report, Year-end edition Vol 11 No 2. 1999.

SOURCE: Centers for Disease Control and Prevention, National Center for HIV, STD, and TB Prevention, Division of HIV/AIDS Prevention—Surveillance and Epidemiology, 1999 special data run.

Table 54 (page 1 of 2). Acquired immunodeficiency syndrome (AIDS) cases, according to race, Hispanic origin, sex, and transmission category for persons 13 years of age and over at diagnosis: United States, selected years 1985–99

[Data are based on reporting by State health departments]

Race, Hispanic origin, sex, and transmission category	All years[1]	All years[1]	1985	1990	1994	1995	1996	1997	1998	January–June 1999
Race and Hispanic origin	Percent distribution[2]	Number, by year of report								
All races	100.0	679,670	8,034	40,778	76,012	69,969	65,595	57,570	45,879	23,109
Men who have sex with men	48.6	330,193	5,356	23,705	35,244	31,009	27,657	21,391	16,659	7,790
Injecting drug use	24.7	167,543	1,390	9,275	21,115	18,780	16,704	14,404	10,494	4,878
Men who have sex with men and injecting drug use	6.4	43,529	656	2,911	4,711	4,005	3,392	2,510	2,027	890
Hemophilia/coagulation disorder	0.7	4,947	71	349	521	467	347	217	174	79
Heterosexual contact[3]	9.6	65,362	151	2,249	8,232	8,364	9,073	8,220	6,634	3,286
Sex with injecting drug user	3.7	25,210	107	1,483	2,970	2,774	2,746	2,280	1,800	841
Transfusion[4]	1.2	8,224	165	772	655	580	507	380	271	128
Undetermined[5]	8.8	59,872	245	1,517	5,534	6,764	7,915	10,448	9,620	6,058
White, non-Hispanic	100.0	309,793	4,896	22,080	32,525	29,193	25,976	19,927	15,966	7,618
Men who have sex with men	68.6	212,661	3,982	16,505	21,695	18,893	16,448	11,873	9,165	4,179
Injecting drug use	11.9	36,837	246	2,052	4,530	4,137	3,694	2,966	2,347	1,079
Men who have sex with men and injecting drug use	7.5	23,237	409	1,627	2,373	2,046	1,710	1,182	967	438
Hemophilia/coagulation disorder	1.2	3,776	59	281	373	327	223	140	104	59
Heterosexual contact[3]	4.9	15,058	34	649	1,934	1,924	1,892	1,651	1,284	631
Sex with injecting drug user	1.9	5,949	19	349	747	689	648	503	385	189
Transfusion[4]	1.6	4,891	125	504	312	276	206	141	104	46
Undetermined[5]	4.3	13,333	41	462	1,308	1,590	1,803	1,974	1,995	1,186
Black, non-Hispanic	100.0	257,050	1,989	12,805	30,260	28,525	28,131	26,553	21,382	11,112
Men who have sex with men	28.0	72,078	785	4,462	8,246	7,455	7,009	6,003	4,675	2,245
Injecting drug use	36.8	94,656	742	5,172	12,078	10,645	9,575	8,394	6,087	2,787
Men who have sex with men and injecting drug use	5.6	14,508	162	932	1,672	1,429	1,240	993	751	337
Hemophilia/coagulation disorder	0.3	651	5	34	80	84	75	44	37	13
Heterosexual contact[3]	14.9	38,323	91	1,214	4,750	4,766	5,551	4,985	4,142	2,078
Sex with injecting drug user	5.6	14,420	65	849	1,676	1,525	1,586	1,332	1,084	495
Transfusion[4]	0.9	2,203	29	163	230	208	206	167	121	58
Undetermined[5]	13.5	34,631	175	828	3,204	3,938	4,475	5,967	5,569	3,594
Hispanic[6]	100.0	104,856	1,089	5,488	12,346	11,390	10,623	10,270	7,820	4,063
Men who have sex with men	39.0	40,876	546	2,454	4,764	4,169	3,757	3,145	2,536	1,239
Injecting drug use	33.5	35,099	395	2,016	4,404	3,875	3,332	2,919	1,963	975
Men who have sex with men and injecting drug use	5.1	5,329	83	328	602	483	395	304	280	106
Hemophilia/coagulation disorder	0.4	412	7	28	55	48	39	25	25	6
Heterosexual contact[3]	10.8	11,323	26	376	1,484	1,590	1,527	1,480	1,141	546
Sex with injecting drug user	4.4	4,634	23	280	522	539	484	424	316	147
Transfusion[4]	0.9	899	6	82	89	76	81	58	36	22
Undetermined[5]	10.4	10,918	26	204	948	1,149	1,492	2,339	1,839	1,169

See footnotes at end of table.

Table 54 (page 2 of 2). Acquired immunodeficiency syndrome (AIDS) cases, according to race, Hispanic origin, sex, and transmission category for persons 13 years of age and over at diagnosis: United States, selected years 1985–99

[Data are based on reporting by State health departments]

Race, Hispanic origin, sex, and transmission category	All years[1]	All years[1]	1985	1990	1994	1995	1996	1997	1998	January–June 1999
Sex	Percent distribution[2]	Number, by year of report								
Male	100.0	570,211	7,511	36,249	62,725	56,957	52,461	45,111	35,404	17,781
Men who have sex with men	57.9	330,193	5,356	23,705	35,244	31,009	27,657	21,391	16,659	7,790
Injecting drug use	21.2	120,981	1,104	6,943	15,133	13,406	11,908	10,132	7,343	3,443
Men who have sex with men and injecting drug use	7.6	43,529	656	2,911	4,711	4,005	3,392	2,510	2,027	890
Hemophilia/coagulation disorder	0.8	4,686	68	333	488	439	322	184	151	72
Heterosexual contact[3]	4.0	22,782	32	713	2,779	2,884	3,240	3,100	2,547	1,290
Sex with injecting drug user	1.4	7,853	25	452	927	877	841	785	622	301
Transfusion[4]	0.8	4,716	102	440	357	323	249	212	146	69
Undetermined[5]	7.6	43,324	193	1,204	4,013	4,891	5,693	7,582	6,531	4,227
Female	100.0	109,459	523	4,529	13,287	13,012	13,134	12,459	10,475	5,328
Injecting drug use	42.5	46,562	286	2,332	5,982	5,374	4,796	4,272	3,151	1,435
Hemophilia/coagulation disorder	0.2	261	3	16	33	28	25	33	23	7
Heterosexual contact[3]	38.9	42,580	119	1,536	5,453	5,480	5,833	5,120	4,087	1,996
Sex with injecting drug user	15.9	17,357	82	1,031	2,043	1,897	1,905	1,495	1,178	540
Transfusion[4]	3.2	3,508	63	332	298	257	258	168	125	59
Undetermined[5]	15.1	16,548	52	313	1,521	1,873	2,222	2,866	3,089	1,831

[1]Includes cases prior to 1985 and through June 30, 1999.
[2]Percents may not sum to 100 percent due to rounding.
[3]Includes persons who have had heterosexual contact with a person with human immunodeficiency virus (HIV) infection or at risk of HIV infection.
[4]Receipt of blood transfusion, blood components, or tissue.
[5]Includes persons for whom risk information is incomplete (because of death, refusal to be interviewed, or loss to followup), persons still under investigation, men reported to have had heterosexual contact only with prostitutes, and interviewed persons for whom no specific risk is identified.
[6]Persons of Hispanic origin may be of any race.

NOTES: The AIDS case reporting definitions were expanded in 1985, 1987, and 1993. See Appendix II, AIDS. Excludes data for U.S. dependencies and possessions and independent nations in free association with the United States. Data for all years have been updated through June 30, 1999, to include temporally delayed case reports and may differ from previous editions of *Health, United States*. Similar data as of December 31, 1999, are available in the Centers for Disease Control and Prevention, HIV/AIDS Surveillance Report, Year-end edition Vol 11 No 2. 1999.

SOURCE: Centers for Disease Control and Prevention, National Center for HIV, STD, and TB Prevention, Division of HIV/AIDS Prevention—Surveillance and Epidemiology, 1999 special data run.

Table 55 (page 1 of 2). Age-adjusted cancer incidence rates for selected cancer sites, according to sex and race: Selected geographic areas, selected years 1973–96

[Data are based on the Surveillance, Epidemiology, and End Results Program's population-based registries in Atlanta, Detroit, Seattle-Puget Sound, San Francisco-Oakland, Connecticut, Iowa, New Mexico, Utah, and Hawaii]

Race, sex, and site	1973	1975	1980	1985	1990	1992	1993	1994	1995	1996
All races, both sexes	Number of new cases per 100,000 population[1]									
All sites	320.0	332.7	345.8	372.5	399.7	425.6	412.1	403.8	395.2	388.6
Oral cavity and pharynx	11.3	11.4	11.6	11.5	11.2	10.5	10.9	10.4	10.0	10.0
Esophagus.	3.4	3.5	3.7	3.8	4.2	3.9	4.0	3.8	3.7	4.0
Stomach	10.2	9.2	8.9	8.1	7.4	7.4	7.2	7.2	6.6	6.6
Colon and rectum	46.4	47.4	50.4	52.8	48.3	46.4	45.3	44.3	42.9	42.7
Colon	31.7	32.6	35.5	37.7	34.6	33.3	32.8	32.1	31.1	30.3
Rectum.	14.7	14.8	14.9	15.1	13.7	13.1	12.5	12.3	11.8	12.5
Pancreas	10.0	9.5	9.3	9.6	9.0	9.3	8.7	9.0	8.7	8.6
Lung and bronchus	42.4	45.3	52.3	56.1	58.6	59.6	57.9	57.1	56.2	54.2
Urinary bladder	14.6	15.5	16.5	16.8	17.1	17.2	17.3	16.9	16.6	16.2
Non-Hodgkin's lymphoma.	8.6	9.4	10.5	12.9	15.3	15.3	15.6	16.3	16.2	15.5
Leukemia.	10.6	10.6	10.7	11.1	10.5	10.6	10.4	10.2	10.5	9.7
Male										
All sites	365.0	378.8	409.2	431.4	479.6	536.3	510.0	483.5	464.9	454.6
Oral cavity and pharynx	17.5	18.0	17.4	17.1	17.0	16.1	16.5	15.7	14.7	14.8
Esophagus.	5.5	5.8	5.9	6.3	7.1	6.7	6.6	6.5	6.0	6.8
Stomach	15.1	13.5	13.5	11.9	10.9	10.7	10.7	10.9	9.9	9.8
Colon and rectum	53.1	54.1	58.7	63.0	58.9	56.3	54.5	53.1	50.5	51.1
Colon	34.2	35.5	39.3	43.2	40.5	39.0	38.4	37.1	35.1	34.9
Rectum.	18.9	18.6	19.4	19.7	18.4	17.3	16.1	16.0	15.3	16.1
Pancreas	12.9	12.5	11.4	11.3	10.4	10.7	10.0	10.6	9.9	10.0
Lung and bronchus	73.2	76.2	84.4	83.8	81.7	81.7	78.7	75.6	74.1	70.0
Prostate gland	64.2	70.6	79.8	88.3	132.5	190.8	171.1	148.4	139.3	135.7
Urinary bladder	25.6	27.1	29.4	28.9	29.8	29.7	29.9	29.2	28.4	27.7
Non-Hodgkin's lymphoma.	10.0	11.0	12.4	15.2	18.9	18.9	19.3	20.3	20.5	19.2
Leukemia.	13.8	13.7	14.2	14.4	13.9	14.0	13.3	13.0	13.5	12.3
Female										
All sites	293.5	307.6	307.1	337.3	348.7	349.3	343.2	347.8	346.3	342.0
Colon and rectum	41.6	42.7	44.5	45.3	40.5	38.9	38.2	37.6	37.0	36.2
Colon.	30.2	30.8	33.0	33.6	30.3	29.1	28.5	28.2	28.0	26.6
Rectum.	11.4	11.9	11.5	11.7	10.1	9.8	9.7	9.3	9.0	9.6
Pancreas	7.7	7.3	7.7	8.2	8.0	8.2	7.6	7.8	7.7	7.4
Lung and bronchus	18.2	21.5	28.1	35.3	41.5	43.2	42.3	43.4	42.7	42.3
Melanoma of skin	5.4	6.3	8.2	9.4	9.9	10.4	10.3	10.5	11.3	11.4
Breast.	82.6	88.1	85.4	104.1	110.4	111.1	108.9	110.8	111.6	110.7
Cervix uteri.	14.2	12.4	10.2	8.5	8.9	8.3	8.1	7.9	7.4	7.7
Corpus uteri	28.4	32.1	24.2	22.1	21.8	21.5	21.0	21.8	21.9	21.1
Ovary	14.1	14.1	13.3	14.3	15.2	15.0	15.0	14.5	14.5	14.1
Non-Hodgkin's lymphoma.	7.4	8.0	8.9	10.9	12.3	12.2	12.4	13.0	12.4	12.2
White										
All sites	319.7	333.9	346.4	375.4	405.1	428.7	412.2	404.2	396.4	387.3
Oral cavity and pharynx	11.2	11.4	11.2	11.4	10.9	10.4	10.6	10.0	9.8	9.5
Esophagus.	3.0	3.0	3.0	3.2	3.6	3.5	3.6	3.5	3.4	3.6
Stomach	9.5	8.4	8.1	7.1	6.3	6.4	6.1	6.1	5.8	5.6
Colon and rectum	46.9	47.8	50.4	53.3	48.2	46.2	44.9	44.0	42.5	42.2
Colon	32.0	32.9	35.4	37.9	34.4	33.1	32.3	31.8	30.7	29.9
Rectum.	14.9	14.9	15.0	15.4	13.8	13.1	12.6	12.2	11.8	12.3
Pancreas	9.8	9.4	8.9	9.2	8.8	9.1	8.3	8.6	8.3	8.2
Lung and bronchus	41.6	45.1	51.2	55.5	58.8	59.1	57.9	57.2	56.4	54.2
Urinary bladder	15.4	16.3	17.4	17.9	18.3	18.5	18.5	18.3	18.0	17.4
Non-Hodgkin's lymphoma.	8.8	9.8	10.8	13.5	16.0	16.0	16.2	16.9	16.6	15.9
Leukemia.	10.8	10.9	11.0	11.4	10.9	10.9	10.6	10.6	11.0	9.8
Black										
All sites	353.1	356.6	390.7	408.6	427.1	470.9	471.8	465.4	442.4	430.9
Oral cavity and pharynx	10.9	11.7	15.3	14.1	14.2	13.3	14.2	14.6	12.2	13.5
Esophagus.	9.0	9.6	11.1	11.3	11.3	9.3	8.9	8.2	7.5	8.3
Stomach	16.7	13.8	12.4	12.9	11.7	11.0	11.3	12.1	10.5	11.5
Colon and rectum	42.4	45.4	55.7	52.2	52.4	52.1	51.7	51.7	48.5	45.7
Colon	30.9	33.7	43.2	40.7	40.7	40.1	40.7	39.6	37.9	34.6
Rectum.	11.5	11.8	12.5	11.5	11.7	12.0	11.0	12.0	10.6	11.2
Pancreas	13.6	13.5	14.8	14.7	12.1	14.1	13.6	14.2	14.2	13.1
Lung and bronchus	58.7	56.5	76.0	79.0	75.3	81.9	74.7	75.9	73.1	69.9
Urinary bladder	7.0	8.7	10.6	10.6	10.3	9.9	10.9	9.7	9.4	9.2
Non-Hodgkin's lymphoma.	7.0	5.6	7.4	8.3	11.3	11.4	11.6	12.0	13.6	12.0
Leukemia.	9.6	9.3	10.0	9.7	8.9	8.9	9.2	7.7	7.9	8.1

See footnotes at end of table.

Table 55 (page 2 of 2). Age-adjusted cancer incidence rates for selected cancer sites, according to sex and race: Selected geographic areas, selected years 1973–96

[Data are based on the Surveillance, Epidemiology, and End Results Program's population-based registries in Atlanta, Detroit, Seattle-Puget Sound, San Francisco-Oakland, Connecticut, Iowa, New Mexico, Utah, and Hawaii]

Race, sex, and site	1973	1975	1980	1985	1990	1992	1993	1994	1995	1996
White male	\multicolumn{10}{c}{Number of new cases per 100,000 population[1]}									
All sites	364.3	379.7	407.5	431.4	483.0	535.6	502.6	476.7	458.1	445.8
Oral cavity and pharynx	17.6	18.3	17.0	16.8	16.4	15.7	16.0	14.8	14.3	14.0
Esophagus	4.8	4.8	4.9	5.3	6.1	6.2	5.9	6.0	5.5	6.2
Stomach	14.0	12.5	12.3	10.5	9.4	9.4	9.1	9.4	8.9	8.4
Colon and rectum	54.2	55.1	58.7	63.5	59.1	56.4	54.2	52.9	49.9	50.7
Colon	34.8	36.1	39.3	43.4	40.4	39.1	38.1	37.0	34.7	34.9
Rectum	19.5	19.0	19.4	20.1	18.7	17.3	16.1	15.8	15.2	15.8
Pancreas	12.8	12.5	11.1	10.7	10.1	10.4	9.6	9.8	9.5	9.5
Lung and bronchus	72.4	75.9	82.2	82.0	80.9	79.3	77.1	74.5	72.3	68.4
Prostate gland	62.6	69.0	78.8	87.2	133.4	188.7	163.9	141.0	132.3	127.8
Urinary bladder	27.3	28.8	31.5	31.2	32.4	31.9	32.0	31.7	30.8	29.9
Non-Hodgkin's lymphoma	10.4	11.5	12.6	15.9	19.7	19.6	20.0	20.7	20.9	19.7
Leukemia	14.3	14.3	14.6	14.8	14.5	14.7	13.8	13.5	14.1	12.4
Black male										
All sites	441.4	438.2	510.4	533.0	561.4	657.2	664.4	636.5	594.8	563.1
Oral cavity and pharynx	16.6	17.2	23.1	22.6	24.5	22.6	22.9	25.0	20.3	21.9
Esophagus	13.3	17.6	16.4	19.4	19.5	15.7	15.2	13.2	12.4	14.0
Stomach	25.9	19.9	21.4	18.8	17.8	15.9	18.5	19.4	14.6	17.6
Colon and rectum	42.8	47.6	63.7	60.8	58.1	61.8	62.0	59.6	54.6	50.9
Colon	31.7	34.7	46.0	47.0	45.0	46.7	47.1	44.2	41.4	36.7
Rectum	11.1	12.9	17.7	13.8	13.1	15.1	14.8	15.3	13.2	14.2
Pancreas	15.9	15.6	17.6	19.7	15.0	15.9	15.4	17.3	16.4	15.9
Lung and bronchus	104.6	101.0	131.0	131.3	115.9	127.6	114.8	112.8	115.2	101.4
Prostate gland	106.3	111.5	126.6	133.8	168.4	258.0	271.6	246.9	218.3	211.3
Urinary bladder	10.6	13.5	14.5	16.3	15.1	16.6	18.1	15.7	14.3	14.0
Non-Hodgkin's lymphoma	8.8	7.0	9.3	10.0	14.0	15.3	15.7	17.7	19.1	15.0
Leukemia	12.0	12.5	13.1	13.0	11.7	11.4	12.2	9.8	10.2	10.1
White female										
All sites	295.1	310.6	311.3	343.9	356.9	356.3	349.6	354.5	354.5	347.1
Colon and rectum	41.7	42.9	44.7	46.0	40.2	38.4	37.7	36.9	36.7	35.5
Colon	30.3	30.9	32.9	34.0	30.1	28.7	27.9	27.7	27.6	25.9
Rectum	11.5	12.0	11.8	12.0	10.1	9.8	9.8	9.2	9.1	9.6
Pancreas	7.5	7.1	7.3	8.1	7.8	8.0	7.3	7.6	7.5	7.1
Lung and bronchus	17.8	21.8	28.2	35.9	42.6	44.3	43.8	44.4	44.5	43.7
Melanoma of skin	5.9	6.9	9.4	10.5	11.4	11.9	11.8	12.1	13.2	13.2
Breast	84.4	90.0	87.8	107.3	114.5	114.2	112.0	114.6	115.3	113.3
Cervix uteri	12.8	11.1	9.1	7.6	8.3	7.9	7.6	7.3	6.6	7.0
Corpus uteri	29.5	33.7	25.3	23.2	23.1	22.7	22.1	22.7	22.8	21.8
Ovary	14.6	14.4	14.0	15.1	16.1	15.8	15.7	15.0	15.4	15.3
Non-Hodgkin's lymphoma	7.6	8.5	9.2	11.4	12.9	12.9	12.8	13.5	12.8	12.7
Black female										
All sites	283.7	296.3	305.0	323.7	337.5	343.5	337.1	344.8	333.0	336.1
Colon and rectum	41.8	43.5	49.6	45.8	48.6	45.8	44.4	46.5	44.2	41.8
Colon	30.0	32.7	41.2	35.9	37.9	36.0	36.2	36.8	35.7	32.9
Rectum	11.8	10.8	8.5	9.9	10.7	9.8	8.2	9.7	8.5	8.9
Pancreas	11.6	11.6	13.0	11.3	10.0	12.8	12.0	11.9	12.4	10.8
Lung and bronchus	20.9	20.6	33.8	40.2	46.3	48.7	45.7	49.0	42.7	47.2
Breast	69.0	78.5	74.5	92.7	96.5	102.2	100.8	102.1	102.4	100.3
Cervix uteri	29.9	27.9	19.0	15.9	13.8	11.1	11.3	11.6	11.3	10.6
Corpus uteri	15.0	17.0	14.1	15.4	14.4	14.6	14.7	15.7	15.8	15.7
Ovary	10.5	10.1	10.1	10.1	10.1	10.6	11.1	12.4	9.9	8.5
Non-Hodgkin's lymphoma	5.5	4.2	6.0	7.0	9.2	8.2	8.1	7.2	9.1	9.5

[1]Age adjusted by the direct method to the 1970 U.S. population. See Appendix II, Age adjustment.

NOTE: Numbers have been revised and differ from previous editions of *Health, United States*.

SOURCE: National Institutes of Health, National Cancer Institute, Cancer Statistics Branch, Bethesda, Maryland 20892.

Table 56. Five-year relative cancer survival rates for selected cancer sites, according to race and sex: Selected geographic areas, 1974–79, 1980–82, 1983–85, 1986–88, and 1989–95

[Data are based on the Surveillance, Epidemiology, and End Results Program's population-based registries in Atlanta, Detroit, Seattle-Puget Sound, San Francisco-Oakland, Connecticut, Iowa, New Mexico, Utah, and Hawaii]

Sex and site	White					Black				
	1974–79	1980–82	1983–85	1986–88	1989–95	1974–79	1980–82	1983–85	1986–88	1989–95
Both sexes					Percent of patients					
All sites	50.8	52.0	53.8	56.6	60.9	39.1	39.7	39.8	42.5	47.7
Oral cavity and pharynx.	54.8	55.4	55.1	55.1	55.5	36.6	30.8	35.1	34.8	33.8
Esophagus.	5.3	7.4	9.3	10.8	13.3	3.3	5.4	6.3	7.3	8.9
Stomach	15.3	16.5	16.3	19.1	19.3	15.8	19.4	18.6	18.9	21.6
Colon	51.8	55.6	58.4	61.5	62.4	47.1	49.2	49.2	52.5	51.8
Rectum	49.8	52.9	55.8	59.1	60.2	40.3	38.2	43.8	51.0	51.2
Pancreas	2.4	2.8	2.9	3.0	4.1	3.2	4.7	5.4	6.2	3.6
Lung and bronchus.	13.1	13.5	13.9	13.5	14.2	11.2	12.2	11.5	11.8	11.3
Urinary bladder.	74.9	78.8	78.2	80.6	81.8	51.6	58.3	59.0	62.0	62.2
Non-Hodgkin's lymphoma . . .	48.2	51.7	54.3	52.8	51.9	49.9	50.0	44.8	49.8	41.3
Leukemia.	36.5	39.3	41.6	43.4	44.4	30.7	33.2	33.4	36.8	33.5
Male										
All sites	43.4	46.6	48.4	51.6	59.2	32.0	34.2	34.6	37.6	46.5
Oral cavity and pharynx.	54.2	54.3	54.3	52.0	51.7	31.2	26.2	29.9	29.6	28.4
Esophagus.	5.0	6.6	7.8	11.4	13.2	2.3	4.6	5.2	7.1	8.0
Stomach	13.9	15.5	14.6	16.1	16.7	15.2	18.5	17.8	14.5	20.6
Colon	50.9	55.9	58.9	62.4	63.0	45.1	46.5	48.3	51.9	51.5
Rectum	49.0	51.4	55.2	58.8	60.0	36.7	36.1	42.7	47.0	52.0
Pancreas	2.7	2.6	2.5	2.9	3.8	2.4	3.6	4.8	6.6	3.2
Lung and bronchus.	11.6	12.2	12.1	12.1	12.7	10.0	11.0	10.4	11.9	9.9
Prostate gland	70.3	74.5	76.2	82.6	93.0	60.6	64.7	64.1	69.0	83.6
Urinary bladder.	75.9	79.8	79.5	82.2	83.9	58.9	62.6	64.2	67.5	66.6
Non-Hodgkin's lymphoma . . .	47.2	50.8	53.3	50.1	47.7	44.2	47.3	43.6	46.6	37.6
Leukemia.	35.6	39.4	41.2	44.8	45.5	30.9	30.2	32.3	35.8	29.7
Female										
All sites	57.3	57.0	58.8	61.3	62.6	46.8	45.9	45.4	47.6	49.1
Colon	52.6	55.3	58.0	60.6	61.9	48.7	51.3	49.9	53.0	52.1
Rectum	50.8	54.5	56.6	59.4	60.6	43.7	40.8	44.8	55.0	50.3
Pancreas	2.1	3.1	3.2	3.2	4.4	4.1	5.7	5.8	5.9	3.9
Lung and bronchus.	16.7	16.2	17.0	15.8	16.4	15.4	15.4	14.1	11.7	14.0
Melanoma of skin	85.8	88.2	89.2	91.0	91.0	69.9	- - -	70.1	- - -	75.2
Breast	75.3	77.1	79.2	83.8	86.0	63.2	65.9	63.5	69.2	71.0
Cervix uteri	69.6	67.9	70.3	71.6	71.4	62.9	61.0	59.9	55.4	58.8
Corpus uteri	87.6	82.8	84.5	84.3	85.4	59.1	54.1	54.0	56.5	56.1
Ovary	37.1	38.6	40.2	41.9	49.9	40.4	38.6	41.7	38.6	47.1
Non-Hodgkin's lymphoma . . .	49.2	52.7	55.4	55.9	57.3	57.3	53.3	46.3	53.9	47.5

- - - Data not available.

NOTES: Rates are based on followup of patients through 1996. The rate is the ratio of the observed survival rate for the patient group to the expected survival rate for persons in the general population similar to the patient group with respect to age, sex, race, and calendar year of observation. It estimates the chance of surviving the effects of cancer. Numbers have been revised and differ from previous editions of *Health, United States*.

SOURCE: National Institutes of Health, National Cancer Institute, Cancer Statistics Branch, Bethesda, Maryland 20892.

Table 57 (page 1 of 3). Limitation of activity caused by chronic conditions, according to selected characteristics: United States, 1997

[Data are based on household interviews of a sample of the civilian noninstitutionalized population]

Characteristic	Percent with any activity limitation[1]
All ages	
Total[2,3]	13.3
Age	
Under 18 years	6.6
Under 5 years	3.5
5–17 years	7.8
18–44 years	7.0
18–24 years	5.1
25–44 years	7.6
45–54 years	14.2
55–64 years	22.2
65 years and over	38.7
65–74 years	30.0
75 years and over	50.2
Sex[3]	
Male	13.1
Female	13.4
Race[3,4]	
White	13.1
Black	17.1
American Indian or Alaska Native	23.1
Asian or Pacific Islander	7.5
Race and Hispanic origin[3]	
White, non-Hispanic	13.2
Black, non-Hispanic	17.0
Hispanic[4]	12.8
Mexican[4]	12.5
Poverty status[3,5]	
Poor	26.8
Near poor	19.0
Nonpoor	10.5
Race and Hispanic origin and poverty status[3,5]	
White, non-Hispanic:	
Poor	29.5
Near poor	20.7
Nonpoor	10.7
Black, non-Hispanic:	
Poor	29.4
Near poor	20.0
Nonpoor	10.7
Hispanic:[4]	
Poor	19.7
Near poor	13.1
Nonpoor	9.8
Geographic region[3]	
Northeast	13.0
Midwest	13.1
South	13.9
West	13.0
Location of residence[3]	
Within MSA[6]	12.7
Outside MSA[6]	15.5

See footnotes at end of table.

[Data are based on household interviews of a sample of the civilian noninstitutionalized population]

Characteristic	Percent with ADL limitation[7]	Percent with IADL limitation[7]
65 years of age and over		
All adults 65 years of age and over[2,8]	6.7	13.7
Age		
65–74 years	3.4	6.9
75 years and over	10.4	21.2
Sex[8]		
Male..	5.2	9.1
Female...	7.7	16.9
Race[4,8]		
White	6.3	13.1
Black	11.7	21.3
American Indian or Alaska Native	*	*
Asian or Pacific Islander.....................................	*	*9.1
Race and Hispanic origin[8]		
White, non-Hispanic..	6.1	13.0
Black, non-Hispanic..	11.7	21.2
Hispanic[4]	10.8	16.3
Mexican[4]	11.4	18.8
Poverty status[5,8]		
Poor..	13.0	26.9
Near poor	7.5	16.3
Nonpoor	5.3	10.1
Race and Hispanic origin and poverty status[5,8]		
White, non-Hispanic:		
Poor	12.7	27.2
Near poor	6.7	15.8
Nonpoor	5.0	10.0
Black, non-Hispanic:		
Poor	12.9	27.4
Near poor	12.0	21.4
Nonpoor	*10.6	*13.0
Hispanic:[4]		
Poor	15.5	25.8
Near poor	11.3	16.5
Nonpoor	*	*9.7

See footnotes at end of table.

Table 57 (page 3 of 3). Limitation of activity caused by chronic conditions according to selected characteristics: United States, 1997

[Data are based on household interviews of a sample of the civilian noninstitutionalized population]

Characteristic	Percent with ADL limitation[7]	Percent with IADL limitation[7]
Geographic region[8]		
Northeast	6.1	12.2
Midwest	5.8	13.1
South	8.2	15.8
West	5.9	12.4
Location of residence[8]		
Within MSA[6]	6.6	13.5
Outside MSA[6]	7.2	14.4

* Data preceded by an asterisk have a relative standard error of 20–30 percent. Data not shown have a relative standard error of greater than 30 percent.
[1]Limitation of activity is assessed by asking respondents a series of questions about limitations in their ability to perform activities usual for their age group because of a physical, mental, or emotional problem. Respondents are asked about limitations in activities of daily living, instrumental activities of daily living, play, school, work, and difficulty in walking and remembering. For reported limitations the condition causing the limitation is determined and respondents are considered limited if the causal conditions are chronic in nature. See Appendix II, Limitation of activity, Activity of daily living, Instrumental activity of daily living.
[2]Includes all other races not shown separately and unknown poverty status.
[3]Estimates for all persons are age adjusted to the year 2000 standard using six age groups: Under 18 years, 18–44 years, 45–54 years, 55–64 years, 65–74 years, and 75 years and over. See Appendix II, Age adjustment.
[4]The race groups, white, black, American Indian or Alaska Native, and Asian or Pacific Islander include persons of Hispanic and non-Hispanic origin; persons of Hispanic origin may be of any race.
[5]Beginning in 1997 poverty status is based on family income, family size, number of children in the family, and, for families with two or fewer adults, the age of the adults in the family. Poor persons are defined as below the poverty threshold. Near poor persons have incomes of 100 percent to less than 200 percent of poverty threshold. Nonpoor persons have incomes of 200 percent or greater than the poverty threshold. See Appendix II, Poverty level. In 1997 poverty status was unknown for 20 percent of persons in the sample.
[6]MSA is metropolitan statistical area.
[7]These estimates are for elderly noninstitutionalized persons. To determine activities of daily living (ADL) limitations respondents were asked "Because of a physical, mental, or emotional problem, does ____ need the help of other persons with personal care needs, such as eating, bathing, dressing, or getting around inside this home?" Instrumental activities of daily living (IADL) were determined by asking respondents "Because of a physical, mental, or emotional problem, does ____ need the help of other persons in handling routine needs, such as everyday household chores, doing necessary business, shopping, or getting around for other purposes?" See Appendix II, Activities of daily living, Instrumental activities of daily living.
[8]Estimates are age adjusted to the year 2000 standard using two age groups: 65–74 years and 75 years and over. See Appendix II, Age adjustment.

SOURCE: Centers for Disease Control and Prevention, National Center for Health Statistics. National Health Interview Survey, family core questionnaire.

Table 58 (page 1 of 2). Respondent-assessed health status according to selected characteristics: United States, 1991, 1995, 1997, and 1998

[Data are based on household interviews of a sample of the civilian noninstitutionalized population]

Characteristic	Percent with fair or poor health[1]			
	1991	1995	1997[2]	1998[2]
Total[3,4]	10.4	10.6	9.2	9.1
Age				
Under 18 years	2.6	2.6	2.1	1.8
Under 6 years	2.7	2.7	1.9	1.5
6–17 years	2.6	2.5	2.1	1.9
18–44 years	6.1	6.6	5.3	5.3
18–24 years	4.8	4.5	3.4	3.2
25–44 years	6.4	7.2	5.9	5.9
45–54 years	13.4	13.4	11.7	11.6
55–64 years	20.7	21.4	18.2	18.0
65 years and over	29.0	28.3	26.7	26.7
65–74 years	26.0	25.6	23.1	23.9
75 years and over	33.6	32.2	31.5	30.4
Sex[3]				
Male	10.0	10.1	8.8	8.8
Female	10.8	11.1	9.7	9.4
Race[3,5]				
White	9.6	9.7	8.3	8.2
Black	16.8	17.2	15.8	15.7
American Indian or Alaska Native	18.3	18.7	17.3	17.6
Asian or Pacific Islander	7.8	9.3	7.8	7.1
Race and Hispanic origin[3]				
White, non-Hispanic	9.1	9.1	8.0	7.8
Black, non-Hispanic	16.8	17.3	15.8	15.8
Hispanic[5]	15.6	15.1	13.0	13.1
Mexican[5]	17.0	16.7	13.1	13.5
Poverty status[3,6]				
Poor	22.8	23.7	21.4	22.2
Near poor	14.7	15.5	14.6	15.6
Nonpoor	6.8	6.7	6.1	5.7
Race and Hispanic origin and poverty status[3,6]				
White, non-Hispanic:				
Poor	21.9	22.8	20.6	21.3
Near poor	14.0	14.8	14.1	15.3
Nonpoor	6.4	6.2	5.7	5.3
Black, non-Hispanic:				
Poor	25.8	27.7	25.6	26.3
Near poor	17.0	19.3	19.5	19.3
Nonpoor	10.9	9.9	9.6	9.0
Hispanic:[5]				
Poor	23.6	22.7	19.8	21.7
Near poor	18.0	16.9	14.0	15.3
Nonpoor	9.3	8.7	8.8	7.9

See footnotes at end of table.

Table 58 (page 2 of 2). Respondent-assessed health status according to selected characteristics: United States, 1991, 1995, 1997, and 1998

[Data are based on household interviews of a sample of the civilian noninstitutionalized population]

Characteristic	Percent with fair or poor health[1]			
	1991	1995	1997[2]	1998[2]
Geographic region[3]				
Northeast	8.3	9.1	8.0	7.9
Midwest	9.1	9.7	8.1	8.0
South..................................	13.1	12.3	10.8	10.9
West	9.7	10.1	8.8	8.4
Location of residence[3]				
Within MSA[7]	9.9	10.1	8.7	8.5
Outside MSA[7]	11.9	12.6	11.1	11.4

[1]See Appendix II, Health status, respondent-assessed.
[2]Data starting in 1997 are not strictly comparable with data for earlier years due to the 1997 questionnaire redesign. See Appendix I, National Health Interview Survey.
[3]Estimates are age adjusted to the year 2000 standard using six age groups: Under 18 years, 18–44 years, 45–54 years, 55–64 years, 65–74 years, and 75 years and over. See Appendix II, Age adjustment.
[4]Includes all other races not shown separately and unknown poverty status.
[5]The race groups white, black, American Indian or Alaska Native, and Asian or Pacific Islander include persons of Hispanic and non-Hispanic origin; persons of Hispanic origin may be of any race.
[6]Prior to 1997 poverty status is based on family income and family size using Bureau of the Census poverty thresholds. Beginning in 1997 poverty status is based on family income, family size, number of children in the family, and for families with two or fewer adults the age of the adults in the family. Poor persons are defined as below the poverty threshold. Near poor persons have incomes of 100 percent to less than 200 percent of poverty threshold. Nonpoor persons have incomes of 200 percent or greater than the poverty threshold. See Appendix II, Poverty level. Missing family income data were imputed for 16–18 percent of persons in 1991 and 1995. See Appendix II, Family income for information on imputation process. Poverty status was unknown for 20 percent of persons in the sample in 1997 and 25 percent in 1998.
[7]MSA is metropolitan statistical area.

SOURCE: Centers for Disease Control and Prevention, National Center for Health Statistics, National Health Interview Survey, family core questionnaire.

Table 59. Current cigarette smoking by persons 18 years of age and over according to sex, race, and age: United States, selected years 1965–98

[Data are based on household interviews of a sample of the civilian noninstitutionalized population]

Sex, race, and age	1965	1974	1979	1983	1985	1990	1992	1993	1994	1995	1997[1]	1998[1]
18 years and over, age adjusted[2]						Percent of persons						
All persons	41.9	37.0	33.3	31.9	29.9	25.3	26.3	24.8	25.3	24.6	24.6	24.0
Male	51.2	42.8	37.0	34.8	32.2	28.0	28.1	27.3	27.6	26.5	27.1	25.9
Female	33.7	32.2	30.1	29.4	27.9	22.9	24.6	22.6	23.1	22.7	22.2	22.1
White male	50.4	41.7	36.4	34.2	31.3	27.6	27.7	26.6	27.1	26.2	26.8	26.0
Black male	58.8	53.6	43.9	41.7	40.2	32.8	33.3	33.7	34.3	29.4	32.4	29.0
White female	33.9	32.0	30.3	29.6	27.9	23.5	25.3	23.4	24.0	23.4	22.8	23.0
Black female	31.8	35.6	30.5	31.3	30.9	20.8	24.5	20.6	21.6	23.5	22.5	21.1
18 years and over, crude												
All persons	42.4	37.1	33.5	32.1	30.1	25.5	26.5	25.0	25.5	24.7	24.7	24.1
Male	51.9	43.1	37.5	35.1	32.6	28.4	28.6	27.7	28.2	27.0	27.6	26.4
Female	33.9	32.1	29.9	29.5	27.9	22.8	24.6	22.5	23.1	22.6	22.1	21.9
White male	51.1	41.9	36.8	34.5	31.7	28.0	28.2	27.0	27.7	26.6	27.2	26.3
Black male	60.4	54.3	44.1	40.6	39.9	32.5	32.2	32.7	33.7	28.5	32.2	29.0
White female	34.0	31.7	30.1	29.4	27.7	23.4	25.1	23.1	23.7	23.1	22.5	22.6
Black female	33.7	36.4	31.1	32.2	31.0	21.2	24.2	20.8	21.7	23.5	22.5	21.0
All males												
18–24 years	54.1	42.1	35.0	32.9	28.0	26.6	28.0	28.8	29.8	27.8	31.7	31.3
25–34 years	60.7	50.5	43.9	38.8	38.2	31.6	32.8	30.2	31.4	29.5	30.3	28.6
35–44 years	58.2	51.0	41.8	41.0	37.6	34.5	32.9	32.0	33.2	31.5	32.1	30.2
45–64 years	51.9	42.6	39.3	35.9	33.4	29.3	28.6	29.2	28.3	27.1	27.6	27.7
65 years and over	28.5	24.8	20.9	22.0	19.6	14.6	16.1	13.5	13.2	14.9	12.8	10.4
White male												
18–24 years	53.0	40.8	34.3	32.5	28.4	27.4	30.0	30.4	31.8	28.4	34.0	34.1
25–34 years	60.1	49.5	43.6	38.6	37.3	31.6	33.5	29.9	32.5	29.9	30.4	29.2
35–44 years	57.3	50.1	41.3	40.8	36.6	33.5	30.9	31.2	32.0	31.2	32.1	29.6
45–64 years	51.3	41.2	38.3	35.0	32.1	28.7	28.1	27.8	26.9	26.3	26.5	27.0
65 years and over	27.7	24.3	20.5	20.6	18.9	13.7	14.9	12.5	11.9	14.1	11.5	10.0
Black male												
18–24 years	62.8	54.9	40.2	34.2	27.2	21.3	*16.2	*19.9	*18.7	*14.6	23.5	19.7
25–34 years	68.4	58.5	47.5	39.9	45.6	33.8	29.5	30.7	29.8	25.1	31.6	25.2
35–44 years	67.3	61.5	48.6	45.5	45.0	42.0	47.5	36.9	44.5	36.3	33.9	36.2
45–64 years	57.9	57.8	50.0	44.8	46.1	36.7	35.4	42.4	41.2	33.9	39.4	37.3
65 years and over	36.4	29.7	26.2	38.9	27.7	21.5	28.3	*27.9	25.6	28.5	26.0	16.3
All females												
18–24 years	38.1	34.1	33.8	35.5	30.4	22.5	24.9	22.9	25.2	21.8	25.7	24.5
25–34 years	43.7	38.8	33.7	32.6	32.0	28.2	30.1	27.3	28.8	26.4	24.8	24.6
35–44 years	43.7	39.8	37.0	33.8	31.5	24.8	27.3	27.4	26.8	27.1	27.2	26.4
45–64 years	32.0	33.4	30.7	31.0	29.9	24.8	26.1	23.0	22.8	24.0	21.5	22.5
65 years and over	9.6	12.0	13.2	13.1	13.5	11.5	12.4	10.5	11.1	11.5	11.5	11.2
White female												
18–24 years	38.4	34.0	34.5	36.5	31.8	25.4	28.5	26.8	28.5	24.9	29.4	28.0
25–34 years	43.4	38.6	34.1	32.2	32.0	28.5	31.5	28.4	30.2	27.3	26.1	26.9
35–44 years	43.9	39.3	37.2	34.8	31.0	25.0	27.6	27.3	27.1	27.0	27.5	26.7
45–64 years	32.7	33.0	30.6	30.6	29.7	25.4	25.8	23.4	23.2	24.3	20.9	22.5
65 years and over	9.8	12.3	13.8	13.2	13.3	11.5	12.6	10.5	11.1	11.7	11.7	11.2
Black female												
18–24 years	37.1	35.6	31.8	32.0	23.7	10.0	10.3	*8.2	11.8	*8.8	11.5	8.3
25–34 years	47.8	42.2	35.2	38.0	36.2	29.1	26.9	24.7	24.8	26.7	22.5	21.5
35–44 years	42.8	46.4	37.7	32.7	40.2	25.5	32.4	31.5	28.2	31.9	30.1	30.0
45–64 years	25.7	38.9	34.2	36.3	33.4	22.6	30.9	21.3	23.5	27.5	28.4	25.3
65 years and over	7.1	*8.9	*8.5	*13.1	14.5	11.1	*11.1	*10.2	13.6	13.3	10.7	11.5

* Data preceded by an asterisk have a relative standard error of 20–30 percent.
[1]See Appendix I, National Health Interview Survey, for discussion of 1997 redesign.
[2]Estimates are age adjusted to the year 2000 standard using five age groups: 18–24 years, 25–34 years, 35–44 years, 45–64 years, 65 years and over. See Appendix II, Age adjustment.

NOTES: The definition of current smoker was revised in 1992 and 1993. See Appendix II, Current smoker. Data for additional years are available (see Appendix III).

SOURCES: Centers for Disease Control and Prevention, National Center for Health Statistics. National Health Interview Survey. Data are from the core questionnaire (1965) and the following questionnaire supplements: hypertension (1974), smoking (1979), alcohol and health practices (1983), health promotion and disease prevention (1985, 1990–91), cancer control and cancer epidemiology (1992), and year 2000 (1993–95). Starting in 1997 data are from the sample adult questionnaire.

Table 60. Age-adjusted prevalence of current cigarette smoking by persons 25 years of age and over, according to sex, race, and education: United States, selected years 1974–98

[Data are based on household interviews of a sample of the civilian noninstitutionalized population]

Sex, race, and education	1974	1979	1983	1985	1990	1992	1993	1994	1995	1997[1]	1998[1]
25 years and over, age adjusted[2]					Percent of persons						
All persons[3]	36.9	33.1	31.6	30.0	25.4	26.3	24.7	24.9	24.5	24.0	23.4
No high school diploma or GED	43.7	40.7	40.7	40.8	36.7	36.6	35.6	37.5	35.6	33.5	34.4
High school diploma or GED	36.2	33.6	33.5	32.0	29.1	30.5	28.4	29.1	29.1	29.9	28.9
Some college, no bachelor's degree	35.9	33.2	30.3	29.5	23.4	24.4	24.3	24.5	22.6	23.7	23.5
Bachelor's degree or higher	27.2	22.6	20.5	18.5	13.9	15.2	13.5	11.9	13.6	11.4	10.9
All males[3]	42.9	37.3	35.1	32.8	28.2	28.1	27.1	27.3	26.4	26.4	25.1
No high school diploma or GED	52.3	47.6	47.1	45.7	42.0	41.4	40.8	43.8	39.7	39.1	37.5
High school diploma or GED	42.4	38.9	37.4	35.5	33.1	33.1	30.4	31.7	32.7	32.2	32.0
Some college, no bachelor's degree	41.8	36.5	33.3	32.9	25.9	25.9	27.2	26.8	23.7	25.5	25.4
Bachelor's degree or higher	28.3	22.7	21.7	19.6	14.5	15.8	14.5	13.4	13.8	12.5	11.0
White males[3]	41.9	36.7	34.4	31.7	27.6	27.3	26.1	26.4	25.9	25.8	24.8
No high school diploma or GED	51.5	47.6	47.7	45.0	41.8	41.5	39.5	42.6	38.7	38.5	37.4
High school diploma or GED	42.0	38.5	37.0	34.8	32.9	32.8	29.7	31.6	32.9	31.8	32.2
Some college, no bachelor's degree	41.6	36.4	32.9	32.2	25.4	25.5	26.6	26.4	23.3	25.6	25.2
Bachelor's degree or higher	27.8	22.5	21.0	19.1	14.4	14.9	14.1	12.8	13.4	12.0	10.9
Black males[3]	53.4	44.4	42.8	42.1	34.5	35.8	35.7	36.6	31.6	33.8	30.4
No high school diploma or GED	58.1	49.7	46.0	50.5	41.6	45.3	46.7	51.7	41.9	44.6	42.9
High school diploma or GED	*50.7	48.6	47.7	41.8	37.4	38.4	36.3	37.8	36.6	39.0	33.0
Some college, no bachelor's degree	*45.3	39.2	44.9	41.8	28.1	28.1	29.7	*29.2	26.4	27.0	28.4
Bachelor's degree or higher	*41.4	*36.8	*31.7	*32.0	*20.8	28.5	*16.1	*26.8	*17.3	14.5	15.3
All females[3]	32.0	29.5	28.5	27.5	22.9	24.6	22.5	22.8	22.9	21.7	21.7
No high school diploma or GED	36.6	34.8	35.2	36.5	31.8	32.2	30.9	31.5	31.7	28.2	31.3
High school diploma or GED	32.2	29.8	30.7	29.5	26.1	28.4	26.8	27.2	26.4	27.9	26.2
Some college, no bachelor's degree	30.1	30.0	27.3	26.3	21.0	23.1	21.7	22.4	21.6	22.0	21.9
Bachelor's degree or higher	25.9	22.5	18.9	17.1	13.3	14.4	12.2	10.2	13.3	10.3	10.7
White females[3]	31.7	29.7	28.6	27.3	23.3	24.9	22.9	23.3	23.1	21.9	22.2
No high school diploma or GED	36.8	35.8	35.6	36.7	33.4	33.0	31.5	33.0	32.4	29.7	33.0
High school diploma or GED	31.9	29.9	30.8	29.4	26.5	29.2	27.7	28.3	26.8	28.3	*27.1
Some college, no bachelor's degree	30.4	30.7	27.8	26.7	21.2	23.4	21.6	22.1	22.2	22.1	22.2
Bachelor's degree or higher	25.5	21.9	18.7	16.5	13.4	14.1	12.4	10.7	13.5	10.5	11.4
Black females[3]	35.6	30.3	31.2	32.0	22.4	26.6	22.4	23.0	25.7	24.1	23.0
No high school diploma or GED	36.1	31.6	36.5	39.4	26.3	32.7	29.8	29.9	32.3	27.1	32.8
High school diploma or GED	40.9	32.6	34.6	32.1	24.1	25.8	24.4	22.6	27.8	29.1	24.3
Some college, no bachelor's degree	32.3	*28.9	*27.1	23.9	22.7	27.2	23.1	28.3	20.8	24.3	21.7
Bachelor's degree or higher	*36.3	*43.3	*36.8	26.6	17.0	25.5	*12.7	*11.1	17.3	12.5	9.0

* Data preceded by an asterisk have a relative standard error of 20–30 percent.

[1] See Appendix I, National Health Interview Survey, for discussion of 1997 redesign.

[2] Estimates are age adjusted to the year 2000 standard using four age groups: 25–34 years, 35–44 years, 45–64 years, 65 years and over. See Appendix II, Age adjustment. For age groups where percent smoking was 0 or 100, the age-adjustment procedure was modified to substitute the percent smoking from the next lower education group.

[3] Includes unknown education. Education categories shown are for 1997 and subsequent years. GED stands for general equivalency diploma. In 1974–95 the following categories based on number of years of school completed were used: less than 12 years, 12 years, 13–15 years, 16 years or more. See Appendix II, Education.

NOTES: The definition of current smoker was revised in 1992 and 1993. See Appendix II, Current smoker. Data for additional years are available (see Appendix III).

SOURCES: Centers for Disease Control and Prevention, National Center for Health Statistics. National Health Interview Survey. Data are from the following questionnaire supplements: hypertension (1974), smoking (1979), alcohol and health practices (1983), health promotion and disease prevention (1985, 1990–91), cancer control and cancer epidemiology (1992), and year 2000 (1993–95). Starting in 1997 data are from the sample adult questionnaire.

Table 61 (page 1 of 2). Current cigarette smoking by adults according to sex, race, Hispanic origin, age, and education: United States, average annual 1990–92 and 1995–98

[Data are based on household interviews of a sample of the civilian noninstitutionalized population]

Characteristic	Male		Female	
	1990–92	1995–98[1]	1990–92	1995–98[1]
18 years of age and over, age adjusted[2]		Percent of persons		
All persons[3]	27.9	26.5	23.7	22.1
White	27.4	26.4	24.3	22.9
Black	33.9	30.7	23.1	21.8
American Indian or Alaska Native	34.2	40.5	36.7	28.9
Asian or Pacific Islander	24.8	18.1	6.3	11.0
White, non-Hispanic	27.7	26.9	25.2	24.1
Black, non-Hispanic	33.9	30.8	23.2	21.9
Hispanic[3]	25.7	24.4	15.8	13.7
Mexican	26.2	24.5	14.8	11.9
18 years of age and over, crude				
All persons[3]	28.4	27.0	23.6	22.0
White	27.8	26.7	24.1	22.6
Black	33.2	30.6	23.3	21.8
American Indian or Alaska Native	35.5	39.2	37.3	31.2
Asian or Pacific Islander	24.9	20.0	6.3	11.1
White, non-Hispanic	28.0	27.0	24.8	23.5
Black, non-Hispanic	33.3	30.6	23.3	21.8
Hispanic[3]	26.5	25.5	16.6	13.8
Mexican	27.1	25.2	15.0	11.6
18–24 years:				
White, non-Hispanic	28.9	35.5	28.7	31.6
Black, non-Hispanic	17.7	21.3	10.8	9.8
Hispanic[3]	19.3	26.5	12.8	12.0
25–34 years:				
White, non-Hispanic	32.7	30.5	30.9	28.5
Black, non-Hispanic	34.6	28.5	29.2	22.0
Hispanic[3]	29.9	25.9	19.2	12.6
35–44 years:				
White, non-Hispanic	32.3	31.5	27.3	28.1
Black, non-Hispanic	44.1	34.8	31.3	30.2
Hispanic[3]	32.1	26.2	19.9	17.6
45–64 years:				
White, non-Hispanic	28.4	26.8	26.1	22.3
Black, non-Hispanic	38.0	38.9	26.1	26.9
Hispanic[3]	26.6	26.8	17.1	14.7
65 years and over:				
White, non-Hispanic	14.2	10.6	12.3	11.5
Black, non-Hispanic	25.2	20.9	10.7	11.2
Hispanic[3]	16.1	14.7	6.6	9.4

See footnotes at end of table.

Table 61 (page 2 of 2). Current cigarette smoking by adults according to sex, race, Hispanic origin, age, and education: United States, average annual 1990–92 and 1995–98

[Data are based on household interviews of a sample of the civilian noninstitutionalized population]

	Male		Female	
Characteristic	1990–92	1995–98[1]	1990–92	1995–98[1]
Education[4], race, and Hispanic origin	Percent of persons			
25 years of age and over, age adjusted[5]				
No high school diploma or GED:				
White, non-Hispanic	46.1	43.9	40.4	40.6
Black, non-Hispanic	45.4	44.6	31.3	30.0
Hispanic[3]	30.2	27.6	15.8	13.2
High school diploma or GED:				
White, non-Hispanic	32.9	32.8	28.4	28.8
Black, non-Hispanic	38.2	35.8	25.4	26.6
Hispanic[3]	29.6	26.7	18.4	16.4
Some college or more:				
White, non-Hispanic	19.3	18.3	18.1	17.2
Black, non-Hispanic	25.6	23.3	22.8	18.9
Hispanic[3]	20.4	16.6	14.3	13.5

[1]Smoking data are for years 1995, 1997, and 1998 (smoking data were not collected in 1996). See Appendix I, National Health Interview Survey, for discussion of 1997 redesign.
[2]Estimates are age adjusted to the year 2000 standard using five age groups: 18–24 years, 25–34 years, 35–44 years, 45–64 years, 65 years and over. See Appendix II, Age adjustment.
[3]The race groups white, black, American Indian or Alaska Native, and Asian or Pacific Islander include persons of Hispanic and non-Hispanic origin; persons of Hispanic origin may be of any race.
[4]Education categories shown are for 1997 and subsequent years. GED stands for general equivalency diploma. In 1990–92 the following categories based on number of years of school completed were used: less than 12 years, 12 years, 13 years or more. See Appendix II, Education.
[5]Estimates are age adjusted to the year 2000 standard using four age groups: 25–34 years, 35–44 years, 45–64 years, 65 years and over. See Appendix II, Age adjustment.

NOTES: The definition of current smoker was revised in 1992 and 1993. See Appendix II, Current smoker. Data for additional years are available (see Appendix III).

SOURCES: Centers for Disease Control and Prevention, National Center for Health Statistics. National Health Interview Survey. Data are from the following questionnaire supplements: health promotion and disease prevention (1990–91), cancer control and cancer epidemiology (1992), and year 2000 (1995). Starting in 1997 data are from the sample adult questionnaire.

Table 62 (page 1 of 2). Use of selected substances in the past month by persons 12 years of age and over, according to age, sex, race, and Hispanic origin: United States, selected years 1979–98

[Data are based on household interviews of a sample of the population 12 years of age and over]

Substance, age, sex, race, and Hispanic origin	1979	1985	1990	1991	1992	1993	1994	1995	1996	1997	1998
Alcohol					Percent of population						
12 years and over	63	60	53	52	49	51	54	52	51	51	52
12–17 years	50	41	33	27	21	24	22	21	19	21	19
12–13 years	---	---	---	---	---	---	9	8	5	7	5
14–15 years	---	---	---	---	---	---	22	21	19	21	21
16–17 years	---	---	---	---	---	---	36	34	31	33	32
18–25 years	75	70	63	63	59	59	63	61	60	58	60
26–34 years	72	71	64	63	62	64	65	63	62	60	61
35 years and over	60	58	50	50	47	50	54	53	52	53	53
12–17 years:											
Male	52	44	34	30	22	24	22	22	19	21	19
Female	47	38	31	24	19	23	21	20	18	20	19
White, non-Hispanic	53	46	37	27	22	26	24	23	20	22	21
Black, non-Hispanic	---	30	21	28	18	18	18	15	15	16	13
Hispanic[1]	---	27	24	28	20	22	18	19	20	19	19
18–25 years:											
Male	---	---	---	---	---	---	71	68	67	66	68
Female	---	---	---	---	---	---	55	55	54	51	52
White, non-Hispanic	---	---	---	---	---	---	68	67	65	64	65
Black, non-Hispanic	---	---	---	---	---	---	52	48	50	47	50
Hispanic[1]	---	---	---	---	---	---	54	49	50	49	51
Binge alcohol[2]											
12 years and over	---	20	14	16	15	15	17	16	15	15	16
12–17 years	---	22	15	13	10	11	8	8	7	8	8
12–13 years	---	---	---	---	---	---	2	2	1	1	1
14–15 years	---	---	---	---	---	---	8	8	6	8	8
16–17 years	---	---	---	---	---	---	16	15	15	16	15
18–25 years	---	34	30	31	30	29	34	30	32	28	32
26–34 years	---	28	21	22	23	22	24	24	23	23	22
35 years and over	---	13	8	10	9	10	12	12	11	12	12
12–17 years:											
Male	---	29	19	17	13	15	9	9	9	10	9
Female	---	14	12	9	7	7	7	6	6	7	7
White, non-Hispanic	---	26	18	16	11	13	10	9	8	9	9
Black, non-Hispanic	---	6	*	6	6	3	3	3	4	4	3
Hispanic[1]	---	15	11	11	9	12	5	7	8	7	6
18–25 years:											
Male	---	---	---	---	---	---	47	41	44	39	43
Female	---	---	---	---	---	---	21	19	21	17	21
White, non-Hispanic	---	---	---	---	---	---	40	34	37	33	38
Black, non-Hispanic	---	---	---	---	---	---	17	16	19	13	16
Hispanic[1]	---	---	---	---	---	---	26	23	25	22	25

See footnotes at end of table.

Table 62 (page 2 of 2). Use of selected substances in the past month by persons 12 years of age and over, according to age, sex, race, and Hispanic origin: United States, selected years 1979–98

[Data are based on household interviews of a sample of the population 12 years of age and over]

Substance, age, sex, race, and Hispanic origin	1979	1985	1990	1991	1992	1993	1994	1995	1996	1997	1998
Marijuana						Percent of population					
12 years and over	13	10	5	5	5	5	5	5	5	5	5
12–17 years	14	10	4	4	3	4	6	8	7	9	8
12–13 years	---	---	---	---	---	---	2	2	1	3	2
14–15 years	---	---	---	---	---	---	5	10	7	9	9
16–17 years	---	---	---	---	---	---	12	13	13	16	15
18–25 years	36	22	13	13	11	11	12	12	13	13	14
26–34 years	20	19	10	8	9	8	7	7	6	6	6
35 years and over	3	3	2	3	2	2	2	2	2	3	3
12–17 years:											
Male	16	11	5	4	4	4	7	9	8	10	9
Female	12	9	4	3	3	4	5	7	7	8	8
White, non-Hispanic	16	12	5	4	4	4	6	8	7	10	9
Black, non-Hispanic	10	6	2	3	2	3	6	8	7	9	8
Hispanic[1]	8	6	3	3	3	4	6	8	7	8	8
18–25 years:											
Male	---	---	---	---	---	---	16	15	17	17	17
Female	---	---	---	---	---	---	9	9	9	8	10
White, non-Hispanic	---	---	---	---	---	---	13	13	14	13	15
Black, non-Hispanic	---	---	---	---	---	---	12	12	14	14	15
Hispanic[1]	---	---	---	---	---	---	8	7	8	8	9
Cocaine											
12 years and over	2.6	3.0	0.9	1.0	0.7	0.7	0.7	0.7	0.8	0.7	0.8
12–17 years	1.5	1.5	0.6	0.4	0.3	0.4	0.3	0.8	0.6	1.0	0.8
18–25 years	9.9	8.1	2.3	2.2	2.0	1.6	1.2	1.3	2.0	1.2	2.0
26–34 years	3.0	6.3	1.9	1.9	1.5	1.0	1.3	1.2	1.5	0.9	1.2
35 years and over	0.2	0.5	0.2	0.5	0.2	0.4	0.4	0.4	0.4	0.5	0.5
12–17 years:											
Male	2.2	1.9	0.8	0.5	0.3	0.5	0.3	0.8	0.4	0.9	0.6
Female	0.8	1.1	0.5	0.3	0.3	0.4	0.3	0.7	0.8	1.1	1.0
White, non-Hispanic	1.4	1.5	0.4	0.3	0.2	0.4	0.3	0.9	0.5	1.1	0.9
Black, non-Hispanic	*	1.3	0.8	0.5	0.3	0.3	0.1	0.1	0.1	0.1	*
Hispanic[1]	2.1	2.6	2.0	1.4	1.3	1.1	0.8	0.8	1.1	1.0	1.4
18–25 years:											
Male	---	---	---	---	---	---	1.9	1.7	2.7	1.9	2.6
Female	---	---	---	---	---	---	0.6	0.9	1.4	0.5	1.3
White, non-Hispanic	---	---	---	---	---	---	1.2	1.5	2.3	1.2	2.2
Black, non-Hispanic	---	---	---	---	---	---	0.7	0.7	1.1	0.9	0.6
Hispanic[1]	---	---	---	---	---	---	2.2	1.1	2.1	1.5	2.7

- - - Data not available.
* Estimates with relative standard error greater than 17.5 percent of the log transformation of the proportion are not shown.
[1]Persons of Hispanic origin may be of any race.
[2]Five or more drinks on the same occasion at least once in the past month.

NOTES: In 1994 the survey underwent major changes. Estimates for 1993 and earlier years are adjusted to be comparable with data from the redesigned survey. See Appendix I, Substance Abuse and Mental Health Services Administration. Estimates of the use of substances from the National Household Survey on Drug Abuse and the Monitoring the Future Study differ because of different methodologies, sampling frames, and tabulation categories. Data for additional years are available (see Appendix III).

SOURCES: Substance Abuse and Mental Health Services Administration, Office of Applied Studies. H–9 National Household Survey on Drug Abuse: Population Estimates 1998; H–10 Summary of Findings from the 1998 National Household Survey on Drug Abuse; and H–11 National Household Survey on Drug Abuse Main Findings 1998.

Table 63 (page 1 of 2). Use of selected substances by high school seniors and eighth-graders, according to sex and race: United States, selected years 1980–99

[Data are based on a survey of high school seniors and eighth-graders in the coterminous United States]

Substance, sex, race, and grade in school	1980	1985	1990	1991	1992	1993	1994	1995	1996	1997	1998	1999
Cigarettes				Percent using substance in the past month								
All seniors	30.5	30.1	29.4	28.3	27.8	29.9	31.2	33.5	34.0	36.5	35.1	34.6
Male	26.8	28.2	29.1	29.0	29.2	30.7	32.9	34.5	34.9	37.3	36.3	35.4
Female	33.4	31.4	29.2	27.5	26.1	28.7	29.2	32.0	32.4	35.2	33.3	33.5
White	31.0	31.7	32.5	31.8	31.8	34.6	35.9	37.3	38.9	42.5	41.0	39.1
Black	25.2	18.7	12.0	9.4	8.2	10.9	11.0	15.0	13.5	14.9	14.9	14.9
All eighth-graders	---	---	---	14.3	15.5	16.7	18.6	19.1	21.0	19.4	19.1	17.5
Male	---	---	---	15.5	14.9	17.2	19.3	18.8	20.6	19.1	18.0	16.7
Female	---	---	---	13.1	15.9	16.3	17.9	19.0	21.1	19.5	19.8	17.7
White	---	---	---	15.0	17.4	18.1	19.8	21.7	23.8	22.0	21.1	19.0
Black	---	---	---	5.3	5.3	7.7	9.6	8.2	11.3	10.4	10.8	10.7
Marijuana												
All seniors	33.7	25.7	14.0	13.8	11.9	15.5	19.0	21.2	21.9	23.7	22.8	23.1
Male	37.8	28.7	16.1	16.1	13.4	18.2	23.0	24.6	25.1	26.4	26.5	26.3
Female	29.1	22.4	11.5	11.2	10.2	12.5	15.1	17.2	18.3	20.3	18.8	19.7
White	34.2	26.4	15.6	15.0	13.1	16.7	20.1	21.5	22.5	24.6	24.2	23.4
Black	26.5	21.7	5.2	6.5	5.6	10.8	15.9	17.8	18.8	18.2	18.3	20.4
All eighth-graders	---	---	---	3.2	3.7	5.1	7.8	9.1	11.3	10.2	9.7	9.7
Male	---	---	---	3.8	3.8	6.1	9.5	9.8	12.1	11.4	10.3	10.5
Female	---	---	---	2.6	3.5	4.1	6.0	8.2	10.2	8.9	8.8	8.8
White	---	---	---	3.0	3.5	4.6	6.7	9.0	11.0	10.2	8.9	8.5
Black	---	---	---	2.1	1.9	3.7	6.2	7.0	9.3	8.7	9.4	10.0
Cocaine												
All seniors	5.2	6.7	1.9	1.4	1.3	1.3	1.5	1.8	2.0	2.3	2.4	2.6
Male	6.0	7.7	2.3	1.7	1.5	1.7	1.9	2.2	2.6	2.8	3.0	3.3
Female	4.3	5.6	1.3	0.9	0.9	0.9	1.1	1.3	1.4	1.6	1.7	1.8
White	5.4	7.0	1.8	1.3	1.2	1.2	1.5	1.7	2.1	2.4	2.7	2.8
Black	2.0	2.7	0.5	0.8	0.5	0.4	0.6	0.4	0.4	0.7	0.4	0.5
All eighth-graders	---	---	---	0.5	0.7	0.7	1.0	1.2	1.3	1.1	1.4	1.3
Male	---	---	---	0.7	0.6	0.9	1.2	1.1	1.2	1.2	1.5	1.4
Female	---	---	---	0.4	0.8	0.6	0.9	1.2	1.4	1.0	1.2	1.2
White	---	---	---	0.4	0.6	0.5	0.9	1.0	1.4	1.0	1.0	1.1
Black	---	---	---	0.4	0.4	0.3	0.3	0.4	0.4	0.3	0.6	0.3
Inhalants												
All seniors	1.4	2.2	2.7	2.4	2.3	2.5	2.7	3.2	2.5	2.5	2.3	2.0
Male	1.8	2.8	3.5	3.3	3.0	3.2	3.6	3.9	3.1	3.3	2.9	2.5
Female	1.0	1.7	2.0	1.6	1.6	1.7	1.9	2.5	2.0	1.8	1.7	1.5
White	1.4	2.4	3.0	2.4	2.4	2.7	2.9	3.7	2.9	3.1	2.6	2.1
Black	1.0	0.8	1.5	1.5	1.5	1.3	1.8	1.1	0.9	0.9	1.0	0.4
All eighth-graders	---	---	---	4.4	4.7	5.4	5.6	6.1	5.8	5.6	4.8	5.0
Male	---	---	---	4.1	4.4	4.9	5.4	5.6	4.8	5.1	4.8	4.6
Female	---	---	---	4.7	4.9	6.0	5.8	6.6	6.6	5.8	4.7	5.3
White	---	---	---	4.5	5.0	5.8	6.1	7.0	6.6	6.4	5.3	5.6
Black	---	---	---	2.3	2.4	2.9	2.6	2.3	1.7	2.2	2.2	2.3

See footnotes at end of table.

Table 63 (page 2 of 2). Use of selected substances by high school seniors and eighth-graders, according to sex and race: United States, selected years 1980–99

[Data are based on a survey of high school seniors and eighth-graders in the coterminous United States]

Substance, sex, race, and grade in school	1980	1985	1990	1991	1992	1993	1994	1995	1996	1997	1998	1999
Alcohol[1]				Percent using substance in the past month								
All seniors	72.0	65.9	57.1	54.0	51.3	48.6	50.1	51.3	50.8	52.7	52.0	51.0
Male	77.4	69.8	61.3	58.4	55.8	54.2	55.5	55.7	54.8	56.2	57.6	55.3
Female	66.8	62.1	52.3	49.0	46.8	43.4	45.2	47.0	46.9	48.9	46.9	46.8
White	75.8	70.2	62.2	57.7	56.0	53.4	54.8	54.8	54.7	57.9	57.6	54.9
Black	47.7	43.6	32.9	34.4	29.5	35.1	33.1	37.4	35.7	33.1	33.6	30.8
All eighth-graders	---	---	---	25.1	26.1	24.3	25.5	24.6	26.2	24.5	23.0	24.0
Male	---	---	---	26.3	26.3	25.3	26.5	25.0	26.6	25.2	24.0	24.8
Female	---	---	---	23.8	25.9	28.7	24.7	24.0	25.8	23.9	21.9	23.3
White	---	---	---	26.0	27.3	25.1	25.4	25.4	27.7	25.7	24.0	25.6
Black	---	---	---	17.8	19.2	17.7	20.2	17.3	19.0	16.9	15.4	16.8
Binge drinking[2]				Percent in last 2 weeks								
All seniors	41.2	36.7	32.2	29.8	27.9	27.5	28.2	29.8	30.2	31.3	31.5	30.8
Male	52.1	45.3	39.1	37.8	35.6	34.6	37.0	36.9	37.0	37.9	39.2	38.1
Female	30.5	28.2	24.4	21.2	20.3	20.7	20.2	23.0	23.5	24.4	24.0	23.6
White	44.6	40.1	36.2	32.9	31.3	31.3	31.7	32.9	34.0	36.1	36.6	34.8
Black	17.0	16.7	11.6	11.8	10.8	14.6	14.2	15.5	15.1	12.0	12.7	11.9
All eighth-graders	---	---	---	12.9	13.4	13.5	14.5	14.5	15.6	14.5	13.7	15.2
Male	---	---	---	14.3	13.9	14.8	16.0	15.1	16.5	15.3	14.4	16.4
Female	---	---	---	11.4	12.8	12.3	13.0	13.9	14.5	13.5	12.7	13.9
White	---	---	---	12.6	12.9	12.4	13.4	14.5	15.7	14.6	13.5	15.2
Black	---	---	---	9.9	9.3	11.9	11.8	10.0	10.9	8.8	9.1	10.8

- - - Data not available.

[1]In 1993 the alcohol question was changed to indicate that a "drink" meant "more than a few sips." 1993 data based on a half sample.
[2]Five or more alcoholic drinks in a row at least once in the prior 2-week period.

NOTES: Monitoring the Future Study excludes high school dropouts (see Appendix I) and absentees (about 16–17 percent of high school seniors, about 9–10 percent of eighth-graders). High school dropouts and absentees have higher drug usage than those included in the survey. Estimates of the use of substances from the National Household Survey on Drug Abuse and the Monitoring the Future Study differ because of different methodologies, sampling frames, and tabulation categories. See Appendix I. Data for additional years are available (see Appendix III).

SOURCE: National Institute on Drug Abuse. Monitoring the Future Study. Annual surveys.

Table 64. Cocaine-related emergency department episodes, according to age, sex, race, and Hispanic origin: United States, selected years 1990–97

[Data are weighted national estimates based on a sample of emergency departments]

Age, sex, race, and Hispanic origin	1990	1991	1992	1993	1994	1995	1996	1997
All races, both sexes[1]				Number of episodes				
All ages[2]	80,355	101,189	119,843	123,423	142,878	135,801	152,433	161,087
6–17 years	1,877	2,210	1,546	1,578	2,068	2,058	2,595	3,642
18–25 years	19,614	21,766	23,883	22,159	25,392	21,116	22,065	25,220
26–34 years	35,639	46,137	52,760	52,658	60,500	54,953	58,732	57,143
35 years and over	23,054	30,582	41,288	46,614	54,238	57,348	68,723	74,602
White, non-Hispanic male								
All ages[2]	15,512	19,385	21,360	21,193	27,216	25,634	28,647	32,780
6–17 years	527	486	264	371	409	493	604	898
18–25 years	3,810	5,284	5,297	5,155	5,877	5,458	4,968	6,466
26–34 years	6,724	8,777	9,175	8,828	11,908	10,426	11,406	11,697
35 years and over	4,432	4,747	6,585	6,818	8,985	9,228	11,647	13,465
Black, non-Hispanic male								
All ages[2]	27,745	36,597	46,064	46,218	51,622	48,875	51,687	54,257
6–17 years	241	244	246	213	273	304	348	388
18–25 years	5,104	5,743	6,308	5,661	6,698	4,735	3,886	4,725
26–34 years	12,160	16,232	19,952	18,542	20,978	18,756	18,559	18,052
35 years and over	10,202	14,110	19,416	21,709	23,533	25,019	28,742	30,850
Hispanic male[3]								
All ages[2]	4,821	6,571	8,683	9,195	9,566	7,889	12,577	11,540
6–17 years	144	201	336	206	518	181	431	402
18–25 years	1,774	1,831	2,535	2,184	2,165	1,892	3,725	3,467
26–34 years	1,758	2,723	3,457	3,893	3,652	2,904	4,342	3,575
35 years and over	1,125	1,801	2,332	2,885	3,222	2,907	4,056	4,077
White, non-Hispanic female								
All ages[2]	8,331	9,541	10,132	11,263	13,230	13,634	15,594	17,595
6–17 years	486	529	204	323	357	495	542	1,021
18–25 years	2,663	2,765	2,817	2,832	3,400	2,966	3,344	3,742
26–34 years	3,636	4,427	4,571	5,472	5,905	6,041	6,540	6,771
35 years and over	1,539	1,808	2,531	2,562	3,566	4,126	5,156	6,045
Black, non-Hispanic female								
All ages[2]	14,833	19,149	22,687	22,186	25,066	24,138	25,713	27,298
6–17 years	177	210	100	134	102	153	89	100
18–25 years	3,820	3,892	4,247	3,674	3,908	3,307	2,803	3,407
26–34 years	7,418	9,481	11,078	10,381	11,551	10,831	11,082	11,004
35 years and over	3,369	5,512	7,198	7,953	9,472	9,823	11,712	12,752
Hispanic female[3]								
All ages[2]	1,719	2,356	3,074	3,466	3,595	3,519	5,044	5,063
6–17 years	64	183	193	166	79	131	250	675
18–25 years	634	616	815	697	955	901	1,297	1,287
26–34 years	663	1,044	1,324	1,529	1,559	1,280	2,116	1,698
35 years and over	357	513	732	1,072	998	1,203	1,378	1,402

[1]Includes other races and unknown race, Hispanic origin, and/or sex.
[2]Includes unknown age.
[3]Persons of Hispanic origin may be of any race.

SOURCE: Substance Abuse and Mental Health Services Administration, Office of Applied Studies, Drug Abuse Warning Network.

Table 65 (page 1 of 2). Alcohol consumption by persons 18 years of age and over, according to sex, race, Hispanic origin, and age: United States, 1997 and 1998

[Data are based on household interviews of a sample of the civilian noninstitutionalized population]

Alcohol consumption, race, Hispanic origin, and age	Both sexes		Male		Female	
	1997	1998	1997	1998	1997	1998
Drinking status[1]			Percent distribution			
All	100.0	100.0	100.0	100.0	100.0	100.0
Lifetime Abstainer	21.1	21.8	14.0	14.5	27.7	28.5
Former drinker	15.5	15.9	15.6	16.2	15.4	15.7
Infrequent	8.9	9.0	7.5	7.4	10.1	10.5
Regular.	6.6	6.9	8.1'	8.8	5.2	5.1
Current drinker	63.4	62.3	70.5	69.3	57.0	55.8
Infrequent	15.0	14.6	11.7	11.0	18.1	17.8
Regular.	48.4	47.7	58.8	58.3	38.8	38.0
Race, Hispanic origin, and age[2]			Percent current drinkers among all persons			
All persons:						
18–44 years.	69.4	68.7	74.8	74.4	64.2	63.1
18–24 years	62.2	60.6	66.7	67.6	57.7	53.5
25–44 years	71.6	71.2	77.2	76.5	66.1	66.0
45 years and over	56.0	54.5	64.7	62.7	48.5	47.5
45–64 years	63.3	61.7	70.8	68.4	56.2	55.4
65 years and over	43.4	41.8	52.7	51.2	36.6	35.0
White, non-Hispanic:						
18–44 years.	75.0	74.5	78.5	78.1	71.4	70.9
18–24 years	69.6	68.2	72.8	73.6	66.5	62.7
25–44 years	76.4	76.2	80.1	79.4	72.8	73.1
45 years and over	58.8	57.2	66.4	64.1	52.2	51.3
45–64 years	66.9	65.1	72.9	70.1	61.2	60.4
65 years and over	45.9	44.3	54.6	52.8	39.5	38.0
Black, non-Hispanic:						
18–44 years.	54.9	53.7	60.9	60.7	49.8	47.9
18–24 years	46.4	38.5	51.4	46.6	42.1	31.6
25–44 years	57.7	59.1	64.3	65.8	52.4	53.6
45 years and over	40.6	41.3	53.7	53.6	30.8	32.2
45–64 years	47.4	48.1	58.7	60.5	38.3	38.5
65 years and over	26.3	26.6	41.7	37.4	16.4	19.7
Hispanic:[2]						
18–44 years.	59.8	58.3	71.7	71.1	46.5	44.1
18–24 years	51.6	53.2	61.6	64.5	40.1	40.4
25–44 years	62.9	60.3	75.7	73.6	48.9	45.5
45 years and over	47.5	46.2	58.7	61.2	37.8	33.0
45–64 years	53.9	52.1	65.5	65.5	43.2	39.4
65 years and over	31.4	30.9	39.2	48.5	25.7	18.1
Level of alcohol consumption in past year for current drinkers[3]			Percent distribution of current drinkers			
All drinking levels.	100.0	100.0	100.0	100.0	100.0	100.0
Light.	69.8	69.8	59.6	59.5	81.4	81.4
Moderate	22.3	22.8	31.7	32.4	11.7	12.0
Heavier.	7.9	7.4	8.8	8.1	6.9	6.6
Number of days in the past year with 5 or more drinks			Percent distribution of current drinkers			
All current drinkers.	100.0	100.0	100.0	100.0	100.0	100.0
No days	65.9	67.2	54.7	56.3	78.6	79.3
At least 1 day	34.1	32.8	45.3	43.7	21.4	20.7
1–11 days	18.5	18.5	22.0	22.3	14.6	14.2
12 or more days.	15.6	14.3	23.4	21.4	6.8	6.4

See footnotes at end of table.

Table 65 (page 2 of 2). Alcohol consumption by persons 18 years of age and over, according to sex, race, Hispanic origin, and age: United States, 1997 and 1998

[Data are based on household interviews of a sample of the civilian noninstitutionalized population]

Alcohol consumption, race, Hispanic origin, and age	Both sexes		Male		Female	
	1997	1998	1997	1998	1997	1998
Race, Hispanic origin, and age[2]	Percent of persons with 5 or more drinks on at least one day among current drinkers					
All persons:						
18–44 years..........................	42.4	41.0	54.6	52.7	28.7	27.9
18–24 years.........................	51.6	53.2	61.5	62.0	40.2	42.3
25–44 years.........................	40.0	37.8	52.8	50.1	25.7	24.5
45 years and over	21.3	20.4	31.0	30.0	10.3	9.6
45–64 years........................	25.3	24.5	36.1	35.6	12.9	12.0
65 years and over...................	11.2	9.7	17.8	15.4	4.4	3.6
White, non-Hispanic:						
18–44 years..........................	44.6	43.2	57.5	55.4	30.8	30.2
18–24 years.........................	55.1	59.1	65.1	69.1	44.2	47.4
25–44 years.........................	42.0	39.2	55.6	51.8	27.5	26.3
45 years and over	20.4	19.7	30.6	29.7	9.4	9.2
45–64 years........................	24.6	24.2	36.0	35.6	12.0	11.7
65 years and over...................	10.8	9.1	17.6	14.8	3.8	3.2
Black, non-Hispanic:						
18–44 years..........................	26.1	28.2	36.4	38.3	15.8	17.8
45 years and over	22.9	22.6	29.0	30.5	15.2	13.4
Hispanic:[2]						
18–44 years..........................	44.9	39.5	55.4	49.9	27.2	21.5
45 years and over	30.4	30.4	39.9	40.5	17.8	14.3

[1]Drinking status categories are based on self-reported responses to questions about alcohol consumption. See Appendix II, Current drinker. Lifetime abstainers had fewer than 12 drinks in their lifetime. Former drinkers had at least 12 drinks in their lifetime and none in the past year. Former infrequent drinkers are former drinkers who had fewer than 12 drinks in any one year. Former regular drinkers are former drinkers who had at least 12 drinks in any one year. Current drinkers had 12 drinks in their lifetime and at least one drink in the past year. Current infrequent drinkers are current drinkers who had fewer than 12 drinks in the past year. Current regular drinkers are current drinkers who had at least 12 drinks in the past year.

[2]Persons of Hispanic origin may be of any race.

[3]Level of alcohol consumption categories are based on self-reported responses to questions about average alcohol consumption and defined as follows: light drinkers: up to 3 drinks per week; moderate drinkers: 4–14 drinks per week for men and 4–7 drinks per week for women; heavier drinkers: more than 14 drinks per week for men and more than 7 drinks per week for women. (In 2000 most drinking guidelines consider more than 7 drinks per week to be a heavier level of consumption for women.)

SOURCE: Centers for Disease Control and Prevention, National Center for Health Statistics. National Health Interview Survey, sample adult questionnaire.

Table 66. Hypertension among persons 20 years of age and over, according to sex, age, race, and Hispanic origin: United States, 1960–62, 1971–74, 1976–80, and 1988–94

[Data are based on physical examinations of a sample of the civilian noninstitutionalized population]

Sex, age, race, and Hispanic origin[1]	1960–62	1971–74	1976–80[2]	1988–94
20–74 years, age adjusted[3]	Percent of population			
Both sexes[4]	36.9	38.3	39.0	23.1
Male	40.0	42.4	44.0	25.3
Female[4]	33.7	34.3	34.0	20.8
White male	39.3	41.7	43.5	24.3
White female[4]	31.7	32.4	32.3	19.3
Black male	48.1	51.8	48.7	34.9
Black female[4]	50.8	50.3	47.5	33.8
White, non-Hispanic male	- - -	- - -	43.9	24.4
White, non-Hispanic female[4]	- - -	- - -	32.1	19.3
Black, non-Hispanic male	- - -	- - -	48.7	35.0
Black, non-Hispanic female[4]	- - -	- - -	47.6	34.2
Mexican male	- - -	- - -	25.0	25.2
Mexican female[4]	- - -	- - -	21.8	22.0
20–74 years, crude				
Both sexes[4]	39.0	39.7	39.7	23.1
Male	41.7	43.3	44.0	24.7
Female[4]	36.6	36.5	35.6	21.5
White male	41.0	42.8	43.8	24.3
White female[4]	34.9	34.9	34.2	20.4
Black male	50.5	52.1	47.4	31.5
Black female[4]	52.0	50.2	46.1	30.6
White, non-Hispanic male	- - -	- - -	44.3	25.0
White, non-Hispanic female[4]	- - -	- - -	34.4	20.9
Black, non-Hispanic male	- - -	- - -	47.5	31.6
Black, non-Hispanic female[4]	- - -	- - -	46.1	31.2
Mexican male	- - -	- - -	18.8	18.0
Mexican female[4]	- - -	- - -	16.7	15.8
Male				
20–34 years	22.8	24.8	28.9	8.6
35–44 years	37.7	39.1	40.5	20.9
45–54 years	47.6	55.0	53.6	34.1
55–64 years	60.3	62.5	61.8	42.9
65–74 years	68.8	67.2	67.1	57.3
75 years and over	- - -	- - -	- - -	64.2
Female[4]				
20–34 years	9.3	11.2	11.1	3.4
35–44 years	24.0	28.2	28.8	12.7
45–54 years	43.4	43.6	47.1	25.1
55–64 years	66.4	62.5	61.1	44.2
65–74 years	81.5	78.3	71.8	60.8
75 years and over	- - -	- - -	- - -	77.3

- - - Data not available.

[1]The race groups, white and black, include persons of Hispanic and non-Hispanic origin. Conversely, persons of Hispanic origin may be of any race.
[2]Data for Mexicans are for 1982–84. See Appendix I.
[3]See Appendix II for age-adjustment procedure.
[4]Excludes pregnant women.

NOTES: A person with hypertension is defined by either having elevated blood pressure (systolic pressure of at least 140 mmHg or diastolic pressure of at least 90 mmHg) or taking antihypertensive medication. Percents are based on a single measurement of blood pressure to provide comparable data across the 4 time periods. In 1976–80, 31.3 percent of persons 20–74 years of age had hypertension, based on the average of 3 blood pressure measurements, in contrast to 39.7 percent when a single measurement is used.

SOURCE: Centers for Disease Control and Prevention, National Center for Health Statistics, Division of Health Examination Statistics. Unpublished data.

Table 67. Serum cholesterol levels among persons 20 years of age and over, according to sex, age, race, and Hispanic origin: United States, 1960–62, 1971–74, 1976–80, and 1988–94

[Data are based on physical examinations of a sample of the civilian noninstitutionalized population]

Sex, age, race, and Hispanic origin[1]	Percent of population with high serum cholesterol				Mean serum cholesterol level, mg/dL			
	1960–62	1971–74	1976–80[2]	1988–94	1960–62	1971–74	1976–80[2]	1988–94
20–74 years, age adjusted[3]								
Both sexes	31.8	27.2	26.3	18.9	220	214	213	203
Male	28.7	25.8	24.6	17.5	217	213	211	202
Female	34.5	28.2	27.6	20.0	222	215	214	204
White male	29.4	25.9	24.6	17.8	218	213	211	202
White female	35.1	28.1	28.0	20.2	223	215	214	205
Black male	24.5	25.1	24.1	15.7	210	212	208	199
Black female	30.7	29.2	24.9	19.4	216	217	213	203
White, non-Hispanic male	- - -	- - -	24.7	17.3	- - -	- - -	211	202
White, non-Hispanic female	- - -	- - -	28.3	20.2	- - -	- - -	214	205
Black, non-Hispanic male	- - -	- - -	24.0	15.7	- - -	- - -	208	200
Black, non-Hispanic female	- - -	- - -	24.9	19.8	- - -	- - -	214	203
Mexican male	- - -	- - -	18.8	17.8	- - -	- - -	207	204
Mexican female	- - -	- - -	20.0	17.5	- - -	- - -	207	203
20–74 years, crude								
Both sexes	33.6	28.2	26.8	18.7	222	216	213	203
Male	30.7	26.8	24.9	17.6	220	214	211	202
Female	36.3	29.6	28.5	19.9	225	217	215	204
White male	31.4	26.9	25.0	18.1	221	215	211	203
White female	37.5	29.8	29.2	20.5	22⁷	217	216	205
Black male	26.7	25.1	23.9	14.4	214	212	208	198
Black female	29.9	28.8	23.7	16.8	216	216	212	199
White, non-Hispanic male	- - -	- - -	25.1	17.9	- - -	- - -	211	203
White, non-Hispanic female	- - -	- - -	29.8	20.9	- - -	- - -	216	206
Black, non-Hispanic male	- - -	- - -	23.7	14.5	- - -	- - -	208	198
Black, non-Hispanic female	- - -	- - -	23.7	17.2	- - -	- - -	212	200
Mexican male	- - -	- - -	16.6	15.5	- - -	- - -	203	200
Mexican female	- - -	- - -	16.5	14.0	- - -	- - -	202	197
Male								
20–34 years	15.1	12.4	11.9	8.2	198	194	192	186
35–44 years	33.9	31.8	27.9	19.4	227	221	217	206
45–54 years	39.2	37.5	36.9	26.6	231	229	227	216
55–64 years	41.6	36.2	36.8	28.0	233	229	229	216
65–74 years	38.0	34.7	31.7	21.9	230	226	221	212
75 years and over	- - -	- - -	- - -	20.4	- - -	- - -	- - -	205
Female								
20–34 years	12.4	10.9	9.8	7.3	194	191	189	184
35–44 years	23.1	19.3	20.7	12.3	214	207	207	195
45–54 years	46.9	38.7	40.5	26.7	237	232	232	217
55–64 years	70.1	53.1	52.9	40.9	262	245	249	235
65–74 years	68.5	57.7	51.6	41.3	266	250	246	233
75 years and over	- - -	- - -	- - -	38.2	- - -	- - -	- - -	229

- - - Data not available.

[1]The race groups, white and black, include persons of Hispanic and non-Hispanic origin. Conversely, persons of Hispanic origin may be of any race.

[2]Data for Mexicans are for 1982–84. See Appendix I.

[3]See Appendix II for age-adjustment procedure.

NOTES: High serum cholesterol is defined as greater than or equal to 240 mg/dL (6.20 mmol/L). Risk levels have been defined by the Second report of the National Cholesterol Education Program Expert Panel on Detection, Evaluation and Treatment of High Blood Cholesterol in Adults. National Heart, Lung, and Blood Institute, National Institutes of Health. September 1993. (Summarized in *JAMA* 269(23):3015–23. June 16, 1993.)

SOURCE: Centers for Disease Control and Prevention, National Center for Health Statistics, Division of Health Examination Statistics. Unpublished data.

Table 68. Healthy weight, overweight, and obesity among persons 20 years of age and over, according to sex, age, race, and Hispanic origin: United States, 1960–62, 1971–74, 1976–80, and 1988–94

[Data are based on measured height and weight of a sample of the civilian noninstitutionalized population]

Sex, age, race, and Hispanic origin[1]	Healthy weight[2]				Overweight[3]				Obesity[4]			
	1960–62	1971–74	1976–80[5]	1988–94	1960–62	1971–74	1976–80[5]	1988–94	1960–62	1971–74	1976–80[5]	1988–94
20–74 years, age adjusted[6]						Percent of population						
Both sexes[7,8]	50.1	48.2	49.1	41.7	43.5	46.0	46.0	54.6	12.8	14.1	14.5	22.6
Male	48.1	44.0	46.0	39.1	48.4	52.7	51.3	59.4	10.4	11.8	12.2	19.9
Female[7]	52.1	52.2	52.1	44.3	38.6	39.7	40.8	49.9	14.9	16.1	16.5	25.1
White male	47.3	43.5	45.2	38.0	49.1	53.4	52.3	60.5	10.1	11.5	12.0	20.3
White female[7]	54.5	54.3	54.3	46.2	36.1	37.6	38.3	48.0	13.6	14.7	14.9	23.5
Black male	53.6	47.4	48.4	40.2	42.7	49.1	48.4	57.0	13.6	15.9	15.1	20.9
Black female[7]	34.3	34.4	34.0	28.9	56.9	57.6	60.6	66.6	24.8	28.6	30.2	37.6
White, non-Hispanic male	- - -	- - -	45.5	38.7	- - -	- - -	52.0	59.9	- - -	- - -	11.9	20.1
White, non-Hispanic female[7]	- - -	- - -	54.9	48.0	- - -	- - -	37.6	45.7	- - -	- - -	14.8	22.5
Black, non-Hispanic male	- - -	- - -	48.5	40.0	- - -	- - -	48.3	57.2	- - -	- - -	15.0	21.1
Black, non-Hispanic female[7]	- - -	- - -	34.4	29.2	- - -	- - -	60.2	66.8	- - -	- - -	29.9	37.7
Mexican male	- - -	- - -	38.3	31.6	- - -	- - -	59.6	67.0	- - -	- - -	15.5	23.1
Mexican female[7]	- - -	- - -	37.0	29.8	- - -	- - -	60.1	67.8	- - -	- - -	25.4	34.6
20–74 years, crude												
Both sexes[7,8]	49.0	47.5	48.7	41.4	45.2	47.0	46.4	55.0	13.5	14.4	14.7	22.7
Male	47.1	43.3	45.8	38.8	49.4	53.5	51.5	59.6	10.7	12.0	12.3	19.9
Female[7]	50.7	51.3	51.5	43.9	41.2	41.0	41.6	50.5	16.1	16.7	16.8	25.5
White male	46.3	42.6	45.0	37.5	50.2	54.3	52.5	61.1	10.4	11.7	12.1	20.4
White female[7]	53.0	53.3	53.6	45.4	38.9	39.1	39.4	49.0	14.7	15.4	15.3	24.0
Black male	53.0	47.3	48.3	40.6	43.9	49.3	48.5	56.7	14.1	16.0	15.0	20.9
Black female[7]	33.2	34.2	34.5	29.7	58.8	58.2	60.0	65.9	26.6	28.7	29.8	37.0
White, non-Hispanic male	- - -	- - -	45.3	37.9	- - -	- - -	52.2	60.8	- - -	- - -	12.0	20.3
White, non-Hispanic female[7]	- - -	- - -	54.0	46.9	- - -	- - -	38.9	47.1	- - -	- - -	15.2	23.1
Black, non-Hispanic male	- - -	- - -	48.4	40.4	- - -	- - -	48.4	57.0	- - -	- - -	14.9	21.1
Black, non-Hispanic female[7]	- - -	- - -	35.0	29.9	- - -	- - -	59.4	66.2	- - -	- - -	29.5	37.2
Mexican male	- - -	- - -	41.0	34.4	- - -	- - -	57.0	64.0	- - -	- - -	14.6	20.7
Mexican female[7]	- - -	- - -	39.4	31.2	- - -	- - -	57.4	66.2	- - -	- - -	23.8	33.6
Male												
20–34 years	54.2	53.9	55.7	50.3	42.7	42.8	41.2	47.5	9.2	9.7	8.9	14.1
35–44 years	44.1	34.5	40.5	33.3	53.5	63.2	57.2	65.5	12.1	13.5	13.5	21.5
45–54 years	43.9	36.7	37.9	33.5	53.9	59.7	60.2	66.1	12.5	13.7	16.7	23.2
55–64 years	43.5	38.1	37.9	28.1	52.2	58.5	60.2	70.5	9.2	14.1	14.1	27.2
65–74 years	44.0	41.4	41.1	29.8	47.8	54.6	54.2	68.5	10.4	10.9	13.2	24.1
75 years and over	- - -	- - -	- - -	40.6	- - -	- - -	- - -	56.5	- - -	- - -	- - -	13.2
Female[7]												
20–34 years	62.6	61.7	61.0	54.3	21.2	25.8	27.9	37.0	7.2	9.7	11.0	18.5
35–44 years	56.2	53.5	53.4	45.5	37.2	40.5	40.7	49.6	14.7	17.7	17.8	25.5
45–54 years	46.1	47.7	47.2	35.6	49.3	49.0	48.7	60.3	20.3	18.9	19.6	32.4
55–64 years	37.2	39.2	42.7	31.2	59.9	54.5	53.7	66.3	24.4	24.1	22.9	33.7
65–74 years	35.5	39.6	36.5	36.0	60.9	55.9	59.5	60.3	23.2	22.0	21.5	26.9
75 years and over	- - -	- - -	- - -	41.0	- - -	- - -	- - -	52.3	- - -	- - -	- - -	19.2

- - - Data not available.

[1]The race groups, white and black, include persons of Hispanic and non-Hispanic origin.
[2]Body mass index (BMI) of 19 to less than 25 kilograms/meter^2 (see Appendix II, Body mass index).
[3]BMI greater than or equal to 25.
[4]BMI greater than or equal to 30.
[5]Data for Mexicans are for 1982–84. See Appendix I.
[6]See Appendix II for age-adjustment procedure.
[7]Excludes pregnant women.
[8]Includes persons of all races and Hispanic origins, not just those shown separately.

NOTES: Percents do not sum to 100 because the percent of persons with BMI less than 19 is not shown and the percent of persons with obesity is a subset of the percent with overweight. Height was measured without shoes; two pounds are deducted from data for 1960–62 to allow for weight of clothing.

SOURCE: Centers for Disease Control and Prevention, National Center for Health Statistics, Division of Health Examination Statistics. Unpublished data.

Table 69. Overweight children and adolescents 6–17 years of age, according to sex, age, race, and Hispanic origin: United States, selected years 1963–65 through 1988–94

[Data are based on physical examinations of a sample of the civilian noninstitutionalized population]

Age, sex, race, and Hispanic origin[1]	1963–65 1966–70[2]	1971–74	1976–80[3]	1988–94[4]
6–11 years of age, age adjusted		Percent of population		
Both sexes	5.0	5.5	7.6	13.6
Boys	4.9	6.5	8.1	14.7
White	5.4	6.6	8.1	14.6
Black	1.7	5.6	8.6	15.1
White, non-Hispanic	- - -	- - -	7.4	13.1
Black, non-Hispanic	- - -	- - -	8.6	14.7
Mexican	- - -	- - -	14.5	18.8
Girls	5.2	4.4	7.1	12.6
White	5.1	4.4	6.5	11.7
Black	5.3	4.5	11.5	17.4
White, non-Hispanic	- - -	- - -	6.2	11.9
Black, non-Hispanic	- - -	- - -	11.6	17.7
Mexican	- - -	- - -	10.7	15.8
12–17 years of age, age adjusted				
Both sexes	5.0	6.2	5.6	11.4
Boys	5.0	5.3	5.3	12.4
White	5.2	5.5	5.3	13.1
Black	3.6	4.4	6.0	12.1
White, non-Hispanic	- - -	- - -	4.5	11.8
Black, non-Hispanic	- - -	- - -	6.1	12.5
Mexican	- - -	- - -	7.7	14.8
Girls[5]	5.0	7.2	6.0	10.5
White	4.8	6.6	5.4	10.0
Black	6.4	10.5	10.2	16.1
White, non-Hispanic	- - -	- - -	5.4	9.3
Black, non-Hispanic	- - -	- - -	10.5	16.0
Mexican	- - -	- - -	9.3	14.1
Boys				
6–8 years	5.1	6.3	8.1	15.4
9–11 years	4.8	6.7	8.1	14.0
12–14 years	5.2	5.4	5.4	11.5
15–17 years	4.8	5.2	5.1	13.1
Girls[5]				
6–8 years	5.1	4.1	7.1	14.6
9–11 years	5.2	4.7	7.1	10.8
12–14 years	5.0	8.6	7.8	13.9
15–17 years	4.9	6.0	4.5	7.5

- - - Data not available.

[1]The race groups, white and black, include persons of Hispanic and non-Hispanic origin. Conversely, persons of Hispanic origin may be of any race.
[2]Data for children 6–11 years of age are for 1963–65; data for adolescents 12–17 years of age are for 1966–70.
[3]Data for Mexicans are for 1982–84. See Appendix I.
[4]Excludes one non-Hispanic white adolescent boy age 12–14 years with an outlier sample weight.
[5]Excludes pregnant women starting with 1971–74. Pregnancy status not available for 1963–65/1966–70.

NOTES: Overweight is defined as body mass index (BMI) at or above the sex- and age-specific 95th percentile BMI cutoff points calculated at 6-month age intervals for children 6–11 years of age from the 1963–65 National Health Examination Survey (NHES) and for adolescents 12–17 years of age from the 1966–70 NHES. Age is at time of examination at mobile examination center. See Appendix II for age-adjustment procedure.

SOURCE: Centers for Disease Control and Prevention, National Center for Health Statistics, Division of Health Examination Statistics. Unpublished data.

Table 70. Persons residing in counties that met national ambient air quality standards throughout the year, by race and Hispanic origin: United States, 1988–96

[Data are based on air quality measurements in counties with monitoring devices]

Type of pollutant, race, and Hispanic origin	1988	1989	1990	1991	1992	1993	1994	1995	1996
All pollutants				Percent of population					
All persons	49.7	65.3	71.0	65.2	78.4	76.5	75.1	67.9	81.3
White	---	---	71.8	66.0	79.1	76.9	76.4	69.7	81.9
Black	---	---	71.5	63.4	76.5	75.2	70.4	59.4	80.8
American Indian or Alaska Native	---	---	76.8	75.2	83.0	82.4	80.0	77.9	83.2
Asian or Pacific Islander	---	---	49.6	46.7	64.4	62.8	55.6	48.2	64.4
Hispanic	---	---	49.3	45.2	56.8	57.7	54.8	44.5	56.3
Ozone									
All persons	53.6	72.6	76.3	71.9	81.9	79.5	79.9	71.6	83.3
White	---	---	76.9	72.7	82.7	79.9	80.0	73.0	83.9
Black	---	---	77.0	69.7	79.8	79.3	75.4	66.1	82.9
American Indian or Alaska Native	---	---	83.0	84.8	88.4	85.5	84.3	81.2	99.9
Asian or Pacific Islander	---	---	58.0	55.2	67.0	64.5	58.5	51.4	65.6
Hispanic	---	---	57.1	53.4	61.2	60.2	58.3	48.5	59.7
Carbon monoxide									
All persons	87.8	86.2	90.8	92.0	94.3	95.4	93.9	95.2	94.9
White	---	---	91.0	92.3	94.4	95.6	94.3	96.4	95.1
Black	---	---	93.4	93.5	95.5	96.0	92.6	96.1	96.0
American Indian or Alaska Native	---	---	88.7	89.9	92.9	95.1	93.2	94.2	93.8
Asian or Pacific Islander	---	---	73.7	78.0	84.7	85.8	84.6	85.9	85.5
Hispanic	---	---	72.5	75.6	79.8	82.2	81.4	82.6	80.9
Particulates (PM–10)[1]									
All persons	89.4	88.8	92.6	91.9	89.6	97.5	94.8	90.2	97.1
White	---	---	92.7	92.1	90.2	97.6	95.6	91.0	97.1
Black	---	---	94.2	93.6	87.9	96.8	94.0	87.1	96.8
American Indian or Alaska Native	---	---	92.4	90.6	89.9	97.4	96.2	90.4	96.8
Asian or Pacific Islander	---	---	82.7	80.8	79.3	98.5	93.2	80.7	96.9
Hispanic	---	---	76.1	76.3	71.3	97.4	91.0	75.2	92.7
Sulfur dioxide									
All persons	99.3	99.9	99.4	97.9	100.0	99.4	100.0	100.0	99.9
White	---	---	99.4	98.3	100.0	99.4	100.0	100.0	99.9
Black	---	---	99.5	95.6	100.0	99.5	100.0	100.0	100.0
American Indian or Alaska Native	---	---	99.8	99.4	100.0	100.0	100.0	100.0	100.0
Asian or Pacific Islander	---	---	99.8	97.4	100.0	99.8	100.0	100.0	100.0
Hispanic	---	---	99.9	96.9	100.0	100.0	100.0	100.0	100.0
Nitrogen dioxide									
All persons	96.6	96.5	96.4	96.4	100.0	100.0	100.0	100.0	100.0
White	---	---	96.8	96.8	100.0	100.0	100.0	100.0	100.0
Black	---	---	96.6	96.6	100.0	100.0	100.0	100.0	100.0
American Indian or Alaska Native	---	---	97.2	97.2	100.0	100.0	100.0	100.0	100.0
Asian or Pacific Islander	---	---	86.7	86.7	100.0	100.0	100.0	100.0	100.0
Hispanic	---	---	85.0	85.0	100.0	100.0	100.0	100.0	100.0
Lead									
All persons	99.3	99.4	94.1	94.1	98.1	97.8	98.3	98.1	98.3
White	---	---	94.9	94.8	98.5	98.2	98.7	98.3	98.6
Black	---	---	91.5	91.1	95.3	94.8	95.9	96.2	96.1
American Indian or Alaska Native	---	---	96.4	96.4	99.4	99.3	99.4	99.3	99.4
Asian or Pacific Islander	---	---	85.5	85.5	99.0	98.9	99.1	98.9	99.1
Hispanic	---	---	83.6	84.0	99.4	99.5	99.5	98.9	99.0

- - - Data not available.

[1] Particulate matter smaller than 10 microns.

NOTES: The race groups, white, black, American Indian or Alaska Native, and Asian or Pacific Islander, include persons of Hispanic and non-Hispanic origin. Conversely, persons of Hispanic origin may be of any race. Standard is met if the concentration of the pollutant does not exceed the criterion value more than once per calendar year. See Appendix II, National ambient air quality standards. 1988–89 data based on 1987 county population estimates; 1990–96 data based on 1990 county population estimates.

SOURCES: U.S. Environmental Protection Agency, Aerometric Information Retrieval System; data computed by the National Center for Health Statistics, Division of Health Promotion Statistics from data compiled by the U.S. Environmental Protection Agency, Office of Air Quality and Standards.

[Data are based on household interviews of a sample of the civilian noninstitutionalized population]

| | Number of health care visits[1] | | | | | | | |
| | None | | 1–3 visits | | 4–9 visits | | 10 or more visits | |
Characteristic	1997	1998	1997	1998	1997	1998	1997	1998
	Percent distribution							
All persons[2,3]	16.5	15.9	46.2	46.8	23.6	23.8	13.7	13.5
Age								
Under 18 years	11.8	11.7	54.1	54.5	25.2	25.6	8.9	8.2
Under 6 years	5.0	4.9	44.9	46.7	37.0	36.6	13.0	11.8
6–17 years	15.3	15.0	58.7	58.4	19.3	20.3	6.8	6.3
18–44 years	21.7	21.6	46.7	47.7	19.0	18.6	12.6	12.2
18–24 years	22.0	22.6	46.8	47.7	20.0	18.5	11.2	11.2
25–44 years	21.6	21.3	46.7	47.6	18.7	18.6	13.0	12.5
45–64 years	16.9	15.9	42.9	43.6	24.7	24.3	15.5	16.2
45–54 years	17.9	17.2	43.9	44.9	23.4	22.5	14.8	15.4
55–64 years	15.3	13.8	41.3	41.6	26.7	27.1	16.7	17.5
65 years and over	8.9	7.3	34.7	34.1	32.5	35.3	23.8	23.4
65–74 years	9.8	8.4	36.9	36.6	31.6	34.3	21.6	20.8
75 years and over	7.7	6.0	31.8	30.8	33.8	36.5	26.6	26.7
Sex[3]								
Male	21.3	20.7	47.1	47.3	20.6	21.2	11.0	10.8
Female	11.8	11.3	45.4	46.4	26.5	26.3	16.3	16.0
Race[3,4]								
White	16.0	15.5	46.1	46.8	23.9	24.1	14.0	13.6
Black	16.8	16.4	46.1	46.5	23.2	23.3	13.9	13.8
American Indian or Alaska Native	17.1	20.0	38.0	39.0	24.2	25.1	20.7	15.9
Asian or Pacific Islander	22.8	21.0	49.1	48.2	19.7	21.3	8.3	9.5
Race and Hispanic origin[3]								
White, non-Hispanic	14.7	14.2	46.6	47.1	24.4	24.6	14.3	14.0
Black, non-Hispanic	16.9	16.5	46.1	46.5	23.1	23.2	13.8	13.8
Hispanic[4]	24.9	24.0	42.3	44.8	20.3	19.7	12.5	11.5
Mexican[4]	28.9	28.5	40.8	41.9	18.5	18.6	11.8	11.0
Respondent-assessed health status[3]								
Fair or poor	7.8	9.7	23.3	23.4	29.0	25.3	39.9	41.6
Good to excellent	17.2	16.6	48.4	49.0	23.3	23.7	11.1	10.8
Poverty status[3,5]								
Poor	20.3	20.9	37.1	37.8	22.7	22.8	19.9	18.5
Near poor	19.9	20.0	42.8	41.4	21.8	22.4	15.5	16.2
Nonpoor	14.0	13.4	48.0	48.6	25.0	25.3	13.0	12.7
Race and Hispanic origin and poverty status[3,5]								
White, non-Hispanic:								
Poor	16.3	17.0	37.7	38.2	24.0	24.0	22.1	20.7
Near poor	17.1	17.1	43.7	41.7	22.3	23.2	17.0	18.0
Nonpoor	13.2	12.8	47.6	48.1	25.7	25.7	13.4	13.4
Black, non-Hispanic:								
Poor	17.8	18.0	37.4	37.9	23.3	25.1	21.5	19.1
Near poor	18.9	20.7	43.0	41.6	23.4	22.5	14.7	15.2
Nonpoor	15.6	13.9	50.5	51.0	23.3	24.6	10.6	10.5
Hispanic:[4]								
Poor	30.6	30.8	33.8	36.6	20.0	17.5	15.6	15.1
Near poor	29.1	26.3	39.0	42.4	20.9	20.4	11.0	11.0
Nonpoor	18.7	17.1	48.6	51.4	20.3	22.0	12.3	9.5

See footnotes at end of table.

Utilization of Health Resources

Table 71 (page 2 of 2). **Health care visits to doctor's offices, emergency departments, and home visits within the past 12 months, according to selected characteristics: United States, 1997 and 1998**

[Data are based on household interviews of a sample of the civilian noninstitutionalized population]

Characteristic	Number of health care visits[1]							
	None		1–3 visits		4–9 visits		10 or more visits	
	1997	1998	1997	1998	1997	1998	1997	1998
Health insurance status[6,7]	Percent distribution							
Under 65 years of age:								
Insured	14.3	- - -	49.0	- - -	23.6	- - -	13.1	- - -
Private	14.8	- - -	50.8	- - -	23.0	- - -	11.4	- - -
Medicaid	9.7	- - -	35.0	- - -	27.1	- - -	28.2	- - -
Uninsured	33.7	- - -	42.8	- - -	15.3	- - -	8.2	- - -
65 years of age and over:								
Private	7.4	- - -	36.0	- - -	33.7	- - -	22.9	- - -
Medicaid	10.2	- - -	21.0	- - -	28.1	- - -	40.7	- - -
Medicare only	13.0	- - -	35.0	- - -	31.0	- - -	21.1	- - -
Poverty status and health insurance status[5,6]								
Under 65 years of age:								
Poor:								
Insured	13.7	- - -	38.8	- - -	24.5	- - -	22.9	- - -
Uninsured	36.7	- - -	38.8	- - -	14.9	- - -	9.5	- - -
Near poor:								
Insured	15.6	- - -	45.5	- - -	22.3	- - -	16.6	- - -
Uninsured	34.5	- - -	41.8	- - -	15.6	- - -	8.1	- - -
Nonpoor:								
Insured	13.4	- - -	50.3	- - -	24.2	- - -	12.1	- - -
Uninsured	29.1	- - -	45.4	- - -	17.0	- - -	8.4	- - -
Geographic region[3]								
Northeast	13.2	12.1	45.9	47.8	26.0	25.4	14.9	14.7
Midwest	15.9	15.6	47.7	46.9	22.8	24.2	13.6	13.3
South	17.2	17.0	46.1	46.7	23.3	23.1	13.5	13.2
West	19.1	18.3	44.8	46.0	22.8	22.9	13.3	12.9
Location of residence[3]								
Within MSA[8]	16.2	15.7	46.4	46.9	23.7	23.9	13.7	13.4
Outside MSA[8]	17.3	16.7	45.4	46.2	23.3	23.4	13.9	13.7

- - - Data not available as of publication date.

[1]This table presents a summary measure of ambulatory and home health care visits during a 12-month period based on the following questions: "During the past 12 months, how many times have you gone to a hospital emergency room about your own health?"; "During the past 12 months, did you receive care at home from a nurse or other health care professional? What was the total number of home visits received?"; "During the past 12 months, how many times have you seen a doctor or other health care professional about your own health at a doctor's office, a clinic, or some other place? Do not include times you were hospitalized overnight, visits to hospital emergency rooms, home visits, or telephone calls." For each question respondents were shown a flashcard with response categories of: 0, 1, 2–3, 4–9, 10–12, or 13 or more visits. For this tabulation responses of 2–3 were recoded to 2 and responses of 4–9 were recoded to 6. The summary measure was constructed by adding recoded responses for these questions and categorizing the sum as: none, 1–3, 4–9, or 10 or more health care visits in the past 12 months. See Appendix II, Health care contacts, Emergency department visits, Home visits.
[2]Includes all other races not shown separately, unknown poverty status, and unknown health insurance status.
[3]Estimates are age adjusted to the year 2000 standard using six age groups: Under 18 years, 18–44 years, 45–54 years, 55–64 years, 65–74 years, and 75 years and over. See Appendix II, Age adjustment.
[4]The race groups white, black, American Indian or Alaska Native, and Asian or Pacific Islander include persons of Hispanic and non-Hispanic origin; persons of Hispanic origin may be of any race.
[5]Poverty status is based on family income, family size, number of children in the family, and for families with two or fewer adults the age of the adults in the family using Bureau of the Census poverty thresholds. Poor persons are defined as below the poverty threshold. Near poor persons have incomes of 100 percent to less than 200 percent of poverty threshold. Nonpoor persons have incomes of 200 percent or greater than the poverty threshold. See Appendix II, Poverty level. Poverty status was unknown for 20, percent of persons in the sample in 1997 and 25 percent in 1998.
[6]Estimates for persons under 65 years of age are age adjusted to the year 2000 standard using four age groups: Under 18 years, 18–44 years, 45–54 years, and 55–64 years of age. Estimates for persons 65 years of age and over are age adjusted to the year 2000 standard using two age groups: 65–74 years and 75 years and over. See Appendix II, Age adjustment.
[7]Health insurance categories are mutually exclusive. Persons who reported both Medicaid and private coverage are classified as having Medicaid coverage. See Appendix II, Health insurance coverage.
[8]MSA is metropolitan statistical area.

NOTES: In 1997 the National Health Interview Survey questionnaire was redesigned. See Appendix I, National Health Interview Survey. Data presented in this table are not comparable with data on physician contacts presented in previous editions of Health, United States.

SOURCE: Centers for Disease Control and Prevention, National Center for Health Statistics. National Health Interview Survey, family core and sample adult questionnaires.

Table 72 (page 1 of 2). Interval since last health care contact among adults 18 years of age and over, according to selected characteristics: United States, 1997 and 1998

[Data are based on household interviews of a sample of the civilian noninstitutionalized population]

Characteristic	Total	1 year or less		More than 1 year to 3 years		More than 3 years	
		1997	1998	1997	1998	1997	1998
		Percent distribution[1]					
All adults 18 years of age and over[2,3]	100.0	82.4	83.1	12.0	11.1	5.6	5.8
Age							
18–44 years	100.0	78.8	79.0	14.6	14.1	6.6	6.9
18–24 years	100.0	78.2	78.9	16.1	14.4	5.7	6.8
25–44 years	100.0	78.9	79.1	14.2	14.0	6.9	6.9
45–64 years	100.0	83.6	84.6	11.0	9.6	5.4	5.7
45–54 years	100.0	82.8	83.8	11.7	10.4	5.5	5.9
55–64 years	100.0	84.9	86.0	9.8	8.5	5.3	5.5
65 years and over	100.0	91.6	93.3	5.4	4.2	3.0	2.5
65–74 years	100.0	90.4	92.2	6.1	4.8	3.5	3.0
75 years and over	100.0	93.1	94.7	4.5	3.5	2.3	1.8
Sex[3]							
Male	100.0	75.3	76.5	16.3	14.7	8.4	8.8
Female	100.0	89.3	89.5	7.8	7.6	2.9	2.9
Race[3,4]							
White	100.0	82.8	83.3	11.8	11.0	5.4	5.7
Black	100.0	83.3	84.7	11.2	10.3	5.4	5.0
American Indian or Alaska Native	100.0	80.4	77.2	11.4	13.0	*8.1	9.8
Asian or Pacific Islander	100.0	76.8	78.0	15.9	13.6	7.3	8.4
Race and Hispanic origin[3]							
White, non-Hispanic	100.0	83.9	84.3	11.5	10.8	4.6	5.0
Black, non-Hispanic	100.0	83.2	84.6	11.4	10.4	5.4	4.9
Hispanic[4]	100.0	74.3	76.1	14.2	12.9	11.5	11.0
Mexican[4]	100.0	69.7	70.8	15.3	14.5	15.0	14.7
Poverty status[3,5]							
Poor	100.0	79.4	78.4	12.0	12.6	8.6	9.0
Near poor	100.0	79.0	79.0	12.8	12.7	8.2	8.3
Nonpoor	100.0	84.5	85.3	11.3	10.3	4.2	4.4
Race and Hispanic origin and poverty status[3,5]							
White, non-Hispanic:							
Poor	100.0	83.3	81.1	10.8	12.3	5.8	6.6
Near poor	100.0	81.4	81.4	12.0	11.7	6.7	7.0
Nonpoor	100.0	85.1	85.8	10.9	10.1	4.0	4.2
Black, non-Hispanic:							
Poor	100.0	83.7	84.2	10.2	10.2	6.1	5.6
Near poor	100.0	81.7	80.3	11.8	13.6	6.4	*6.1
Nonpoor	100.0	84.5	86.1	11.2	9.8	4.3	4.1
Hispanic:[4]							
Poor	100.0	67.4	68.4	15.7	15.2	16.9	16.4
Near poor	100.0	69.6	73.1	15.5	14.5	14.9	12.4
Nonpoor	100.0	79.8	82.0	13.7	11.6	6.5	6.4
Health insurance status[6,7]							
18–64 years of age:							
Insured	100.0	84.2	- - -	11.7	- - -	4.1	- - -
Private	100.0	83.5	- - -	12.3	- - -	4.2	- - -
Medicaid	100.0	91.5	- - -	5.2	- - -	3.3	- - -
Uninsured	100.0	63.5	- - -	20.8	- - -	15.8	- - -
65 years of age and over:							
Private	100.0	93.3	- - -	4.6	- - -	2.2	- - -
Medicaid	100.0	91.2	- - -	5.6	- - -	*3.1	- - -
Medicare only	100.0	86.9	- - -	7.8	- - -	5.3	- - -

See footnotes at end of table.

Table 72 (page 2 of 2). Interval since last health care contact among adults 18 years of age and over, according to selected characteristics: United States, 1997 and 1998

[Data are based on household interviews of a sample of the civilian noninstitutionalized population]

Characteristic	Total	1 year or less		More than 1 year to 3 years		More than 3 years	
		1997	1998	1997	1998	1997	1998
Poverty status and health insurance status[5,6]			Percent distribution[1]				
18–64 years of age:							
Poor:							
Insured	100.0	86.5	- - -	9.3	- - -	4.1	- - -
Uninsured	100.0	62.4	- - -	19.2	- - -	18.4	- - -
Near poor:							
Insured	100.0	83.8	- - -	10.6	- - -	5.6	- - -
Uninsured	100.0	61.4	- - -	21.9	- - -	16.6	- - -
Nonpoor:							
Insured	100.0	84.5	- - -	11.8	- - -	3.7	- - -
Uninsured	100.0	66.8	- - -	20.0	- - -	13.3	- - -
Geographic region[3]							
Northeast	100.0	85.6	86.0	10.1	9.3	4.4	4.6
Midwest	100.0	82.8	83.2	12.3	11.4	4.8	5.4
South	100.0	81.9	82.7	12.3	11.3	5.9	6.0
West	100.0	79.7	81.0	12.8	12.0	7.5	7.0
Location of residence[3]							
Within MSA[8]	100.0	82.7	83.4	11.7	10.9	5.6	5.7
Outside MSA[8]	100.0	81.4	82.4	12.9	11.7	5.7	5.9

* Data preceded by an asterisk have a relative standard error of 20–30 percent.

- - - Data not available as of publication date.

[1]Respondents were asked "About how long has it been since you last saw or talked to a doctor or other health care professional about your own health? Include doctors seen while a patient in a hospital." See Appendix II, Health care contacts.

[2]Includes all other races not shown separately, unknown poverty status, and unknown health insurance status.

[3]Estimates are for persons 18 years of age and over and are age adjusted to the year 2000 standard using five age groups: 18–44 years, 45–54 years, 55–64 years, 65–74 years, and 75 years and over. See Appendix II, Age adjustment.

[4]The race groups white, black, American Indian or Alaska Native, and Asian or Pacific Islander include persons of Hispanic and non-Hispanic origin; persons of Hispanic origin may be of any race.

[5]Poverty status is based on family income, family size, number of children in the family, and for families with two or fewer adults the age of the adults in the family using Bureau of the Census poverty thresholds. Poor persons are defined as below the poverty threshold. Near poor persons have incomes of 100 percent to less than 200 percent of poverty threshold. Nonpoor persons have incomes of 200 percent or greater than the poverty threshold. See Appendix II, Poverty level. Poverty status was unknown for 22 percent of adults in the sample in 1997 and 27 percent in 1998.

[6]Estimates for persons 18–64 years of age are age adjusted to the year 2000 standard using three age groups: 18–44 years, 45–54 years, and 55–64 years of age. Estimates for persons 65 years of age and over are age adjusted to the year 2000 standard using two age groups: 65–74 years and 75 years and over. See Appendix II, Age adjustment.

[7]Health insurance categories are mutually exclusive. Persons who reported both Medicaid and private coverage are classified as having Medicaid coverage. See Appendix II, Health insurance coverage.

[8]MSA is metropolitan statistical area.

NOTES: In 1997 the National Health Interview Survey questionnaire was redesigned. See Appendix I, National Health Interview Survey. Data presented in this table are not comparable with data on interval since last physician contact presented in previous editions of Health, United States.

SOURCE: Centers for Disease Control and Prevention, National Center for Health Statistics. National Health Interview Survey, family core and sample adult questionnaires.

Table 73. Vaccinations of children 19–35 months of age for selected diseases, according to race, Hispanic origin, poverty status, and residence in metropolitan statistical area (MSA): United States, 1994–98

[Data are based on telephone interviews of a sample of the civilian noninstitutionalized population supplemented by a survey of immunization providers for interview participants]

| Vaccination and year | All | Race and Hispanic origin | | | | | Poverty status | | Location of residence | | |
| | | Non-Hispanic | | | | Hispanic[2] | Below poverty | At or above poverty | Inside MSA[1] | | Outside MSA |
		White	Black	American Indian or Alaska Native	Asian or Pacific Islander				Central city	Remaining areas	
Combined series (4:3:1:3):[3]				Percent of children 19–35 months of age							
1994	69	72	67	82	60	62	61	72	68	70	70
1995	74	77	70	70	75	69	67	77	73	76	75
1996	77	79	74	80	78	71	69	80	74	78	77
1997	76	79	73	72	70	72	71	79	74	78	77
1998	79	82	73	78	79	75	74	82	77	81	81
DTP (4 doses or more):[4]											
1994	76	80	72	84	84	70	69	79	75	77	78
1995	79	81	74	73	82	75	71	81	77	80	79
1996	81	83	79	83	84	77	73	84	80	83	81
1997	81	84	78	80	80	77	76	84	80	83	81
1998	84	87	77	83	89	81	80	86	82	85	85
Polio (3 doses or more):											
1994	83	85	79	90	92	81	78	85	83	84	83
1995	88	89	84	87	89	87	84	89	87	88	89
1996	91	92	90	89	90	89	88	92	89	92	92
1997	91	92	90	91	88	90	90	92	90	91	92
1998	91	92	88	85	93	89	90	92	89	91	93
Measles-containing:[5]											
1994	89	90	86	90	95	88	87	90	90	90	87
1995	90	91	86	88	95	88	85	91	89	91	90
1996	91	92	89	87	94	88	87	92	90	92	91
1997	91	92	90	92	89	88	86	92	90	91	90
1998	92	93	89	91	92	91	90	93	92	92	93
Hib (3 doses or more):[6]											
1994	86	87	85	90	70	84	81	88	86	87	86
1995	92	93	89	92	91	90	88	93	91	92	92
1996	92	93	90	90	92	89	88	93	90	93	92
1997	93	94	92	87	89	90	90	94	92	94	94
1998	93	95	90	90	92	92	91	95	92	94	94
Hepatitis B (3 doses or more):											
1994	37	40	29	43	39	33	25	41	36	40	28
1995	68	68	65	55	80	69	64	69	68	71	60
1996	82	82	82	78	84	80	78	83	81	83	80
1997	84	85	83	83	88	81	80	85	82	85	85
1998	87	88	84	82	89	86	85	88	85	88	87

| Vaccination and year | White, non-Hispanic | | Black, non-Hispanic | | Hispanic[2] | |
	Below poverty	At or above poverty	Below poverty	At or above poverty	Below poverty	At or above poverty
Combined series (4:3:1:3):[3]	Percent of children 19–35 months of age					
1995	68	79	66	75	65	72
1996	68	81	70	78	68	74
1997	70	76	72	80	71	77
1998	77	83	72	74	73	79

[1]Metropolitan statistical area.
[2]Persons of Hispanic origin may be of any race.
[3]The 4:3:1:3 combined series consists of 4 doses of diphtheria-tetanus-pertussis (DTP) vaccine, 3 doses of polio vaccine, 1 dose of a measles-containing vaccine, and 3 doses of *Haemophilus influenzae* type b (Hib) vaccine.
[4]Diphtheria-tetanus-pertussis vaccine.
[5]Respondents were asked about measles-containing or MMR (measles-mumps-rubella) vaccines.
[6]*Haemophilus influenzae* type b (Hib) vaccine.

NOTES: Final estimates of data from the National Immunization Survey include an adjustment for children with missing immunization provider data. Poverty status is based on family income and family size using Bureau of the Census poverty thresholds. Children missing information about poverty status were omitted from analysis by poverty level. In 1998, 15.6 percent of all children, 20.7 percent of Hispanic, 13.8 percent of non-Hispanic white, and 17.8 percent of non-Hispanic black children were missing information about poverty status and were omitted. See Appendix II.

SOURCE: Centers for Disease Control and Prevention, National Center for Health Statistics and National Immunization Program. Data from the National Immunization Survey.

Table 74 (page 1 of 2). Vaccination coverage among children 19–35 months of age according to geographic division, State, and selected urban areas: United States, 1994–98

[Data are based on telephone interviews of a sample of the civilian noninstitutionalized population supplemented by a survey of immunization providers for interview participants]

Geographic division and State	1994	1995	1996	1997	1998
	Percent of children 19–35 months of age with 4:3:1:3 series[1]				
United States	69	74	77	76	79
New England:					
Maine	75	87	85	84	86
New Hampshire	78	86	83	84	82
Vermont	82	84	85	84	86
Massachusetts	77	80	86	86	87
Rhode Island	78	82	85	81	86
Connecticut	81	83	87	85	90
Middle Atlantic:					
New York.	72	77	79	76	85
New Jersey	67	72	77	76	82
Pennsylvania	71	76	79	80	83
East North Central:					
Ohio	70	73	77	73	78
Indiana	69	75	70	72	78
Illinois	60	79	75	74	78
Michigan	55	67	74	75	78
Wisconsin	70	74	76	79	78
West North Central:					
Minnesota	74	76	83	78	82
Iowa	75	82	80	76	82
Missouri.	59	75	74	77	85
North Dakota	73	81	81	82	79
South Dakota	67	79	80	76	74
Nebraska	62	75	80	75	76
Kansas	76	70	73	82	82
South Atlantic:					
Delaware	77	72	80	79	79
Maryland	75	78	78	80	77
District of Columbia	67	67	78	73	71
Virginia	76	71	77	72	80
West Virginia	62	71	71	80	82
North Carolina	75	80	77	80	83
South Carolina	78	80	84	79	88
Georgia	75	77	80	79	80
Florida.	72	75	77	77	79
East South Central:					
Kentucky	74	79	76	79	82
Tennessee	68	73	77	77	82
Alabama	70	75	75	85	82
Mississippi	79	81	79	80	84
West South Central:					
Arkansas	64	73	72	77	73
Louisiana	66	76	79	76	78
Oklahoma	70	73	73	71	75
Texas	65	73	72	74	74
Mountain:					
Montana	69	71	77	74	82
Idaho	58	64	66	70	76
Wyoming	71	71	77	72	80
Colorado	66	77	76	72	76
New Mexico	66	76	79	75	71
Arizona	70	70	70	73	76
Utah	62	66	63	69	76
Nevada	63	65	70	71	76
Pacific:					
Washington	68	77	78	79	81
Oregon	64	72	70	72	76
California.	67	69	76	74	76
Alaska.	65	72	69	75	81
Hawaii	78	78	77	79	79

See footnotes at end of table.

Table 74 (page 2 of 2). Vaccination coverage among children 19–35 months of age according to geographic division, State, and selected urban areas: United States, 1994–98

[Data are based on telephone interviews of a sample of the civilian noninstitutionalized population supplemented by a survey of immunization providers for interview participants]

Geographic division and urban areas	1994	1995	1996	1997	1998
	Percent of children 19–35 months of age with 4:3:1:3 series[1]				
New England:					
Boston, Massachusetts	87	87	84	86	89
Middle Atlantic:					
New York City, New York.	73	78	75	75	81
Newark, New Jersey.	46	67	62	66	64
Philadelphia, Pennsylvania	67	67	75	78	80
East North Central:					
Cuyahoga County (Cleveland), Ohio.	82	71	80	73	75
Franklin County (Columbus), Ohio	71	74	78	74	78
Marion County (Indianapolis), Indiana.	72	75	72	81	78
Chicago, Illinois	55	69	74	68	64
Detroit, Michigan	45	57	63	65	70
Milwaukee County (Milwaukee), Wisconsin	72	68	70	70	73
South Atlantic:					
Baltimore, Maryland	74	75	81	83	81
District of Columbia	67	67	78	73	71
Fulton/DeKalb Counties (Atlanta), Georgia	72	79	74	75	71
Dade County (Miami), Florida	73	77	76	75	75
Duval County (Jacksonville), Florida.	69	71	76	70	79
East South Central:					
Davidson County (Nashville), Tennessee	65	73	77	77	80
Shelby County (Memphis), Tennessee	67	68	70	70	71
Jefferson County (Birmingham), Alabama	72	85	77	82	85
West South Central:					
Orleans Parish (New Orleans), Louisiana	59	75	71	69	79
Bexar County (San Antonio), Texas	60	74	74	79	79
Dallas County (Dallas), Texas	62	70	71	74	71
El Paso County (El Paso), Texas	78	77	62	65	78
Houston, Texas	57	70	68	64	61
Mountain:					
Maricopa County (Phoenix), Arizona.	71	69	71	72	77
Pacific:					
King County (Seattle), Washington.	70	82	81	77	86
Los Angeles County (Los Angeles), California . .	65	70	79	71	76
San Diego County (San Diego), California	68	73	77	78	77
Santa Clara County (Santa Clara), California . .	78	74	79	73	84

[1]The 4:3:1:3 combined series consists of 4 doses of diphtheria-tetanus-pertussis (DTP) vaccine, 3 doses of polio vaccine, 1 dose of a measles-containing vaccine, and 3 doses of *Haemophilus influenzae* type b (Hib) vaccine.

NOTES: Urban areas were chosen because they were high risk for under-vaccination. Final estimates of data from the National Immunization Survey include an adjustment for children with missing immunization provider data.

SOURCES: Centers for Disease Control and Prevention, National Center for Health Statistics and National Immunization Program. National, State, and Urban Area Vaccination Coverage Levels Among Children Aged 19–35 Months-United States, 1994–1998, data are available on the CDC Web site at www.cdc.gov/nip/coverage/data.htm.

Table 75 (page 1 of 2). No health care visits to an office or clinic within the past 12 months among children under 18 years of age according to selected characteristics: United States, 1997 and 1998

[Data are based on household interviews of a sample of the civilian noninstitutionalized population]

Characteristic	Under 18 years of age		Under 6 years of age		6–17 years of age	
	1997	1998	1997	1998	1997	1998
	Percent of children without a health care visit[1]					
All children[2]	12.8	12.8	5.7	5.7	16.4	16.3
Race[3]						
White	12.2	12.2	5.6	5.3	15.6	15.5
Black	13.8	14.9	5.2	7.8	18.1	18.2
American Indian or Alaska Native	*15.7	*	*	*	*19.8	*
Asian or Pacific Islander	16.0	16.7	*	*	21.5	22.9
Race and Hispanic origin						
White, non-Hispanic	10.7	10.7	4.4	4.3	13.7	13.7
Black, non-Hispanic	14.1	15.0	5.1	8.0	18.4	18.2
Hispanic[3]	19.5	19.1	10.5	8.9	25.2	25.4
Poverty status[4]						
Poor	17.6	17.9	7.3	9.0	24.4	23.3
Near poor	16.9	15.2	7.4	6.6	21.8	19.7
Nonpoor	9.7	9.7	4.1	3.6	12.4	12.6
Race and Hispanic origin and poverty status[4]						
White, non-Hispanic:						
Poor	14.3	13.2	*5.7	*	20.0	18.9
Near poor	14.3	13.8	*6.5	*5.4	18.2	17.9
Nonpoor	9.1	9.1	3.5	3.3	11.7	11.6
Black, non-Hispanic:						
Poor	15.4	16.9	*	*10.2	21.7	20.4
Near poor	19.3	13.8	*	*	24.9	16.9
Nonpoor	11.5	13.1	*	*	14.4	17.0
Hispanic:[3]						
Poor	23.5	23.3	11.5	12.1	31.7	30.7
Near poor	20.7	19.6	9.8	8.9	27.6	27.0
Nonpoor	13.3	12.5	*9.4	*4.9	15.5	16.9
Health insurance status[5]						
Insured	10.2	---	4.4	---	13.2	---
Private	10.4	---	4.4	---	13.1	---
Medicaid	9.3	---	4.5	---	13.4	---
Uninsured	29.0	---	14.7	---	35.0	---
Poverty status and health insurance status[4]						
Poor:						
Insured	12.5	---	5.0	---	18.0	---
Uninsured	36.4	---	19.2	---	42.9	---
Near poor:						
Insured	13.7	---	5.0	---	18.3	---
Uninsured	28.2	---	*16.9	---	32.9	---
Nonpoor:						
Insured	8.7	---	3.7	---	11.1	---
Uninsured	22.6	---	*	---	27.7	---

See footnotes at end of table.

Table 75 (page 2 of 2). No health care visits to an office or clinic within the past 12 months among children under 18 years of age according to selected characteristics: United States, 1997 and 1998

[Data are based on household interviews of a sample of the civilian noninstitutionalized population]

Characteristic	Under 18 years of age		Under 6 years of age		6–17 years of age	
	1997	1998	1997	1998	1997	1998
Geographic region	Percent of children without a health care visit[1]					
Northeast	7.1	6.9	*3.0	*3.2	9.3	8.6
Midwest	11.8	12.7	5.7	6.2	14.7	15.9
South	14.8	13.7	5.3	5.9	19.5	17.6
West.	16.0	16.7	8.8	7.0	19.8	21.6
Location of residence						
Within MSA[6]	12.3	12.3	5.3	5.6	16.1	15.7
Outside MSA[6]	14.6	14.7	7.6	6.2	17.4	18.6

* Data preceded by an asterisk have a relative standard error of 20–30 percent. Data not shown have a relative standard error of greater than 30 percent.

\- - - Data not available as of publication date.

[1]Respondents were asked how many times a doctor or other health care professional was seen in the past 12 months at a doctor's office, clinic, or some other place. Excluded are visits to emergency rooms, hospitalizations, home visits, and telephone calls. This table presents the percent of children with no visits in the past 12 months. See Appendix II, Health care contact.

[2]Includes all other races not shown separately, unknown poverty status, and unknown health insurance status.

[3]The race groups white, black, American Indian or Alaska Native, and Asian or Pacific Islander include persons of Hispanic and non-Hispanic origin; persons of Hispanic origin may be of any race.

[4]Poverty status is based on family income, family size, number of children in the family, and for families with two or fewer adults the age of the adults in the family, using Bureau of the Census poverty thresholds. Poor persons are defined as below the poverty threshold. Near poor persons have incomes of 100 percent to less than 200 percent of poverty threshold. Nonpoor persons have incomes of 200 percent or greater than the poverty threshold. See Appendix II, Poverty level. Poverty status was unknown for 17 percent of children in the sample in 1997 and 21 percent in 1998.

[5]Health insurance categories are mutually exclusive. Persons who reported both Medicaid and private coverage are classified as having Medicaid coverage. See Appendix II, Health insurance coverage.

[6]MSA is metropolitan statistical area.

NOTES: In 1997 the National Health Interview Survey questionnaire was redesigned. See Appendix I, National Health Interview Survey. Data presented in this table are not comparable with data on percent of children without a physician contact within the past 12 months presented in *Health, United States*, 1996–97, 1998, and 1999.

SOURCE: Centers for Disease Control and Prevention, National Center for Health Statistics. National Health Interview Survey, family core and sample child questionnaires.

Table 76 (page 1 of 2). No usual source of health care among children under 18 years of age according to selected characteristics: United States, average annual 1993–94, 1995–96, and 1997–98

[Data are based on household interviews of a sample of the civilian noninstitutionalized population]

Characteristic	Under 18 years of age			Under 6 years of age			6–17 years of age		
	1993–94	1995–96	1997–98[1]	1993–94	1995–96	1997–98[1]	1993–94	1995–96	1997–98[1]
	Percent of children without a usual source of health care[2]								
All children[3]	7.7	6.4	6.7	5.2	4.4	4.5	9.0	7.4	7.8
Race[4]									
White	7.0	6.1	5.8	4.7	4.3	4.1	8.3	7.0	6.7
Black	10.3	7.5	8.9	7.6	5.2	5.6	11.9	8.7	10.4
American Indian or Alaska Native	*9.3	*5.2	*10.8	*	*	*	*8.7	*6.6	*
Asian or Pacific Islander	9.7	8.4	10.7	*3.4	*	*	13.5	10.8	14.4
Race and Hispanic origin									
White, non-Hispanic	5.7	4.6	4.5	3.7	3.2	3.4	6.7	5.3	5.0
Black, non-Hispanic	10.2	7.5	8.8	7.7	5.3	5.4	11.6	8.7	10.4
Hispanic[4]	14.3	13.2	13.2	9.3	8.7	7.6	17.7	16.1	16.7
Poverty status[5]									
Poor	13.9	10.7	12.4	9.4	7.2	8.2	16.8	12.9	15.0
Near poor	9.8	9.0	10.1	6.7	6.1	6.5	11.6	10.5	12.0
Nonpoor	3.7	3.4	3.5	1.8	2.1	2.0	4.6	4.0	4.2
Race and Hispanic origin and poverty status[5]									
White, non-Hispanic:									
Poor	10.2	9.2	11.4	6.5	6.7	10.7	12.7	10.7	11.9
Near poor	8.7	6.7	6.7	6.3	4.6	4.5	10.1	7.8	7.7
Nonpoor	3.4	2.9	2.8	1.6	1.8	1.6	4.2	3.5	3.3
Black, non-Hispanic:									
Poor	13.7	8.4	9.1	10.9	6.6	*5.4	15.5	9.6	11.2
Near poor	9.1	9.9	12.5	*6.0	5.8	*7.2	10.8	12.0	15.0
Nonpoor	4.6	3.9	6.4	*	*2.2	*4.0	5.8	4.6	7.4
Hispanic:[4]									
Poor	19.6	15.0	16.9	12.7	9.0	8.4	24.8	19.2	22.7
Near poor	15.3	16.2	16.0	9.9	11.8	10.2	18.9	18.9	19.9
Nonpoor	5.0	7.1	5.7	*2.7	4.7	*3.1	6.5	8.5	7.3
Health insurance status[6]									
Insured	5.0	3.9	3.8	3.3	2.6	3.0	5.9	4.5	4.2
Private	3.8	3.1	3.3	2.0	1.7	2.4	4.6	3.7	3.7
Medicaid	8.5	6.2	5.1	6.0	4.4	4.0	10.8	7.7	6.1
Uninsured	23.5	22.3	27.6	18.0	17.5	17.3	26.0	24.4	32.1
Poverty status and health insurance status[5]									
Poor:									
Insured	9.1	6.2	6.2	6.0	4.5	*5.0	11.5	7.4	7.1
Uninsured	29.4	27.1	37.6	25.0	22.5	27.4	31.5	28.9	41.4
Near poor:									
Insured	6.0	5.0	5.6	4.0	3.3	*4.2	7.2	6.0	6.3
Uninsured	22.9	22.5	25.9	18.0	17.9	12.1	25.3	24.5	31.8
Nonpoor:									
Insured	2.9	2.6	2.6	1.5	1.5	1.8	3.6	3.1	3.0
Uninsured	14.5	15.3	19.0	6.4	11.2	*9.3	18.1	17.5	23.2

See footnotes at end of table.

Table 76 (page 2 of 2). No usual source of health care among children under 18 years of age according to selected characteristics: United States, average annual 1993–94, 1995–96, and 1997–98

[Data are based on household interviews of a sample of the civilian noninstitutionalized population]

Characteristic	Under 18 years of age			Under 6 years of age			6–17 years of age		
	1993–94	1995–96	1997–98[1]	1993–94	1995–96	1997–98[1]	1993–94	1995–96	1997–98[1]
	Percent of children without a usual source of health care[2]								
Geographic region									
Northeast	4.1	3.2	3.1	2.9	2.3	*2.5	4.8	3.7	3.5
Midwest	5.2	4.3	4.6	4.1	3.3	4.0	5.9	4.8	4.9
South	10.9	7.9	8.4	7.3	5.1	5.3	12.7	9.3	9.9
West	8.6	9.3	9.8	5.3	6.4	5.5	10.6	10.8	12.0
Location of residence									
Within MSA[7]	7.7	6.5	6.8	5.0	4.5	4.4	9.2	7.5	8.0
Outside MSA[7]	7.8	6.1	6.4	6.0	4.0	4.7	8.7	7.1	7.2

* Data preceded by an asterisk have a relative standard error of 20–30 percent. Data not shown have a relative standard error of greater than 30 percent.

[1]Percents by health insurance status are for 1997 only. 1998 data on health insurance coverage were not available as of publication date. Data starting in 1997 are not strictly comparable with data for earlier years due to the 1997 questionnaire redesign. See Appendix I, National Health Interview Survey.

[2]Persons who report the emergency department as the place of their usual source of care are defined as having no usual source of care. See Appendix II, Usual source of care. The computation of percent without a usual source of care for 1993–96 was revised slightly from the previous edition of *Health, United States*.

[3]Includes all other races not shown separately, unknown poverty status, and unknown health insurance status.

[4]The race groups white, black, American Indian or Alaska Native, and Asian or Pacific Islander include persons of Hispanic and non-Hispanic origin; persons of Hispanic origin may be of any race.

[5]Prior to 1997 poverty status is based on family income and family size using Bureau of the Census poverty thresholds. Beginning in 1997 poverty status is based on family income, family size, number of children in the family, and for families with two or fewer adults the age of the adults in the family. Poor persons are defined as below the poverty threshold. Near poor persons have incomes of 100 percent to less than 200 percent of poverty threshold. Nonpoor persons have incomes of 200 percent or greater than the poverty threshold. See Appendix II, Poverty level. Missing family income data were imputed for 14 percent of children in 1993–96. See Appendix II, Family income for information on imputation. Poverty status was unknown for 17 percent of children in the sample in 1997 and 21 percent in 1998.

[6]Health insurance categories are mutually exclusive. Persons who reported both Medicaid and private coverage are classified as having Medicaid coverage. In 1993–96 health insurance status was unknown for 8–9 percent of children in the sample. In 1997 health insurance status was unknown for 1 percent of children in the sample. See Appendix II, Health insurance coverage.

[7]MSA is metropolitan statistical area.

SOURCES: Centers for Disease Control and Prevention, National Center for Health Statistics. National Health Interview Survey, access to care and health insurance supplements (1993–96). Starting in 1997 data are from the family core and sample child questionnaires.

[Data are based on household interviews of a sample of the civilian noninstitutionalized population]

Characteristic	Under 18 years of age		Under 6 years of age		6–17 years of age	
	1997	1998	1997	1998	1997	1998
	Percent of children with 1 or more emergency department visits[1]					
All children[2]	19.9	20.2	24.3	25.2	17.7	17.8
Race[3]						
White	19.4	19.8	22.6	24.6	17.8	17.4
Black	24.0	24.0	33.1	29.8	19.4	21.2
American Indian or Alaska Native	*24.1	29.0	*24.3	*40.7	*24.0	*22.8
Asian or Pacific Islander	12.6	11.0	20.8	15.6	8.6	*8.1
Race and Hispanic origin						
White, non-Hispanic	19.2	20.0	22.2	24.5	17.7	17.8
Black, non-Hispanic	23.6	24.0	32.7	29.8	19.2	21.4
Hispanic[3]	21.1	19.0	25.7	25.5	18.1	14.9
Poverty status[4]						
Poor	25.4	27.1	29.9	33.8	22.5	22.9
Near poor	22.6	22.9	28.8	27.5	19.4	20.5
Nonpoor	17.4	17.6	21.0	21.0	15.8	16.0
Race and Hispanic origin and poverty status[4]						
White, non-Hispanic:						
Poor	26.3	30.6	28.0	33.6	25.1	28.4
Near poor	23.0	22.4	26.5	27.9	21.2	19.7
Nonpoor	17.4	18.2	20.6	21.8	15.9	16.6
Black, non-Hispanic:						
Poor	29.8	29.7	40.9	38.0	22.8	25.5
Near poor	23.6	25.7	33.6	29.5	19.1	23.9
Nonpoor	17.8	18.8	23.8	21.3	15.5	17.7
Hispanic:[3]						
Poor	22.0	20.9	24.8	29.6	20.1	15.3
Near poor	20.8	21.2	28.9	25.4	15.6	18.2
Nonpoor	20.3	15.4	22.7	20.1	18.9	12.7
Health insurance status[5]						
Insured	19.8	---	24.4	---	17.5	---
Private	17.2	---	20.6	---	15.8	---
Medicaid	28.4	---	33.2	---	24.3	---
Uninsured	20.2	---	23.0	---	18.9	---
Poverty status and health insurance status[4]						
Poor:						
Insured	26.6	---	31.4	---	23.2	---
Uninsured	20.9	---	20.9	---	20.9	---
Near poor:						
Insured	22.7	---	29.2	---	19.2	---
Uninsured	22.2	---	27.3	---	20.1	---
Nonpoor:						
Insured	17.3	---	20.8	---	15.7	---
Uninsured	18.8	---	23.7	---	16.7	---
Geographic region						
Northeast	18.5	18.5	20.7	20.4	17.4	17.5
Midwest	19.5	20.1	26.0	25.3	16.4	17.5
South	21.8	22.9	25.6	28.8	19.9	20.0
West	18.5	17.6	23.5	23.4	15.9	14.7
Location of residence						
Within MSA[6]	19.7	19.5	23.9	24.0	17.4	17.3
Outside MSA[6]	20.8	22.7	26.2	29.8	18.6	19.4

See footnotes at end of table.

[Data are based on household interviews of a sample of the civilian noninstitutionalized population]

Characteristic	Under 18 years of age		Under 6 years of age		6–17 years of age	
	1997	1998	1997	1998	1997	1998
	Percent of children with 2 or more emergency department visits[1]					
All children[2]	7.1	6.9	9.6	9.3	5.8	5.8
Race[3]						
White	6.6	6.3	8.4	8.2	5.7	5.4
Black	9.6	10.0	14.9	14.7	6.9	7.8
American Indian or Alaska Native	*	*11.3	*	*	*	*
Asian or Pacific Islander..............	*5.7	*5.4	*12.9	*	*	*
Race and Hispanic origin						
White, non-Hispanic.................	6.2	6.2	7.8	8.0	5.5	5.4
Black, non-Hispanic	9.3	10.0	14.6	14.6	6.8	7.8
Hispanic[3]	8.9	7.0	11.8	9.3	7.0	5.5
Poverty status[4]						
Poor............................	11.2	11.7	14.4	15.6	9.1	9.4
Near poor	8.6	9.0	12.7	10.5	6.4	8.1
Nonpoor	5.2	4.7	6.7	6.3	4.6	4.0
Race and Hispanic origin and poverty status[4]						
White, non-Hispanic:						
Poor	11.0	12.4	12.4	*13.7	10.1	11.6
Near poor	8.4	8.7	11.8	10.0	6.6	8.0
Nonpoor......................	5.0	4.7	6.0	6.4	4.5	3.9
Black, non-Hispanic:						
Poor	12.9	13.9	19.6	21.5	*8.7	10.1
Near poor	9.5	10.8	*14.0	*13.9	*7.5	9.3
Nonpoor......................	5.1	5.2	*8.1	*7.2	*4.0	*4.4
Hispanic:[3]						
Poor	10.6	8.1	13.9	11.5	8.4	*5.9
Near poor	8.1	7.4	12.2	8.3	*5.4	6.7
Nonpoor......................	7.4	6.1	8.2	*6.6	7.0	5.8
Health insurance status[5]						
Insured........................	7.0	---	9.6	---	5.7	---
Private........................	5.0	---	6.6	---	4.4	---
Medicaid	13.2	---	16.2	---	10.6	---
Uninsured	7.7	---	9.8	---	6.8	---
Poverty status and health insurance status[4]						
Poor:						
Insured	12.0	---	15.4	---	9.6	---
Uninsured	8.0	---	*8.7	---	*7.7	---
Near poor:						
Insured	8.6	---	12.7	---	6.4	---
Uninsured	8.3	---	*12.2	---	6.8	---
Nonpoor:						
Insured	5.1	---	6.4	---	4.5	---
Uninsured	7.1	---	*11.8	---	*5.0	---

See footnotes at end of table.

Table 77 (page 3 of 3). Emergency department visits within the past 12 months among children under 18 years of age, according to selected characteristics: United States, 1997 and 1998

[Data are based on household interviews of a sample of the civilian noninstitutionalized population]

Characteristic	Under 18 years of age		Under 6 years of age		6–17 years of age	
	1997	1998	1997	1998	1997	1998
Geographic region	Percent of children with 2 or more emergency department visits[1]					
Northeast	6.2	5.8	7.6	6.6	5.4	5.4
Midwest	6.6	7.1	10.4	10.3	4.8	5.5
South	8.0	8.0	10.1	11.1	6.9	6.6
West	7.1	6.0	10.0	7.6	5.6	5.1
Location of residence						
Within MSA[6]	7.2	6.6	9.6	8.8	5.9	5.4
Outside MSA[6]	6.8	8.2	9.7	11.0	5.6	6.9

* Data preceded by an asterisk have a relative standard error of 20–30 percent. Data not shown have a relative standard error of greater than 30 percent.

- - - Data not available as of publication date.

[1]See Appendix II, Emergency department visit.

[2]Includes all other races not shown separately, unknown poverty status, and unknown health insurance status.

[3]The race groups white, black, American Indian or Alaska Native, and Asian or Pacific Islander include persons of Hispanic and non-Hispanic origin; persons of Hispanic origin may be of any race.

[4]Poverty status is based on family income, family size, number of children in the family, and for families with two or fewer adults the age of the adults in the family, using Bureau of the Census poverty thresholds. Poor persons are defined as below the poverty threshold. Near poor persons have incomes of 100 percent to less than 200 percent of poverty threshold. Nonpoor persons have incomes of 200 percent or greater than the poverty threshold. See Appendix II, Poverty level. Poverty status was unknown for 17 percent of children in the sample in 1997 and 21 percent in 1998.

[5]Health insurance categories are mutually exclusive. Persons who reported both Medicaid and private coverage are classified as having Medicaid coverage. See Appendix II, Health insurance coverage.

[6]MSA is metropolitan statistical area.

SOURCE: Centers for Disease Control and Prevention, National Center for Health Statistics. National Health Interview Survey, family core and sample child questionnaires.

Table 78 (page 1 of 2). No usual source of health care among adults 18–64 years of age, according to selected characteristics: United States, average annual 1993–94, 1995–96, and 1997–98

[Data are based on household interviews of a sample of the civilian noninstitutionalized population]

Characteristic	1993–94	1995–96	1997–98[1]
	Percent of adults without a usual source of health care[2]		
All adults 18–64 years of age[3,4]	18.5	16.6	17.5
Age			
18–44 years	21.7	19.6	21.0
18–24 years	26.6	22.6	27.0
25–44 years	20.3	18.8	19.3
45–64 years	12.8	11.3	11.2
45–54 years	14.1	12.2	12.6
55–64 years	11.1	9.8	9.0
Sex[4]			
Male	23.3	21.0	23.2
Female	13.9	12.5	11.9
Race[4,5]			
White	18.2	16.3	16.9
Black	19.2	17.6	18.7
American Indian or Alaska Native	19.1	15.9	20.7
Asian or Pacific Islander	24.0	20.7	21.1
Race and Hispanic origin[4]			
White, non-Hispanic	17.0	15.0	15.4
Black, non-Hispanic	18.9	17.4	18.6
Hispanic[5]	28.8	26.2	28.6
Mexican[5]	30.5	28.1	33.4
Poverty status[4,6]			
Poor	28.2	24.9	28.0
Near poor	24.6	22.3	25.3
Nonpoor	14.8	13.5	13.8
Race and Hispanic origin and poverty status[4,6]			
White, non-Hispanic:			
Poor	27.1	22.8	24.6
Near poor	22.7	20.3	22.6
Nonpoor	14.4	13.0	13.2
Black, non-Hispanic:			
Poor	23.8	21.1	22.9
Near poor	21.6	21.2	25.5
Nonpoor	14.6	13.6	14.0
Hispanic:[5]			
Poor	38.0	32.6	41.0
Near poor	35.7	31.6	32.7
Nonpoor	18.3	18.2	18.7
Health insurance status[4,7]			
Insured	13.3	11.4	12.1
Private	13.1	11.3	12.3
Medicaid	14.8	12.0	10.5
Uninsured	41.5	40.9	44.8
Poverty status and health insurance status[4,6]			
Poor:			
Insured	16.8	13.6	14.4
Uninsured	45.7	43.1	52.4
Near poor:			
Insured	15.3	13.1	15.0
Uninsured	42.9	41.5	46.9
Nonpoor:			
Insured	12.3	10.8	11.5
Uninsured	37.0	39.4	40.2

See footnotes at end of table.

Table 78 (page 2 of 2). No usual source of health care among adults 18–64 years of age, according to selected characteristics: United States, average annual 1993–94, 1995–96, and 1997–98

[Data are based on household interviews of a sample of the civilian noninstitutionalized population]

Characteristic	1993–94	1995–96	1997–98[1]
Geographic region[4]	Percent of adults without a usual source of health care[2]		
Northeast	14.5	13.3	13.2
Midwest	15.8	14.5	14.8
South	21.6	18.4	20.5
West	20.5	19.5	19.8
Location of residence[4]			
Within MSA[8]	18.8	16.9	17.6
Outside MSA[8]	17.4	15.4	17.0

[1]Percents by health insurance status are for 1997 only. 1998 data on health insurance coverage were not available as of publication date. Data starting in 1997 are not strictly comparable with data for earlier years due to the 1997 questionnaire redesign. See Appendix I, National Health Interview Survey.
[2]Persons who report the emergency department as the place of their usual source of care are defined as having no usual source of care. See Appendix II, Usual source of care. The computation of percent without a usual source of care for 1993–96 was revised slightly from the previous edition of *Health, United States.*
[3]Includes all other races not shown separately, unknown poverty status, and unknown health insurance status.
[4]Estimates are for persons 18–64 years of age and are age adjusted to the year 2000 standard using three age groups: 18–44 years, 45–54 years, and 55–64 years of age. See Appendix II, Age adjustment.
[5]The race groups white, black, American Indian or Alaska Native, and Asian or Pacific Islander include persons of Hispanic and non-Hispanic origin; persons of Hispanic origin may be of any race.
[6]Prior to 1997 poverty status is based on family income and family size using Bureau of the Census poverty thresholds. Beginning in 1997 poverty status is based on family income, family size, number of children in the family, and for families with two or fewer adults the age of the adults in the family. Poor persons are defined as below the poverty threshold. Near poor persons have incomes of 100 percent to less than 200 percent of poverty threshold. Nonpoor persons have incomes of 200 percent or greater than the poverty threshold. See Appendix II, Poverty level. Missing family income data were imputed for 16 percent of adults in 1993–96. See Appendix II, Family income for information on imputation process. Poverty status was unknown for 22 percent of adults in the sample in 1997 and 27 percent in 1998.
[7]Health insurance categories are mutually exclusive. Persons who reported both Medicaid and private coverage are classified as having Medicaid coverage. In 1993–96 health insurance coverage was unknown for 8–9 percent of adults in the sample. In 1997 health insurance coverage was unknown for 1 percent of adults in the sample. See Appendix II, Health insurance coverage.
[8]MSA is metropolitan statistical area.

SOURCE: Centers for Disease Control and Prevention, National Center for Health Statistics, National Health Interview Survey, access to care and health insurance supplements (1993–96). Starting in 1997 data are from the family core and sample adult questionnaires.

Table 79 (page 1 of 2). Emergency department visits within the past 12 months among adults 18 years of age and over, according to selected characteristics: United States, 1997 and 1998

[Data are based on household interviews of a sample of the civilian noninstitutionalized population]

Characteristic	1 or more emergency department visits		2 or more emergency department visits	
	1997	1998	1997	1998
	Percent of adults with emergency department visit[1]			
All adults 18 years of age and over[2,3]	19.6	19.7	6.7	6.7
Age				
18–44 years	20.7	20.4	6.8	7.0
18–24 years	26.3	24.7	9.1	8.3
25–44 years	19.0	19.1	6.2	6.7
45–64 years	16.2	17.1	5.6	5.6
45–54 years	15.7	17.0	5.5	6.0
55–64 years	16.9	17.2	5.7	5.2
65 years and over	22.0	21.9	8.1	7.3
65–74 years	20.3	20.0	7.1	6.8
75 years and over	24.3	24.3	9.3	8.0
Sex[3]				
Male	19.1	19.4	5.9	6.1
Female	20.2	19.9	7.5	7.3
Race[3,4]				
White	19.0	19.1	6.2	6.1
Black	25.9	25.3	11.1	10.7
American Indian or Alaska Native	24.8	28.6	13.1	12.4
Asian or Pacific Islander	11.6	14.4	*2.9	5.8
Race and Hispanic origin[3]				
White, non-Hispanic	19.1	19.2	6.2	6.1
Black, non-Hispanic	25.9	25.2	11.0	10.6
Hispanic[4]	19.2	18.6	7.4	6.6
Mexican[4]	17.8	16.3	6.4	5.7
Poverty status[3,5]				
Poor	29.2	28.0	13.7	13.4
Near poor	24.9	24.4	10.0	10.1
Nonpoor	17.5	18.0	5.0	5.2
Race and Hispanic origin and poverty status[3,5]				
White, non-Hispanic:				
Poor	30.8	30.1	14.1	13.9
Near poor	25.5	24.8	9.8	10.3
Nonpoor	17.2	17.8	4.8	4.9
Black, non-Hispanic:				
Poor	35.5	32.7	17.9	17.9
Near poor	30.8	29.6	12.9	13.5
Nonpoor	20.7	22.4	7.8	8.0
Hispanic:[4]				
Poor	22.9	19.6	10.2	8.1
Near poor	19.2	20.4	8.4	6.9
Nonpoor	17.9	17.4	5.5	4.8
Health insurance status[6,7]				
18–64 years of age:				
Insured	18.8	- - -	6.1	- - -
Private	16.9	- - -	4.7	- - -
Medicaid	36.9	- - -	19.5	- - -
Uninsured	20.0	- - -	7.5	- - -
65 years of age and over:				
Private	21.4	- - -	6.7	- - -
Medicaid	32.3	- - -	18.0	- - -
Medicare only	20.9	- - -	8.8	- - -

See footnotes at end of table.

Table 79 (page 2 of 2). **Emergency department visits within the past 12 months among adults 18 years of age and over, according to selected characteristics: United States, 1997 and 1998**

[Data are based on household interviews of a sample of the civilian noninstitutionalized population]

Characteristic	1 or more emergency department visits		2 or more emergency department visits	
	1997	1998	1997	1998
Poverty status and health insurance status[5,6]	Percent of adults with emergency department visit[1]			
18–64 years of age:				
Poor:				
Insured	32.1	- - -	15.9	- - -
Uninsured	24.4	- - -	10.0	- - -
Near poor:				
Insured	26.6	- - -	10.3	- - -
Uninsured	21.3	- - -	9.1	- - -
Nonpoor:				
Insured	16.6	- - -	4.5	- - -
Uninsured	18.7	- - -	5.5	- - -
Geographic region[3]				
Northeast.	19.5	19.6	6.9	6.1
Midwest.	19.3	18.9	6.2	6.3
South	20.9	21.2	7.3	7.6
West	17.7	18.0	6.0	5.9
Location of residence[3]				
Within MSA[8].	19.1	19.0	6.4	6.4
Outside MSA[8]	21.5	22.3	7.8	7.7

* Data preceded by an asterisk have a relative standard error of 20–30 percent.

- - - Data not available as of publication date.

[1]See Appendix II, Emergency department visit.

[2]Includes all other races not shown separately, unknown poverty status, and unknown health insurance status.

[3]Estimates are for persons 18 years of age and over and are age adjusted to the year 2000 standard using five age groups: 18–44 years, 45–54 years, 55–64 years, 65–74 years, and 75 years and over. See Appendix II, Age adjustment.

[4]The race groups white, black, American Indian or Alaska Native, and Asian or Pacific Islander include persons of Hispanic and non-Hispanic origin; persons of Hispanic origin may be of any race.

[5]Poverty status is based on family income, family size, number of children in the family, and for families with two or fewer adults the age of the adults in the family, using Bureau of the Census poverty thresholds. Poor persons are defined as below the poverty threshold. Near poor persons have incomes of 100 percent to less than 200 percent of poverty threshold. Nonpoor persons have incomes of 200 percent or greater than the poverty threshold. See Appendix II, Poverty level. Poverty status was unknown for 22 percent of adults in the sample in 1997 and 27 percent in 1998.

[6]Estimates for persons 18–64 years of age are age adjusted to the year 2000 standard using three age groups: 18–44 years, 45–54 years, and 55–64 years of age. Estimates for persons 65 years of age and over are age adjusted to the year 2000 standard using two age groups: 65–74 years and 75 years and over. See Appendix II, Age adjustment.

[7]Health insurance categories are mutually exclusive. Persons who reported both Medicaid and private coverage are classified as having Medicaid coverage. See Appendix II, Health insurance coverage.

[8]MSA is metropolitan statistical area.

SOURCE: Centers for Disease Control and Prevention, National Center for Health Statistics. National Health Interview Survey, family core and sample adult questionnaires.

Table 80. Dental visits in the past year according to selected patient characteristics: United States, 1997 and 1998

[Data are based on household interviews of a sample of the civilian noninstitutionalized population]

Characteristic	2 years of age and over[1]		2–17 years of age		18–64 years of age		65 years of age and over[2]	
	1997	1998	1997	1998	1997	1998	1997	1998
	Percent of persons with a dental visit in the past year[3]							
Total[4]	64.9	66.2	72.7	73.5	64.1	65.6	54.8	56.4
Sex								
Male	62.6	63.6	72.3	72.0	60.4	61.7	55.4	57.8
Female	67.2	68.8	73.0	75.1	67.7	69.2	54.4	55.4
Race[5]								
White	66.5	67.8	74.0	74.9	65.7	67.2	56.8	58.2
Black	56.5	58.0	68.8	69.8	57.0	58.3	35.4	36.9
American Indian or Alaska Native	51.5	56.1	66.8	72.6	49.9	53.7	*	*41.1
Asian or Pacific Islander	61.8	65.5	69.9	67.8	60.3	63.4	53.9	67.4
Race and Hispanic origin								
White, non-Hispanic	68.2	69.5	76.4	77.1	67.5	68.9	57.2	58.7
Black, non-Hispanic	56.5	58.0	68.8	69.8	56.9	58.1	35.3	37.3
Hispanic[5]	52.9	54.1	61.0	62.4	50.8	52.2	47.8	46.8
Poverty status[6]								
Poor	47.2	48.3	62.0	63.5	46.4	47.1	30.3	32.6
Near poor	48.9	50.5	61.6	61.2	46.4	49.0	39.6	41.8
Nonpoor	72.3	73.2	79.7	80.4	71.1	72.0	66.3	66.8
Race and Hispanic origin and poverty status[6]								
White, non-Hispanic:								
Poor	49.9	51.8	63.3	64.1	50.3	51.8	31.1	34.0
Near poor	51.0	52.6	64.8	63.5	48.2	51.4	41.2	43.0
Nonpoor	73.6	74.4	80.7	81.5	72.5	73.3	67.6	67.7
Black, non-Hispanic:								
Poor	46.7	47.1	66.7	67.7	44.5	46.6	26.2	22.5
Near poor	44.9	47.8	60.1	61.3	44.7	46.4	23.6	33.9
Nonpoor	65.4	65.4	75.5	76.1	66.2	65.5	48.9	48.4
Hispanic:[5]								
Poor	41.9	41.7	56.8	58.7	39.0	37.4	33.0	36.3
Near poor	46.2	45.3	54.1	53.1	42.6	43.7	49.2	40.3
Nonpoor	65.1	67.2	74.8	75.5	62.5	65.4	56.5	59.4
Geographic region								
Northeast	69.6	70.4	77.5	80.5	69.6	69.6	55.5	56.3
Midwest	68.3	69.4	76.4	76.9	67.4	69.2	57.6	56.2
South	60.0	62.2	68.0	69.1	59.4	61.2	49.0	53.9
West	64.9	65.6	71.5	70.1	62.9	64.7	61.9	61.2
Location of residence								
Within MSA[7]	66.5	67.9	73.6	74.6	65.7	67.2	57.6	59.1
Outside MSA[7]	59.1	60.3	69.3	69.6	58.0	59.5	46.1	47.6

* Data preceded by an asterisk have a relative standard error of 20–30 percent. Data not shown have a relative standard error greater than 30 percent.
[1] Estimates are age adjusted to the year 2000 standard using six age groups: 2–17 years, 18–44 years, 45–54 years, 55–64 years, 65–74 years, and 75 years and over. See Appendix II, Age adjustment.
[2] Estimates for the elderly present the percent of persons 65 years of age and over with a dental visit in the past year. Data from the 1997 and 1998 National Health Interview Survey estimate that 29–30 percent of persons 65 years of age and over were edentulous (having lost all their natural teeth). In 1997 and 1998, 70–71 percent of elderly dentate persons compared with 18 percent of elderly edentate persons had a dental visit in the past year.
[3] Respondents were asked "About how long has it been since you last saw or talked to a dentist? Include all types of dentists, such as orthodontists, oral surgeons, and all other dental specialists as well as dental hygienists." This question was not asked for children under two years of age. This table presents the percent of persons with a visit in the past one year or less.
[4] Includes all other races not shown separately and unknown poverty status.
[5] The race groups white, black, American Indian or Alaska Native, and Asian or Pacific Islander include persons of Hispanic and non-Hispanic origin; persons of Hispanic origin may be of any race.
[6] Poverty status is based on family income, family size, number of children in the family, and for families with two or fewer adults the age of the adults in the family, using Bureau of the Census poverty thresholds. Poor persons are defined as below the poverty threshold. Near poor persons have incomes of 100 percent to less than 200 percent of poverty threshold. Nonpoor persons have incomes of 200 percent or greater than the poverty threshold. See Appendix II, Poverty level. Poverty status was unknown for 20 percent of persons in 1997 and 25 percent in 1998 in the sample.
[7] MSA is metropolitan statistical area.

NOTES: In 1997 the National Health Interview Survey questionnaire was redesigned. See Appendix I, National Health Interview Survey.

SOURCE: Centers for Disease Control and Prevention, National Center for Health Statistics. National Health Interview Survey, sample child and sample adult questionnaires.

[Data are based on dental examinations of a sample of the civilian noninstitutionalized population]

Sex, race and Hispanic origin, and poverty status	2–5 years			6–17 years			18–64 years			65–74 years		
	1971–74	1982–84	1988–94	1971–74	1982–84	1988–94	1971–74	1982–84	1988–94	1971–74	1982–84	1988–94
	Percent of persons with at least one untreated dental caries											
Total[1]	24.4	- - -	18.7	55.0	- - -	23.1	48.4	- - -	28.2	29.7	- - -	25.4
Sex												
Male	26.1	- - -	19.2	54.8	- - -	22.6	48.4	- - -	31.2	30.2	- - -	29.9
Female	22.7	- - -	18.1	55.2	- - -	23.7	48.5	- - -	25.3	28.3	- - -	21.5
Race and Hispanic origin[2]												
White, non-Hispanic	23.7	- - -	14.4	52.3	- - -	18.9	45.2	- - -	23.6	28.1	- - -	22.7
Black, non-Hispanic	28.2	- - -	25.1	70.9	- - -	33.0	68.1	- - -	47.9	41.5	- - -	46.7
Mexican	- - -	23.1	34.9	- - -	42.8	37.2	- - -	45.4	39.9	- - -	44.3	43.8
Poverty status[3]												
Poor	30.7	- - -	28.8	70.4	- - -	36.3	63.6	- - -	47.3	34.3	- - -	46.7
Near poor	29.8	- - -	24.3	60.2	- - -	29.2	56.3	- - -	42.7	35.6	- - -	39.3
Nonpoor	17.5	- - -	9.7	46.3	- - -	14.5	43.1	- - -	19.5	26.2	- - -	19.4
Race, Hispanic origin, and poverty status[2,3]												
White, non-Hispanic:												
Poor	31.9	- - -	25.4	68.1	- - -	32.5	58.4	- - -	42.3	33.3	- - -	39.0
Near poor and nonpoor	22.1	- - -	12.4	50.3	- - -	16.7	44.3	- - -	21.6	28.0	- - -	22.7
Black, non-Hispanic:												
Poor	29.0	- - -	27.5	73.4	- - -	35.6	73.1	- - -	59.0	39.8	- - -	50.1
Near poor and nonpoor	26.5	- - -	23.0	67.4	- - -	31.2	65.8	- - -	43.4	41.1	- - -	43.6
Mexican:												
Poor	- - -	22.6	38.5	- - -	46.4	45.8	- - -	56.3	52.4	- - -	54.4	55.5
Near poor and nonpoor	- - -	22.0	30.5	- - -	39.3	27.6	- -	41.0	31.5	- - -	30.8	35.6

- - - Data not available.

[1]Includes all other races not shown separately and unknown poverty status.

[2]In 1971–74, data are for white persons and black persons. Persons of Hispanic origin may be of any race.

[3]Poverty status is based on family income and family size. Poor persons are defined as below the poverty threshold. Near poor persons have incomes of 100 percent to less than 200 percent of poverty threshold. Nonpoor persons have incomes of 200 percent or greater than the poverty threshold. Persons with unknown poverty status are excluded (4 percent in 1971–74, 8 percent in 1982–84, and 6 percent in 1988–94). See Appendix II, Poverty level.

NOTES: Excludes edentulous persons (persons without teeth) of all ages. The majority of edentulous persons are 65 years of age and over. Estimates of edentulism among the elderly are 46 percent in 1971–74, 37 percent in 1982–84, and 33 percent in 1988–94

SOURCES: Centers for Disease Control and Prevention, National Center for Health Statistics. National Health and Nutrition Examination Survey (NHANES) I, Hispanic Health and Nutrition Examination Survey, and NHANES III.

Table 82 (page 1 of 2). Use of mammography for women 40 years of age and over according to selected characteristics: United States, selected years 1987–98

[Data are based on household interviews of a sample of the civilian noninstitutionalized population]

Characteristic	1987	1990	1991	1993	1994	1998
Age	Percent of women having a mammogram within the past 2 years[1]					
40 years and over	28.7	51.4	54.6	59.7	60.9	66.9
40–49 years	31.9	55.1	55.6	59.9	61.3	63.4
50 years and over	27.4	49.7	54.1	59.7	60.6	68.9
50–64 years	31.7	56.0	60.3	65.1	66.5	73.7
65 years and over	22.8	43.4	48.1	54.2	55.0	63.8
Age, race, and Hispanic origin						
40 years and over:						
White, non-Hispanic	30.3	52.7	56.0	60.6	61.3	68.0
Black, non-Hispanic	23.8	46.0	47.7	59.2	64.4	66.0
Hispanic[2]	18.3	45.2	49.2	50.9	51.9	60.2
40–49 years:						
White, non-Hispanic	34.3	57.0	58.1	61.6	62.0	64.3
Black, non-Hispanic	27.9	48.4	48.0	55.6	67.2	65.0
Hispanic[2]	15.3	45.1	44.0	52.6	47.5	55.3
50 years and over:						
White, non-Hispanic	28.8	50.7	55.1	60.2	61.0	69.8
Black, non-Hispanic	21.5	44.6	47.6	61.4	62.4	66.7
Hispanic[2]	20.0	45.2	53.7	49.7	54.7	63.9
50–64 years:						
White, non-Hispanic	33.6	58.1	61.5	66.2	67.5	75.3
Black, non-Hispanic	26.4	48.4	52.4	65.5	63.6	71.2
Hispanic[2]	23.0	47.5	61.7	59.2	60.1	67.2
65 years and over:						
White, non-Hispanic	24.0	43.8	49.1	54.7	54.9	64.3
Black, non-Hispanic	14.1	39.7	41.6	56.3	61.0	60.7
Hispanic[2]	*13.7	41.1	40.9	35.7	48.0	59.0
Age and poverty status[3]						
40 years and over:						
Below poverty	15.0	28.7	36.5	40.8	44.4	50.5
At or above poverty	31.0	54.8	58.4	62.7	64.8	69.3
40–49 years:						
Below poverty	19.0	33.2	33.7	35.8	44.0	44.2
At or above poverty	33.4	57.3	58.8	62.6	64.7	65.0
50 years and over:						
Below poverty	13.8	27.0	37.6	42.9	44.5	53.0
At or above poverty	29.9	53.5	58.2	62.8	64.9	71.9
50–64 years:						
Below poverty	14.5	25.6	39.6	45.3	47.0	54.2
At or above poverty	34.1	59.5	64.3	67.8	70.3	76.7
65 years and over:						
Below poverty	13.4	28.0	36.0	41.2	43.2	52.2
At or above poverty	25.0	46.6	51.5	57.3	58.7	66.2

See footnotes at end of table.

[Data are based on household interviews of a sample of the civilian noninstitutionalized population]

Characteristic	1987	1990	1991	1993	1994	1998
Age and education[4]	Percent of women having a mammogram within the past 2 years[1]					
40 years of age and over:						
No high school diploma or GED	17.8	36.4	40.0	46.4	48.2	54.5
High school diploma or GED.......	31.3	52.7	55.8	59.0	61.0	66.7
Some college or more	37.7	62.8	65.2	69.5	69.7	72.8
40–49 years of age:						
No high school diploma or GED...	15.1	38.5	40.8	43.6	50.4	47.3
High school diploma or GED	32.6	53.1	52.0	56.6	55.8	59.1
Some college or more...........	39.2	62.3	63.7	66.1	68.7	68.3
50 years of age and over:						
No high school diploma or GED...	18.4	36.0	39.9	46.9	47.7	56.1
High school diploma or GED	30.6	52.6	57.7	60.1	63.6	70.1
Some college or more...........	36.8	63.2	66.3	72.5	70.5	76.8
50–64 years of age:						
No high school diploma or GED .	21.2	41.0	43.6	51.4	51.6	58.7
High school diploma or GED....	33.8	56.5	60.8	62.4	67.8	73.3
Some college or more	40.5	68.0	72.7	78.5	74.7	79.9
65 years of age and over:						
No high school diploma or GED .	16.5	33.0	37.7	44.2	45.6	54.7
High school diploma or GED....	25.9	47.5	54.0	57.4	59.1	66.8
Some college or more	32.3	56.7	57.9	64.8	64.3	71.3

* Relative standard error greater than 30 percent.

[1]Questions concerning use of mammography differed slightly on the National Health Interview Survey across the years for which data are shown. In 1987 and 1990 women were asked to report when they had their last mammogram. In 1991 women were asked whether they had a mammogram in the past 2 years. In 1993 and 1994 women were asked whether they had a mammogram within the past year, between 1 and 2 years ago, or over 2 years ago. In 1998 women were asked whether they had a mammogram a year ago or less, more than 1 year but not more than 2 years, or more than 2 years ago.

[2]Persons of Hispanic origin may be of any race.

[3]Poverty status is based on family income and family size using Bureau of the Census poverty thresholds. See Appendix II, Poverty level.

[4]Education categories shown are for 1998. GED stands for general equivalency diploma. In years prior to 1998 the following categories based on number of years of school completed were used: Less than 12 years, 12 years, 13 years or more. See Appendix II, Education.

SOURCE: Centers for Disease Control and Prevention, National Center for Health Statistics, National Health Interview Survey.

Table 83 (page 1 of 2). Ambulatory care visits to physician offices and hospital outpatient and emergency departments by selected patient characteristics: United States, selected years 1995–98

[Data are based on reporting by a sample of office-based physicians and hospital outpatient and emergency departments]

Age, sex, and race	All places[1]			Physician offices		
	1995	1997	1998	1995	1997	1998
	Number of visits in thousands					
Total	860,858	959,300	1,005,101	697,082	787,372	829,280
Under 18 years	194,643	203,843	213,505	150,351	158,423	168,520
18–44 years	285,184	311,879	328,480	219,065	245,127	260,379
45–64 years	188,319	226,064	237,700	159,531	192,753	203,296
45–54 years	104,891	124,377	132,146	88,266	105,511	112,316
55–64 years	83,429	101,687	105,555	71,264	87,243	90,979
65 years and over	192,712	217,514	225,416	168,135	191,069	197,085
65–74 years	102,605	112,593	115,526	90,544	99,714	102,306
75 years and over	90,106	104,922	109,890	77,591	91,355	94,779
	Number of visits per 100 persons					
Total, age adjusted[2]	334	365	378	271	300	312
Total, crude	329	360	373	266	295	308
Under 18 years	275	285	297	213	222	235
18–44 years	264	288	303	203	226	240
45–64 years	364	412	419	309	351	358
45–54 years	339	372	384	286	316	327
55–64 years	401	473	473	343	406	407
65 years and over	612	678	697	534	596	609
65–74 years	560	623	643	494	552	569
75 years and over	683	750	764	588	653	659
Sex and age						
Male, age adjusted[2]	290	313	321	232	255	261
Male, crude	277	301	310	220	243	251
Under 18 years	274	289	303	209	225	239
18–44 years	190	196	202	139	145	149
45–54 years	275	302	302	229	251	251
55–64 years	351	433	435	300	370	379
65–74 years	508	583	608	445	516	538
75 years and over	711	744	739	616	653	640
Female, age adjusted[2]	377	414	431	309	344	360
Female, crude	378	416	433	310	345	362
Under 18 years	277	282	291	217	219	231
18–44 years	336	378	401	265	306	328
45–54 years	400	438	462	339	377	399
55–64 years	446	510	506	382	439	433
65–74 years	603	656	672	534	581	595
75 years and over	666	753	780	571	652	671
Race and age						
White, age adjusted[2]	339	368	376	282	310	316
White, crude	338	368	376	281	310	317
Under 18 years	295	301	293	238	243	235
18–44 years	267	290	305	211	234	248
45–54 years	334	372	380	286	324	328
55–64 years	397	469	462	345	410	406
65–74 years	557	613	639	496	547	572
75 years and over	689	745	768	598	653	669
Black, age adjusted[2]	309	377	400	204	260	281
Black, crude	281	342	373	178	228	259
Under 18 years	193	247	315	100	145	217
18–44 years	260	296	317	158	186	207
45–54 years	387	422	426	281	294	310
55–64 years	414	542	561	294	396	411
65–74 years	553	711	660	429	582	511
75 years and over	534	764	725	395	607	537

See notes at end of table.

Table 83 (page 2 of 2). Ambulatory care visits to physician offices and hospital outpatient and emergency departments by selected patient characteristics: United States, selected years 1995–98

[Data are based on reporting by a sample of office-based physicians and hospital outpatient and emergency departments]

Age, sex, and race	Hospital outpatient departments			Hospital emergency departments		
	1995	1997	1998	1995	1997	1998
	Number of visits in thousands					
Total	67,232	76,993	75,412	96,545	94,936	100,408
Under 18 years	17,636	21,078	18,551	26,656	24,342	26,433
18–44 years	24,299	26,592	26,032	41,820	40,160	42,068
45–64 years	14,811	17,682	17,980	13,978	15,629	16,425
45–54 years	8,029	9,597	9,859	8,595	9,270	9,970
55–64 years	6,782	8,085	8,120	5,383	6,359	6,455
65 years and over	10,487	11,640	12,849	14,090	14,805	15,482
65–74 years	6,004	6,677	6,869	6,057	6,201	6,350
75 years and over	4,482	4,963	5,979	8,033	8,604	9,132
	Number of visits per 100 persons					
Total, age adjusted[2]	26	29	28	37	36	37
Total, crude	26	29	28	37	36	37
Under 18 years	25	30	26	38	34	37
18–44 years	23	25	24	39	37	39
45–64 years	29	32	32	27	28	29
45–54 years	26	29	29	28	28	29
55–64 years	33	38	36	26	30	29
65 years and over	33	36	40	45	46	48
65–74 years	33	37	38	33	34	35
75 years and over	34	35	42	61	61	64
Sex and age						
Male, age adjusted[2]	21	24	23	37	35	37
Male, crude	21	24	23	36	34	36
Under 18 years	25	29	26	40	35	39
18–44 years	14	16	16	37	34	37
45–54 years . . . . :	20	23	23	26	27	28
55–64 years	26	33	28	25	30	28
65–74 years	29	33	35	34	34	35
75 years and over	34	31	42	61	60	57
Female, age adjusted[2]	31	34	33	37	37	38
Female, crude	31	34	33	37	37	38
Under 18 years	25	30	26	36	33	35
18–44 years	31	33	32	40	40	41
45–54 years	32	34	34	29	28	30
55–64 years	38	42	44	26	30	30
65–74 years	36	40	41	32	34	35
75 years and over	34	38	42	61	62	67
Race and age						
White, age adjusted[2] •	23	26	25	34	33	35
White, crude	23	26	25	34	33	35
Under 18 years	23	26	23	35	32	34
18–44 years	20	22	21	36	34	36
45–54 years	23	23	25	25	25	27
55–64 years	28	33	30	24	26	26
65–74 years	29	33	33	32	32	33
75 years and over	31	31	38	60	61	61
Black, age adjusted[2]	48	57	55	58	61	63
Black, crude	45	54	52	58	60	62
Under 18 years	39	50	43	53	53	55
18–44 years	38	44	44	64	66	67
45–54 years	55	72	63	51	55	54
55–64 years	73	*83	91	47	63	59
65–74 years	*77	75	86	47	54	64
75 years and over	66	*81	85	73	76	103

* Data preceded by an asterisk have a relative standard error of 20–30 percent.
[1]All places includes visits to physician offices and hospital outpatient and emergency departments.
[2]Estimates are age adjusted to the year 2000 standard using six age groups: Under 18 years, 18–44 years, 45–54 years, 55–64 years, 65–74 years, and 75 years and over. See Appendix II, Age adjustment.

NOTES: Rates are based on the civilian noninstitutionalized population as of July 1. Population figures are adjusted for net underenumeration using the 1990 National Population Adjustment Matrix from the U.S. Bureau of the Census. Rates will be overestimated to the extent that visits by institutionalized persons are counted in the numerator (for example, hospital emergency department visits by nursing home residents) and institutionalized persons are omitted from the denominator.

SOURCES: Centers for Disease Control and Prevention, National Center for Health Statistics. Division Health Care Statistics. National Ambulatory Medical Care Survey and the National Hospital Ambulatory Medical Care Survey.

Table 84 (page 1 of 2). Injury-related visits to hospital emergency departments by sex, age, intent and mechanism of injury: United States, average annual 1995–96 and 1997–98

[Data are based on reporting by a sample of hospital emergency departments]

Sex, age, and intent and mechanism of injury[1]	Visits in thousands		Visits per 10,000 persons	
	1995–96	1997–98	1995–96	1997–98
Both sexes				
All ages[2,3]	36,081	36,122	1,360.9	1,344.6
Male				
All ages[2,3]	20,030	19,844	1,530.7	1,500.5
Under 18 years[2]	6,238	6,060	1,720.2	1,653.0
Unintentional injuries	5,478	5,196	1,510.5	1,417.2
Falls	1,402	1,241	386.5	338.6
Struck by or against objects or persons .	1,011	1,472	278.9	401.5
Motor vehicle traffic.	453	405	125.0	110.6
Cut or pierce	493	482	136.0	131.5
Intentional injuries	290	229	80.0	62.4
18–24 years[2]	2,980	2,807	2,396.9	2,224.3
Unintentional injuries	2,423	2,171	1,948.7	1,720.6
Falls	299	255	240.8	202.1
Struck by or against objects or persons .	387	459	311.0	363.5
Motor vehicle traffic.	347	404	279.4	320.2
Cut or pierce	304	310	244.8	245.7
Intentional injuries	335	269	269.2	213.1
25–44 years[2]	7,245	6,788	1,767.4	1,660.4
Unintentional injuries	5,757	5,122	1,404.3	1,252.8
Falls	817	779	199.4	190.5
Struck by or against objects or persons .	619	849	151.0	207.8
Motor vehicle traffic.	912	831	222.6	203.2
Cut or pierce	860	741	209.8	181.1
Intentional injuries	701	526	171.0	128.8
45–64 years[2]	2,240	2,755	883.4	1,020.4
Unintentional injuries . . . :	1,845	2,108	727.6	781.0
Falls	445	512	175.6	189.5
Struck by or against objects or persons .	186	202	73.3	74.8
Motor vehicle traffic.	244	312	96.3	115.6
Cut or pierce	203	290	79.9	107.4
Intentional injuries	86	107	33.8	39.7
65 years and over[2].	1,327	1,434	1,000.7	1,056.6
Unintentional injuries	1,009	1,109	760.6	817.2
Falls	505	492	380.9	362.3
Struck by or against objects or persons .	*39	*84	*29.4	*61.9
Motor vehicle traffic.	99	124	74.7	91.7
Cut or pierce	*81	117	*61.1	86.4
Intentional injuries	*	*	*	*

See footnotes at end of table.

Table 84 (page 2 of 2). Injury-related visits to hospital emergency departments by sex, age, intent and mechanism of injury: United States, average annual 1995–96 and 1997–98

[Data are based on reporting by a sample of hospital emergency departments]

Sex, age, and intent and mechanism of injury[1]	Visits in thousands		Visits per 10,000 persons	
	1995–96	1997–98	1995–96	1997–98
Female				
All ages[2,3]	16,051	16,278	1,186.4	1,183.5
Under 18 years[2]	4,372	4,105	1,263.9	1,173.6
Unintentional injuries	3,760	3,400	1,087.0	972.1
Falls	1,040	826	300.7	236.1
Struck by or against objects or persons .	477	704	137.9	201.4
Motor vehicle traffic	447	403	129.3	115.4
Cut or pierce	253	265	73.0	75.9
Intentional injuries	220	178	63.6	50.9
18–24 years[2]	1,900	2,025	1,523.4	1,606.2
Unintentional injuries	1,430	1,494	1,146.7	1,185.3
Falls	268	222	214.5	176.2
Struck by or against objects or persons .	134	180	107.4	143.1
Motor vehicle traffic	373	473	298.8	374.9
Cut or pierce	131	121	105.3	96.0
Intentional injuries	239	227	191.7	179.9
25–44 years[2]	5,098	5,050	1,205.8	1,194.2
Unintentional injuries	3,877	3,720	916.8	879.9
Falls	817	830	193.3	196.2
Struck by or against objects or persons .	380	447	89.8	105.7
Motor vehicle traffic	872	821	206.2	194.3
Cut or pierce	338	381	79.8	90.0
Intentional injuries	422	400	99.8	94.7
45–64 years[2]	2,369	2,649	873.7	919.1
Unintentional injuries	1,857	1,980	685.2	686.8
Falls	600	659	221.5	228.5
Struck by or against objects or persons .	160	224	58.8	77.6
Motor vehicle traffic	343	331	126.5	114.7
Cut or pierce	127	192	46.9	66.6
Intentional injuries	*64	88	*23.5	30.4
65 years and over[2]	2,313	2,449	1,256.1	1,314.2
Unintentional injuries	1,931	2,009	1,049.0	1,078.0
Falls	1,230	1,239	667.9	664.7
Struck by or against objects or persons .	82	146	44.8	78.2
Motor vehicle traffic	169	163	91.6	87.5
Cut or pierce	*42	*68	*22.7	*36.7
Intentional injuries	*	*	*	*

* Data preceded by an asterisk have a relative standard error of 20–30 percent. Data not shown have a relative standard error of greater than 30 percent.

[1]Intent and mechanism of injury are based on the first-listed external cause of injury code (E code). See Appendix II, First-listed external cause of injury and Appendix II, table VI for listing of E codes.

[2]An emergency department visit was considered injury related if the checkbox for injury was indicated. In addition, injury visits were identified if the physician's diagnosis or the patient's reason for visit were injury related. All injury-related visits include visits with undetermined intent; unintentional injury-related visits include visits with mechanism of injury not shown in table. See Appendix II, Injury-related visit.

[3]Age adjusted to year 2000 standard using six age groups: Under 18 years of age, 18–24 years, 25–44 years, 45–64 years, 65–74 years, and 75 years and over. See Appendix II, Age adjustment.

NOTE: Rates are based on the civilian noninstitutionalized population adjusted for net underenumeration using the 1990 National Population Adjustment Matrix from the Bureau of the Census.

SOURCE: Centers for Disease Control and Prevention, National Center for Health Statistics. National Hospital Ambulatory Medical Care Survey.

Table 85 (page 1 of 2). Ambulatory care visits to primary care and specialist physicians, according to selected patient characteristics and type of physician: United States, 1980, 1990, and 1998

[Data are based on reporting by a sample of office-based physicians]

Age, sex, and race	Type of primary care physician[1]											
	All primary care			General and family practice			Internal medicine			Pediatrics		
	1980	1990	1998	1980	1990	1998	1980	1990	1998	1980	1990	1998
	Percent of all physician office visits											
Total	56.6	54.9	52.7	33.5	29.9	24.2	12.1	13.8	17.1	10.9	11.2	11.4
Under 18 years...........	76.6	78.3	81.9	26.1	26.5	22.5	2.0	2.9	*4.4	48.5	48.9	55.0
18–44 years.............	43.6	44.3	42.3	34.3	31.9	26.3	8.6	11.8	15.4	0.7	0.7	*0.7
45–64 years.............	56.0	50.9	48.8	36.3	32.1	24.7	19.5	18.6	24.0	*	*	*
45–54 years	54.6	49.4	48.7	37.4	32.0	26.2	17.1	17.1	22.3	*	*	*
55–64 years	57.3	52.4	48.9	35.4	32.1	22.7	21.8	20.0	26.1	*	*	*
65 years and over.........	60.3	51.5	45.4	37.5	28.1	22.3	22.7	23.3	23.0	*	*	*
65–74 years	59.5	51.2	46.0	37.4	28.1	23.2	22.1	23.0	22.8	*	*	*
75 years and over	61.3	51.8	44.8	37.6	28.0	21.4	23.5	23.7	23.3	*	*	*
Sex and age												
Male:												
Under 18 years	77.1	77.9	82.8	25.6	24.1	22.5	2.0	3.0	*	49.4	50.7	56.5
18–44 years	50.5	51.7	53.1	38.0	35.9	32.8	11.5	15.0	19.4	*	*	*
45–64 years	55.0	50.5	51.3	34.4	31.0	25.2	20.5	19.2	25.9	*	*	*
65 years and over	57.9	51.1	43.5	35.6	27.7	20.6	22.3	23.3	22.8	*	*	*
Female:												
Under 18 years	76.0	78.8	81.0	26.6	29.1	22.5	2.0	2.8	*5.0	47.4	46.9	53.4
18–44 years	40.4	41.0	37.6	32.5	30.0	23.4	7.3	10.3	13.7	*	*	*
45–64 years	56.7	51.1	47.1	37.7	32.8	24.3	18.9	18.2	22.7	*	*	*
65 years and over	61.8	51.7	46.7	38.7	28.3	23.4	22.9	23.3	23.2	*	*	*
Race and age												
White:												
Under 18 years	76.5	78.2	80.3	26.4	27.1	25.4	2.0	2.3	*5.2	48.2	48.8	49.8
18–44 years	43.8	43.2	43.0	34.5	31.9	27.7	8.6	10.6	14.7	*	*	*
45–64 years	55.4	49.4	48.0	36.0	31.5	25.7	19.2	17.6	22.1	*	*	*
65 years and over	60.0	50.7	44.5	36.6	27.5	22.1	23.3	23.1	22.4	*	*	*
Black:												
Under 18 years	77.1	82.1	85.7	23.7	20.2	*	*	*	*	51.2	52.1	74.5
18–44 years	41.4	50.4	36.6	31.7	31.9	*17.3	9.0	18.1	18.6	*	*	*
45–64 years	61.3	58.2	49.8	38.6	31.2	*15.5	22.6	26.9	34.3	*	*	*
65 years and over	63.3	57.8	51.5	49.0	28.9	*23.1	14.2	28.7	28.4	*	*	*

See footnotes at end of table.

Table 85 (page 2 of 2). Ambulatory care visits to primary care and specialist physicians, according to selected patient characteristics and type of physician: United States, 1980, 1990, and 1998

[Data are based on reporting by a sample of office-based physicians]

Age, sex, and race	Type of specialist physician[1]								
	All specialists			Obstetrics and gynecology			All other specialists		
	1980	1990	1998	1980	1990	1998	1980	1990	1998
	Percent of all physician office visits								
Total	43.4	45.1	47.3	9.6	9.0	10.1	33.8	36.1	37.2
Under 18 years..........	23.4	21.7	18.1	1.3	1.2	1.4	22.2	20.5	16.7
18–44 years.............	56.4	55.7	57.7	21.7	21.5	24.8	34.7	34.1	32.8
45–64 years.............	44.0	49.1	51.2	4.2	4.8	6.3	39.8	44.3	44.9
45–54 years............	45.4	50.6	51.3	5.6	6.5	7.8	39.8	44.2	43.4
55–64 years...........	42.7	47.6	51.1	2.9	3.2	4.4	39.8	44.4	46.7
65 years and over........	39.7	48.5	54.6	1.4	1.2	2.0	38.4	47.3	52.6
65–74 years...........	40.5	48.8	54.0	1.7	1.6	2.5	38.8	47.2	51.5
75 years and over	38.7	48.2	55.2	1.0	*0.7	*1.5	37.7	47.5	53.7
Sex and age									
Male:									
Under 18 years.........	22.9	22.1	17.2	...	...	...	22.7	21.9	17.1
18–44 years...........	49.5	48.3	46.9	...	...	...	49.2	48.2	45.8
45–64 years...........	45.0	49.5	48.7	...	...	...	44.4	49.4	48.7
65 years and over	42.1	48.9	56.5	...	...	...	41.8	48.8	56.3
Female:									
Under 18 years.........	24.0	21.2	19.0	2.5	2.3	2.7	21.5	18.9	16.3
18–44 years...........	59.6	59.0	62.4	31.7	31.4	35.3	27.9	27.6	27.1
45–64 years...........	43.3	48.9	52.9	6.7	7.9	10.6	36.6	40.9	42.3
65 years and over	38.2	48.3	53.3	2.1	1.9	3.2	36.1	46.4	50.1
Race and age									
White:									
Under 18 years.........	23.5	21.8	19.7	1.1	1.0	1.3	22.4	20.8	18.4
18–44 years...........	56.2	56.8	57.0	21.0	21.8	24.0	35.2	35.0	33.0
45–64 years...........	44.6	50.6	52.0	4.1	4.9	6.5	40.4	45.7	45.5
65 years and over	40.0	49.3	55.5	1.4	1.3	1.9	38.6	48.1	53.5
Black:									
Under 18 years.........	22.9	17.9	*14.3	2.8	*3.4	*	20.1	14.5	*12.4
18–44 years...........	58.6	49.6	63.4	27.1	18.6	31.8	31.5	31.0	31.6
45–64 years...........	38.7	41.8	50.2	4.8	4.0	*5.5	33.9	37.9	44.8
65 years and over	36.7	42.2	48.5	*	*	*	35.4	41.3	45.5

* Data preceded by an asterisk have a relative standard error of 20–30 percent. Data not shown have a relative standard error of greater than 30 percent.
. . . Category not applicable.
[1]This table presents data on ambulatory care visits to physician offices and excludes ambulatory care visits to other sites such as hospital outpatient and emergency departments. Type of physician is based on physician's self-designated primary area of practice. Primary care physicians are defined as practitioners in the fields of general and family practice, general internal medicine, and general pediatrics. Primary care physicians in general and family practice exclude specialists such as sports medicine and geriatrics. Primary care internal medicine physicians exclude all internal medicine specialists such as allergists, cardiologists, endocrinologists, etc. Primary care pediatrics exclude all pediatric specialists such as adolescent medicine, neonatologists, pediatric allergists, pediatric cardiologists, etc. Specialist physicians include obstetricians and gynecologists in addition to specialists not included in general and family practice, internal medicine, pediatrics, and all other specialists.

NOTES: In 1980 the survey excluded Alaska and Hawaii. Data for all other years include all 50 states. Excludes visits with type of physician unknown. Data for additional years are available (see Appendix III).

SOURCE: Centers for Disease Control and Prevention, National Center for Health Statistics. National Ambulatory Medical Care Survey.

Table 86. Substance abuse clients in specialty treatment units according to substance abused, geographic division, and State: United States, 1996–98

[Data are based on a 1-day census of treatment providers]

Geographic division and State	All clients			Clients with both alcoholism and drug abuse			Alcoholism only clients			Drug abuse only clients		
	1996	1997[1,2]	1998[1]	1996	1997[1,2]	1998[1]	1996	1997[1,2]	1998[1]	1996	1997[1,2]	1998[1]
	Clients per 100,000 population											
United States	423.0	415.3	460.6	183.7	170.7	228.4	117.5	109.0	109.0	121.8	135.7	123.2
New England	517.9	589.9	704.3	253.2	245.2	366.5	124.5	153.1	160.1	140.2	191.6	177.6
Maine	574.6	776.3	807.9	280.9	374.3	406.3	203.2	260.2	288.7	90.5	141.8	112.8
New Hampshire	367.5	255.3	340.5	203.7	104.7	176.0	132.8	103.3	132.8	31.0	47.4	31.7
Vermont	370.3	326.5	513.6	169.9	143.7	282.4	151.0	139.9	168.4	49.4	42.9	62.8
Massachusetts	568.8	647.6	823.8	310.3	272.6	461.6	126.5	175.5	170.9	132.0	199.5	191.3
Rhode Island	635.6	616.1	770.9	207.2	229.5	357.5	173.1	156.1	154.9	255.3	230.6	258.5
Connecticut	445.4	570.3	585.4	181.7	217.6	259.1	68.1	89.4	100.0	195.6	263.3	226.3
Middle Atlantic	547.5	578.2	553.6	221.0	195.4	259.7	101.1	124.1	86.2	225.4	258.6	207.7
New York	773.6	849.1	767.8	298.9	234.7	328.3	127.5	185.7	113.1	347.2	428.7	326.4
New Jersey	364.1	308.4	365.1	145.5	137.0	178.0	61.9	52.7	55.6	156.8	118.7	131.5
Pennsylvania	331.6	356.7	360.5	154.8	176.0	212.1	87.4	80.3	66.5	89.3	100.3	81.8
East North Central	456.0	452.0	472.2	201.1	195.1	224.1	147.1	147.0	140.0	107.8	109.9	108.1
Ohio	453.5	432.2	454.3	240.3	223.2	255.3	134.1	123.9	119.7	79.0	85.0	79.4
Indiana	341.8	375.3	343.9	128.6	154.5	151.1	126.6	132.7	117.4	86.5	88.1	75.4
Illinois	433.9	398.6	463.7	202.6	183.5	229.1	109.5	104.5	112.2	121.8	110.7	122.3
Michigan	598.7	627.4	601.3	228.7	228.4	244.4	213.2	220.9	193.7	156.8	178.1	163.2
Wisconsin	377.6	381.4	433.3	144.0	146.1	190.3	161.4	174.0	172.0	72.2	61.3	71.0
West North Central	262.1	261.4	357.2	130.2	126.7	201.5	85.2	86.7	97.4	46.7	48.0	58.3
Minnesota	182.5	195.1	265.5	94.8	93.0	141.7	58.4	69.3	66.8	29.3	32.8	57.1
Iowa	219.7	223.1	303.1	112.2	107.1	151.9	78.7	79.9	108.4	28.8	36.1	42.8
Missouri	246.7	246.3	388.9	136.6	128.6	250.7	52.2	56.9	73.7	57.8	60.8	64.5
North Dakota	313.9	384.1	560.6	135.0	157.6	264.9	143.8	181.9	227.0	35.1	44.6	68.7
South Dakota	419.1	305.5	455.7	159.4	120.1	207.2	238.7	148.2	215.0	21.0	37.2	33.5
Nebraska	309.6	304.6	400.3	139.5	155.3	222.7	123.3	117.1	123.3	46.8	32.2	54.4
Kansas	398.3	384.8	410.7	185.7	181.4	231.1	127.3	127.5	108.0	85.3	76.0	71.6
South Atlantic	341.5	365.8	382.2	155.4	164.0	192.2	97.0	93.1	93.8	89.1	108.8	96.2
Delaware	552.9	580.4	604.5	293.6	367.1	307.3	110.4	111.8	127.1	148.9	101.5	170.1
Maryland	572.2	559.3	561.5	274.4	237.1	258.5	109.8	113.7	117.2	187.9	208.4	185.8
District of Columbia	974.1	1,806.2	1,449.3	403.5	599.5	881.8	220.7	318.5	198.7	349.9	888.2	368.9
Virginia	286.4	371.5	367.1	138.3	191.4	186.5	78.5	95.2	102.7	69.6	84.9	77.9
West Virginia	287.6	299.2	299.2	65.8	73.7	104.7	182.1	177.9	143.5	39.6	47.6	51.0
North Carolina	324.8	280.4	405.7	155.0	134.9	217.0	108.9	90.3	116.1	60.9	55.3	72.7
South Carolina	427.8	349.0	301.4	145.7	126.7	114.6	188.9	141.6	110.2	93.2	80.7	76.5
Georgia	158.7	262.4	251.2	63.4	118.8	115.3	46.9	64.1	64.8	48.4	79.5	71.1
Florida	336.9	339.6	363.7	165.9	157.9	198.6	80.3	68.4	69.5	90.7	113.3	95.6
East South Central	304.6	301.7	330.3	107.6	110.4	153.3	121.6	84.4	89.5	75.5	106.9	87.6
Kentucky	697.6	368.8	445.2	217.7	124.5	200.9	348.6	141.8	161.8	131.3	102.4	82.4
Tennessee	211.2	290.3	283.8	66.5	134.8	112.7	66.4	65.8	72.1	78.3	89.7	99.0
Alabama	159.3	295.1	245.6	81.4	66.0	117.7	29.6	68.4	47.4	48.4	160.7	80.6
Mississippi	149.1	237.4	392.8	70.3	111.9	222.7	46.9	63.6	86.7	31.9	61.9	83.4
West South Central	264.4	270.2	327.5	128.6	106.3	185.3	50.3	72.3	63.0	85.6	91.5	79.2
Arkansas	212.0	194.8	331.6	109.3	77.9	194.2	43.5	41.9	67.2	59.1	74.9	70.2
Louisiana	343.0	340.8	471.9	180.1	175.5	268.6	58.2	64.8	87.7	104.7	100.6	115.6
Oklahoma	312.8	275.0	314.6	121.6	91.2	125.6	76.4	96.1	95.8	114.8	87.7	93.2
Texas	244.9	263.4	296.7	120.6	97.0	175.8	44.7	74.0	51.2	79.6	92.4	69.7
Mountain	438.1	432.1	589.9	182.4	166.3	281.0	159.3	139.1	176.0	96.4	126.8	132.9
Montana	263.9	305.5	332.9	131.3	150.9	179.0	95.2	90.5	110.9	37.3	64.1	43.0
Idaho	382.9	244.3	288.3	180.8	170.3	185.5	134.0	38.4	59.7	68.1	35.7	43.1
Wyoming	509.3	506.7	425.0	265.2	204.7	202.7	192.8	232.9	166.4	51.3	69.1	56.0
Colorado	608.1	418.2	732.5	275.3	136.3	331.7	224.6	149.4	270.4	108.2	132.5	130.4
New Mexico	522.2	456.4	732.5	217.9	174.7	305.0	217.1	201.7	281.6	87.2	80.1	145.8
Arizona	334.3	340.7	520.4	82.3	119.0	231.4	137.8	94.1	134.3	114.3	127.7	154.7
Utah	467.4	846.9	712.1	234.2	358.8	355.9	137.2	257.5	146.3	96.0	230.6	209.9
Nevada	310.4	380.4	558.3	141.7	122.3	328.7	72.0	102.6	118.2	96.7	155.5	111.5
Pacific	558.8	436.1	515.1	233.3	195.8	252.3	166.6	92.6	117.3	158.8	147.7	145.5
Washington	775.1	671.6	676.4	425.8	371.6	400.0	250.5	205.7	182.4	98.8	94.4	94.0
Oregon	619.8	830.9	659.7	337.4	394.1	351.6	150.1	247.6	139.3	132.3	189.3	168.8
California	522.7	347.4	477.6	191.0	142.4	217.9	153.3	50.1	102.7	178.3	155.0	157.0
Alaska	703.8	1,070.1	598.6	309.8	427.4	296.7	340.9	460.9	257.3	53.1	181.8	44.6
Hawaii	251.5	218.9	304.6	116.4	89.8	172.2	82.1	50.3	65.3	53.0	78.8	67.0

[1]Beginning in 1997 the scope of the universe was expanded to include all substance abuse treatment facilities whereas previously only State-sanctioned facilities were included.
[2]Data for 1997 exclude facilities that served only driving under the influence or driving while intoxicated (DUI/DWI) clients.

NOTES: Rates are based on the resident population 12 years of age and over as of July 1. Client data are as of October 1. Treatment rates at the State level can vary from year to year for a variety of reasons, including failure of large facilities to respond to the survey in some years, and normal variation in the number of people in treatment on a given day.

SOURCE: Substance Abuse and Mental Health Services Administration, Office of Applied Studies. Uniform Facility Data Set (UFDS), 1996–98.

Table 87. Additions to mental health organizations according to type of service and organization: United States, selected years 1983–94

[Data are based on inventories of mental health organizations]

Service and organization	Additions in thousands				Additions per 100,000 civilian population			
	1983	1990	1992	1994	1983	1990	1992	1994
Inpatient and residential treatment								
All organizations	1,633	2,036	2,092	2,197	701.4	833.5	830.0	840.3
State and county mental hospitals	339	276	275	236	146.0	113.2	109.3	91.2
Private psychiatric hospitals	165	407	470	480	70.9	166.5	186.4	185.5
Non-Federal general hospital psychiatric services	786	960	951	1,067	336.8	393.2	377.4	411.9
Department of Veterans Affairs psychiatric services[1]	149	198	181	172	64.3	81.2	71.6	61.5
Residential treatment centers for emotionally disturbed children	17	42	36	39	7.1	17.0	14.4	15.0
All other[2]	177	153	179	203	76.3	62.4	70.9	75.2
Outpatient treatment								
All organizations	2,665	3,005	2,883	3,242	1,147.5	1,230.9	1,180.6	1,252.8
State and county mental hospitals	84	43	46	38	36.3	17.5	18.6	14.8
Private psychiatric hospitals	78	121	141	145	33.4	49.7	57.7	56.1
Non-Federal general hospital psychiatric services	469	605	429	443	202.1	247.8	175.8	171.0
Department of Veterans Affairs psychiatric services[1]	103	164	145	120	44.5	67.2	59.2	46.5
Residential treatment centers for emotionally disturbed children	33	86	113	156	14.1	35.3	46.2	60.3
Freestanding psychiatric outpatient clinics	538	462	464	567	231.7	189.3	190.3	218.9
All other[2]	1,360	1,524	1,545	1,773	585.4	624.1	632.8	685.2
Partial care treatment								
All organizations	177	293	281	273	76.3	120.2	115.8	105.3
State and county mental hospitals	4	5	4	3	1.6	2.2	1.7	1.3
Private psychiatric hospitals	6	42	65	68	2.4	17.2	26.8	26.4
Non-Federal general hospital psychiatric services	46	54	50	55	19.8	21.9	20.7	21.1
Department of Veterans Affairs psychiatric services[1]	10	19	14	12	4.4	8.0	5.9	4.6
Residential treatment centers for emotionally disturbed children	3	13	8	12	1.5	5.5	3.5	4.3
Freestanding psychiatric outpatient clinics[3]	5	...	...	...	2.3	...	...	...
All other[2,3,4]	103	160	140	123	44.3	65.4	57.2	47.6

... Category not applicable.

[1]Includes Department of Veterans Affairs neuropsychiatric hospitals, general hospital psychiatric services, and psychiatric outpatient clinics.
[2]Includes other multiservice mental health organizations with inpatient and residential treatment services that are not elsewhere classified.
[3]Beginning in 1986 outpatient psychiatric clinics providing partial care are counted as multiservice mental health organizations in the "all other" category.
[4]Includes freestanding psychiatric partial care organizations.

NOTES: See Appendix II for definition of Addition. Outpatient and partial care treatment exclude office-based mental health care (psychiatrists, psychologists, licensed clinical social workers, and psychiatric nurses). Data for additional years are available (see Appendix III).

SOURCES: Survey and Analysis Branch, Division of State and Community Systems Development, Center for Mental Health Services. Manderscheid RW, Sonnenschein MA. *Mental Health, United States, 1996*. DHHS. 1996. Unpublished data.

Table 88 (page 1 of 2). Home health care and hospice patients, according to selected characteristics: United States, selected years 1992–96

[Data are based on a survey of current home health care and hospice patients]

Type of patient and characteristic	1992	1994	1996
Home health care patients	Number of current patients		
Total.	1,232,200	1,889,327	2,427,483
	Patients per 10,000 population		
Total.	47.8	71.8	90.6
Age at interview:			
Under 65 years, crude	12.6	21.0	27.8
65 years and over, crude.	295.4	424.9	526.3
65 years and over, age adjusted[1]	315.8	449.6	546.6
65–74 years	151.7	209.1	240.1
75–84 years	398.3	542.2	753.6
85 years and over	775.9	1,206.1	1,253.4
Sex:			
Male, total	32.6	47.8	60.9
Under 65 years, crude.	10.9	17.8	22.1
65 years and over, crude	219.2	303.1	386.4
65 years and over, age adjusted[1]	255.8	350.0	438.3
65–74 years	121.8	169.9	187.0
75–84 years	322.0	427.5	598.7
85 years and over	635.2	893.1	1,044.3
Female, total	62.4	94.7	118.9
Under 65 years, crude	14.3	24.2	33.6
65 years and over, crude	347.4	508.9	623.9
65 years and over, age adjusted[1]	351.5	506.6	615.0
65–74 years	175.3	240.6	283.2
75–84 years	445.3	614.5	854.0
85 years and over	830.7	1,327.6	1,337.0
	Percent distribution		
Age at interview:[2]			
Under 65 years	23.1	25.7	27.0
65 years and over	76.9	74.3	73.0
65–74 years	22.6	20.6	18.4
75–84 years	33.9	31.2	35.3
85 years and over	20.4	22.4	19.4
Sex:			
Male	33.2	32.5	32.9
Female	66.8	67.5	67.1
Primary admission diagnosis:[3]			
Malignant neoplasms	5.7	5.7	4.8
Diabetes	7.7	8.1	8.5
Diseases of the nervous system and sense organs	6.3	8.0	5.8
Diseases of the circulatory system	25.9	27.2	25.6
Diseases of heart	12.6	14.3	10.9
Cerebrovascular diseases	5.8	6.1	7.8
Diseases of the respiratory system.	6.6	6.1	7.7
Decubitus ulcers.	1.9	1.1	1.0
Diseases of the musculoskeletal system and connective tissue. .	9.4	8.3	8.8
Osteoarthritis	2.5	2.8	3.2
Fractures, all sites	3.8	3.7	3.3
Fracture of neck of femur (hip)	1.4	1.7	1.3
Other	32.7	31.8	34.6

See footnotes at end of table.

Table 88 (page 2 of 2). Home health care and hospice patients, according to selected characteristics: United States, selected years 1992–96

[Data are based on a survey of current home health care and hospice patients]

Type of patient and characteristic	1992	1994	1996
Hospice patients	Number of current patients		
Total.	52,100	60,783	59,363
	Patients per 10,000 population		
Total.	2.0	2.3	2.2
Age at interview:			
Under 65 years, crude	0.5	0.8	0.5
65 years and over, crude.	13.1	12.9	13.9
65 years and over, age adjusted[1].	13.7	13.6	14.4
65–74 years	7.8	7.3	7.8
75–84 years	19.2	16.9	16.9
85 years and over	23.4	30.6	34.7
Sex:			
Male, total	1.9	2.1	2.0
Under 65 years, crude	0.5	0.9	0.5
65 years and over, crude	13.9	12.5	14.8
65 years and over, age adjusted[1]	16.0	14.4	16.1
65–74 years	6.3	7.0	10.4
75–84 years	25.8	18.2	18.5
85 years and over	28.8	34.8	33.9
Female, total	2.1	2.5	2.4
Under 65 years, crude	0.4	0.7	0.6
65 years and over, crude	12.6	13.2	13.2
65 years and over, age adjusted[1]	12.6	13.2	12.9
65–74 years	8.9	7.5	5.8
75–84 years . . . . , ...	15.1	16.1	15.9
85 years and over	21.4	29.0	35.0
	Percent distribution		
Age at interview:[2]			
Under 65 years	19.5	30.1	21.3
65 years and over	80.5	69.9	78.7
65–74 years	27.3	22.2	24.5
75–84 years	38.6	30.1	32.4
85 years and over	14.6	17.6	21.9
Sex:			
Male	46.1	44.7	44.9
Female	53.9	55.3	55.1
Primary admission diagnosis:[3]			
Malignant neoplasms	65.7	57.2	58.3
Malignant neoplasms of large intestine and rectum.	9.0	8.0	4.0
Malignant neoplasms of trachea, bronchus, and lung	21.1	12.5	15.8
Malignant neoplasm of breast.	3.9	4.8	6.2
Malignant neoplasm of prostate	6.0	5.9	6.6
Diseases of heart	10.2	9.3	8.3
Diseases of the respiratory system.	4.3	6.6	7.3
Other	19.8	27.0	26.1

[1]Age adjusted by the direct method to the year 2000 standard population using the following three age groups: 65–74 years, 75–84 years, and 85 years and over. See Appendix II, Age adjustment.
[2]Denominator excludes persons with unknown age.
[3]Denominator excludes persons with unknown diagnosis.

NOTES: Current home health care and hospice patients are those who were under the care of their agency on any given day during the survey period. Rates are based on the civilian population as of July 1. Population figures are adjusted for net underenumeration using the 1990 National Population Adjustment Matrix from the U.S. Bureau of the Census. Diagnostic categories are based on the *International Classification of Diseases, 9th Revision, Clinical Modification.* For a listing of the code numbers, see Appendix II, table VIII. The number of home health care patients in 1994 has been revised and differs from the previous edition of *Health, United States.* Data are presented for age at interview and replace data for age at admission shown in the previous edition of *Health, United States.*

SOURCE: Centers for Disease Control and Prevention, National Center for Health Statistics. National Home and Hospice Care Survey.

[Data are based on household interviews of a sample of the civilian noninstitutionalized population]

Characteristic	Discharges[1]		Days of care[1]		Average length of stay[1]	
	1997	1998	1997	1998	1997	1998
	Number per 1,000 population				Number of days	
Total[2,3]	124.3	123.8	601.2	611.0	4.5	4.6
Age						
Under 18 years	90.8	81.9	319.0	315.6	3.7	3.9
Under 6 years	203.5	192.1	632.6	645.1	3.3	3.4
6–17 years	34.0	27.3	163.1	152.6	4.9	5.6
18–44 years	96.8	93.1	358.8	380.5	3.8	4.1
45–64 years	124.9	134.0	631.1	678.6	5.1	5.2
45–54 years	99.2	105.5	527.5	530.8	5.4	5.2
55–64 years	164.8	177.9	792.4	906.1	4.9	5.2
65 years and over	274.4	283.4	1,852.5	1,789.7	6.9	6.6
65–74 years	249.1	244.3	1,595.2	1,496.6	6.5	6.2
75 years and over	307.3	333.0	2,188.4	2,160.8	7.3	7.0
Under 65 years of age						
All persons under 65 years of age[2,4]	102.2	100.2	416.4	437.0	4.1	4.3
Sex[4]						
Male	79.1	80.6	374.9	422.7	5.0	5.4
Female	124.7	119.2	456.6	450.4	3.8	3.8
Race[4,5]						
White	100.8	98.6	385.8	417.4	3.9	4.2
Black	126.3	117.3	688.6	608.6	5.3	4.9
American Indian or Alaska Native	111.9	186.4	*494.3	*	3.7	*
Asian or Pacific Islander	61.7	75.4	*268.6	313.5	*4.4	4.4
Race and Hispanic origin[4]						
White, non-Hispanic	99.6	97.8	382.7	408.7	3.9	4.2
Black, non-Hispanic	125.7	116.6	692.6	609.3	5.4	4.9
Hispanic[5]	109.9	103.5	416.7	468.5	3.8	4.6
Poverty status[4,6]						
Poor	196.8	174.7	971.0	968.0	4.8	5.3
Near poor	125.5	125.5	553.7	649.9	4.3	5.1
Nonpoor	85.6	87.4	312.1	342.0	3.7	3.8
Race and Hispanic origin and poverty status[4,6]						
White, non-Hispanic:						
Poor	222.2	181.7	1,053.4	1,004.8	4.8	5.3
Near poor	132.8	127.6	539.1	626.7	3.9	4.9
Nonpoor	85.7	88.5	306.8	340.2	3.6	3.8
Black, non-Hispanic:						
Poor	195.9	183.4	*1,260.0	964.9	5.8	4.6
Near poor	142.0	161.0	819.2	969.2	5.3	5.5
Nonpoor	92.3	79.3	389.0	407.8	4.2	4.8
Hispanic:[5]						
Poor	163.9	158.6	625.1	*	3.8	*
Near poor	93.9	85.9	421.4	342.9	4.7	3.9
Nonpoor	95.4	81.6	297.9	287.7	3.1	3.5
Health insurance status[4,7]						
Insured	108.1	- - -	442.5	- - -	4.2	- - -
Private	84.3	- - -	302.7	- - -	3.6	- - -
Medicaid	310.3	- - -	1,554.8	- - -	5.1	- - -
Uninsured	75.3	- - -	296.3	- - -	3.9	- - -
Poverty status and health insurance status[4,6]						
Poor:						
Insured	243.9	- - -	1,272.5	- - -	5.1	- - -
Uninsured	110.0	- - -	459.4	- - -	4.1	- - -
Near poor:						
Insured	149.2	- - -	663.8	- - -	4.3	- - -
Uninsured	73.4	- - -	302.1	- - -	3.9	- - -
Nonpoor:						
Insured	88.1	- - -	316.0	- - -	3.6	- - -
Uninsured	*59.8	- - -	*253.5	- - -	4.2	- - -

See footnotes at end of table.

Table 89 (page 2 of 2). Discharges, days of care, and average length of stay in short-stay hospitals, according to selected characteristics: United States, 1997 and 1998

[Data are based on household interviews of a sample of the civilian noninstitutionalized population]

Characteristic	Discharges[1]		Days of care[1]		Average length of stay[1]	
	1997	1998	1997	1998	1997	1998
Geographic region[4]	Number per 1,000 population				Number of days	
Northeast	96.0	94.9	455.4	502.5	4.9	5.1
Midwest	108.7	103.4	384.4	441.9	3.6	4.3
South	111.8	107.3	466.1	456.7	4.2	4.2
West	82.9	88.3	327.2	330.0	4.0	3.7
Location of residence[4]						
Within MSA[8]	99.3	97.9	411.8	431.8	4.2	4.3
Outside MSA[8]	113.2	109.2	435.9	458.7	3.9	4.3
65 years of age and over						
All persons 65 years of age and over[2,9]	276.9	286.6	1,878.4	1,813.8	6.9	6.6
Sex[9]						
Male	291.6	283.5	2,077.4	1,855.7	7.2	6.6
Female	265.2	288.1	1,727.4	1,793.4	6.7	6.7
Race and Hispanic origin[9]						
White, non-Hispanic	274.8	268.6	1,808.2	1,752.0	6.7	6.6
Black, non-Hispanic	290.8	372.7	2,423.5	2,476.5	8.5	7.0
Hispanic[5]	312.7	295.1	2,512.1	1,907.1	8.1	7.0
Poverty status[6,9]						
Poor	357.4	337.4	2,690.9	2,034.3	7.7	6.1
Near poor	329.6	330.6	2,498.3	2,378.0	7.7	7.2
Nonpoor	256.6	285.4	1,680.3	1,648.9	6.4	6.3
Health insurance status[7,9]						
Medicare and Private[10]	266.3	- - -	1,719.8	- - -	6.5	- - -
Medicare and Medicaid[10]	516.2	- - -	3,697.9	- - -	7.3	- - -
Medicare only	231.1	- - -	1,623.9	- - -	7.3	- - -
Geographic region[9]						
Northeast	265.0	252.7	1,828.5	1,814.6	6.9	7.4
Midwest	285.2	276.6	1,971.1	1,619.0	7.1	5.8
South	298.1	312.3	2,140.2	2,107.7	7.4	6.9
West	237.2	285.7	1,299.2	1,493.6	5.4	6.2
Location of residence[9]						
Within MSA[8]	271.3	258.6	1,875.9	1,736.8	7.0	6.8
Outside MSA[8]	295.1	378.8	1,893.6	2,068.9	6.6	6.3

- - - Data not available as of publication.
* Data preceded by an asterisk have a relative standard error of 20–30 percent. Data not shown have a relative standard error of greater than 30 percent.
[1]See Appendix II, Discharge, Days of care, Average length of stay.
[2]Includes all other races not shown separately, unknown poverty status, and unknown health insurance status.
[3]Estimates for all persons are age adjusted to the year 2000 standard using six age groups: Under 18 years, 18–44 years, 45–54 years, 55–64 years, 65–74 years, and 75 years of age and over. See Appendix II, Age adjustment.
[4]Estimates are for persons under 65 years of age and are age adjusted to the year 2000 standard using four age groups: Under 18 years, 18–44 years, 45–54 years, and 55–64 years of age. See Appendix II, Age adjustment.
[5]The race groups white, black, American Indian or Alaska Native, and Asian or Pacific Islander include persons of Hispanic and non-Hispanic origin; persons of Hispanic origin may be of any race.
[6]Poverty status is based on family income, family size, number of children in the family, and for families with two or fewer adults the age of the adults in the family, using Bureau of the Census poverty thresholds. Poor persons are defined as below the poverty threshold. Near poor persons have incomes of 100 percent to less than 200 percent of poverty threshold. Nonpoor persons have incomes of 200 percent or greater than the poverty threshold. See Appendix II, Poverty level. Poverty status was missing for 20 percent of persons in the sample in 1997 and 25 percent in 1998.
[7]Health insurance categories are mutually exclusive. Persons who reported both Medicaid and private coverage are classified as having Medicaid coverage. See Appendix II, Health insurance coverage.
[8]MSA is metropolitan statistical area.
[9]Estimates are for persons 65 years of age and over and are age adjusted to the year 2000 standard using two age groups: 65–74 years and 75 years and over. See Appendix II, Age adjustment.
[10]Includes some persons who do not have Medicare coverage.

NOTES: Hospital utilization data starting in 1997 are not comparable with data for earlier years due to the 1997 redesign. See Appendix I, National Health Interview Survey. Estimates of hospital utilization presented in this table are for all discharges. Previous estimates of hospital utilization from the National Health Interview Survey (NHIS) in *Health, United States* excluded hospitalizations for newborns and delivery. Estimates of hospital utilization from the NHIS and the National Hospital Discharge Survey (NHDS) may differ because NHIS data are based on household interviews of the civilian noninstitutionalized population, whereas NHDS data are based on hospital discharge records of all persons (NHDS tables presented in *Health, United States* exclude estimates for newborn infants). See Appendix I, National Hospital Discharge Survey. NHDS includes records for persons discharged alive or deceased and institutionalized persons; differences in the two surveys are particularly evident for children and the elderly.

SOURCE: Centers for Disease Control and Prevention, National Center for Health Statistics. National Health Interview Survey, family core questionnaire.

Table 90 (page 1 of 2). Discharges, days of care, and average length of stay in non-Federal short-stay hospitals, according to selected characteristics: United States, selected years 1980–98

[Data are based on a sample of hospital records]

Characteristic	1980[1]	1985[1]	1990	1992	1994	1996	1997	1998
	Discharges per 1,000 population							
Total[2]	158.5	137.7	113.0	110.5	106.5	102.3	101.4	103.0
Age								
Under 15 years	71.6	57.7	44.6	45.2	39.2	38.2	38.7	38.3
15–44 years	150.1	125.0	101.6	96.0	93.2	87.0	82.5	85.1
45–64 years	194.8	170.8	135.0	131.0	124.1	117.2	115.4	117.3
65 years and over	383.7	369.8	330.9	336.5	341.6	346.1	361.1	365.3
65–74 years	315.8	297.2	259.1	264.5	261.6	257.3	265.9	267.6
75 years and over	489.3	475.6	429.9	432.7	445.3	455.2	474.0	477.4
Sex[2]								
Male	140.3	124.4	100.9	98.6	94.2	89.7	88.9	89.0
Female	177.0	151.8	126.0	123.2	119.1	115.3	114.4	117.1
Geographic region[2]								
Northeast	147.6	129.1	121.0	123.9	121.3	112.6	111.6	112.9
Midwest	175.4	143.4	115.1	105.3	102.6	99.6	100.1	100.6
South	165.1	143.5	119.2	116.3	111.8	105.7	106.5	110.2
West	136.9	130.3	92.1	93.7	87.6	90.3	85.4	85.0
	Days of care per 1,000 population							
Total[2]	1,129.0	872.1	705.0	659.3	594.0	520.6	502.1	508.1
Age								
Under 15 years	315.7	263.0	215.4	219.6	189.2	174.4	164.6	178.0
15–44 years	786.8	603.3	465.3	416.1	390.4	333.9	305.5	316.1
45–64 years	1,596.9	1,201.6	911.5	827.1	727.5	624.3	601.9	603.9
65 years and over	4,098.4	3,228.0	2,867.7	2,771.7	2,516.3	2,263.7	2,285.6	2,264.2
65–74 years	3,147.0	2,437.3	2,067.7	2,040.8	1,798.8	1,603.8	1,599.3	1,596.1
75 years and over	5,578.7	4,381.4	3,970.7	3,747.8	3,445.7	3,074.7	3,099.6	3,030.8
Sex[2]								
Male	1,076.0	848.2	690.4	656.3	580.8	511.8	481.5	487.2
Female	1,187.1	902.0	725.3	667.5	609.5	531.6	524.5	530.3
Geographic region[2]								
Northeast	1,204.7	953.5	878.0	838.6	774.9	666.9	634.0	627.2
Midwest	1,296.2	952.0	713.4	626.2	553.9	484.4	467.7	466.6
South	1,105.5	848.9	704.1	676.2	618.0	532.2	528.8	544.2
West	836.2	713.2	509.9	483.1	420.3	402.5	373.6	385.1
	Average length of stay in days							
Total[2]	7.1	6.3	6.2	6.0	5.6	5.1	5.0	4.9
Age								
Under 15 years	4.4	4.6	4.8	4.9	4.8	4.6	4.3	4.6
15–44 years	5.2	4.8	4.6	4.3	4.2	3.8	3.7	3.7
45–64 years	8.2	7.0	6.8	6.3	5.9	5.3	5.2	5.1
65 years and over	10.7	8.7	8.7	8.2	7.4	6.5	6.3	6.2
65–74 years	10.0	8.2	8.0	7.7	6.9	6.2	6.0	6.0
75 years and over	11.4	9.2	9.2	8.7	7.7	6.8	6.5	6.3
Sex[2]								
Male	7.7	6.8	6.8	6.7	6.2	5.7	5.4	5.5
Female	6.7	5.9	5.8	5.4	5.1	4.6	4.6	4.5

See footnotes at end of table.

Table 90 (page 2 of 2). Discharges, days of care, and average length of stay in non-Federal short-stay hospitals, according to selected characteristics: United States, selected years 1980–98

[Data are based on a sample of hospital records]

Characteristic	1980[1]	1985[1]	1990	1992	1994	1996	1997	1998
Geographic region[2]				Average length of stay in days				
Northeast	8.2	7.4	7.3	6.8	6.4	5.9	5.7	5.6
Midwest	7.4	6.6	6.2	5.9	5.4	4.9	4.7	4.6
South	6.7	5.9	5.9	5.8	5.5	5.0	5.0	4.9
West	6.1	5.5	5.5	5.2	4.8	4.5	4.4	4.5

[1]Comparisons of data from 1980–85 with data from later years should be made with caution as estimates of change may reflect improvements in the design (see Appendix I) rather than true changes in hospital use.
[2]Age adjusted. See Appendix II, Age adjustment.

NOTES: Rates are based on the civilian population as of July 1. In 1993 children's hospitals had a high rate of nonresponse that may have resulted in underestimates of hospital utilization by children. Beginning with data year 1997, population figures are adjusted for net underenumeration using the 1990 National Population Adjustment Matrix from the U.S. Bureau of the Census. Comparisons of selected estimates based on matrix-adjusted populations with those based on nonadjusted populations for data years 1995 and 1996 show little difference between the two sets of estimates. Estimates of hospital utilization from the National Health Interview Survey (NHIS) and the National Hospital Discharge Survey (NHDS) may differ because NHIS data are based on household interviews of the civilian noninstitutionalized population, whereas NHDS data are based on hospital discharge records of all persons. NHDS includes records for persons discharged alive or deceased and institutionalized persons, and excludes newborn infants. Differences in hospital utilization estimated by the two surveys are particularly evident for children and the elderly. See Appendix I. Data for additional years are available (see Appendix III).

SOURCE: Centers for Disease Control and Prevention, National Center for Health Statistics, Division of Health Care Statistics. Data from the National Hospital Discharge Survey.

Table 91. Discharges, days of care, and average length of stay in non-Federal short-stay hospitals for discharges with the diagnosis of human immunodeficiency virus (HIV) and for all discharges: United States, selected years 1986–98

[Data are based on a sample of hospital records]

Type of discharge, sex, and age	1986[1]	1987[1]	1988	1990	1992	1993	1995[2]	1996[2]	1997[2]	1998[2]
					Discharges in thousands					
Discharges with diagnosis of HIV	44	67	95	146	194	225	249	227	178	189
Male, 20–49 years	35	51	73	102	141	158	162	141	107	113
Female, 20–49 years	*	*	13	27	31	44	55	52	46	51
All discharges	34,256	33,387	31,146	30,788	30,951	30,825	30,722	30,545	30,914	31,827
Male, 20–49 years	4,300	4,075	3,670	3,649	3,529	3,619	3,360	3,248	3,116	3,154
Female, 20–49 years	9,027	8,980	8,169	8,228	7,942	7,901	7,593	7,457	7,322	7,639
					Discharges per 1,000 population					
Discharges with diagnosis of HIV	0.18	0.28	0.39	0.59	0.76	0.88	0.94	0.85	0.66	0.69
Male, 20–49 years	0.67	0.96	1.36	1.84	2.47	2.76	2.72	2.34	1.77	1.88
Female, 20–49 years	*	*	0.23	0.47	0.54	0.74	0.91	0.86	0.76	0.84
All discharges	143.7	138.8	128.3	124.3	122.1	120.2	115.7	114.0	114.3	116.5
Male, 20–49 years	82.2	76.8	68.2	65.8	62.0	63.1	56.5	54.0	51.8	52.6
Female, 20–49 years	166.7	163.6	147.1	144.5	136.1	134.6	125.9	122.8	120.8	125.2
					Days of care in thousands					
Discharges with diagnosis of HIV	714	936	1,277	2,188	2,136	2,561	2,326	2,123	1,448	1,503
Male, 20–49 years	573	724	914	1,645	1,422	1,696	1,408	1,401	855	892
Female, 20–49 years	*	*	233	341	455	619	559	457	364	365
All discharges	218,496	214,942	203,678	197,422	190,386	184,601	164,627	159,883	157,458	160,914
Male, 20–49 years	26,488	26,295	22,697	22,539	21,614	21,348	17,984	17,818	15,529	16,085
Female, 20–49 years	40,620	39,356	34,800	34,473	30,886	29,555	26,596	25,368	24,955	25,976
					Days of care per 1,000 population					
Discharges with diagnosis of HIV	2.99	3.89	5.26	8.83	8.43	9.99	8.76	7.92	5.35	5.50
Male, 20–49 years	10.95	13.64	16.97	29.68	24.97	29.57	23.70	23.29	14.22	14.86
Female, 20–49 years	*	*	4.19	5.99	7.80	10.54	9.27	7.52	6.00	5.98
All discharges	916.5	893.6	838.8	796.9	751.0	719.9	620.2	596.5	582.3	589.2
Male, 20–49 years	506.4	495.2	421.5	406.6	379.5	372.2	302.7	296.2	258.3	268.0
Female, 20–49 years	750.2	717.1	626.5	605.4	529.3	503.4	441.0	417.8	411.7	425.8
					Average length of stay in days					
Discharges with diagnosis of HIV	16.4	14.1	13.4	14.9	11.0	11.4	9.3	9.4	8.1	8.0
Male, 20–49 years	16.4	14.1	12.5	16.2	10.1	10.7	8.7	9.9	8.0	8.0
Female, 20–49 years	*	*	18.0	12.6	14.6	14.2	10.2	8.7	7.9	7.1
All discharges	6.4	6.4	6.5	6.4	6.2	6.0	5.4	5.2	5.1	5.1
Male, 20–49 years	6.2	6.5	6.2	6.2	6.1	5.9	5.4	5.5	5.0	5.1
Female, 20–49 years	4.5	4.4	4.3	4.2	3.9	3.7	3.5	3.4	3.4	3.4

* Statistics based on fewer than 5,000 estimated discharges are not shown.

[1]Comparisons of data from 1986 and 1987 with data from later years should be made with caution as estimates of change may reflect improvements in the design (see Appendix I) rather than true changes in hospital use.

[2]Beginning with data year 1995, population figures are adjusted for net underenumeration using the 1990 National Population Adjustment Matrix from the U.S. Bureau of the Census. Comparisons of selected estimates based on matrix-adjusted populations with those based on nonadjusted populations for data years 1995 and 1996 show little difference between the two sets of estimates.

NOTES: Excludes newborn infants. Rates are based on the civilian population as of July 1. Discharges with diagnosis of HIV have at least one HIV diagnosis listed on the face sheet of the medical record and are not limited to the first-listed diagnosis, See Appendix II, Human immunodeficiency virus (HIV) infection. Data for additional years are available (see Appendix III).

SOURCE: Centers for Disease Control and Prevention, National Center for Health Statistics, Division of Health Care Statistics. Data from the National Hospital Discharge Survey.

Table 92 (page 1 of 3). Rates of discharges and days of care in non-Federal short-stay hospitals, according to sex, age, and selected first-listed diagnoses: United States, 1985, 1990, 1996, and 1997

[Data are based on a sample of hospital records]

Sex, age, and first-listed diagnosis	Discharges				Days of care			
	1985[1]	1990	1996	1997	1985[1]	1990	1996	1997
Both sexes	Number per 1,000 population							
Total[2,3]	137.7	113.0	102.3	101.4	872.1	705.0	520.6	502.1
Male								
All ages[2,3]	124.4	100.9	89.7	88.9	848.2	690.4	511.8	481.5
Under 15 years[3]	64.4	49.2	42.0	43.0	289.9	234.1	193.2	183.8
Bronchitis	1.7	0.8	0.5	0.5	5.4	2.4	1.6	1.3
Pneumonia	5.7	6.3	6.0	7.3	23.6	26.3	21.8	25.2
Asthma	3.5	3.9	4.2	4.4	12.0	11.0	11.6	10.7
Injuries and poisoning	9.3	5.9	4.8	4.2	36.8	26.0	17.1	16.6
Fracture, all sites	3.2	2.0	1.7	1.5	16.7	7.9	6.1	6.3
15–44 years[3]	75.3	57.8	47.7	44.1	458.2	353.6	263.2	218.7
Psychoses	3.0	3.5	4.7	4.3	43.7	50.3	44.6	36.5
Diseases of heart	3.0	2.9	2.8	2.6	16.6	15.4	10.5	11.9
Intervertebral disc disorders	2.9	2.4	1.5	1.4	18.7	10.0	4.3	3.2
Injuries and poisoning	17.9	13.4	9.3	8.3	98.7	66.7	43.9	35.9
Fracture, all sites	5.2	4.1	3.1	3.0	34.6	22.9	15.0	13.3
45–64 years[3]	177.6	140.2	120.8	117.9	1,229.0	943.6	658.7	622.5
Malignant neoplasms	13.1	10.6	7.7	7.3	120.6	99.1	55.8	47.6
Trachea, bronchus, lung	3.6	2.7	1.4	1.3	31.9	19.1	9.7	10.8
Diabetes	3.4	2.9	3.2	3.4	26.5	21.2	24.4	21.6
Diseases of heart	36.9	31.7	30.5	28.8	239.2	185.0	139.3	123.8
Ischemic heart disease	27.1	22.6	21.8	19.9	171.1	128.2	97.7	81.8
Acute myocardial infarction	9.2	7.4	7.7	6.9	82.4	55.8	42.9	35.8
Congestive heart failure	2.5	3.0	3.2	3.3	18.9	19.7	18.5	16.8
Cerebrovascular diseases	5.0	4.1	4.1	4.2	51.0	40.7	25.1	22.3
Pneumonia	3.4	3.5	3.2	3.3	27.4	27.4	22.1	21.2
Injuries and poisoning	15.0	11.6	10.4	10.2	99.1	82.6	56.1	54.3
Fracture, all sites	4.0	3.3	2.9	2.8	29.9	24.2	15.9	14.5
65–74 years[3]	325.5	285.9	270.6	273.8	2,622.0	2,237.2	1,675.3	1,630.9
Malignant neoplasms	38.8	27.7	23.5	22.3	352.8	275.8	171.0	153.1
Large intestine and rectum	3.9	3.0	2.8	2.1	54.9	34.0	26.3	18.3
Trachea, bronchus, lung	10.8	6.3	4.7	4.6	89.5	55.4	33.6	36.3
Prostate	6.6	5.0	4.8	4.4	48.2	32.9	21.3	16.7
Diabetes	4.3	4.3	4.6	5.0	42.6	39.6	36.0	38.7
Diseases of heart	69.9	69.0	73.5	75.7	520.2	484.1	396.2	386.2
Ischemic heart disease	43.2	41.7	44.8	43.1	317.2	283.4	240.2	213.5
Acute myocardial infarction	17.6	13.9	16.4	14.8	160.4	121.7	105.1	89.2
Congestive heart failure	9.8	11.3	11.9	15.3	76.4	89.6	73.6	91.0
Cerebrovascular diseases	18.5	13.7	15.3	17.0	182.0	114.0	92.0	91.9
Pneumonia	10.9	11.3	13.0	13.1	104.9	107.1	89.2	90.8
Hyperplasia of prostate	13.5	14.3	5.0	5.6	84.8	64.6	14.6	16.4
Osteoarthritis	3.4	5.0	6.7	6.9	36.9	44.6	31.4	30.7
Injuries and poisoning	16.0	17.5	15.8	15.4	131.7	138.1	103.3	93.4
Fracture, all sites	4.5	4.5	3.5	4.0	42.8	45.6	25.6	24.1
Fracture of neck of femur (hip)	1.4	1.5	1.4	1.3	21.6	18.0	10.6	11.1
75 years and over[3]	529.1	476.3	476.6	498.6	4,682.0	4,211.9	3,160.4	3,183.4
Malignant neoplasms	55.7	40.8	28.0	31.5	545.9	406.4	199.5	235.9
Large intestine and rectum	6.9	5.4	4.2	5.2	84.7	80.3	41.0	56.0
Trachea, bronchus, lung	10.4	5.3	5.6	6.5	99.0	53.1	43.2	44.7
Prostate	15.3	9.7	3.5	3.8	116.5	65.3	13.9	16.9
Diabetes	6.4	4.6	6.7	6.4	66.6	50.9	55.6	43.5
Diseases of heart	108.6	105.7	114.3	113.9	841.2	851.7	616.5	611.2
Ischemic heart disease	51.3	48.9	53.2	48.6	413.2	396.2	299.4	260.4
Acute myocardial infarction	23.8	23.0	22.4	20.6	230.5	226.5	153.1	131.0
Congestive heart failure	27.8	30.9	31.4	35.0	220.5	241.2	172.0	198.2
Cerebrovascular diseases	37.9	30.0	33.4	32.9	380.7	296.9	228.3	181.8
Pneumonia	30.1	38.4	38.3	46.0	305.7	391.8	291.7	323.7
Hyperplasia of prostate	19.7	17.8	7.8	8.4	141.0	108.7	34.0	31.1
Osteoarthritis	4.4	5.7	7.7	6.0	49.4	60.4	43.9	30.0
Injuries and poisoning	31.8	31.1	33.2	34.3	358.8	339.7	239.2	225.1
Fracture, all sites	14.3	13.7	14.2	16.4	223.9	144.4	116.7	117.6
Fracture of neck of femur (hip)	8.4	8.5	9.2	10.3	161.3	97.4	77.3	79.4

See footnotes at end of table.

Table 92 (page 2 of 3). Rates of discharges and days of care in non-Federal short-stay hospitals, according to sex, age, and selected first-listed diagnoses: United States, 1985, 1990, 1996, and 1997

[Data are based on a sample of hospital records]

Sex, age, and first-listed diagnosis	Discharges				Days of care			
	1985[1]	1990	1996	1997	1985[1]	1990	1996	1997
Female	Number per 1,000 population							
All ages[2,3]	151.8	126.0	115.3	114.4	902.0	725.3	531.6	524.5
Under 15 years[3]	50.6	39.7	34.3	34.1	234.8	195.8	154.6	144.5
Bronchitis	1.2	0.7	0.4	0.3	3.6	3.0	1.2	0.8
Pneumonia	4.7	4.8	5.0	5.2	20.9	20.5	18.5	18.4
Asthma	2.1	2.3	2.5	2.7	7.5	7.2	6.4	6.5
Injuries and poisoning	6.1	3.9	2.9	2.9	23.0	15.1	12.4	11.7
Fracture, all sites	1.9	1.3	0.7	0.9	8.9	6.0	2.7	4.2
15–44 years[3]	173.5	144.7	126.1	121.1	744.8	575.4	404.4	392.8
Delivery	67.9	68.5	64.2	62.5	222.6	191.0	140.2	150.6
Psychoses	3.2	3.8	5.0	5.1	50.7	56.3	48.2	40.1
Diseases of heart	1.5	1.3	1.4	1.5	8.8	6.8	6.2	6.3
Intervertebral disc disorders	1.8	1.4	1.1	1.0	13.5	6.8	3.2	2.3
Injuries and poisoning	9.2	6.9	5.3	5.2	48.0	36.5	20.1	20.8
Fracture, all sites	1.9	1.6	1.3	1.4	13.8	10.8	5.5	6.3
45–64 years[3]	164.6	130.2	113.8	113.0	1,176.5	881.9	592.0	582.5
Malignant neoplasms	15.4	12.6	9.0	7.6	128.8	106.8	53.3	51.7
Trachea, bronchus, lung	2.4	1.7	1.3	0.8	22.3	14.7	7.9	6.1
Breast	3.9	2.8	1.9	1.5	25.2	12.0	5.3	5.1
Diabetes	3.8	2.9	2.8	2.9	31.6	25.7	17.8	14.4
Diseases of heart	18.0	16.5	16.4	15.4	121.4	100.5	75.8	72.9
Ischemic heart disease	10.6	9.9	9.7	8.5	71.1	57.1	40.9	36.5
Acute myocardial infarction	3.0	2.8	2.9	2.6	33.5	21.5	16.6	15.5
Congestive heart failure	1.8	2.1	2.5	3.0	12.7	15.8	14.4	16.8
Cerebrovascular diseases	3.7	3.0	2.9	3.2	44.9	31.9	21.9	18.5
Pneumonia	3.3	3.3	3.4	3.4	29.2	26.4	20.9	19.8
Injuries and poisoning	12.2	9.4	7.8	7.6	82.4	62.9	39.8	40.7
Fracture, all sites	4.1	3.1	2.8	2.3	30.0	24.8	13.7	12.2
65–74 years[3]	275.5	238.2	246.6	259.4	2,294.9	1,935.3	1,546.3	1,573.6
Malignant neoplasms	29.1	20.6	19.8	18.5	274.8	187.5	133.9	141.7
Large intestine and rectum	3.2	2.4	2.4	2.3	41.8	34.5	22.4	21.1
Trachea, bronchus, lung	3.6	2.6	3.0	2.8	34.9	26.6	22.2	24.0
Breast	5.1	3.9	3.3	2.7	44.6	17.4	9.6	6.4
Diabetes	6.8	5.8	6.0	6.0	65.5	46.3	38.2	41.8
Diseases of heart	49.4	44.6	53.4	49.8	375.1	313.1	298.5	267.9
Ischemic heart disease	27.5	24.1	27.0	23.7	205.1	151.9	148.9	122.8
Acute myocardial infarction	8.6	7.4	9.0	7.6	88.7	57.3	57.1	52.1
Congestive heart failure	8.2	9.1	11.2	11.5	67.9	80.8	72.6	69.0
Cerebrovascular diseases	15.0	11.2	12.0	14.8	155.1	94.8	76.9	83.0
Pneumonia	7.0	8.6	10.8	12.2	65.2	80.8	79.5	100.1
Osteoarthritis	4.3	6.8	9.5	10.1	45.2	68.1	47.7	49.3
Injuries and poisoning	19.7	17.6	20.2	19.3	178.8	164.2	135.3	109.4
Fracture, all sites	9.3	8.3	9.7	8.7	97.7	96.2	61.6	50.1
Fracture of neck of femur (hip)	3.5	3.5	4.7	3.1	48.0	58.8	34.4	20.0

See footnotes at end of table.

Table 92 (page 3 of 3). Rates of discharges and days of care in non-Federal short-stay hospitals, according to sex, age, and selected first-listed diagnoses: United States, 1985, 1990, 1996, and 1997

[Data are based on a sample of hospital records]

Sex, age, and first-listed diagnosis	Discharges				Days of care			
	1985[1]	1990	1996	1997	1985[1]	1990	1996	1997
Female—Con.			Number per 1,000 population					
75 years and over[3]	446.8	404.6	442.8	459.6	4,219.1	3,838.9	3,025.3	3,050.4
Malignant neoplasms	26.1	21.8	18.8	19.8	282.9	254.1	148.7	153.9
Large intestine and rectum	5.3	4.6	3.8	3.7	69.3	68.9	43.4	34.9
Trachea, bronchus, lung	1.8	2.1	2.2	2.2	24.9	20.3	16.6	16.7
Breast	4.1	3.8	2.2	2.7	37.0	21.7	6.6	8.3
Diabetes	6.6	4.6	6.3	6.3	69.7	54.6	40.8	46.4
Diseases of heart	91.6	83.5	95.7	95.8	773.1	664.4	576.8	571.4
Ischemic heart disease	40.9	33.3	36.8	33.5	341.4	250.0	220.0	210.1
Acute myocardial infarction	17.0	12.9	15.2	13.9	170.3	124.3	112.6	99.1
Congestive heart failure	24.5	27.6	30.8	32.1	208.3	233.7	198.3	193.7
Cerebrovascular diseases	33.7	29.2	30.0	30.3	368.1	298.3	207.6	186.6
Pneumonia	18.4	23.6	28.1	30.5	184.8	256.9	199.5	215.1
Osteoarthritis	4.8	5.2	9.9	9.3	64.4	53.4	56.2	65.1
Injuries and poisoning	47.8	45.8	47.0	49.1	541.4	483.2	315.0	323.7
Fracture, all sites	31.9	31.1	32.6	32.2	402.9	348.4	226.8	222.3
Fracture of neck of femur (hip)	18.9	18.6	21.3	20.1	270.8	233.4	156.6	148.2

[1]Comparisons of data from 1985 with data from later years should be made with caution as estimates of change may reflect improvements in the design (see Appendix I) rather than true changes in hospital use.
[2]Age adjusted. See Appendix II for age-adjustment procedure.
[3]Includes discharges with first-listed diagnoses not shown in table.

NOTES: Excludes newborn infants. Rates are based on the civilian population as of July 1. Beginning with data year 1997, population figures are adjusted for net underenumeration using the 1990 National Population Adjustment Matrix from the U.S. Bureau of the Census. Comparisons of selected estimates based on matrix adjusted populations with those based on nonadjusted populations for data years 1995 and 1996 show little difference between the two sets of estimates. Diagnostic categories are based on the *International Classification of Diseases, Ninth Revision, Clinical Modification.* For a listing of the code numbers, see Appendix II, table VIII. Data for additional years are available (see Appendix III).

SOURCE: Centers for Disease Control and Prevention, National Center for Health Statistics, Division of Health Care Statistics. Data from the National Hospital Discharge Survey.

Table 93 (page 1 of 3). Discharges and average length of stay in non-Federal short-stay hospitals, according to sex, age, and selected first-listed diagnoses: United States, 1985, 1990, 1996, and 1997

[Data are based on a sample of hospital records]

Sex, age, and first-listed diagnosis	Discharges				Average length of stay			
	1985[1]	1990	1996	1997	1985[1]	1990	1996	1997
Both sexes	Number in thousands				Number of days			
Total[2,3]	35,056	30,788	30,545	30,914	6.3	6.2	5.1	4.4
Male								
All ages[2,3]	14,160	12,280	12,110	12,268	6.8	6.8	5.7	4.9
Under 15 years[3]	1,698	1,362	1,240	1,316	4.5	4.8	4.6	4.3
Bronchitis	45	22	15	16	3.2	3.1	3.2	2.4
Pneumonia	150	174	178	223	4.2	4.2	3.6	3.5
Asthma	93	107	123	136	3.4	2.8	2.8	2.4
Injuries and poisoning	245	164	142	128	4.0	4.4	3.6	4.0
Fracture, all sites	85	54	51	47	5.2	4.0	3.6	4.1
15–44 years[3]	4,153	3,330	2,831	2,688	6.1	6.1	5.5	5.0
Psychoses	167	200	277	264	14.4	14.5	9.5	8.4
Diseases of heart	165	166	166	157	5.5	5.3	3.7	4.6
Intervertebral disc disorders	161	138	90	85	6.4	4.2	2.8	2.3
Injuries and poisoning	988	772	550	508	5.5	5.0	4.7	4.3
Fracture, all sites	290	238	185	185	6.6	5.5	4.8	4.4
45–64 years[3]	3,776	3,115	3,138	3,161	6.9	6.7	5.5	5.3
Malignant neoplasms	279	235	200	195	9.2	9.4	7.3	6.5
Trachea, bronchus, lung	76	60	36	36	8.9	7.1	6.9	8.0
Diabetes	71	65	83	91	7.9	7.3	7.6	6.3
Diseases of heart	784	704	793	771	6.5	5.8	4.6	4.3
Ischemic heart disease	577	502	567	533	6.3	5.7	4.5	4.1
Acute myocardial infarction	197	165	200	185	8.9	7.5	5.6	5.2
Congestive heart failure	53	66	84	88	7.6	6.7	5.7	5.1
Cerebrovascular diseases	107	91	105	112	10.2	10.0	6.2	5.4
Pneumonia	73	77	82	90	8.0	7.9	7.0	6.3
Injuries and poisoning	320	257	269	274	6.6	7.2	5.4	5.3
Fracture, all sites	85	74	76	76	7.5	7.2	5.4	5.1
65–74 years[3]	2,389	2,268	2,253	2,250	8.1	7.8	6.2	6.0
Malignant neoplasms	284	220	196	184	9.1	9.9	7.3	6.9
Large intestine and rectum	29	24	23	17	14.0	11.4	9.4	8.9
Trachea, bronchus, lung	79	50	39	37	8.3	8.7	7.2	8.0
Prostate	49	40	40	36	7.3	6.5	4.4	3.8
Diabetes	31	34	38	41	9.9	9.1	7.8	7.8
Diseases of heart	513	547	612	622	7.4	7.0	5.4	5.1
Ischemic heart disease	317	331	373	354	7.3	6.8	5.4	5.0
Acute myocardial infarction	129	110	137	122	9.1	8.8	6.4	6.0
Congestive heart failure	72	90	99	126	7.8	7.9	6.2	6.0
Cerebrovascular diseases	136	108	127	140	9.8	8.3	6.0	6.0
Pneumonia	80	90	108	108	9.6	9.5	6.9	6.9
Hyperplasia of prostate	99	113	42	46	6.3	4.5	2.9	2.9
Osteoarthritis	25	39	56	57	10.9	9.0	4.7	4.4
Injuries and poisoning	118	139	132	127	8.2	7.9	6.5	6.1
Fracture, all sites	33	36	29	33	9.5	10.2	7.2	6.1
Fracture of neck of femur (hip)	10	12	12	11	15.2	11.8	7.6	8.4
75 years and over[3]	2,144	2,203	2,648	2,852	8.8	8.8	6.6	6.4
Malignant neoplasms	226	189	155	180	9.8	10.0	7.1	7.5
Large intestine and rectum	28	25	23	30	12.3	15.0	9.8	10.8
Trachea, bronchus, lung	42	25	31	37	9.5	10.0	7.8	6.9
Prostate	62	45	20	22	7.6	6.8	4.0	4.4
Diabetes	26	21	37	37	10.5	11.0	8.3	6.8
Diseases of heart	440	489	635	651	7.7	8.1	5.4	5.4
Ischemic heart disease	208	226	296	278	8.1	8.1	5.6	5.4
Acute myocardial infarction	97	106	125	118	9.7	9.9	6.8	6.4
Congestive heart failure	113	143	174	200	7.9	7.8	5.5	5.7
Cerebrovascular diseases	154	139	186	188	10.0	9.9	6.8	5.5
Pneumonia	122	178	213	263	10.2	10.2	7.6	7.0
Hyperplasia of prostate	80	82	43	48	7.2	6.1	4.4	3.7
Osteoarthritis	18	27	43	34	11.3	10.5	5.7	5.0
Injuries and poisoning	129	144	184	196	11.3	10.9	7.2	6.6
Fracture, all sites	58	63	79	94	15.6	10.6	8.2	7.2
Fracture of neck of femur (hip)	34	39	51	59	19.2	11.5	8.4	7.7

See footnotes at end of table.

[Data are based on a sample of hospital records]

Sex, age, and first-listed diagnosis	Discharges				Average length of stay			
	1985[1]	1990	1996	1997	1985[1]	1990	1996	1997
Female	Number in thousands				Number of days			
All ages[2,3]	20,896	18,508	18,435	18,647	5.9	5.8	4.6	4.2
Under 15 years[3]	1,274	1,049	967	995	4.6	4.9	4.5	4.2
Bronchitis	30	19	11	8	3.0	4.0	2.9	2.9
Pneumonia	119	125	142	152	4.4	4.3	3.7	3.5
Asthma	52	62	72	78	3.6	3.1	2.5	2.4
Injuries and poisoning	153	102	81	85	3.8	3.9	4.3	4.0
Fracture, all sites	47	33	21	25	4.8	4.8	3.6	4.9
15–44 years[3]	9,813	8,469	7,495	7,341	4.3	4.0	3.2	3.2
Delivery	3,838	4,008	3,817	3,791	3.3	2.8	2.2	2.4
Psychoses	180	222	299	311	15.9	14.9	9.6	7.8
Diseases of heart	85	73	86	92	5.8	5.4	4.3	4.2
Intervertebral disc disorders	104	85	66	58	7.4	4.7	2.9	2.4
Injuries and poisoning	521	402	315	313	5.2	5.3	3.8	4.0
Fracture, all sites	108	93	78	82	7.2	6.8	4.2	4.7
45–64 years[3]	3,834	3,129	3,156	3,216	7.1	6.8	5.2	5.2
Malignant neoplasms	359	303	249	215	8.4	8.5	5.9	6.8
Trachea, bronchus, lung	56	41	36	23	9.3	8.6	6.0	7.5
Breast	91	67	54	42	6.5	4.3	2.7	3.5
Diabetes	88	70	78	81	8.3	8.9	6.3	5.0
Diseases of heart	420	397	455	438	6.7	6.1	4.6	4.7
Ischemic heart disease	248	237	268	242	6.7	5.8	4.2	4.3
Acute myocardial infarction	71	68	82	75	11.0	7.6	5.7	5.9
Congestive heart failure	43	51	69	85	6.9	7.4	5.8	5.7
Cerebrovascular diseases	85	72	82	90	12.2	10.7	7.5	5.9
Pneumonia	76	80	93	96	8.9	7.9	6.2	5.8
Injuries and poisoning	283	225	215	216	6.8	6.7	5.1	5.4
Fracture, all sites	96	75	78	65	7.3	7.9	4.9	5.3
65–74 years[3]	2,623	2,421	2,551	2,621	8.3	8.1	6.3	6.1
Malignant neoplasms	277	210	205	187	9.4	9.1	6.8	7.6
Large intestine and rectum	31	24	25	24	13.0	14.5	9.3	9.0
Trachea, bronchus, lung	35	26	31	28	9.6	10.2	7.3	8.7
Breast	49	40	34	27	8.7	4.5	2.9	2.4
Diabetes	64	59	62	60	9.7	8.0	6.4	7.0
Diseases of heart	470	453	553	503	7.6	7.0	5.6	5.4
Ischemic heart disease	262	245	280	239	7.5	6.3	5.5	5.2
Acute myocardial infarction	82	75	93	76	10.3	7.8	6.4	6.9
Congestive heart failure	78	92	116	116	8.3	8.9	6.5	6.0
Cerebrovascular diseases	143	114	125	149	10.3	8.5	6.4	5.6
Pneumonia	66	87	111	123	9.4	9.4	7.4	8.2
Osteoarthritis	40	69	98	102	10.6	10.0	5.0	4.9
Injuries and poisoning	188	179	209	196	9.1	9.3	6.7	5.7
Fracture, all sites	88	85	100	88	10.6	11.5	6.4	5.8
Fracture of neck of femur (hip)	33	36	49	31	13.9	16.7	7.3	6.5

See footnotes at end of table.

Table 93 (page 3 of 3). Discharges and average length of stay in non-Federal short-stay hospitals, according to sex, age, and selected first-listed diagnoses: United States, 1985, 1990, 1996, and 1997

[Data are based on a sample of hospital records]

Sex, age, and first-listed diagnosis	Discharges				Average length of stay			
	1985[1]	1990	1996	1997	1985[1]	1990	1996	1997
Female—Con.	Number in thousands				Number of days			
75 years and over[3]	3,352	3,440	4,266	4,472	9.4	9.5	6.8	6.6
Malignant neoplasms	196	185	181	193	10.8	11.7	7.9	7.8
Large intestine and rectum	40	39	37	36	13.1	15.1	11.3	9.5
Trachea, bronchus, lung	13	18	21	21	13.9	9.9	7.6	7.6
Breast	31	33	21	26	9.1	5.7	3.0	3.0
Diabetes	49	39	60	61	10.6	11.9	6.5	7.4
Diseases of heart	688	711	922	932	8.4	8.0	6.0	6.0
Ischemic heart disease	307	283	354	326	8.3	7.5	6.0	6.3
Acute myocardial infarction	127	110	146	135	10.0	9.6	7.4	7.1
Congestive heart failure	184	235	296	312	8.5	8.5	6.4	6.0
Cerebrovascular diseases	253	249	289	294	10.9	10.2	6.9	6.2
Pneumonia	138	201	270	297	10.1	10.9	7.1	7.1
Osteoarthritis	36	45	95	90	13.5	10.2	5.7	7.0
Injuries and poisoning	358	389	453	477	11.3	10.6	6.7	6.6
Fracture, all sites	240	265	314	313	12.6	11.2	7.0	6.9
Fracture of neck of femur (hip)	142	158	205	196	14.3	12.5	7.4	7.4

[1]Comparisons of data from 1985 with data from later years should be made with caution as estimates of change may reflect improvements in the design (see Appendix I) rather than true changes in hospital use.
[2]Average length of stay is age-adjusted. See Appendix II for age-adjustment procedure.
[3]Includes discharges with first-listed diagnoses not shown in table.

NOTES: Excludes newborn infants. Diagnostic categories are based on the *International Classification of Diseases, Ninth Revision, Clinical Modification.* For a listing of the code numbers, see Appendix II, table VIII. Data for additional years are available (see Appendix III).

SOURCE: Centers for Disease Control and Prevention, National Center for Health Statistics, Division of Health Care Statistics. Data from the National Hospital Discharge Survey.

Table 94 (page 1 of 3). **Ambulatory and inpatient procedures according to place, sex, age, and type of procedure: United States, 1994–97**

[Data are based on a sample of inpatient and ambulatory surgery records]

Sex, age, and procedure category	Total			Ambulatory[1]			Inpatient[2]			
	1994	1995	1996	1994	1995	1996	1994	1995	1996	1997
Both sexes	Procedures per 1,000 population									
Total[3,4]	239.2	239.1	244.8	98.8	103.3	109.0	140.5	135.8	135.8	133.2
Male										
All ages[3,4]	214.7	215.6	222.3	93.5	97.8	104.0	121.2	117.8	118.3	114.2
Under 15 years[4]	85.3	85.2	86.3	48.7	45.9	48.0	36.6	39.3	38.3	35.8
Myringotomy with insertion of tube	11.6	10.8	10.5	11.0	10.3	10.1	0.5	0.4	0.4	*0.2
Tonsillectomy, with or without adenoidectomy	4.6	5.3	4.6	4.1	4.8	4.2	0.5	0.5	0.4	*0.2
Reduction of fracture	2.2	1.8	2.3	0.9	0.8	1.1	1.3	1.0	1.3	1.0
15–44 years[4]	119.9	118.9	119.4	57.9	60.3	62.4	62.1	58.6	57.0	52.4
Cardiac catheterization	1.5	1.4	1.7	0.5	*0.3	0.5	1.1	1.1	1.1	1.0
Endoscopy of small or large intestine with or without biopsy	6.8	6.7	7.0	4.9	4.9	5.5	1.9	1.7	1.5	1.7
Cholecystectomy	0.7	0.8	0.8	*0.2	*0.3	0.4	0.5	0.5	0.4	0.5
Reduction of fracture	3.6	3.7	3.9	1.1	1.1	1.5	2.5	2.5	2.5	2.6
Arthroscopy of the knee	4.2	4.3	3.6	3.6	4.0	3.4	0.5	0.4	0.2	*0.2
Excision or destruction of intervertebral disc	1.7	1.6	1.6	*	*	*0.2	1.5	1.4	1.3	1.2
Angiocardiography with contrast material	2.3	2.1	2.2	0.7	0.4	0.6	1.6	1.7	1.6	1.3
45–64 years[4]	321.7	327.4	341.8	132.7	146.7	155.9	189.0	180.7	185.9	176.4
Coronary angioplasty	5.9	5.8	6.7	*	*	*	5.6	5.6	6.4	5.6
Coronary artery bypass graft[5]	6.7	7.6	7.2	–	–	–	6.7	7.6	7.2	6.9
Cardiac catheterization	14.9	15.5	18.1	3.3	3.8	5.4	11.7	11.7	12.7	11.2
Endoscopy of small or large intestine with or without biopsy	27.4	27.7	28.3	20.2	21.1	21.8	7.2	6.5	6.4	5.6
Cholecystectomy	2.6	2.6	3.2	*0.5	*0.7	1.1	2.1	1.8	2.1	1.6
Prostatectomy	2.7	2.5	2.1	*	*	*	2.5	2.2	1.9	2.3
Reduction of fracture	2.9	3.1	2.8	*0.6	*0.8	0.8	2.3	2.3	2.0	1.9
Arthroscopy of the knee	3.9	4.6	4.6	3.7	4.5	4.4	*0.3	*	*	*
Excision or destruction of intervertebral disc	2.8	2.3	3.0	*	*	*	2.6	2.2	2.6	2.5
Angiocardiography with contrast material	20.6	20.8	24.2	4.6	5.1	6.4	16.0	15.8	17.7	15.2
65–74 years[4]	693.7	697.7	729.6	269.9	280.8	314.5	423.8	416.9	415.1	413.1
Coronary angioplasty	10.1	9.8	12.4	*	*	*	9.9	9.3	11.6	10.8
Extraction of lens	32.5	34.1	37.2	31.4	33.2	36.7	*	*	*	*
Insertion of prosthetic lens (pseudophakos)	26.7	26.7	30.0	25.6	25.8	29.4	*	*	*	*
Coronary artery bypass graft[5]	15.3	18.1	19.1	–	–	–	15.3	18.1	19.1	18.5
Cardiac catheterization	27.9	30.5	33.1	5.7	7.1	10.2	22.2	23.4	22.9	23.7
Pacemaker insertion or replacement	5.7	5.0	6.3	*	*	*	5.6	4.7	5.7	5.9
Carotid endarterectomy	3.2	4.2	3.9	*	–	*	3.2	4.2	3.9	3.8
Endoscopy of small or large intestine with or without biopsy	60.6	58.9	56.5	42.4	42.5	40.0	18.2	16.4	16.5	16.2
Cholecystectomy	5.0	5.3	4.9	*	*	*	4.4	4.4	3.9	4.2
Prostatectomy	14.9	13.2	11.7	*	*	*1.5	14.1	12.3	10.2	10.4
Reduction of fracture	3.3	2.8	3.1	*	*	*	2.7	2.4	2.4	2.2
Total hip replacement	1.6	2.5	2.3	–	–	–	1.6	2.5	2.3	2.3
Angiocardiography with contrast material	39.8	39.5	43.0	9.0	9.2	13.4	30.8	30.3	29.5	29.4
75 years and over[4]	919.6	918.6	953.9	337.9	353.7	377.2	581.8	564.9	576.7	595.0
Coronary angioplasty	6.6	8.1	8.5	–	–	*	6.4	8.1	7.4	7.4
Extraction of lens	62.6	73.0	72.1	61.5	71.3	71.3	*	*	*	*
Insertion of prosthetic lens (pseudophakos)	48.8	55.0	55.5	47.7	53.4	54.9	*	*	*	*
Coronary artery bypass graft[5]	10.7	12.5	11.5	–	–	–	10.7	12.5	11.5	11.1
Cardiac catheterization	21.8	23.8	26.6	*3.8	4.7	7.0	18.0	19.1	19.6	18.0
Pacemaker insertion or replacement	16.0	16.3	18.1	*	*	*	15.3	15.3	16.3	13.5
Carotid endarterectomy	3.6	4.6	4.6	*	–	–	3.6	4.6	4.6	5.3
Endoscopy of small or large intestine with or without biopsy	78.7	79.4	83.8	43.0	43.2	48.7	35.7	36.2	35.1	35.1
Cholecystectomy	6.5	6.5	6.7	*	*	*	6.2	5.5	5.7	5.1
Prostatectomy	18.1	17.4	14.5	*2.1	*2.2	*2.2	16.1	15.2	12.3	13.1
Reduction of fracture	6.5	6.9	6.8	*	*	*	6.4	6.3	6.5	6.6
Total hip replacement	2.2	2.1	2.2	–	–	–	2.2	2.1	2.2	2.7
Angiocardiography with contrast material	27.9	29.4	36.0	*3.8	5.5	10.3	24.1	23.9	25.8	24.4

See footnotes at end of table.

[Data are based on a sample of inpatient and ambulatory surgery records]

Sex, age, and procedure category	Total			Ambulatory[1]			Inpatient[2]			
	1994	1995	1996	1994	1995	1996	1994	1995	1996	1997
Female	Procedures per 1,000 population									
All ages[3,4]	265.8	264.3	269.4	104.5	109.1	114.4	161.2	155.2	155.0	153.9
Under 15 years[4]	64.0	64.5	63.2	35.0	33.9	34.2	29.0	30.5	29.0	27.2
Myringotomy with insertion of tube	8.6	8.0	7.1	8.2	7.6	6.8	0.4	*0.3	*0.3	*
Tonsillectomy, with or without adenoidectomy	5.4	5.3	5.3	4.9	4.8	4.9	0.5	0.4	0.4	*0.2
Reduction of fracture	1.2	1.3	1.3	*0.6	0.7	0.8	0.7	0.6	0.5	0.5
15–44 years[4]	290.7	282.8	287.4	92.0	93.7	98.6	198.7	189.2	188.9	184.5
Cardiac catheterization	0.6	0.6	0.6	*	*0.2	*0.2	0.4	0.4	0.4	0.4
Endoscopy of small or large intestine with or without biopsy	8.3	8.8	9.8	6.3	7.1	7.9	1.9	1.8	1.8	1.6
Cholecystectomy	3.5	4.0	4.0	1.4	1.7	2.1	2.1	2.3	1.9	1.9
Bilateral destruction or occlusion of fallopian tubes	11.3	11.5	11.0	5.2	6.0	5.3	6.1	5.5	5.7	5.3
Hysterectomy	5.2	5.7	5.4	*	*0.3	*0.2	5.0	5.5	5.2	5.0
Cesarean section[6]	14.5	13.2	14.0	–	–	–	14.5	13.2	14.0	13.4
Repair of current obstetrical laceration	15.3	16.2	17.8	*	*	*	15.3	16.2	17.8	17.8
Reduction of fracture	1.5	1.7	1.6	0.4	0.5	0.5	1.1	1.2	1.1	1.1
Arthroscopy of the knee	2.1	2.2	2.2	1.9	2.1	2.0	0.2	*0.1	*0.1	*0.1
Excision or destruction of intervertebral disc	1.2	0.9	1.0	*	*	*	1.1	0.8	0.9	0.8
Lumpectomy	2.5	2.0	2.1	2.4	1.9	2.1	*0.1	*0.1	*	*
Mastectomy	0.3	0.3	0.2	*	*	*	0.2	0.2	0.2	0.2
45–64 years[4]	327.1	326.7	333.7	154.7	165.0	172.3	172.4	161.7	161.4	157.9
Coronary angioplasty	2.1	2.1	2.3	`	*	*	2.1	2.0	2.0	1.7
Coronary artery bypass graft[5]	2.0	1.7	2.0	–	–	–	2.0	1.7	2.0	2.0
Cardiac catheterization	8.2	7.4	8.4	2.2	2.0	2.4	6.0	5.3	6.0	5.3
Endoscopy of small or large intestine with or without biopsy	28.5	30.3	28.3	22.0	24.2	22.8	6.5	6.2	5.5	5.8
Cholecystectomy	5.5	5.8	6.7	1.8	2.3	3.3	3.7	3.5	3.4	3.1
Hysterectomy	7.4	7.3	8.1	*	*	*	7.1	7.1	7.8	8.1
Reduction of fracture	2.8	2.9	3.1	*0.7	*0.7	0.8	2.2	2.2	2.3	1.9
Arthroscopy of the knee	2.9	3.5	3.6	2.8	3.4	3.5	*	*	*	*
Excision or destruction of intervertebral disc	2.1	1.7	2.0	*	*	*	2.0	1.6	1.8	2.0
Lumpectomy	5.4	5.4	4.9	4.9	5.0	4.5	0.5	0.4	*0.4	*0.3
Mastectomy	1.8	1.8	1.7	*	*	*0.4	1.6	1.5	1.3	1.2
Angiocardiography with contrast material	11.5	10.8	11.7	3.0	2.7	3.3	8.5	8.1	8.4	7.4
65–74 years[4]	576.0	591.6	618.8	251.5	269.3	288.4	324.4	322.3	330.4	351.8
Coronary angioplasty	5.0	4.7	5.9	*	*	*	4.8	4.6	5.6	5.3
Extraction of lens	42.4	48.6	47.7	41.3	47.7	47.2	*	*	*	*
Insertion of prosthetic lens (pseudophakos)	34.1	36.1	35.9	33.1	35.3	35.4	*	*	*	*
Coronary artery bypass graft[5]	5.0	6.1	6.6	–	*	–	5.0	6.1	6.6	7.5
Cardiac catheterization	15.8	15.8	19.9	3.3	3.6	5.4	12.5	12.2	14.6	14.5
Pacemaker insertion or replacement	4.5	3.9	3.8	*	*	*	4.2	3.8	3.6	3.3
Carotid endarterectomy	1.7	2.3	2.1	–	–	–	1.7	2.3	2.1	2.8
Endoscopy of small or large intestine with or without biopsy	54.5	58.5	59.4	38.6	40.6	44.9	15.9	17.9	14.5	17.3
Cholecystectomy	6.4	6.1	6.9	*1.3	*1.6	2.3	5.1	4.5	4.6	5.0
Hysterectomy	4.7	4.3	3.8	*	*	*	4.6	4.3	3.7	4.5
Reduction of fracture	5.3	5.1	5.9	*	*	*	4.6	4.3	5.0	5.4
Total hip replacement	2.6	2.6	2.9	–	–	*	2.6	2.6	2.8	3.3
Lumpectomy	4.8	5.1	5.5	4.4	4.6	4.9	*	*	*0.6	*0.5
Mastectomy	3.0	2.7	2.7	*	*	*	2.7	2.3	2.3	2.3
Angiocardiography with contrast material	22.6	22.3	26.9	4.8	4.9	6.8	17.8	17.3	20.1	19.8

See footnotes at end of table.

[Data are based on a sample of inpatient and ambulatory surgery records]

Sex, age, and procedure category	Total			Ambulatory[1]			Inpatient[2]			
	1994	1995	1996	1994	1995	1996	1994	1995	1996	1997
	Procedures per 1,000 population									
75 years and over[4]	742.5	764.0	779.1	271.1	301.2	315.8	471.4	462.8	463.3	479.0
Coronary angioplasty	4.0	4.3	4.8	*	*	*	3.9	4.2	4.3	4.7
Extraction of lens	72.1	83.4	82.4	69.8	81.1	81.7	*	*	*	*
Insertion of prosthetic lens (pseudophakos)	56.1	62.8	61.4	53.9	60.6	60.7	*	*	*	*
Coronary artery bypass graft[5]	3.3	4.1	4.6	–	–	–	3.3	4.1	4.6	4.9
Cardiac catheterization	11.8	12.9	15.0	*1.5	*1.8	3.5	10.3	11.1	11.5	12.2
Pacemaker insertion or replacement	11.9	10.6	12.3	*	*	*1.1	11.4	10.0	11.2	10.2
Carotid endarterectomy	2.0	2.0	2.3	*	*	–	2.0	2.0	2.3	2.2
Endoscopy of small or large intestine with or without biopsy	69.7	73.4	71.0	34.1	38.8	38.2	35.6	34.6	32.8	34.3
Cholecystectomy	4.9	6.4	6.1	*	*	*1.2	4.2	5.5	5.0	5.2
Hysterectomy	2.4	2.4	2.8	*	*	*	2.4	2.4	2.6	2.3
Reduction of fracture	14.6	15.5	17.3	*	*	*	13.8	14.5	16.7	15.6
Total hip replacement	3.2	3.3	3.6	–	*	*	3.2	3.3	3.5	3.2
Lumpectomy	3.2	3.2	3.2	2.7	2.5	2.8	*	*0.7	*	*
Mastectomy	2.6	2.9	2.1	*	*	*	2.4	2.5	1.8	2.2
Angiocardiography with contrast material	16.6	17.5	20.8	2.3	*2.1	5.4	14.4	15.4	15.4	16.7

* Rates for all places or inpatient hospitals based on fewer than 5,000 estimated procedures are unreliable and are not shown; those based on 5,000–9,999 estimated procedures are preceded by an asterisk and may have low reliability. Rates for ambulatory surgery based on fewer than 10,000 estimated procedures are unreliable and are not shown: those based on 10,000–19,999 estimated procedures are preceded by an asterisk.

– Quantity zero.

[1]Data are from the National Survey of Ambulatory Surgery (conducted from 1994–96) and exclude ambulatory surgery procedures for patients who became inpatients. See Appendix II, Ambulatory surgery.

[2]Data are from the National Hospital Discharge Survey and exclude newborn infants.

[3]See Appendix II for age-adjustment procedure.

[4]Includes procedures not listed in table.

[5]Data in the main body of the table are for all-listed coronary artery bypass grafts. Often, more than one coronary bypass procedure is performed during a single operation. The following table gives additional information based on the number of inpatient discharges with one or more coronary artery bypass grafts.

Sex and age	1994	1995	1996	1997
	Inpatient discharges per 1,000 population			
Males:				
45–64 years	4.1	4.5	4.2	4.0
65–74 years	9.3	11.2	11.4	11.1
75 years and over	7.6	8.9	7.6	6.9
Females:				
45–64 years	1.3	1.0	1.2	1.2
65–74 years	3.3	3.8	4.1	4.5
75 years and over	2.3	3.0	3.3	3.4

[6]Cesarean sections accounted for 22.0 percent of deliveries in 1994, 20.8 percent in 1995, 21.8 percent in 1996, and 21.5 percent in 1997.

NOTES: Data in this table are for up to four procedures for inpatients and for up to six procedures for ambulatory surgery patients. See Appendix II, Procedure. Procedure categories are based on the *International Classification of Diseases, Ninth Revision, Clinical Modification.* For a listing of the code numbers, see Appendix II, table IX. Rates are based on the civilian population as of July 1. Beginning with data year 1997, population figures are adjusted for net underenumeration using the 1990 National Population Adjustment Matrix from the U.S. Bureau of the Census. Comparisons of selected estimates based on matrix-adjusted populations with those based on non-adjusted populations for data years 1995 and 1996 show little difference between the two sets of estimates.

SOURCES: Centers for Disease Control and Prevention, National Center for Health Statistics, Division of Health Care Statistics. Data from the National Hospital Discharge Survey and the National Survey of Ambulatory Surgery.

Table 95. Hospital admissions, average length of stay, and outpatient visits, according to type of ownership and size of hospital, and percent outpatient surgery: United States, selected years 1975–98

[Data are based on reporting by a census of hospitals]

Type of ownership and size of hospital	1975	1980	1985	1990	1995	1996	1997	1998
Admissions			Number in thousands					
All hospitals	36,157	38,892	36,304	33,774	33,282	33,307	33,624	33,766
Federal	1,913	2,044	2,103	1,759	1,559	1,422	1,249	1,133
Non-Federal[1]	34,243	36,848	34,201	32,015	31,723	31,885	32,375	32,633
Community[2]	33,435	36,143	33,449	31,181	30,945	31,099	31,577	31,812
Nonprofit	23,722	25,566	24,179	22,878	22,557	22,542	22,905	23,282
For profit	2,646	3,165	3,242	3,066	3,428	3,684	3,953	3,971
State-local government	7,067	7,413	6,028	5,236	4,961	4,873	4,720	4,559
6–24 beds	174	159	102	95	124	117	139	139
25–49 beds	1,431	1,254	1,009	870	944	925	933	965
50–99 beds	3,675	3,700	2,953	2,474	2,299	2,280	2,311	2,265
100–199 beds	7,017	7,162	6,487	5,833	6,288	6,456	6,416	6,656
200–299 beds	6,174	6,596	6,371	6,333	6,495	6,426	6,352	6,230
300–399 beds	4,739	5,358	5,401	5,091	4,693	4,856	5,099	5,021
400–499 beds	3,689	4,401	3,723	3,644	3,413	3,481	3,360	3,390
500 beds or more	6,537	7,513	7,401	6,840	6,690	6,558	6,967	7,146
Average length of stay			Number of days					
All hospitals	11.4	9.9	9.1	9.1	7.8	7.5	7.3	7.2
Federal	20.3	16.8	14.8	14.9	13.1	13.4	14.3	14.4
Non-Federal[1]	10.9	9.6	8.8	8.8	7.5	7.2	7.0	6.9
Community[2]	7.7	7.6	7.1	7.2	6.5	6.2	6.1	6.0
Nonprofit	7.8	7.7	7.2	7.3	6.4	6.1	6.0	5.9
For profit	6.6	6.5	6.1	6.4	5.8	5.6	5.5	5.5
State-local government	7.6	7.3	7.2	7.7	7.4	7.2	7.1	7.0
6–24 beds	5.6	5.3	5.0	5.4	5.5	4.9	4.8	4.6
25–49 beds	6.0	5.8	5.3	6.1	5.7	5.3	5.2	5.2
50–99 beds	6.8	6.7	6.5	7.2	7.0	6.9	6.8	6.9
100–199 beds	7.1	7.0	6.7	7.1	6.4	6.2	6.0	5.9
200–299 beds	7.5	7.4	6.8	6.9	6.2	5.9	5.9	5.8
300–399 beds	7.8	7.6	7.0	7.0	6.1	5.9	5.7	5.7
400–499 beds	8.1	7.9	7.3	7.3	6.3	6.1	6.1	5.9
500 beds or more	9.1	8.7	8.1	8.1	7.1	6.7	6.6	6.5
Outpatient visits[3]			Number in thousands					
All hospitals	254,844	262,951	282,140	368,184	483,195	505,455	520,600	545,481
Federal	51,957	50,566	52,342	58,527	59,934	56,593	60,757	63,642
Non-Federal[1]	202,887	212,385	229,798	309,657	423,261	448,861	459,843	481,838
Community[2]	190,672	202,310	218,716	301,329	414,345	439,863	450,140	474,193
Nonprofit	131,435	142,156	158,953	221,073	303,851	320,746	330,215	352,114
For profit	7,713	9,696	12,378	20,110	31,940	37,347	40,919	42,072
State-local government	51,525	50,459	47,386	60,146	78,554	81,770	79,007	80,008
6–24 beds	915	1,155	829	1,471	3,644	3,622	3,920	4,278
25–49 beds	5,855	6,227	6,623	10,812	19,465	20,960	21,682	22,694
50–99 beds	16,303	17,976	18,716	27,582	38,597	41,003	40,882	42,161
100–199 beds	35,156	36,453	41,049	58,940	91,312	99,999	100,838	107,966
200–299 beds	32,772	36,073	40,515	60,561	84,080	86,958	83,826	85,494
300–399 beds	29,169	30,495	33,773	43,699	54,277	60,190	64,741	67,070
400–499 beds	22,127	25,501	23,950	33,394	44,284	47,241	46,579	49,022
500 beds or more	48,375	48,430	53,262	64,870	78,685	79,891	87,672	95,508
Outpatient surgery			Percent of total surgeries[4]					
Community hospitals[2]	- - -	16.3	34.6	50.5	58.1	59.5	60.7	61.6

- - - Data not available.

[1]The category of non-Federal hospitals is comprised of psychiatric, tuberculosis and other respiratory diseases hospitals, and long-term and short-term hospitals.
[2]Community hospitals are short-term hospitals excluding hospital units in institutions such as prison and college infirmaries, facilities for the mentally retarded, and alcoholism and chemical dependency hospitals.
[3]Outpatient visits include visits to the emergency department, outpatient department, referred visits (pharmacy, EKG, radiology), and outpatient surgery.
[4]The American Hospital Association defines surgery as a surgical episode in the operating or procedure room. During a single episode, multiple surgical procedures may be performed. In contrast the National Hospital Discharge Survey codes up to 4 procedures and the National Survey of Ambulatory Surgery codes up to 6 procedures that are performed in a single surgical episode. See Appendix II, Ambulatory surgery and Outpatient surgery.

NOTE: Data for additional years are available (see Appendix III).

SOURCES: American Hospital Association: Hospital Statistics, 1976, 1981, 1986, 1991–99 Editions. Chicago, 1976, 1981, 1986, 1991–99. (Copyrights 1976, 1981, 1986, 1991–99: Used with the permission of the American Hospital Association (AHA) and Health Forum, an AHA company.)

Table 96. Nursing home residents 65 years of age and over according to age, sex, and race: United States, 1973–74, 1985, 1995, and 1997

[Data are based on a sample of nursing home residents]

Age, sex, and race	Residents				Residents per 1,000 population			
	1973–74	1985	1995	1997	1973–74	1985	1995	1997
Age								
65 years and over, age adjusted[1]	...	...	...	...	58.5	54.0	45.9	45.3
65 years and over, crude	961,500	1,318,300	1,422,600	1,465,000	44.7	46.2	42.4	43.4
65–74 years	163,100	212,100	190,200	198,400	12.3	12.5	10.1	10.8
75–84 years	384,900	509,000	511,900	528,300	57.7	57.7	45.9	45.5
85 years and over	413,600	597,300	720,400	738,300	257.3	220.3	198.6	192.0
Male								
65 years and over, age adjusted[1]	...	...	...	...	42.5	38.8	32.8	32.0
65 years and over, crude	265,700	334,400	356,800	372,100	30.0	29.0	26.1	26.7
65–74 years	65,100	80,600	79,300	80,800	11.3	10.8	9.5	9.8
75–84 years	102,300	141,300	144,300	159,300	39.9	43.0	33.3	34.6
85 years and over	98,300	112,600	133,100	132,000	182.7	145.7	130.8	119.0
Female								
65 years and over, age adjusted[1]	...	...	...	...	67.5	61.5	52.3	51.9
65 years and over, crude	695,800	983,900	1,065,800	1,092,900	54.9	57.9	53.7	55.1
65–74 years	98,000	131,500	110,900	117,700	13.1	13.8	10.6	11.6
75–84 years	282,600	367,700	367,600	368,900	68.9	66.4	53.9	52.7
85 years and over	315,300	484,700	587,300	606,300	294.9	250.1	224.9	221.6
White								
65 years and over, age adjusted[1]	...	...	...	...	61.2	55.5	45.4	44.5
65 years and over, crude	920,600	1,227,400	1,271,200	1,294,900	46.9	47.7	42.3	43.0
65–74 years	150,100	187,800	154,400	160,800	12.5	12.3	9.3	10.0
75–84 years	369,700	473,600	453,800	464,400	60.3	59.1	44.9	44.2
85 years and over	400,800	566,000	663,000	669,700	270.8	228.7	200.7	192.4
Black								
65 years and over, age adjusted[1]	...	...	...	...	28.2	41.5	50.4	54.4
65 years and over, crude	37,700	82,000	122,900	137,400	22.0	35.0	45.2	49.4
65–74 years	12,200	22,500	29,700	31,400	11.1	15.4	18.4	19.2
75–84 years	13,400	30,600	47,300	51,900	26.7	45.3	57.2	60.6
85 years and over	12,100	29,000	45,800	54,100	105.7	141.5	167.1	186.0

... Category not applicable.

[1]Age adjusted by the direct method to the year 2000 population standard using the following three age groups: 65–74 years, 75–84 years, and 85 years and over.

NOTES: Excludes residents in personal care or domiciliary care homes. Age refers to age at time of interview. Rates are based on the resident population as of July 1. In 1997 population figures are adjusted for net underenumeration using the 1990 National Population Adjustment Matrix from the U.S. Bureau of the Census.

SOURCES: Centers for Disease Control and Prevention: Hing E, Sekscenski E, Strahan G. The National Nursing Home Survey: 1985 summary for the United States. National Center for Health Statistics. Vital Health Stat 13(97). 1989; and unpublished data from the 1995 and 1997 National Nursing Home Surveys.

Table 97. Nursing home residents 65 years of age and over, according to selected functional status and age, sex, and race: United States, 1985, 1995, and 1997

[Data are based on a sample of nursing home residents]

Age, sex, and race	Functional status[1]											
	Dependent mobility			Incontinent			Dependent eating			Dependent mobility, eating, and incontinent		
	1985	1995	1997	1985	1995	1997	1985	1995	1997	1985	1995	1997
All persons						Percent						
65 years and over, age adjusted[2]	75.7	79.0	79.3	55.0	63.8	64.9	40.9	44.9	45.1	32.5	36.5	35.7
65 years and over, crude	74.8	79.0	79.4	54.5	63.8	64.9	40.5	44.9	45.1	32.1	36.5	35.6
65–74 years	61.2	73.0	73.1	42.9	61.9	59.2	33.5	43.8	42.1	25.7	35.8	30.7
75–84 years	70.5	76.5	77.1	55.1	62.5	64.3	39.4	45.2	44.8	30.6	35.3	34.5
85 years and over	83.3	82.4	82.6	58.1	65.3	66.9	43.9	45.0	46.1	35.6	37.5	37.8
Male												
65 years and over, age adjusted[2]	71.2	76.6	76.3	54.2	63.8	65.0	36.0	42.1	42.8	28.0	34.3	33.6
65 years and over, crude	67.8	75.8	75.6	51.9	63.9	64.5	34.9	42.7	42.9	26.9	34.8	33.7
65–74 years	55.8	70.6	72.3	38.8	63.4	60.1	32.8	44.2	42.7	24.1	36.9	32.9
75–84 years	65.7	76.6	75.1	54.4	64.6	65.9	32.6	44.1	43.7	25.5	35.5	34.6
85 years and over	79.2	78.2	78.3	58.1	63.4	65.6	39.2	40.2	42.1	30.9	32.7	33.0
Female												
65 years and over, age adjusted[2]	77.3	79.7	80.2	55.4	63.6	64.8	42.4	45.6	45.6	33.9	36.9	35.9
65 years and over, crude	77.1	80.1	80.6	55.4	63.8	65.1	42.4	45.6	45.8	33.8	37.0	36.3
65–74 years	64.5	74.8	73.7	45.4	60.9	58.6	34.0	43.6	41.6	26.7	35.0	29.2
75–84 years	72.3	76.5	78.0	55.3	61.7	63.6	42.0	45.7	45.3	32.6	35.2	34.4
85 years and over	84.3	83.3	83.5	58.1	65.7	67.2	45.0	46.0	46.9	36.7	38.6	38.8
White												
65 years and over, age adjusted[2]	75.2	78.5	78.9	54.6	63.2	64.4	40.4	44.2	44.2	32.1	35.7	34.8
65 years and over, crude	74.3	78.7	79.0	54.2	63.3	64.5	40.1	44.2	44.2	31.7	35.7	34.8
65–74 years	60.2	71.4	72.3	42.2	60.2	59.6	32.6	41.9	40.2	24.9	33.8	29.3
75–84 years	69.6	76.4	76.1	54.2	61.8	63.4	38.9	44.9	43.9	30.1	34.7	33.5
85 years and over	83.1	81.9	82.6	58.2	65.0	66.4	43.5	44.3	45.4	35.5	36.9	37.1
Black												
65 years and over, age adjusted[2]	83.4	83.2	82.7	61.0	69.3	71.0	49.2	52.2	53.3	38.2	44.0	44.1
65 years and over, crude	81.1	82.1	82.0	59.9	69.1	69.2	47.9	51.7	53.3	37.7	43.7	43.2
65–74 years	70.9	79.6	75.9	48.6	68.3	55.8	43.1	51.2	53.2	33.8	43.1	38.4
75–84 years	82.5	77.8	84.1	70.1	68.9	72.4	47.9	49.5	52.9	40.6	42.3	42.0
85 years and over	87.4	88.0	83.5	57.9	69.8	74.0	51.7	54.3	53.6	37.6	45.5	47.2

[1]Nursing home residents who are dependent in mobility and eating require the assistance of a person or special equipment. Nursing home residents who are incontinent have difficulty in controlling bowels and/or bladder or have an ostomy or indwelling catheter.
[2]Age adjusted by the direct method to the 1995 National Nursing Home Survey population using the following three age groups: 65–74 years, 75–84 years, and 85 years and over.

NOTES: Age refers to age at time of interview. Excludes residents in personal care or domiciliary care homes.

SOURCES: Centers for Disease Control and Prevention: Hing E, Sekscenski E, Strahan G. The National Nursing Home Survey: 1985 summary for the United States. National Center for Health Statistics. Vital Health Stat 13(97). 1989; and unpublished data from the 1995 and 1997 National Nursing Home Surveys.

Table 98. Additions to selected inpatient psychiatric organizations according to sex, age, and race: United States, 1975, 1980, and 1986

[Data are based on a sample survey of patients]

Sex, age, and race	State and county mental hospitals			Private psychiatric hospitals			Non-Federal general hospitals[1]		
	1975	1980	1986	1975	1980	1986	1975	1980	1986
Both sexes				Additions in thousands					
Total	385	369	343	130	141	222	516	564	851
Under 18 years	25	17	17	15	17	43	43	44	50
18–24 years	72	77	61	19	23	25	93	98	126
25–44 years	166	177	200	47	56	99	220	249	425
45–64 years	102	78	50	35	32	34	121	123	156
65 years and over	21	20	15	13	14	21	38	50	94
White	296	265	230	119	123	183	451	469	659
All other	89	104	113	10	18	39	65	95	192
Male									
Total	249	239	217	56	67	115	212	255	398
Under 18 years	16	11	10	8	9	23	20	20	22
18–24 years	52	56	41	10	13	16	45	52	59
25–44 years	107	119	134	20	27	56	85	115	222
45–64 years	61	43	25	14	13	14	48	46	66
65 years and over	13	11	7	5	5	6	14	21	29
White	191	171	145	51	58	89	184	213	292
All other	58	68	72	5	9	26	27	42	106
Female									
Total	136	130	126	74	74	107	304	309	453
Under 18 years	9	5	7	8	7	20	23	23	28
18–24 years	20	22	20	9	10	8	48	45	67
25–44 years	59	58	66	28	29	44	135	135	203
45–64 years	41	35	24	21	18	20	74	77	90
65 years and over	8	9	8	8	9	15	24	29	65
White	105	94	85	69	65	94	267	256	367
All other	31	36	41	5	9	13	37	53	86
Both sexes				Additions per 100,000 civilian population					
Total	182.2	163.6	143.4	61.4	62.6	92.5	243.8	250.0	355.4
Under 18 years	38.1	26.1	26.9	23.3	26.3	67.5	64.4	68.5	78.7
18–24 years	271.8	264.6	225.6	73.7	79.6	91.6	352.8	334.2	467.0
25–44 years	314.1	282.9	267.0	89.3	89.1	132.7	416.8	399.0	566.8
45–64 years	233.5	175.7	110.9	80.1	71.0	75.2	278.5	276.4	346.2
65 years and over	91.8	78.0	52.5	57.7	54.1	71.4	170.3	195.4	323.6
White	161.1	136.8	113.2	64.9	63.4	90.1	245.4	241.8	324.7
All other	321.9	328.0	311.4	37.9	57.5	106.1	233.3	300.0	526.2
Male									
Total	243.7	219.8	187.8	54.5	61.9	99.3	207.1	233.8	343.6
Under 18 years	48.3	35.4	32.2	22.5	28.9	69.8	59.1	62.6	67.5
18–24 years	409.0	387.9	307.5	78.0	92.2	124.2	350.8	365.3	446.2
25–44 years	418.4	388.1	363.0	76.6	86.8	151.2	332.8	374.7	602.9
45–64 years	291.5	202.3	118.6	66.8	63.2	65.5	228.6	219.1	306.1
65 years and over	136.4	105.3	59.4	50.3	47.3	52.1	152.0	203.4	245.6
White	214.2	182.2	147.2	57.0	61.7	90.3	206.9	226.3	296.4
All other	444.5	457.8	419.7	38.1	62.7	151.2	209.1	281.1	614.2
Female									
Total	124.7	111.1	101.8	67.8	63.3	86.2	278.1	265.1	366.4
Under 18 years	27.5	16.4	21.4	24.1	23.6	65.0	70.0	74.6	90.3
18–24 years	143.1	145.8	146.6	69.6	67.4	60.2	354.6	304.4	487.1
25–44 years	215.9	182.3	174.1	101.2	91.2	114.9	495.8	422.2	531.9
45–64 years	180.5	151.7	103.8	92.3	78.1	84.0	324.3	328.2	382.8
65 years and over	60.8	59.6	47.8	62.8	58.8	84.6	182.9	190.0	376.7
White	111.2	94.1	81.1	72.5	65.0	90.0	281.7	256.4	351.5
All other	212.0	212.6	214.2	37.7	52.8	65.5	254.9	316.7	447.0

[1]Non-Federal general hospitals include public and nonpublic facilities.

NOTES: An addition is a new admission, a readmission, a return from long-term leave, or a transfer. See Appendix II, Addition.

SOURCES: National Institute of Mental Health. Taube CA, Barrett SA. *Mental Health, United States, 1985.* DHHS. 1985; Manderscheid RW, Sonnenschein MA. *Mental Health, United States, 1992.* DHHS. 1992. Unpublished data.

Table 99. Additions to selected inpatient psychiatric organizations, according to selected primary diagnoses and age: United States, 1975, 1980, and 1986

[Data are based on a sample survey of patients]

Primary diagnosis and age	State and county mental hospitals			Private psychiatric hospitals			Non-Federal general hospitals[1]		
	1975	1980	1986	1975	1980	1986	1975	1980	1986
All diagnoses[2]				Additions per 100,000 civilian population					
All ages	182.2	163.6	143.4	61.4	62.6	92.5	243.8	250.0	355.4
Under 25 years	104.8	101.2	86.3	37.7	43.1	74.7	146.7	152.2	194.7
25–44 years	314.1	282.9	267.0	89.3	89.1	132.7	416.8	399.0	566.8
45–64 years	233.5	175.7	110.9	80.1	71.0	75.2	278.5	276.4	346.2
65 years and over	91.8	78.0	52.5	57.7	54.1	71.4	170.3	195.4	323.6
Alcohol related									
All ages	50.4	35.5	23.8	5.1	5.8	6.6	17.0	18.8	42.4
Under 25 years	10.7	12.4	16.8	0.4	1.4	2.2	2.4	4.4	13.7
25–44 years	86.2	64.0	45.4	7.6	9.3	10.0	31.0	34.3	94.8
45–64 years	110.0	57.7	15.3	12.5	10.9	11.0	34.5	30.6	32.9
65 years and over	14.8	11.5	*3.2	4.3	4.4	4.5	10.2	12.8	11.3
Drug related									
All ages	6.8	7.8	9.1	1.5	1.8	6.1	8.4	7.4	20.8
Under 25 years	7.2	9.4	6.3	1.5	1.8	7.5	7.7	7.8	18.8
25–44 years	12.6	12.9	14.8	2.3	3.0	9.3	13.8	9.3	42.0
45–64 years	*0.6	1.4	10.5	0.1	1.0	*1.8	6.5	7.1	*2.2
65 years and over	*3.5	*0.7	*0.8	0.4	0.6	- - -	*2.6	*2.0	*1.2
Organic disorders[3]									
All ages	9.6	6.8	4.5	2.5	2.2	2.0	9.0	7.4	10.7
Under 25 years	2.2	1.2	*0.2	0.7	0.5	*0.5	1.1	*0.8	1.7
25–44 years	6.4	4.7	3.0	1.1	0.9	*0.3	5.4	5.6	6.9
45–64 years	12.2	8.1	7.3	1.7	2.7	*1.5	9.3	6.9	6.8
65 years and over	43.3	30.0	17.2	14.5	10.8	11.7	49.3	36.4	54.5
Affective disorders									
All ages	21.3	22.0	23.6	26.0	26.8	45.4	91.9	79.2	135.9
Under 25 years	7.5	9.1	9.9	9.5	13.5	31.6	35.3	32.2	55.9
25–44 years	40.6	36.9	45.2	39.4	38.9	67.1	160.9	123.7	190.4
45–64 years	29.4	32.4	25.5	43.3	36.3	38.5	135.6	113.8	165.7
65 years and over	16.8	14.3	7.9	29.6	29.2	42.9	78.5	81.0	197.4
Schizrenia									
All ages	61.2	62.1	53.2	13.4	13.3	11.0	58.9	59.9	66.2
Under 25 years	35.9	36.6	19.6	11.1	10.6	5.7	42.0	38.3	30.8
25–44 years	125.8	125.0	115.3	23.8	22.5	22.6	118.0	114.5	124.2
45–64 years	63.5	54.8	38.8	11.3	11.6	8.5	50.3	53.6	73.7
65 years and over	9.3	13.9	19.9	2.7	3.6	*1.8	5.6	16.3	15.3

* Based on 5 or fewer sample additions.
- - - Data not available.
[1]Non-Federal general hospitals include public and nonpublic facilities.
[2]Includes all other diagnoses not listed separately.
[3]Excludes alcohol- and drug-related diagnoses.

NOTES: An addition is a new admission, a readmission, a return from long-term leave, or a transfer. See Appendix II, Addition. Primary diagnosis categories are based on the then current *International Classification of Diseases* and *Diagnostic and Statistical Manual of Mental Disorders*. For a listing of the code numbers, see Appendix II, table X.

SOURCES: National Institute of Mental Health. Taube CA, Barrett SA. *Mental Health, United States, 1985*. DHHS. 1985; Manderscheid RW, Sonnenschein MA. *Mental Health, United States, 1992*. DHHS. 1992. Unpublished data.

Table 100. Persons employed in health service sites: United States, selected years 1970–99

[Data are based on household interviews of a sample of the civilian noninstitutionalized population]

Site	1970	1975	1980	1985	1990	1993	1994[1]	1995[1]	1996[1]	1997[1]	1998[1]	1999[1]
	Number of persons in thousands											
All employed civilians.........	76,805	85,846	99,303	107,150	117,914	119,306	123,060	124,900	126,708	129,558	131,463	133,488
All health service sites........	4,246	5,945	7,339	7,910	9,447	10,553	10,587	10,928	11,199	11,525	11,504	11,646
Offices and clinics of physicians...........	477	618	777	894	1,098	1,450	1,404	1,512	1,501	1,559	1,581	1,624
Offices and clinics of dentists.............	222	331	415	480	580	567	596	644	614	662	666	694
Offices and clinics of chiropractors[2]..........	19	30	40	59	90	116	105	99	99	118	127	142
Hospitals.................	2,690	3,441	4,036	4,269	4,690	5,032	5,009	4,961	5,041	5,130	5,116	5,117
Nursing and personal care facilities................	509	891	1,199	1,309	1,543	1,752	1,692	1,718	1,765	1,755	1,801	1,786
Other health service sites	330	634	872	899	1,446	1,635	1,781	1,995	2,178	2,301	2,213	2,283
	Percent of employed civilians											
All health service sites........	5.5	6.9	7.4	7.4	8.0	8.8	8.6	8.7	8.8	8.9	8.8	8.7
	Percent distribution											
All health service sites........	100.0	100.0	100.0	100.0	100.0	100.0	100.0	100.0	100.0	100.0	100.0	100.0
Offices and clinics of physicians...........	11.2	10.4	10.6	11.3	11.6	13.7	13.3	13.8	13.4	13.5	13.7	13.9
Offices and clinics of dentists.............	5.2	5.6	5.7	6.1	6.1	5.4	5.6	5.9	5.5	5.7	5.8	6.0
Offices and clinics of chiropractors[2]..........	0.4	0.5	0.5	0.7	1.0	1.1	1.0	0.9	0.9	1.0	1.1	1.2
Hospitals.................	63.4	57.9	55.0	54.0	49.6	47.7	47.3	45.4	45.0	44.5	44.5	43.9
Nursing and personal care facilities................	12.0	15.0	16.3	16.5	16.3	16.6	16.0	15.7	15.8	15.2	15.7	15.3
Other health service sites	7.8	10.7	11.9	11.4	15.3	15.5	16.8	18.3	19.4	20.0	19.2	19.6

[1]Data for 1994 and later years are not strictly comparable with data from previous years due to a redesign of the Current Population Survey. See Appendix I, Department of Commerce.

[2]Data for 1980 are from the American Chiropractic Association; data for all other years are from the U.S. Bureau of Labor Statistics.

NOTES: Employment is full- or part-time work. Totals exclude persons in health-related occupations who are working in nonhealth industries, as classified by the U.S. Bureau of the Census, such as pharmacists employed in drugstores, school nurses, and nurses working in private households. Totals include Federal, State, and county health workers. In 1970–82, employed persons were classified according to the industry groups used in the 1970 Census of Population. In 1983–91, persons were classified according to the system used in the 1980 Census of Population. Beginning in 1992 persons were classified according to the system used in the 1990 Census of Population. Data for additional years are available (see Appendix III).

SOURCES: U.S. Bureau of the Census: 1970 Census of Population, occupation by industry. Subject Reports. Final Report PC(2)–7C. Washington. U.S. Government Printing Office, Oct. 1972; U.S. Bureau of Labor Statistics: Labor Force Statistics Derived from the Current Population Survey: A Databook, Vol. I. Washington. U.S. Government Printing Office, Sept. 1982; Employment and Earnings, January issue 1986, 1991–2000. U.S. Government Printing Office, Jan. 1986, 1991–2000; American Chiropractic Association: Unpublished data.

Health Care Resources

Table 101 (page 1 of 2). Active non-Federal physicians and doctors of medicine in patient care, according to geographic division and State: United States, 1975, 1985, 1995, and 1998

[Data are based on reporting by physicians]

Geographic division and State	Total physicians[1]				Doctors of medicine in patient care[2]			
	1975	1985	1995[3]	1998[4]	1975	1985	1995	1998
	Number per 10,000 civilian population							
United States	15.3	20.7	24.2	25.5	13.5	18.0	21.3	22.5
New England	19.1	26.7	32.5	34.0	16.9	22.9	28.8	30.2
Maine	12.8	18.7	22.3	24.7	10.7	15.6	18.2	20.0
New Hampshire	14.3	18.1	21.5	23.6	13.1	16.7	19.8	21.6
Vermont	18.2	23.8	26.9	29.9	15.5	20.3	24.2	26.8
Massachusetts	20.8	30.2	37.5	38.4	18.3	25.4	33.2	34.2
Rhode Island	17.8	23.3	30.4	33.6	16.1	20.2	26.7	29.7
Connecticut	19.8	27.6	32.8	34.0	17.7	24.3	29.5	30.5
Middle Atlantic	19.5	26.1	32.4	34.0	17.0	22.2	28.0	29.2
New York	22.7	29.0	35.3	37.1	20.2	25.2	31.6	33.1
New Jersey	16.2	23.4	29.3	30.6	14.0	19.8	24.9	25.8
Pennsylvania	16.6	23.6	30.1	31.5	13.9	19.2	24.6	25.6
East North Central	13.9	19.3	23.3	24.4	12.0	16.4	19.8	20.7
Ohio	14.1	19.9	23.8	25.1	12.2	16.8	20.0	21.0
Indiana	10.6	14.7	18.4	19.6	9.6	13.2	16.6	17.6
Illinois	14.5	20.5	24.8	25.8	13.1	18.2	22.1	22.9
Michigan	15.4	20.8	24.8	25.9	12.0	16.0	19.0	19.8
Wisconsin	12.5	17.7	21.5	22.5	11.4	15.9	19.6	20.5
West North Central	13.3	18.3	21.8	22.6	11.4	15.6	18.9	19.6
Minnesota	14.9	20.5	23.4	24.1	13.7	18.5	21.5	22.1
Iowa	11.4	15.6	19.2	19.6	9.4	12.4	15.1	15.4
Missouri	15.0	20.5	23.9	24.7	11.6	16.3	19.7	20.3
North Dakota	9.7	15.8	20.5	22.0	9.2	14.9	18.9	20.4
South Dakota	8.2	13.4	16.7	18.4	7.7	12.3	15.7	17.2
Nebraska	12.1	15.7	19.8	21.2	10.9	14.4	18.3	19.7
Kansas	12.8	17.3	20.8	21.4	11.2	15.1	18.0	18.4
South Atlantic	14.0	19.7	23.4	24.6	12.6	17.6	21.0	22.1
Delaware	14.3	19.7	23.4	24.2	12.7	17.1	19.7	20.6
Maryland	18.6	30.4	34.1	35.4	16.5	24.9	29.9	31.3
District of Columbia	39.6	55.3	63.6	68.5	34.6	45.6	53.6	59.5
Virginia	12.9	19.5	22.5	23.4	11.9	17.8	20.8	21.6
West Virginia	11.0	16.3	21.0	22.9	10.0	14.6	17.9	19.3
North Carolina	11.7	16.9	21.1	22.3	10.6	15.0	19.4	20.5
South Carolina	10.0	14.7	18.9	20.1	9.3	13.6	17.6	18.6
Georgia	11.5	16.2	19.7	20.6	10.6	14.7	18.0	18.8
Florida	15.2	20.2	22.9	24.3	13.4	17.8	20.3	21.5
East South Central	10.5	15.0	19.2	20.6	9.7	14.0	17.8	19.0
Kentucky	10.9	15.1	19.2	20.4	10.1	13.9	18.0	19.0
Tennessee	12.4	17.7	22.5	23.9	11.3	16.2	20.8	22.1
Alabama	9.2	14.2	18.4	19.4	8.6	13.1	17.0	17.8
Mississippi	8.4	11.8	13.9	16.2	8.0	11.1	13.0	14.9
West South Central	11.9	16.4	19.5	20.6	10.5	14.5	17.3	18.3
Arkansas	9.1	13.8	17.3	18.9	8.5	12.8	16.0	17.5
Louisiana	11.4	17.3	21.7	23.6	10.5	16.1	20.3	22.2
Oklahoma	11.6	16.1	18.8	19.6	9.4	12.9	14.7	15.3
Texas	12.5	16.8	19.4	20.4	11.0	14.7	17.3	18.1
Mountain	14.3	17.8	20.2	20.8	12.6	15.7	17.8	18.2
Montana	10.6	14.0	18.4	19.1	10.1	13.2	17.1	17.7
Idaho	9.5	12.1	13.9	15.6	8.9	11.4	13.1	14.4
Wyoming	9.5	12.9	15.3	16.9	8.9	12.0	13.9	15.4
Colorado	17.3	20.7	23.7	24.3	15.0	17.7	20.6	21.2
New Mexico	12.2	17.0	20.2	21.0	10.1	14.7	18.0	18.6
Arizona	16.7	20.2	21.4	21.3	14.1	17.1	18.2	18.0
Utah	14.1	17.2	19.2	19.6	13.0	15.5	17.6	17.7
Nevada	11.9	16.0	16.7	17.9	10.9	14.5	14.6	15.8

See footnotes at end of table.

Table 101 (page 2 of 2). Active non-Federal physicians and doctors of medicine in patient care, according to geographic division and State: United States, 1975, 1985, 1995, and 1998

[Data are based on reporting by physicians]

Geographic division and State	Total physicians[1]				Doctors of medicine in patient care[2]			
	1975	1985	1995[3]	1998[4]	1975	1985	1995	1998
	Number per 10,000 civilian population							
Pacific	17.9	22.5	23.3	23.5	16.3	20.5	21.2	21.3
Washington	15.3	20.2	22.5	23.2	13.6	17.9	20.2	20.8
Oregon	15.6	19.7	21.6	22.4	13.8	17.6	19.5	20.2
California	18.8	23.7	23.7	23.7	17.3	21.5	21.7	21.6
Alaska	8.4	13.0	15.7	16.8	7.8	12.1	14.2	15.2
Hawaii	16.2	21.5	24.8	26.1	14.7	19.8	22.8	23.8

[1]Includes active non-Federal doctors of medicine and active doctors of osteopathy.
[2]Excludes doctors of osteopathy; States with large numbers are Florida, Michigan, Missouri, New Jersey, Ohio, Pennsylvania, and Texas. Excludes doctors of medicine in medical teaching, administration, research, and other nonpatient care activities.
[3]Data for doctors of osteopathy are as of July 1996.
[4]Data for doctors of osteopathy are as of December 1998.

NOTES: Data for doctors of medicine are as of December 31. See Appendix II for physician definitions.

SOURCES: American Medical Association (AMA). Physician distribution and medical licensure in the U.S., 1975; Physician characteristics and distribution in the U.S., 1986 edition; 1996–97 edition; 1999 edition; 2000 edition. Department of Data Survey and Planning, Division of Survey and Data Resources, AMA. (Copyrights 1976, 1986, 1997, 1999, 2000: Used with the permission of the AMA); American Osteopathic Association: 1975–76 Yearbook and Directory of Osteopathic Physicians, 1985–86 Yearbook and Directory of Osteopathic Physicians; Rockville, Md. American Association of Colleges of Osteopathic Medicine: Annual Statistical Report, 1996 and 1998.

Table 102. Physicians, according to activity and place of medical education: United States and outlying U.S. areas, selected years 1975–98

[Data are based on reporting by physicians]

Activity and place of medical education	1975	1985	1990	1995	1996	1997	1998
				Number of physicians			
Doctors of medicine	393,742	552,716	615,421	720,325	737,764	756,710	777,859
Professionally active[1]	340,280	497,140	547,310	625,443	643,955	664,556	667,000
Place of medical education:							
U.S. medical graduates	- - -	392,007	432,884	481,137	495,463	509,942	509,524
International medical graduates[2]	- - -	105,133	114,426	144,306	148,492	154,614	157,476
Activity:[3]							
Non-Federal	312,089	475,573	526,835	604,364	623,526	645,203	648,009
Patient care	287,837	431,527	487,796	564,074	580,706	603,684	606,425
Office-based practice	213,334	329,041	359,932	427,275	445,765	458,209	468,788
General and family practice	46,347	53,862	57,571	59,932	61,760	62,022	64,588
Cardiovascular diseases	5,046	9,054	10,670	13,739	14,304	15,026	15,112
Dermatology	3,442	5,325	5,996	6,959	7,234	7,353	7,641
Gastroenterology	1,696	4,135	5,200	7,300	7,580	7,938	7,948
Internal medicine	28,188	52,712	57,799	72,612	77,929	81,352	83,270
Pediatrics	12,687	22,392	26,494	33,890	35,453	36,846	38,359
Pulmonary diseases	1,166	3,035	3,659	4,964	4,892	4,965	4,927
General surgery	19,710	24,708	24,498	24,086	25,425	27,865	27,509
Obstetrics and gynecology	15,613	23,525	25,475	29,111	29,872	30,063	31,194
Ophthalmology	8,795	12,212	13,055	14,596	14,931	15,118	15,560
Orthopedic surgery	8,148	13,033	14,187	17,136	17,637	18,482	18,479
Otolaryngology	4,297	5,751	6,360	7,139	7,152	7,378	7,498
Plastic surgery	1,706	3,299	3,835	4,612	5,012	5,257	5,303
Urological surgery	5,025	7,081	7,392	7,991	8,229	8,383	8,424
Anesthesiology	8,970	15,285	17,789	23,770	24,929	25,569	26,218
Diagnostic radiology	1,978	7,735	9,806	12,751	13,313	14,142	14,241
Emergency medicine	- - -	- - -	8,402	11,700	12,348	12,450	13,253
Neurology	1,862	4,691	5,587	7,623	7,898	8,199	8,458
Pathology, anatomical/clinical	4,195	6,877	7,269	9,031	9,661	10,229	9,970
Psychiatry	12,173	18,521	20,048	23,334	24,400	24,541	24,962
Radiology	6,970	7,355	6,056	5,994	6,276	6,297	6,353
Other specialty	15,320	28,453	22,784	29,005	29,530	28,734	29,521
Hospital-based practice	74,503	102,486	127,864	136,799	134,941	145,318	137,637
Residents and interns[4]	53,527	72,159	89,913	93,650	90,592	95,808	92,332
Full-time hospital staff	20,976	30,327	37,951	43,149	44,349	49,510	45,305
Other professional activity[5]	24,252	44,046	39,039	40,290	42,820	41,519	41,584
Federal[6]	28,191	21,567	20,475	21,079	20,429	19,353	18,991
Patient care	24,100	17,293	15,632	18,057	18,218	16,947	15,311
Office-based practice	2,095	1,156	1,063	. . .	. . .	. . .	. . .
Hospital-based practice	22,005	16,137	14,569	18,057	18,218	16,945	15,311
Residents and interns	4,275	3,252	1,725	2,702	5,749	4,068	660
Full-time hospital staff	17,730	12,885	12,844	15,355	12,469	12,877	14,651
Other professional activity[5]	4,091	4,274	4,843	3,022	2,211	2,406	3,680
Inactive	21,449	38,646	52,653	72,326	72,510	71,106	69,889
Not classified	26,145	13,950	12,678	20,579	19,998	20,049	40,032
Unknown address	5,868	2,980	2,780	1,977	1,311	999	938

- - - Data not available.
. . . Category not applicable.
[1]Excludes inactive, not classified, and address unknown.
[2]International medical graduates received their medical education in schools outside the United States and Canada.
[3]Specialty information based on the physician's self-designated primary area of practice. Categories include generalists and specialists.
[4]Beginning in 1990 clinical fellows are included in this category. In prior years clinical fellows were included in other professional activity.
[5]Includes medical teaching, administration, research, and other. Prior to 1990 this category included clinical fellows, also.
[6]Beginning in 1993 data collection for Federal physicians was revised.

NOTES: Data for doctors of medicine are as of December 31, except for 1990–94 data, which are as of January 1. See Appendix II for discussion of physician specialties. Outlying areas include Puerto Rico, Virgin Islands, and the Pacific islands of Canton, Caroline, Guam, Mariana, Marshall, American Samoa, and Wake. Data for additional years are available (see Appendix III).

SOURCES: American Medical Association (AMA). Distribution of physicians in the United States, 1970; Physician distribution and medical licensure in the U.S., 1975; Physician characteristics and distribution in the U.S., 1981 edition; 1986 edition; 1989 edition; 1990 edition; 1992 edition; 1993 edition; 1994 edition; 1995–96 edition; 1996–97 edition; 1997–98 edition; 1999 edition; 2000–2001 edition. Department of Data Survey and Planning, Division of Survey and Data Resources, AMA. (Copyrights 1971, 1976, 1982, 1986, 1989, 1990, 1992, 1993, 1994, 1996, 1997, 1997, 1999, 2000: Used with the permission of the AMA.)

Table 103. Primary care doctors of medicine, according to specialty: United States and outlying U.S. areas, selected years 1949–98

[Data are based on reporting by physicians]

Specialty	1949[1]	1960[1]	1970	1980	1990	1994	1995	1996	1997	1998
					Number					
Total[2]	201,277	260,484	334,028	467,679	615,421	684,414	720,325	737,764	756,710	777,859
Active doctors of medicine[3]	191,577	247,257	310,845	414,916	547,310	605,468	625,443	643,955	664,556	667,000
Primary care generalists	113,222	125,359	115,822	146,093	183,294	200,020	207,810	216,446	216,598	218,421
General/family practice	95,980	88,023	57,948	60,049	70,480	73,163	75,976	78,910	78,258	79,769
Internal medicine.	12,453	26,209	39,924	58,462	76,295	84,951	88,240	92,321	93,797	93,227
Pediatrics	4,789	11,127	17,950	27,582	36,519	41,906	43,594	45,215	44,543	45,425
Primary care specialists	- - -	- - -	2,817	14,949	27,434	33,927	35,290	39,315	32,918	34,299
Internal medicine.	- - -	- - -	1,948	13,069	22,054	26,476	26,928	29,804	24,582	25,365
Pediatrics	- - -	- - -	869	1,880	5,380	'7,451	8,362	9,511	8,336	8,934
					Percent of active doctors of medicine					
Primary care generalists	59.1	50.7	37.3	35.2	33.5	33.0	33.2	33.6	32.6	32.7
General/family practice	50.1	35.6	18.6	14.5	12.9	12.1	12.1	12.3	11.8	12.0
Internal medicine.	6.5	10.6	12.8	14.1	13.9	14.0	14.1	14.3	14.1	14.0
Pediatrics	2.5	4.5	5.8	6.6	6.7	6.9	7.0	7.0	6.7	6.8
Primary care specialists	- - -	- - -	0.9	3.6	5.0	5.6	5.6	6.1	5.0	5.1
Internal medicine.	- - -	- - -	0.6	3.1	4.0	4.4	4.3	4.6	3.7	3.8
Pediatrics	- - -	- - -	0.3	0.5	1.0	1.2	1.3	1.5	1.3	1.3

- - - Data not available.

[1]Estimated by the Bureau of Health Professions, Health Resources Administration. Active doctors of medicine (M.D.'s) include those with address unknown and primary specialty not classified.

[2]Includes M.D.'s engaged in Federal and non-Federal patient care (office-based or hospital-based) and other professional activities.

[3]Beginning in 1970, M.D.'s who are inactive, have unknown address, or primary specialty not classified are excluded.

NOTES: See Appendix II for definitions of physician specialties. Data are as of December 31 except for 1990–94 data, which are as of January 1, and 1949 data, which are as of midyear. Outlying areas include Puerto Rico, Virgin Islands, and the Pacific islands of Canton, Caroline, Guam, Mariana, Marshall, American Samoa, and Wake.

SOURCES: Health Manpower Source Book: Medical Specialists, USDHEW, 1962; American Medical Association (AMA). Distribution of physicians in the United States, 1970; Physician characteristics and distribution in the U.S., 1981 edition; 1992 edition; 1995–96 edition; 1996–97 edition; 1997–98 edition; 1999 edition; 2000–2001 edition. Department of Data Survey and Planning, Division of Survey and Data Resources, AMA. (Copyrights 1971, 1982, 1992, 1996, 1997, 1997, 1999, 2000: Used with the permission of the AMA.)

Table 104. Active health personnel according to occupation: United States, 1980–97

[Data are compiled by the Bureau of Health Professions]

Occupation	1980	1985[1]	1990	1995	1997[2]
		Number of active health personnel			
Chiropractors	25,600	- - -	41,500	47,200	- - -
Dentists[3]	121,240	135,500	146,600	- - -	159,500
Nutritionists/Dieticians	32,000	- - -	67,000	- - -	69,000
Nurses, registered	1,272,900	1,531,200	1,789,600	2,115,800	2,161,700
Associate and diploma	908,300	1,016,700	1,107,300	1,235,000	1,252,600
Baccalaureate	297,300	419,200	549,000	673,200	693,200
Masters and doctorate	67,300	95,300	133,300	207,500	215,900
Occupational therapists	25,000	- - -	34,000	- - -	45,000
Optometrists	22,330	23,900	26,000	28,900	29,500
Pharmacists	142,780	159,200	161,900	182,300	185,000
Physical therapists	50,000	- - -	92,000	- - -	107,000
Physicians	427,122	542,653	567,611	672,859	723,507
Federal	17,642	23,305	20,784	21,153	20,619
Doctors of medicine[4]	16,585	21,938	19,166	19,830	19,353
Doctors of osteopathy	1,057	1,367	1,618	1,323	1,266
Non-Federal	409,480	519,348	546,826	651,706	702,888
Doctors of medicine[4]	393,407	497,473	520,450	617,362	665,252
Doctors of osteopathy	16,073	21,875	26,376	34,344	37,636
Podiatrists[5]	7,000	9,700	10,600	10,300	- - -
Speech therapists	50,000	- - -	65,000	- - -	97,000
		Number per 100,000 population			
Chiropractors	11.2	- - -	16.5	17.8	- - -
Dentists[3]	53.5	56.9	58.8	- - -	58.2
Nutritionists/Dieticians	14.0	- - -	26.7	- - -	25.9
Nurses, registered	560.0	641.4	713.7	797.6	814.9
Associate and diploma	399.9	425.8	441.6	465.5	472.2
Baccalaureate	130.9	175.6	218.9	253.8	261.3
Masters and doctorate	29.6	39.9	53.2	78.2	81.4
Occupational therapists	10.9	- - -	13.5	- - -	16.9
Optometrists	9.8	9.9	10.4	10.9	11.1
Pharmacists	62.5	66.3	64.4	68.9	69.4
Physical therapists	21.8	- - -	36.6	- - -	40.1
Physicians	189.8	221.3	230.2	255.9	265.9
Federal	7.8	9.5	8.4	8.0	7.6
Doctors of medicine[4]	7.4	8.9	7.7	7.5	7.1
Doctors of osteopathy	0.5	0.6	0.7	0.5	0.5
Non-Federal	182.0	211.8	221.8	247.9	258.3
Doctors of medicine[4]	174.9	202.9	211.1	234.8	244.5
Doctors of osteopathy	7.1	8.9	10.7	13.1	13.8
Podiatrists[5]	3.0	4.2	4.2	3.9	- - -
Speech therapists	21.8	- - -	25.9	- - -	36.4

- - - Data not available.

[1]Osteopath data are for 1986 and podiatric data are for 1984.
[2]All physician data are for 1997, other occupations are for 1996.
[3]Excludes dentists in military service, U.S. Public Health Service, and Department of Veterans Affairs.
[4]Excludes physicians with unknown addresses and those who do not practice or practice less than 20 hours per week.
[5]Podiatrists in patient care.

NOTES: Ratios for physicians and dentists are based on civilian population; ratios for all other health occupations are based on resident population. From 1989 to 1994 data for doctors of medicine are as of January 1; in other years these data are as of December 31. See Appendix II for physician definitions.

SOURCES: Division of Health Professions Analysis, Bureau of Health Professions: Supply and Characteristics of Selected Health Personnel. DHHS Pub. No. (HRA) 81–20. Health Resources Administration. Hyattsville, Md., June 1981 and unpublished data; American Medical Association. Physician characteristics and distribution in the U.S., 1981, 1992, and 1997/98 editions. Chicago, 1982, 1992, and 1997; American Osteopathic Association. 1980–81 Yearbook and Directory of Osteopathic Physicians. Chicago, 1980. American Association of Colleges of Osteopathic Medicine. Annual statistical report, 1990, 1997, and 1998 editions. Rockville, Md., 1990, 1997, and 1998.

Table 105 (page 1 of 2). Full-time equivalent patient care staff in mental health organizations, according to type of organization and staff discipline: United States, selected years 1984–94

[Data are based on inventories of mental health organizations]

Organization and discipline	1984	1990	1992	1994	1984	1990	1992	1994
All organizations	Number				Percent distribution			
All patient care staff	313,243	416,282	434,620	457,503	100.0	100.0	100.0	100.0
Professional patient care staff	202,474	273,758	306,688	326,952	64.6	65.8	70.6	71.5
Psychiatrists	18,482	18,846	22,821	24,069	5.9	4.5	5.3	5.3
Psychologists	21,052	22,888	25,021	21,798	6.7	5.5	5.8	4.8
Social workers	36,397	53,487	57,201	55,493	11.6	12.8	13.2	12.1
Registered nurses	54,406	77,686	78,625	105,410	17.4	18.7	18.1	23.0
Other professional staff[1]	72,137	100,851	123,020	120,182	23.0	24.2	28.3	26.3
Other mental health workers	110,769	142,524	127,932	130,551	35.4	34.2	29.4	28.5
State and county mental hospitals								
All patient care staff	117,630	114,198	110,874	102,153	100.0	100.0	100.0	100.0
Professional patient care staff	51,290	50,035	56,953	41,359	43.6	43.8	51.4	40.5
Psychiatrists	4,108	3,849	4,457	3,177	3.5	3.4	4.0	3.1
Psychologists	3,239	3,324	3,620	2,697	2.8	2.9	3.3	2.6
Social workers	6,175	7,013	7,378	5,450	5.2	6.1	6.7	5.3
Registered nurses	16,051	20,848	21,119	17,685	13.6	18.3	19.0	17.3
Other professional staff[1]	21,717	15,001	20,379	12,350	18.5	13.1	18.4	12.1
Other mental health workers	66,340	64,163	53,921	60,794	56.4	56.2	48.6	59.5
Private psychiatric hospitals								
All patient care staff	26,359	57,200	56,877	58,262	100.0	100.0	100.0	100.0
Professional patient care staff	19,524	45,669	44,206	45,669	74.1	79.8	77.7	78.4
Psychiatrists	1,447	1,582	2,081	2,183	5.5	2.8	3.7	3.7
Psychologists	1,461	1,977	1,656	2,003	5.5	3.5	2.9	3.4
Social workers	2,179	4,044	4,587	5,473	8.3	7.1	8.1	9.4
Registered nurses	6,818	14,819	15,086	15,939	25.9	25.9	26.5	27.4
Other professional staff[1]	7,619	23,247	20,796	20,071	28.9	40.6	36.6	34.4
Other mental health workers	6,835	11,531	12,671	12,593	25.9	20.2	22.3	21.6
Non-Federal general hospitals' psychiatric services								
All patient care staff	59,848	72,214	72,880	87,304	100.0	100.0	100.0	100.0
Professional patient care staff	46,335	57,019	58,544	76,558	77.4	79.0	80.3	87.7
Psychiatrists	6,679	6,500	6,160	4,336	11.2	9.0	8.5	5.0
Psychologists	3,283	3,951	4,182	2,441	5.5	5.5	5.7	2.8
Social workers	4,898	7,241	7,985	5,355	8.2	10.0	11.0	6.1
Registered nurses	20,454	28,473	28,355	54,647	34.2	39.4	38.9	62.6
Other professional staff[1]	11,021	10,854	11,862	9,779	18.4	15.0	16.3	11.2
Other mental health workers	13,513	15,195	14,336	10,746	22.6	21.0	19.7	12.3
Department of Veterans Affairs psychiatric services								
All patient care staff	22,948	22,080	20,834	21,671	100.0	100.0	100.0	100.0
Professional patient care staff	16,265	14,619	16,274	18,393	70.9	66.2	78.1	84.9
Psychiatrists	2,463	2,103	3,403	6,272	10.7	9.5	16.3	28.9
Psychologists	1,247	1,476	2,479	587	5.4	6.7	11.9	2.7
Social workers	1,545	1,855	2,244	1,773	6.7	8.4	10.8	8.2
Registered nurses	5,699	5,888	5,485	8,475	24.8	26.7	26.3	39.1
Other professional staff[1]	5,311	3,297	2,663	1,286	23.1	14.9	12.8	5.9
Other mental health workers	6,683	7,461	4,560	3,278	29.1	33.8	21.9	15.1
Residential treatment centers for emotionally disturbed children								
All patient care staff	15,297	40,969	42,801	44,146	100.0	100.0	100.0	100.0
Professional patient care staff	10,551	26,032	30,207	31,079	69.0	63.5	70.6	70.4
Psychiatrists	240	498	748	840	1.6	1.2	1.7	1.9
Psychologists	820	1,492	1,641	1,707	5.4	3.6	3.8	3.9
Social workers	2,283	5,636	6,506	6,635	14.9	13.8	15.2	15.0
Registered nurses	485	1,238	1,367	1,468	3.2	3.0	3.2	3.3
Other professional staff[1]	6,723	17,168	19,945	20,429	43.9	41.9	46.6	46.3
Other mental health workers	4,746	14,937	12,594	13,067	31.0	36.5	29.4	29.6

See footnotes at end of table.

Table 105 (page 2 of 2). Full-time equivalent patient care staff in mental health organizations, according to type of organization and staff discipline: United States, selected years 1984–94

[Data are based on inventories of mental health organizations]

Organization and discipline	1984	1990	1992	1994	1984	1990	1992	1994
All other organizations[2]	Number				Percent distribution			
All patient care staff	71,161	109,621	130,354	143,967	100.0	100.0	100.0	100.0
Professional patient care staff	58,509	80,384	100,504	113,894	82.2	73.3	77.1	79.1
Psychiatrists	3,545	4,314	5,972	7,261	5.0	3.9	4.6	5.0
Psychologists	11,002	10,668	11,443	12,363	15.5	9.7	8.8	8.6
Social workers	19,317	27,698	28,501	30,807	27.1	25.3	21.9	21.4
Registered nurses	4,899	6,420	7,213	7,196	6.9	5.9	5.5	5.0
Other professional staff[1]	19,746	31,284	47,375	56,267	27.7	28.5	36.3	39.1
Other mental health workers	12,652	29,237	29,850	30,073	17.8	26.7	22.9	20.9

[1]Includes occupational therapists, recreation therapists, vocational rehabilitation counselors, and teachers.
[2]Includes freestanding outpatient clinics, freestanding day–night organizations, multiservice organizations, and other residential organizations.

NOTES: Full-time equivalent figures presented in this table combine staffing data for inpatient, residential, outpatient, and partial care treatment programs. Some mental health organizations provide a mixture of inpatient and outpatient care (for example Private psychiatric hospitals and Department of Veterans Affairs), while others provide predominantly inpatient (State and county mental hospitals) or outpatient (All other organizations) care. Caution should be exercised in comparing levels of FTE staff between different types of mental health organizations due to the different types of care provided. Figures for nonpatient care staff (administrative, clerical, and maintenance staff) are not shown. Data for additional years are available (see Appendix III).

SOURCES: Survey and Analysis Branch, Division of State and Community Systems Development, Center for Mental Health Services. Manderscheid RW, Sonnenschein MA. *Mental Health, United States, 1996*. DHHS. 1996; Unpublished data.

Table 106. First-year enrollment and graduates of health professions schools and number of schools, according to profession: United States, selected years 1980–99

[Data are based on reporting by health professions schools]

Profession	1980	1985	1990	1995	1996	1997	1998	1999
First-year enrollment								
Chiropractic[1]	- - -	1,383	1,485	- - -	- - -	- - -	- - -	- - -
Dentistry	6,132	5,047	3,979	4,121	4,237	4,255	4,347	4,268
Medicine (Allopathic)	16,930	16,997	16,756	17,085	17,058	16,935	16,867	- - -
Medicine (Osteopathic)	1,426	1,750	1,844	2,217	2,274	2,535	2,692	- - -
Nursing:								
Licensed practical	56,316	47,034	52,969	57,906	- - -	- - -	- - -	- - -
Registered, total	105,952	118,224	108,580	127,184	119,205	- - -	- - -	- - -
Baccalaureate	35,414	39,573	29,858	43,451	40,048	- - -	- - -	- - -
Associate degree	53,633	63,776	68,634	76,016	72,930	- - -	- - -	- - -
Diploma	16,905	14,875	10,088	7,717	6,227	- - -	- - -	- - -
Optometry	1,202	1,187	1,258	1,390	1,438	1,362	- - -	- - -
Pharmacy	8,035	6,986	8,033	9,157	8,740	8,790	8,571	8,346
Podiatry	718	782	599	652	630	616	676	623
Public Health[2]	3,348	3,836	4,087	5,332	5,342	5,083	5,376	- - -
Graduates								
Chiropractic	2,049	- - -	1,661	- - -	- - -	- - -	- - -	- - -
Dentistry	5,256	5,353	4,233	3,908	3,810	3,930	4,041	- - -
Medicine (Allopathic)	15,135	16,319	15,336	15,911	16,029	15,904	- - -	- - -
Medicine (Osteopathic)	1,059	1,474	1,529	1,843	1,932	2,009	- - -	- - -
Nursing:								
Licensed practical	41,892	36,955	35,417	44,234	- - -	- - -	- - -	- - -
Registered, total	75,523	82,075	66,088	97,052	94,757	- - -	- - -	- - -
Baccalaureate	24,994	24,975	18,571	31,254	32,413	- - -	- - -	- - -
Associate degree	36,034	45,208	42,318	58,749	56,641	- - -	- - -	- - -
Diploma	14,495	11,892	5,199	7,049	5,703	- - -	- - -	- - -
Occupational therapy	- - -	- - -	2,424	3,473	4,270	4,223	- - -	- - -
Optometry	1,073	1,114	1,115	1,219	1,210	- - -	- - -	- - -
Pharmacy	7,432	5,735	6,956	7,837	8,003	7,772	7,400	- - -
Physical therapy	- - -	- - -	- - -	- - -	- - -	4,746	- - -	- - -
Podiatry	577	586	671	558	680	645	592	- - -
Public Health	3,326	3,047	3,549	4,636	5,064	5,100	5,308	- - -
Schools[3]								
Chiropractic	14	17	17	- - -	- - -	- - -	- - -	- - -
Dentistry	60	60	56	54	54	54	55	- - -
Medicine (Allopathic)	126	127	126	125	125	125	125	- - -
Medicine (Osteopathic)	14	15	15	16	17	17	19	- - -
Nursing:								
Licensed practical	1,299	1,165	1,154	1,210	- - -	- - -	- - -	- - -
Registered, total	1,385	1,473	1,470	1,516	1,508	- - -	- - -	- - -
Baccalaureate	377	441	489	521	523	- - -	- - -	- - -
Associate degree	697	776	829	876	876	- - -	- - -	- - -
Diploma	311	256	152	119	109	- - -	- - -	- - -
Occupational therapy	50	61	69	98	105	116	- - -	- - -
Optometry	16	17	17	17	17	17	17	- - -
Pharmacy	72	72	74	75	79	81	81	- - -
Physical therapy	- - -	- - -	- - -	- - -	- - -	154	- - -	- - -
Podiatry	5	7	7	7	7	7	7	7
Public Health	21	23	25	27	28	28	28	29
Speech therapy	- - -	- - -	194	222	223	223	- - -	- - -

- - - Data not available.

[1]Chiropractic first-year enrollment data are partial data from eight reporting schools.
[2]These are students entering Schools of Public Health for the first time.
[3]Some nursing schools offer more than one type of program. Numbers shown for nursing are number of nursing programs.

NOTES: Some numbers in this table have been revised and differ from previous editions of *Health, United States*. Data on the number of schools are reported as of the beginning of the academic year while data on first-year enrollment and number of graduates are reported as of the end of the academic year. Data on first-year enrollment for occupational, physical, and speech therapy were not available.

SOURCES: Association of American Medical Colleges: AAMC Data Book, Statistical Information Related to Medical Education. Washington, DC. 1999; Bureau of Health Professions: Health Personnel in the United States, Eighth Report to Congress, 1991. Health Resources and Services Administration. DHHS Pub. No. HRS-P-OD-92-1, Rockville, Maryland. 1992 and unpublished data; National League for Nursing: Nursing data source, 1997 and unpublished data; American Nurses Association: Facts About Nursing, 1951 and 1961; American Dental Association: 1997/98 Survey of predoctoral dental educational institutions, Chicago. 1998; American Medical Association: Medical education in the United States. *JAMA* 278(9). September 3, 1997; American Association of Colleges of Osteopathic Medicine. Annual statistical report 1998. Rockville, Maryland. 1998; American Chiropractic Association: unpublished data; Association of Schools of Public Health: 1998 Annual Data Report. Washington, DC. 1999; Association of Schools and Colleges of Optometry: unpublished data; American Association of Colleges of Pharmacy: Profile of pharmacy students 1997, and unpublished data; American Association of Colleges of Podiatric Medicine: unpublished data.

Table 107 (page 1 of 2). Total enrollment of minorities in schools for selected health occupations, according to detailed race and Hispanic origin: United States, academic years 1970–71, 1980–81, 1990–91, and 1997–98

[Data are based on reporting by health professions associations]

Occupation, detailed race, and Hispanic origin	1970–71[1]	1980–81	1990–91	1997–98[2]	1970–71[1]	1980–81	1990–91	1997–98[2]
Dentistry[3]	Number of students				Percent distribution of students			
All races	19,187	22,842	15,951	16,926	100.0	100.0	100.0	100.0
White, non-Hispanic[4]	17,531	20,208	11,185	11,246	91.4	88.5	70.1	66.4
Black, non-Hispanic	872	1,022	940	883	4.5	4.5	5.9	5.2
Hispanic	185	519	1,254	825	1.0	2.3	7.9	4.9
American Indian	28	53	53	96	0.1	0.2	0.3	0.6
Asian	490	1,040	2,519	3,876	2.6	4.6	15.8	22.9
Medicine (Allopathic)								
All races[4]	40,238	65,189	65,163	66,900	100.0	100.0	100.0	100.0
White, non-Hispanic	37,944	55,434	47,893	44,310	94.3	85.0	73.5	66.2
Black, non-Hispanic	1,509	3,708	4,241	5,303	3.8	5.7	6.5	7.9
Hispanic	196	2,761	3,538	4,423	0.5	4.2	5.4	6.6
Mexican	---	951	1,109	1,838	---	1.5	1.7	2.7
Mainland Puerto Rican	---	329	457	476	---	0.5	0.7	0.7
Other Hispanic[5]	---	1,481	1,972	2,109	---	2.3	3.0	3.2
American Indian	18	221	277	561	0.0	0.3	0.4	0.8
Asian	571	1,924	8,436	12,303	1.4	3.0	12.9	18.4
Medicine (Osteopathic)								
All races	2,304	4,940	6,792	9,434	100.0	100.0	100.0	100.0
White, non-Hispanic[4]	2,241	4,688	5,680	7,404	97.3	94.9	83.6	78.5
Black, non-Hispanic	27	94	217	386	1.2	1.9	3.2	4.1
Hispanic	19	52	277	378	0.8	1.1	4.1	4.0
American Indian	6	19	36	82	0.3	0.4	0.5	0.9
Asian	11	87	582	1,184	0.5	1.8	8.6	12.6
Nursing, registered[3,6]								
All races	211,239	230,966	221,170	238,244	---	---	100.0	100.0
White, non-Hispanic[4]	---	---	183,102	193,061	---	---	82.8	81.0
Black, non-Hispanic	---	---	23,094	23,611	---	---	10.4	9.9
Hispanic	---	---	6,580	9,227	---	---	3.0	3.9
American Indian	---	---	1,803	1,816	---	---	0.8	0.8
Asian	---	---	6,591	10,529	---	---	3.0	4.4
Optometry[3]								
All races	3,094	4,540	4,650	5,075	100.0	100.0	100.0	100.0
White, non-Hispanic[4]	2,913	4,148	3,706	3,705	94.1	91.4	79.7	73.0
Black, non-Hispanic	32	57	134	120	1.0	1.3	2.9	2.4
Hispanic	30	80	186	200	1.0	1.8	4.0	3.9
American Indian	2	12	21	23	0.1	0.3	0.5	0.5
Asian	117	243	603	1,027	3.8	5.4	13.0	20.2
Pharmacy[3,7]								
All races	17,909	21,628	22,764	32,529	100.0	100.0	100.0	100.0
White, non-Hispanic[4]	16,222	19,153	18,325	22,166	90.6	88.6	80.5	68.1
Black, non-Hispanic	659	945	1,301	2,632	3.7	4.4	5.7	8.1
Hispanic	254	459	945	1,130	1.4	2.1	4.2	3.5
American Indian	29	36	63	150	0.2	0.2	0.3	0.5
Asian	672	1,035	2,130	6,451	3.8	4.8	9.4	19.8

See footnotes at end of table.

Table 107 (page 2 of 2). Total enrollment of minorities in schools for selected health occupations, according to detailed race and Hispanic origin: United States, academic years 1970–71, 1980–81, 1990–91, and 1997–98

[Data are based on reporting by health professions associations]

Occupation, detailed race, and Hispanic origin	1970–71[1]	1980–81	1990–91	1997–98[2]	1970–71[1]	1980–81	1990–91	1997–98[2]
Podiatry	Number of students				Percent distribution of students			
All races	1,268	2,577	2,226	2,471	100.0	100.0	100.0	100.0
White, non-Hispanic[4]	1,228	2,353	1,671	1,820	96.8	91.3	75.1	73.7
Black, non-Hispanic	27	110	237	148	2.1	4.3	10.6	6.0
Hispanic	5	39	148	92	0.4	1.5	6.6	3.7
American Indian	1	6	7	9	0.1	0.2	0.3	0.4
Asian	7	69	163	402	0.6	2.7	7.3	16.3

- - - Data not available.

[1]Data for osteopathic medicine, podiatry, and optometry are for 1971–72. Data for pharmacy and registered nurses are for 1972–73.
[2]Data for podiatry exclude New York College of Podiatric Medicine. Data for registered nurses and optometry are for 1996–97.
[3]Excludes Puerto Rican schools.
[4]Includes race and ethnicity unspecified.
[5]Includes Puerto Rican Commonwealth students.
[6]In 1990 the National League for Nursing developed a new system for analyzing minority data. In evaluating the former system, much underreporting was noted. Therefore, race-specific data before 1990 would not be comparable and are not shown. Additional changes in the minority data question were introduced for academic years 1992–93 and 1993–94 resulting in a discontinuity in the trend.
[7]Prior to 1992–93 pharmacy total enrollment data are for students in the final 3 years of pharmacy education. Beginning in 1992–93 pharmacy data are for all students.

NOTES: Total enrollment data are collected at the beginning of the academic year. Data for chiropractic students and occupational, physical, and speech therapy students were not available for this table.

SOURCES: Association of American Medical Colleges: AAMC Data Book: Statistical Information Related to Medical Education. Washington, DC. 1999; American Association of Colleges of Osteopathic Medicine: 1998 Annual statistical report. Rockville, Maryland. 1998; Bureau of Health Professions: Minorities and women in the health fields, 1990 Edition; American Dental Association: 1997/98 Survey of predoctoral dental educational institutions, Chicago. 1998; Association of Schools and Colleges of Optometry: Unpublished data; American Association of Colleges of Pharmacy: Profile of pharmacy students 1997, and unpublished data; American Association of Colleges of Podiatric Medicine: Unpublished data; National League for Nursing: Nursing datasource, 1997; Nursing data book. New York. 1982.

Table 108. First-year and total enrollment of women in schools for selected health occupations, according to detailed race and Hispanic origin: United States, academic years 1971–72, 1980–81, 1990–91, and 1997–98

[Data are based on reporting by health professions associations]

Enrollment, occupation, detailed race, and Hispanic origin	Both sexes				Women			
	1971–72[1]	1980–81	1990–91	1997–98[2]	1971–72[1]	1980–81	1990–91	1997–98[2]
First-year enrollment	Number of students				Percent of students			
Dentistry	4,705	5,964	3,961	4,347	3.1	19.8	37.9	37.0
Medicine (Allopathic)[3]	12,361	17,186	16,876	16,935	13.7	28.9	38.8	42.9
White, non-Hispanic	- - -	14,262	11,830	10,916	- - -	27.4	37.7	40.4
Black, non-Hispanic	881	1,128	1,263	1,423	22.7	45.5	55.3	60.5
Hispanic	- - -	818	933	1,207	- - -	31.5	42.0	44.9
Mexican	118	258	285	501	8.5	30.6	39.3	44.3
Mainland Puerto Rican	40	95	120	150	15.0	43.2	43.3	50.7
Other Hispanic[4]	- - -	465	528	556	- - -	29.7	43.3	43.9
American Indian	23	67	76	149	34.8	35.8	40.8	50.3
Asian	217	572	2,527	3,039	19.4	31.5	40.3	42.3
Medicine (Osteopathic)	670	1,496	1,950	2,692	4.3	22.0	34.2	39.8
Nurses, registered[5]	93,344	110,201	113,526	119,205	94.5	92.7	89.3	87.5
Optometry[5]	906	1,174	1,207	1,323	5.3	25.3	50.6	53.4
Pharmacy[5,6]	6,532	7,442	8,009	8,571	25.8	48.4	- - -	64.1
Podiatry	399	695	622	676	- - -	- - -	- - -	35.2
Public Health	- - -	3,348	4,289	5,376	- - -	- - -	62.1	66.5
Total enrollment								
Dentistry	16,553	22,842	15,951	16,926	- - -	17.0	34.4	37.3
Medicine (Allopathic)[3]	43,650	65,189	65,163	66,900	10.9	26.5	37.3	42.6
White, non-Hispanic	- - -	55,434	47,893	44,310	- - -	25.0	35.4	- - -
Black, non-Hispanic	2,055	3,708	4,241	5,303	20.4	44.3	55.8	- - -
Hispanic	- - -	2,761	3,538	4,423	- - -	30.1	39.0	- - -
Mexican	252	951	1,109	1,838	9.5	26.4	38.5	- - -
Mainland Puerto Rican	76	329	457	476	17.1	35.9	43.1	- - -
Other Hispanic[4]	- - -	1,481	1,972	2,109	- - -	31.1	38.4	- - -
American Indian	42	221	277	561	23.8	28.5	42.6	- - -
Asian	647	1,924	8,436	12,303	17.9	30.4	37.7	- - -
Medicine (Osteopathic)	2,304	4,940	6,792	9,434	3.4	19.7	32.7	38.1
Nurses, registered[5]	211,239	230,966	221,170	238,244	95.5	94.3	- - -	87.9
Optometry[5]	3,094	4,540	4,650	5,075	- - -	- - -	47.3	52.9
Pharmacy[5]	16,476	26,617	29,797	32,529	24.0	47.4	62.4	64.2
Podiatry	1,268	2,577	2,226	2,471	1.2	11.9	- - -	31.4
Public Health	- - -	8,486	11,386	14,736	- - -	55.2	62.5	65.3

- - - Data not available.

[1]Total enrollments for registered nurse students are for 1972–73.
[2]First-year enrollments for allopathic medicine, registered nurses, and optometry and total enrollments for registered nurses and optometry are for 1996–97.
[3]Includes race and ethnicity unspecified.
[4]Includes Puerto Rican Commonwealth students.
[5]Excludes Puerto Rican schools.
[6]Pharmacy first-year enrollment data are for students in the first year of the final 3 years of pharmacy education.

NOTES: Some numbers in this table have been revised and differ from previous editions of *Health, United States*. Total enrollment data are collected at the beginning of the academic year while first-year enrollment data are collected during the academic year. Data for chiropractic students and occupational, physical, and speech therapy students were not available for this table.

SOURCES: Association of American Medical Colleges: AAMC Data Book: Statistical Information Related to Medical Education. Washington, DC. 1999 and unpublished data; American Association of Colleges of Osteopathic Medicine: 1998 Annual Statistical Report. Rockville, Maryland. 1998; Bureau of Health Professions: Minorities and women in the health fields, 1990 edition; American Dental Association: 1997/98 Survey of predoctoral dental educational institutions, Chicago. 1998; Association of Schools and Colleges of Optometry: Unpublished data; American Association of Colleges of Pharmacy: unpublished data; American Association of Colleges of Podiatric Medicine: Unpublished data; National League for Nursing: Nursing datasource. New York. 1997; Nursing data book. New York. 1982; State-Approved Schools of Nursing-RN. New York. 1973; Association of Schools of Public Health: 1998 Annual Data Report. Washington, DC. 1999.

Table 109. Hospitals, beds, and occupancy rates, according to type of ownership and size of hospital: United States, selected years 1975–98

[Data are based on reporting by a census of hospitals]

Type of ownership and size of hospital	1975	1980	1985	1990	1995	1996	1997	1998
Hospitals				Number				
All hospitals	7,156	6,965	6,872	6,649	6,291	6,201	6,097	6,021
Federal	382	359	343	337	299	290	285	275
Non-Federal[1]	6,774	6,606	6,529	6,312	5,992	5,911	5,812	5,746
Community[2]	5,875	5,830	5,732	5,384	5,194	5,134	5,057	5,015
Nonprofit	3,339	3,322	3,349	3,191	3,092	3,045	3,000	3,026
For profit	775	730	805	749	752	759	797	771
State-local government	1,761	1,778	1,578	1,444	1,350	1,330	1,260	1,218
6–24 beds	299	259	208	226	278	262	281	293
25–49 beds	1,155	1,029	982	935	922	906	890	900
50–99 beds	1,481	1,462	1,399	1,263	1,139	1,128	1,111	1,085
100–199 beds	1,363	1,370	1,407	1,306	1,324	1,338	1,289	1,304
200–299 beds	678	715	739	739	718	692	679	644
300–399 beds	378	412	439	408	354	361	367	352
400–499 beds	230	266	239	222	195	196	185	183
500 beds or more	291	317	319	285	264	251	255	254
Beds								
All hospitals	1,465,828	1,364,516	1,317,630	1,213,327	1,080,601	1,061,688	1,035,390	1,012,582
Federal	131,946	117,328	112,023	98,255	77,079	73,171	61,937	56,698
Non-Federal[1]	1,333,882	1,247,188	1,205,607	1,115,072	1,003,522	988,517	973,453	955,884
Community[2]	941,844	988,387	1,000,678	927,360	872,736	862,352	853,287	839,988
Nonprofit	658,195	692,459	707,451	656,755	609,729	598,162	590,636	587,658
For profit	73,495	87,033	103,921	101,377	105,737	109,197	115,074	112,975
State-local government	210,154	208,895	189,306	169,228	157,270	154,993	147,577	139,355
6–24 beds	5,615	4,932	4,031	4,427	5,085	4,770	5,128	5,351
25–49 beds	41,783	37,478	36,833	35,420	34,352	33,814	33,138	33,510
50–99 beds	106,776	105,278	101,680	90,394	82,024	81,185	79,837	78,035
100–199 beds	192,438	192,892	199,690	183,867	187,381	189,630	182,284	186,118
200–299 beds	164,405	172,390	180,165	179,670	175,240	168,977	165,197	156,978
300–399 beds	127,728	139,434	151,919	138,938	121,136	123,822	126,307	120,512
400–499 beds	101,278	117,724	106,653	98,833	86,459	86,913	82,250	81,247
500 beds or more	201,821	218,259	219,707	195,811	181,059	173,241	179,146	178,237
Occupancy rate				Percent of beds occupied				
All hospitals	76.7	77.7	69.0	69.5	65.7	64.5	65.0	65.4
Federal	80.7	80.1	76.3	72.9	72.6	71.4	79.1	78.9
Non-Federal[1]	76.3	77.4	68.4	69.2	65.1	64.0	64.1	64.6
Community[2]	75.0	75.6	64.8	66.8	62.8	61.5	61.8	62.5
Nonprofit	77.5	78.2	67.2	69.3	64.5	63.3	63.6	64.2
For profit	65.9	65.2	52.1	52.8	51.8	51.6	52.0	53.2
State-local government	70.4	71.1	62.9	65.3	63.7	61.7	62.3	62.7
6–24 beds	48.0	46.8	34.7	32.3	36.9	33.2	35.4	33.2
25–49 beds	56.7	52.8	40.0	41.3	42.6	40.0	40.3	41.2
50–99 beds	64.7	64.2	51.8	53.8	54.1	53.1	54.2	54.7
100–199 beds	71.2	71.4	59.7	61.5	58.8	57.8	58.2	58.4
200–299 beds	77.1	77.4	65.7	67.1	63.1	62.0	61.8	62.9
300–399 beds	79.7	79.7	68.4	70.0	64.8	63.6	63.2	64.7
400–499 beds	81.1	81.2	70.1	73.5	68.1	67.4	68.0	67.3
500 beds or more	80.9	82.1	74.6	77.3	71.4	69.7	69.8	70.9

[1]The category of non-Federal hospitals is comprised of psychiatric, tuberculosis and other respiratory disease hospitals, and long-term and short-term hospitals.
[2]Community hospitals are short-term hospitals excluding hospital units in institutions such as prison and college infirmaries, facilities for the mentally retarded, and alcoholism and chemical dependency hospitals.

NOTE: Data for additional years are available (see Appendix III).

SOURCES: American Hospital Association: Hospital Statistics, 1976, 1981, 1986, 1991–2000 Editions. Chicago, 1976, 1981, 1986, 1991–2000. (Copyrights 1976, 1981, 1986, 1991–2000: Used with the permission of the American Hospital Association (AHA) and Health Forum, an AHA company.)

Table 110. Inpatient and residential mental health organizations and beds, according to type of organization: United States, selected years 1984–94

[Data are based on inventories of mental health organizations]

Type of organization	1984	1986	1988	1990	1992	1994
	Number of mental health organizations					
All organizations	2,849	3,039	3,231	3,430	3,415	3,319
State and county mental hospitals	277	285	285	273	273	256
Private psychiatric hospitals	220	314	444	462	475	430
Non-Federal general hospital psychiatric services	1,259	1,287	1,425	1,571	1,517	1,531
Department of Veterans Affairs psychiatric services[1]	124	124	125	130	133	135
Residential treatment centers for emotionally disturbed children	322	437	440	501	497	459
All other[2]	647	592	512	493	520	508
	Number of beds					
All organizations	262,673	267,613	271,923	272,253	270,867	252,333
State and county mental hospitals	130,411	119,033	107,109	98,789	93,058	79,294
Private psychiatric hospitals	21,474	30,201	42,255	44,871	43,684	41,195
Non-Federal general hospital psychiatric services	46,045	45,808	48,421	53,479	52,059	52,984
Department of Veterans Affairs psychiatric services[1]	23,546	26,874	25,742	21,712	22,466	21,146
Residential treatment centers for emotionally disturbed children	16,745	24,547	25,173	29,756	30,089	32,110
All other[2]	24,452	21,150	23,223	23,646	29,511	25,604
	Beds per 100,000 civilian population					
All organizations	112.9	111.7	111.4	111.6	107.4	97.5
State and county mental hospitals	56.1	49.7	44.0	40.5	36.9	30.6
Private psychiatric hospitals	9.2	12.6	17.3	18.4	17.3	15.9
Non-Federal general hospital psychiatric services	19.8	19.1	19.8	21.9	20.7	20.5
Department of Veterans Affairs psychiatric services[1]	10.1	11.2	10.5	8.9	8.9	8.2
Residential treatment centers for emotionally disturbed children	7.2	10.3	10.3	12.2	11.9	12.4
All other[2]	10.5	8.8	9.5	9.7	11.7	9.9

[1]Includes Department of Veterans Affairs neuropsychiatric hospitals and general hospital psychiatric services.

[2]Includes other multiservice mental health organizations with inpatient and residential treatment services that are not elsewhere classified. See Appendix I.

SOURCES: Survey and Analysis Branch, Division of State and Community Systems Development, Center for Mental Health Services. Manderscheid RW, Sonnenschein MA. *Mental Health, United States, 1996*. DHHS. 1996.

Table 111. Community hospital beds and average annual percent change, according to geographic division and State: United States, selected years 1940–98

[Data are based on reporting by facilities]

Geographic division and State	Beds per 1,000 civilian population							Average annual percent change				
	1940[1,2]	1950[1,2]	1960[2,3]	1970[2]	1980[2]	1990[4]	1998[4]	1940–60[1,2,3]	1960–70[2,3]	1970–80[2]	1980–90[5]	1990–98[4]
United States	3.2	3.3	3.6	4.3	4.5	3.7	3.1	0.6	1.8	0.5	−1.9	−2.2
New England	4.4	4.2	3.9	4.1	4.1	3.4	2.6	−0.6	0.5	0.0	−1.9	−3.3
Maine	3.0	3.2	3.4	4.7	4.7	3.7	3.0	0.6	3.3	0.0	−2.4	−2.6
New Hampshire	4.2	4.2	4.4	4.0	3.9	3.1	2.4	0.2	−0.9	−0.3	−2.3	−3.1
Vermont	3.3	4.0	4.5	4.5	4.4	3.0	2.8	1.6	0.0	−0.2	−3.8	−0.9
Massachusetts	5.1	4.8	4.2	4.4	4.4	3.6	2.7	−1.0	0.5	0.0	−2.0	−3.5
Rhode Island	3.9	3.8	3.7	4.0	3.8	3.2	2.6	−0.3	0.8	−0.5	−1.7	−2.6
Connecticut	3.7	3.6	3.4	3.4	3.5	2.9	2.1	−0.4	0.0	0.3	−1.9	−4.0
Middle Atlantic	3.9	3.8	4.0	4.4	4.6	4.1	3.6	0.1	1.0	0.4	−1.1	−1.6
New York	4.3	4.1	4.3	4.6	4.5	4.1	3.8	0.0	0.7	−0.2	−0.9	−0.9
New Jersey	3.5	3.2	3.1	3.6	4.2	3.7	3.2	−0.6	1.5	1.6	−1.3	−1.8
Pennsylvania	3.5	3.8	4.1	4.7	4.8	4.4	3.7	0.8	1.4	0.2	−0.9	−2.1
East North Central	3.2	3.2	3.6	4.4	4.7	3.9	3.1	0.6	2.0	0.7	−1.8	−2.8
Ohio	2.7	2.9	3.4	4.2	4.7	4.0	3.1	1.2	2.1	1.1	−1.6	−3.1
Indiana	2.3	2.6	3.1	4.0	4.5	3.9	3.3	1.5	2.6	1.2	−1.4	−2.1
Illinois	3.4	3.6	4.0	4.7	5.1	4.0	3.3	0.8	1.6	0.8	−2.4	−2.4
Michigan	4.0	3.3	3.3	4.3	4.4	3.7	2.8	−1.0	2.7	0.2	−1.7	−3.4
Wisconsin	3.4	3.7	4.3	5.2	4.9	3.8	3.2	1.2	1.9	−0.6	−2.5	−2.1
West North Central	3.1	3.7	4.3	5.7	5.8	4.9	4.1	1.6	2.9	0.2	−1.7	−2.2
Minnesota	3.9	4.4	4.8	6.1	5.7	4.4	3.5	1.0	2.4	−0.7	−2.6	−2.8
Iowa	2.7	3.2	3.9	5.6	5.7	5.1	4.3	1.9	3.7	0.2	−1.1	−2.1
Missouri	2.9	3.3	3.9	5.1	5.7	4.8	3.8	1.5	2.7	1.1	−1.7	−2.9
North Dakota	3.5	4.3	5.2	6.8	7.4	7.0	6.2	2.0	2.7	0.8	−0.6	−1.5
South Dakota	2.8	4.4	4.5	5.6	5.5	6.1	6.0	2.4	2.2	−0.2	1.0	−0.2
Nebraska	3.4	4.2	4.4	6.2	6.0	5.5	4.9	1.3	3.5	−0.3	−0.9	−1.4
Kansas	2.8	3.4	4.2	5.4	5.8	4.8	4.2	2.0	2.5	0.7	−1.9	−1.7
South Atlantic	2.5	2.8	3.3	4.0	4.5	3.7	3.1	1.4	1.9	1.2	−1.9	−2.2
Delaware	4.4	3.9	3.7	3.7	3.6	3.0	2.7	−0.9	0.0	−0.3	−1.8	−1.3
Maryland	3.9	3.6	3.3	3.1	3.6	2.8	2.5	−0.8	−0.6	1.5	−2.5	−1.4
District of Columbia	5.5	5.5	5.9	7.4	7.3	7.6	6.8	0.4	2.3	−0.1	0.4	−1.4
Virginia	2.2	2.5	3.0	3.7	4.1	3.3	2.6	1.6	2.1	1.0	−2.1	−2.9
West Virginia	2.7	3.1	4.1	5.4	5.5	4.7	4.5	2.1	2.8	0.2	−1.6	−0.5
North Carolina	2.2	2.6	3.4	3.8	4.2	3.3	3.1	2.2	1.1	1.0	−2.4	−0.8
South Carolina	1.8	2.4	2.9	3.7	3.9	3.3	3.0	2.4	2.5	0.5	−1.7	−1.2
Georgia	1.7	2.0	2.8	3.8	4.6	4.0	3.3	2.5	3.1	1.9	−1.4	−2.4
Florida	2.8	2.9	3.1	4.4	5.1	3.9	3.3	0.5	3.6	1.5	−2.6	−2.1
East South Central	1.7	2.1	3.0	4.4	5.1	4.7	4.0	2.9	3.9	1.5	−0.8	−2.0
Kentucky	1.8	2.2	3.0	4.0	4.5	4.3	3.9	2.6	2.9	1.2	−0.5	−1.2
Tennessee	1.9	2.3	3.4	4.7	5.5	4.8	3.8	3.0	3.3	1.6	−1.4	−2.9
Alabama	1.5	2.0	2.8	4.3	5.1	4.6	3.9	3.2	4.4	1.7	−1.0	−2.0
Mississippi	1.4	1.7	2.9	4.4	5.3	5.0	4.7	3.7	4.3	1.9	−0.6	−0.8
West South Central	2.1	2.7	3.3	4.3	4.7	3.8	3.2	2.3	2.7	0.9	−2.1	−2.1
Arkansas	1.4	1.6	2.9	4.2	5.0	4.6	3.9	3.7	3.8	1.8	−0.8	−2.0
Louisiana	3.1	3.8	3.9	4.2	4.8	4.6	4.1	1.2	0.7	1.3	−0.4	−1.4
Oklahoma	1.9	2.5	3.2	4.5	4.6	4.0	3.3	2.6	3.5	0.2	−1.4	−2.4
Texas	2.0	2.7	3.3	4.3	4.7	3.5	2.9	2.5	2.7	0.9	−2.9	−2.3
Mountain	3.6	3.8	3.5	4.3	3.8	3.1	2.4	−0.1	2.1	−1.2	−2.0	−3.1
Montana	4.9	5.3	5.1	5.8	5.9	5.8	5.0	0.2	1.3	0.2	−0.2	−1.8
Idaho	2.6	3.4	3.2	4.0	3.7	3.2	2.8	1.0	2.3	−0.8	−1.4	−1.7
Wyoming	3.5	3.9	4.6	5.5	3.6	4.8	4.0	1.4	1.8	−4.1	2.9	−2.3
Colorado	3.9	4.2	3.8	4.6	4.2	3.2	2.3	−0.1	1.9	−0.9	−2.7	−4.0
New Mexico	2.7	2.2	2.9	3.5	3.1	2.8	2.0	0.4	1.9	−1.2	−1.0	−4.1
Arizona	3.4	4.0	3.0	4.1	3.6	2.7	2.3	−0.6	3.2	−1.3	−2.8	−2.0
Utah	3.2	2.9	2.8	3.6	3.1	2.6	1.9	−0.7	2.5	−1.5	−1.7	−3.8
Nevada	5.0	4.4	3.9	4.2	4.2	2.8	2.0	−1.2	0.7	0.0	−4.0	−4.1
Pacific	4.1	3.2	3.1	3.7	3.5	2.7	2.2	−1.4	1.8	−0.6	−2.6	−2.5
Washington	3.4	3.6	3.3	3.5	3.1	2.5	1.9	−0.1	0.6	−1.2	−2.1	−3.4
Oregon	3.5	3.1	3.5	4.0	3.5	2.8	2.1	0.0	1.3	−1.3	−2.2	−3.5
California	4.4	3.3	3.0	3.8	3.6	2.7	2.3	−1.9	2.4	−0.5	−2.8	−2.0
Alaska	...	...	2.4	2.3	2.7	2.3	2.0	...	−0.4	1.6	−1.6	−1.7
Hawaii	...	...	3.7	3.4	3.1	2.7	2.3	...	−0.8	−0.9	−1.4	−2.0

0.0 Quantity more than zero but less than 0.05.   ... Category not applicable.

[1]1940 and 1950 data are estimated based on published figures.
[2]Data exclude facilities for the mentally retarded. See Appendix II, Hospital.   [3]1960 data include hospital units of institutions.
[4]Starting with 1990, data exclude hospital units of institutions, facilities for the mentally retarded, and alcoholism and chemical dependency hospitals. See Appendix II.
[5]1990 data used in this calculation (not shown in table) exclude only facilities for the mentally retarded, consistent with exclusions from 1980 data.

NOTE: Data for additional years are available (see Appendix III).

SOURCES: American Medical Association (AMA): Hospital service in United States. *JAMA* 116(11):1055–1144, 1941 and 146(2):109–184, 1951 (Copyright 1941, 1951: Used with permission of AMA); American Hospital Association (AHA): Hospitals. *JAHA* 35(15):383–430, 1961 (Copyright 1961: Used with permission of AHA); National Center for Health Statistics, Division of Health Care Statistics and AHA annual surveys for 1970, 1980; Hospital Statistics 1991–92, 2000 Editions. Chicago (Copyrights 1971, 1981, 1991, 2000: Used with permission of AHA and Health Forum, an AHA company).

Table 112. Occupancy rates in community hospitals and average annual percent change, according to geographic division and State: United States, selected years 1940–98

[Data are based on reporting by facilities]

Geographic division and State	Percent of beds occupied						Average annual percent change				
	1940[1,2]	1960[2,3]	1970[2]	1980[2]	1990[4]	1998[4]	1940–60[1,2,3]	1960–70[2,3]	1970–80[2]	1980–90[5]	1990–98[4]
United States	69.9	74.7	77.3	75.2	66.8	62.4	0.3	0.3	–0.3	–1.2	–0.8
New England	72.5	75.2	79.7	80.1	74.0	67.9	0.2	0.6	0.1	–0.8	–1.1
Maine	72.4	73.2	73.0	74.5	71.5	61.4	0.1	–0.0	0.2	–0.4	–1.9
New Hampshire	65.3	66.5	73.4	73.2	66.8	63.5	0.1	1.0	–0.0	–0.9	–0.6
Vermont	68.8	68.5	76.3	73.7	67.3	64.5	–0.0	1.1	–0.3	–0.9	–0.5
Massachusetts	71.8	75.8	80.3	81.7	74.2	69.5	0.3	0.6	0.2	–1.0	–0.8
Rhode Island	77.7	75.7	82.9	85.9	79.4	70.1	–0.1	0.9	0.4	–0.8	–1.5
Connecticut	75.9	78.2	82.6	80.4	77.0	69.3	0.1	0.5	–0.3	–0.4	–1.3
Middle Atlantic	75.5	78.1	82.4	83.2	80.5	72.4	0.2	0.5	0.1	–0.3	–1.3
New York	78.9	79.4	82.9	85.9	86.0	76.7	0.0	0.4	0.4	–0.0	–1.4
New Jersey	72.4	78.4	82.5	82.8	80.2	70.6	0.4	0.5	0.0	–0.3	–1.6
Pennsylvania	71.3	76.0	81.5	79.5	72.9	66.9	0.3	0.7	–0.2	–0.9	–1.1
East North Central	71.0	78.4	79.5	76.9	64.6	59.4	0.5	0.1	–0.3	–1.7	–1.0
Ohio	72.1	81.3	81.8	79.2	64.7	56.8	0.6	0.1	–0.3	–2.0	–1.6
Indiana	68.5	79.6	80.3	77.6	60.6	57.6	0.8	0.1	–0.3	–2.4	–0.6
Illinois	73.1	76.0	79.3	74.9	65.7	60.4	0.2	0.4	–0.6	–1.3	–1.0
Michigan	71.5	80.5	80.6	78.2	65.5	64.3	0.6	0.0	–0.3	–1.8	–0.2
Wisconsin	65.2	73.9	73.2	73.6	64.6	56.5	0.6	–0.1	0.1	–1.3	–1.7
West North Central	65.7	71.8	73.6	71.2	61.8	59.9	0.4	0.2	–0.3	–1.4	–0.4
Minnesota	71.0	72.3	73.9	73.7	66.8	68.3	0.1	0.2	–0.0	–1.0	0.3
Iowa	63.6	72.6	71.9	68.7	61.7	56.7	0.7	–0.1	–0.5	–1.1	–1.1
Missouri	68.6	75.8	79.3	75.1	61.8	57.3	0.5	0.5	–0.5	–1.9	–0.9
North Dakota	61.9	71.3	67.1	68.6	64.2	60.2	0.7	–0.6	0.2	–0.7	–0.8
South Dakota	59.1	66.0	66.3	60.6	62.1	64.3	0.6	0.0	–0.9	0.2	0.4
Nebraska	59.0	65.6	69.9	67.4	57.6	59.9	0.5	0.6	–0.4	–1.6	0.5
Kansas	60.4	69.1	71.4	68.8	55.6	53.9	0.7	0.3	–0.4	–2.1	–0.4
South Atlantic	66.7	74.8	77.9	75.5	67.4	63.2	0.6	0.4	–0.3	–1.1	–0.8
Delaware	59.2	70.2	78.8	81.8	76.5	70.5	0.9	1.2	0.4	–0.7	–1.0
Maryland	74.6	73.9	79.3	84.0	78.6	68.0	–0.0	0.7	0.6	–0.7	–1.8
District of Columbia	76.2	80.8	77.7	83.0	75.3	75.4	0.3	–0.4	0.7	–1.0	0.0
Virginia	70.0	78.0	81.1	77.8	67.4	62.6	0.5	0.4	–0.4	–1.4	–0.9
West Virginia	62.1	74.5	79.3	76.5	62.7	60.0	0.9	0.6	–0.5	–1.9	–0.5
North Carolina	64.6	73.9	78.5	77.8	73.2	68.4	0.7	0.6	–0.1	–0.6	–0.8
South Carolina	69.1	76.9	76.4	77.0	70.9	65.7	0.5	–0.1	0.1	–0.8	–0.9
Georgia	62.7	71.7	76.5	70.4	65.8	59.4	0.7	0.7	–0.8	–0.7	–1.3
Florida	57.5	73.9	76.2	71.7	61.8	60.3	1.3	0.3	–0.6	–1.5	–0.3
East South Central	62.6	71.8	78.2	74.6	62.6	58.4	0.7	0.9	–0.5	–1.7	–0.9
Kentucky	61.6	73.4	79.6	77.4	62.4	57.1	0.9	0.8	–0.3	–2.1	–1.1
Tennessee	65.5	75.9	78.2	75.9	64.4	56.9	0.7	0.3	–0.3	–1.6	–1.5
Alabama	59.0	70.8	80.0	73.3	62.5	58.7	0.9	1.2	–0.9	–1.6	–0.8
Mississippi	63.8	62.8	73.6	70.5	59.4	62.1	–0.1	1.6	–0.4	–1.7	0.6
West South Central	62.5	68.7	73.2	69.7	57.8	56.3	0.5	0.6	–0.5	–1.9	–0.3
Arkansas	55.6	70.0	74.4	69.6	62.0	58.5	1.2	0.6	–0.7	–1.1	–0.7
Louisiana	75.0	67.9	73.6	69.7	57.4	54.8	–0.5	0.8	–0.5	–1.9	–0.6
Oklahoma	54.5	71.0	72.5	68.1	57.7	53.9	1.3	0.2	–0.6	–1.6	–0.8
Texas	59.6	68.2	73.0	70.1	57.2	56.8	0.7	0.7	–0.4	–2.0	–0.1
Mountain	60.9	69.9	71.2	69.6	60.5	59.6	0.7	0.2	–0.2	–1.4	–0.2
Montana	62.8	60.3	65.9	66.1	61.2	67.7	–0.2	0.9	0.0	–0.8	1.3
Idaho	65.4	55.9	66.1	65.2	55.7	56.0	–0.8	1.7	–0.1	–1.6	0.1
Wyoming	47.5	61.1	63.1	57.2	53.8	53.9	1.3	0.3	–1.0	–0.6	0.0
Colorado	62.1	80.6	74.0	71.6	64.0	56.0	1.3	–0.9	–0.3	–1.1	–1.7
New Mexico	47.8	65.1	69.8	66.2	57.5	55.5	1.6	0.7	–0.5	–1.4	–0.4
Arizona	61.2	74.2	73.3	74.2	61.8	60.7	1.0	–0.1	0.1	–1.8	–0.2
Utah	65.8	70.0	73.7	70.0	58.7	60.5	0.3	0.5	–0.5	–1.7	0.4
Nevada	67.9	70.7	72.7	68.8	60.2	65.0	0.2	0.3	–0.5	–1.3	1.0
Pacific . . . . :	69.7	71.4	71.0	69.0	63.8	61.3	0.1	–0.1	–0.3	–0.8	–0.5
Washington	67.5	63.4	69.7	71.7	62.7	58.6	–0.3	1.0	0.3	–1.3	–0.8
Oregon	71.2	65.8	69.3	69.3	56.7	56.4	–0.4	0.5	0.0	–2.0	–0.1
California	69.9	74.3	71.3	68.5	64.1	61.3	0.3	–0.4	–0.4	–0.7	–0.6
Alaska	. . .	53.8	59.1	58.3	49.5	83.6	. . .	0.9	–0.1	–1.6	6.8
Hawaii	. . .	61.5	75.7	74.7	85.1	76.2	. . .	2.1	–0.1	1.3	–1.4

0.0 Quantity more than zero but less than 0.05. –0.0 Quantity is between 0 and –0.05. . . . Category not applicable.

[1] 1940 data are estimated based on published figures.
[2] Data exclude facilities for the mentally retarded. See Appendix II, Hospital. [3] 1960 data include hospital units of institutions.
[4] Starting with 1990, data exclude hospital units of institutions, facilities for the mentally retarded, and alcoholism and chemical dependency hospitals. See Appendix II.
[5] 1990 data used in this calculation (not shown in table) exclude only facilities for the mentally retarded, consistent with exclusions from 1980 data.

NOTES: Occupancy rates exclude data for newborns from the numerator. Data for additional years are available (see Appendix III).

SOURCES: American Medical Association (AMA): Hospital service in United States. JAMA 116(11):1055–1144, 1941. (Copyright 1941: Used with permission of AMA); American Hospital Association (AHA): Hospitals. JAHA 35(15):383–430, 1961. (Copyright 1961: Used with permission of AHA); National Center for Health Statistics, Division of Health Care Statistics, and AHA annual surveys for 1970 and 1980; Hospital Statistics 1991–92, 2000 Editions. Chicago (Copyrights 1971, 1981, 1991, 2000: Used with permission of AHA and Health Forum, an AHA company).

Table 113 (page 1 of 2). Nursing homes, beds, occupancy, and residents, according to geographic division and State: United States, 1995–98

[Data are based on a census of certified nursing facilities]

Geographic division and State	Nursing homes				Beds			
	1995	1996	1997	1998	1995	1996	1997	1998
United States	16,389	16,706	17,121	17,259	1,751,302	1,780,772	1,827,615	1,812,056
New England	1,140	1,131	1,183	1,185	115,488	115,718	121,854	122,317
Maine	132	129	135	132	9,243	9,168	9,363	9,227
New Hampshire	74	80	81	83	7,412	7,972	8,107	7,929
Vermont	23	43	44	45	1,862	3,548	3,739	3,792
Massachusetts	550	528	563	564	54,532	53,109	57,774	58,215
Rhode Island	94	90	100	102	9,612	9,594	10,190	10,361
Connecticut	267	261	260	259	32,827	32,327	32,681	32,793
Middle Atlantic	1,650	1,703	1,744	1,819	244,342	247,445	255,366	265,659
New York	624	606	621	660	107,750	104,663	109,538	118,273
New Jersey	300	320	331	359	43,967	46,951	49,402	50,796
Pennsylvania	726	777	792	800	92,625	95,831	96,426	96,590
East North Central	3,171	3,278	3,324	3,332	367,879	384,310	390,907	375,380
Ohio	943	1,004	1,014	1,011	106,884	118,193	121,330	104,766
Indiana	556	569	577	572	59,538	60,887	62,086	61,465
Illinois	827	858	866	877	103,230	107,482	108,406	109,898
Michigan	432	430	444	447	49,473	49,919	51,287	51,572
Wisconsin	413	417	423	425	48,754	47,829	47,798	47,679
West North Central	2,258	2,314	2,350	2,333	200,109	206,525	209,055	200,562
Minnesota	432	444	449	448	43,865	45,140	45,271	45,202
Iowa	419	464	469	470	39,959	45,710	45,359	37,859
Missouri	546	544	570	568	52,679	52,252	55,472	55,466
North Dakota	87	88	88	88	7,125	7,128	7,108	7,087
South Dakota	114	112	114	114	8,296	8,046	8,080	8,034
Nebraska	231	234	237	239	18,169	18,207	18,227	18,354
Kansas	429	428	423	406	30,016	30,042	29,538	28,560
South Atlantic	2,215	2,249	2,348	2,417	243,069	243,174	253,621	261,036
Delaware	42	43	43	44	4,739	4,883	4,890	5,158
Maryland	218	220	248	257	28,394	27,929	30,851	31,510
District of Columbia	19	19	21	21	3,206	2,764	3,097	3,093
Virginia	271	265	271	280	30,070	29,653	29,915	30,757
West Virginia	129	132	136	140	10,903	10,928	11,203	11,368
North Carolina	391	398	402	404	38,322	39,197	39,508	39,959
South Carolina	166	170	176	176	16,682	16,878	17,463	17,732
Georgia	352	351	354	360	38,097	37,872	39,016	39,377
Florida	627	651	697	735	72,656	73,070	77,678	82,082
East South Central	1,014	1,061	1,090	1,095	99,707	102,835	106,104	107,018
Kentucky	288	308	315	315	23,221	24,535	25,282	25,489
Tennessee	322	336	348	354	37,074	37,891	39,009	39,433
Alabama	221	223	224	223	23,353	24,083	24,787	25,017
Mississippi	183	194	203	203	16,059	16,326	17,026	17,079
West South Central	2,264	2,248	2,313	2,303	224,695	224,239	229,469	225,277
Arkansas	256	263	261	265	29,952	31,769	31,088	25,903
Louisiana	337	345	339	331	37,769	38,850	38,043	37,834
Oklahoma	405	401	413	411	33,918	33,568	34,460	34,246
Texas	1,266	1,239	1,300	1,296	123,056	120,052	125,878	127,294
Mountain	800	817	843	848	70,134	71,545	74,058	74,668
Montana	100	103	103	105	7,210	7,389	7,521	7,657
Idaho	76	80	86	84	5,747	5,991	6,515	6,390
Wyoming	37	38	38	40	3,035	3,125	3,120	3,158
Colorado	219	220	225	229	19,912	19,714	20,150	20,397
New Mexico	83	86	85	83	6,969	7,265	7,245	7,329
Arizona	152	158	165	163	16,162	16,983	17,761	17,703
Utah	91	90	96	95	7,101	7,070	7,568	7,596
Nevada	42	42	45	49	3,998	4,008	4,178	4,438
Pacific	1,877	1,905	1,926	1,927	185,879	184,981	187,181	180,139
Washington	285	284	285	284	28,464	27,428	27,656	27,290
Oregon	161	164	163	163	13,885	14,101	14,030	14,073
California	1,382	1,398	1,419	1,421	140,203	138,796	140,837	134,085
Alaska	15	16	16	15	814	829	828	811
Hawaii	34	43	43	44	2,513	3,827	3,830	3,880

See footnotes at end of table.

[Data are based on a census of certified nursing facilities]

Geographic division and State	Occupancy rate[1]				Resident rate[2]			
	1995	1996	1997	1998	1995	1996	1997	1998
United States	84.5	83.1	82.2	83.5	404.5	393.3	388.3	373.6
New England	91.6	91.5	90.4	90.1	474.2	462.2	468.4	453.2
Maine	92.9	89.4	88.0	86.4	417.9	391.4	386.0	364.3
New Hampshire	92.8	91.8	90.5	92.4	434.1	450.1	441.8	420.9
Vermont	96.2	94.6	94.9	90.0	207.0	379.7	392.6	362.9
Massachusetts	91.3	90.0	89.2	89.5	477.3	447.8	470.9	462.0
Rhode Island	91.8	93.7	92.2	90.3	476.9	470.2	475.4	459.1
Connecticut	91.2	93.4	92.2	91.6	541.7	528.8	510.4	489.9
Middle Atlantic	93.6	93.0	92.4	92.1	384.0	376.5	376.2	374.2
New York	96.0	95.5	94.9	94.4	371.8	352.1	358.1	370.8
New Jersey	91.9	92.6	91.2	90.9	351.6	364.6	364.0	358.9
Pennsylvania	91.6	90.4	90.3	89.8	419.2	416.8	408.0	387.5
East North Central	80.0	77.5	76.6	79.5	476.1	471.2	463.5	439.9
Ohio	73.9	69.3	68.7	79.5	499.5	507.4	506.3	485.0
Indiana	74.5	73.7	72.0	71.2	548.9	543.9	530.1	496.8
Illinois	81.1	78.8	78.5	77.8	495.3	490.0	480.9	458.6
Michigan	87.5	86.3	85.9	85.4	345.0	333.8	332.6	316.0
Wisconsin	90.2	90.6	88.6	87.5	518.9	501.7	481.1	450.9
West North Central	82.3	80.1	80.0	82.1	489.6	485.6	483.6	460.5
Minnesota	93.8	92.4	92.3	91.3	537.4	535.9	528.0	499.2
Iowa	68.8	65.8	67.3	80.2	458.0	496.1	497.9	477.6
Missouri	75.7	74.0	73.5	72.8	432.8	414.1	430.0	415.8
North Dakota	96.4	95.4	95.3	92.9	522.0	505.0	491.0	459.4
South Dakota	95.5	94.5	94.9	92.8	543.3	515.0	512.5	477.5
Nebraska	89.0	87.4	85.8	84.9	501.4	488.5	475.1	461.1
Kansas	83.8	82.2	81.3	81.0	528.9	513.6	492.9	456.0
South Atlantic	89.4	89.0	88.0	87.4	335.4	322.4	321.3	311.4
Delaware	80.6	82.5	79.0	74.7	448.7	455.1	419.8	396.1
Maryland	87.0	86.5	84.4	82.4	432.7	407.8	423.6	405.8
District of Columbia	80.3	87.8	94.8	95.0	297.6	279.0	335.1	324.5
Virginia	93.5	92.3	90.5	90.2	385.2	363.2	348.1	340.7
West Virginia	93.7	93.9	92.3	91.2	355.2	349.1	344.0	332.8
North Carolina	92.7	93.2	93.8	92.5	401.1	399.7	392.9	366.7
South Carolina	87.3	87.3	85.7	87.1	366.0	356.7	349.2	339.6
Georgia	94.3	93.7	91.9	92.2	496.0	474.1	463.3	442.1
Florida	85.1	84.0	83.8	83.4	228.2	217.6	222.3	221.9
East South Central	91.8	90.9	90.3	90.8	416.6	415.1	415.5	408.6
Kentucky	89.1	88.5	88.2	89.1	391.9	401.3	401.7	400.8
Tennessee	91.5	90.7	89.6	89.7	479.6	473.5	469.1	458.9
Alabama	92.9	92.0	91.7	92.5	370.1	370.0	370.2	363.4
Mississippi	94.9	93.1	93.2	93.1	405.3	394.9	403.0	394.5
West South Central	75.2	73.2	71.6	72.2	486.1	460.2	448.6	426.5
Arkansas	69.5	65.3	65.9	78.3	508.3	498.6	484.0	462.3
Louisiana	86.0	82.4	81.3	80.2	639.3	616.3	581.6	551.2
Oklahoma	77.8	76.2	73.7	72.6	499.1	475.9	464.3	441.6
Texas	72.6	71.5	69.6	68.5	439.9	409.8	405.0	385.4
Mountain	83.8	83.9	81.2	80.8	335.9	327.4	313.0	296.2
Montana	89.0	87.2	83.0	81.8	491.4	471.6	437.0	423.7
Idaho	81.7	80.0	73.4	75.7	321.7	315.0	301.5	283.1
Wyoming	87.7	83.5	84.6	83.9	468.2	447.5	440.5	422.9
Colorado	85.7	87.2	83.8	83.8	420.6	408.5	386.2	373.1
New Mexico	86.8	84.5	84.6	84.2	332.0	323.3	309.4	294.1
Arizona	76.6	79.6	77.8	77.5	233.3	241.6	234.5	218.7
Utah	82.1	82.6	78.0	77.4	323.5	309.0	298.3	283.0
Nevada	91.2	87.7	90.3	83.2	312.0	275.4	272.1	244.3
Pacific	80.4	79.1	78.3	81.4	302.4	285.3	275.1	261.3
Washington	87.7	85.1	82.9	82.1	362.5	325.0	306.1	283.8
Oregon	84.1	80.9	80.6	79.1	244.9	231.3	221.3	206.8
California	78.3	77.6	76.8	81.2	302.9	286.9	277.9	265.9
Alaska	77.9	75.5	74.8	76.3	348.0	321.5	297.7	273.4
Hawaii	96.0	85.0	91.6	92.0	178.5	224.5	227.4	217.4

[1]Percent of beds occupied.
[2]Number of nursing home residents (all ages) per 1,000 resident population 85 years of age and over.

NOTE: Annual numbers of nursing homes, beds, and residents are based on a 15-month OSCAR reporting cycle and may differ from annual numbers shown in previous editions of Health, United States (see Appendix I).

SOURCES: Cowles CM, 1995 Nursing Home Statistical Yearbook. 1996 Nursing Home Statistical Yearbook. 1997 Nursing Home Statistical Yearbook. Anacortes, WA: Cowles Research Group, 1995; 1997; 1998; and Cowles CM, 1998 Nursing Home Statistical Yearbook. Washington, DC: American Association of Homes and Services for the Aging, 1999. Based on data from the Health Care Financing Administrations Online Survey Certification and Reporting (OSCAR) database.

Table 114. Total health expenditures as a percent of gross domestic product and per capita health expenditures in dollars: Selected countries and years 1960–97

[Data compiled by the Organization for Economic Cooperation and Development]

Country	1960	1965	1970	1975	1980	1985	1990	1994	1995	1996	1997[1]
	Health expenditures as a percent of gross domestic product										
Australia	4.9	5.1	5.7	7.5	7.3	7.7	8.2	8.5	8.4	8.6	8.4
Austria	4.3	4.6	5.3	7.2	7.7	6.7	7.2	8.1	8.0	8.0	8.3
Belgium	3.4	3.9	4.1	5.9	6.5	7.3	7.5	8.0	7.9	7.8	7.6
Canada	5.4	5.9	7.0	7.2	7.7	8.3	9.2	9.8	9.4	9.3	9.2
Czech Republic	---	---	---	---	3.8	4.5	5.4	7.5	7.5	7.2	7.2
Denmark	3.6	---	5.9	6.3	9.3	8.7	8.3	8.3	8.1	8.1	8.0
Finland	3.9	4.9	5.7	6.4	6.5	7.3	8.0	7.9	7.7	7.8	7.4
France	4.2	5.2	5.8	7.0	7.6	8.5	8.9	9.7	9.8	9.8	9.6
Germany	4.8	5.1	6.3	8.8	8.8	9.3	8.7	10.0	10.4	10.8	10.7
Greece	3.1	---	5.7	---	6.6	---	7.6	8.3	8.4	8.4	8.6
Hungary	---	---	---	---	---	---	6.1	7.3	7.0	6.6	6.5
Iceland	3.3	3.9	5.0	5.8	6.2	7.3	7.9	8.1	8.2	8.2	7.9
Ireland	3.8	4.2	5.3	7.7	8.7	7.9	6.7	7.3	7.0	6.4	6.3
Italy	3.6	4.3	5.2	6.2	7.0	7.1	8.1	8.4	7.7	7.8	7.6
Japan	3.0	4.5	4.6	5.6	6.5	6.7	6.1	6.9	7.2	7.1	7.2
Korea	---	---	2.3	2.3	3.7	4.3	5.2	5.4	5.4	5.9	6.0
Luxembourg	---	---	3.7	5.1	6.2	6.1	6.6	6.5	6.7	6.8	7.0
Mexico	---	---	---	---	---	---	3.6	4.7	4.9	4.6	4.7
Netherlands	3.8	4.3	5.9	7.5	7.9	7.9	8.3	8.8	8.8	8.7	8.5
New Zealand	4.3	---	5.2	6.7	6.0	5.3	7.0	7.3	7.3	7.3	7.6
Norway	2.9	3.5	4.5	6.0	7.0	6.7	7.8	8.0	8.0	7.8	7.5
Poland	---	---	---	---	---	---	4.4	4.4	4.5	4.9	5.2
Portugal	---	---	2.8	5.6	5.8	6.3	6.4	7.5	7.8	7.9	7.9
Spain	1.5	2.6	3.7	4.9	5.6	5.7	6.9	7.4	7.3	7.4	7.4
Sweden	4.7	5.5	7.1	7.9	9.4	9.0	8.8	8.7	8.5	8.6	8.6
Switzerland	3.1	3.6	4.9	6.6	6.9	7.7	8.3	9.5	9.6	10.1	10.0
Turkey	---	---	2.4	2.7	3.3	2.2	3.6	3.6	3.3	3.8	4.0
United Kingdom	3.9	4.1	4.5	5.5	5.6	5.9	6.0	6.9	6.9	6.9	6.8
United States	5.1	5.7	7.1	8.0	8.9	10.3	12.2	13.6	13.7	13.6	13.4
	Per capita health expenditures[2]										
Australia	$ 94	$122	$207	$438	$ 663	$ 998	$1,320	$1,627	$1,778	$1,874	$1,909
Austria	64	88	159	357	663	814	1,205	1,613	1,675	1,773	1,905
Belgium	53	82	130	305	578	882	1,247	1,656	1,698	1,725	1,768
Canada	109	157	262	433	716	1,201	1,695	2,006	2,106	2,112	2,175
Czech Republic	---	---	---	---	---	---	575	805	898	918	943
Denmark	67	121	216	344	832	1,173	1,424	1,765	1,855	1,973	2,042
Finland	54	91	163	304	510	849	1,292	1,295	1,414	1,486	1,525
France	72	120	206	389	701	1,082	1,539	1,869	1,984	2,005	2,047
Germany	90	125	224	476	824	1,242	1,602	1,973	2,178	2,288	2,364
Greece	21	---	100	---	345	---	702	978	1,054	1,113	1,196
Hungary	---	---	---	---	---	---	510	606	625	611	642
Iceland	50	84	137	288	577	949	1,374	1,579	1,826	1,918	1,981
Ireland	35	52	98	234	455	592	759	1,156	1,246	1,189	1,293
Italy	49	80	154	287	579	830	1,321	1,562	1,534	1,615	1,613
Japan	26	64	131	263	524	820	1,082	1,463	1,637	1,713	1,760
Korea	---	---	15	28	87	180	401	593	688	801	870
Luxembourg	---	---	147	310	605	892	1,495	1,956	2,120	2,147	2,303
Mexico	---	---	---	---	---	---	210	328	335	330	363
Netherlands	67	98	202	399	679	929	1,326	1,653	1,777	1,832	1,933
New Zealand	90	---	174	354	458	587	937	1,188	1,244	1,267	1,357
Norway	46	73	131	297	632	915	1,365	1,746	1,860	2,010	2,017
Poland	---	---	---	---	---	---	216	239	296	338	386
Portugal	---	---	43	145	260	381	614	941	1,046	1,086	1,148
Spain	14	36	82	185	325	454	815	1,015	1,063	1,122	1,183
Sweden	89	145	270	465	850	1,172	1,492	1,533	1,623	1,701	1,762
Switzerland	87	128	252	483	801	1,250	1,760	2,294	2,464	2,548	2,611
Turkey	---	---	23	41	75	74	171	191	188	227	259
United Kingdom	74	98	144	271	444	669	955	1,213	1,253	1,358	1,391
United States	141	202	341	582	1,052	1,735	2,689	3,501	3,637	3,772	3,912

--- Data not available.

[1] Preliminary figures.

[2] Per capita health expenditures for each country have been adjusted to U.S. dollars using gross domestic product purchasing power parities for each year.

NOTE: Some numbers in this table have been revised and differ from previous editions of Health, United States.

SOURCES: Schieber GJ, Poullier JP, and Greenwald LG. U.S. health expenditure performance: An international comparison and data update. Health Care Financing Review vol 13 no 4. Washington: Health Care Financing Administration. September 1992; Anderson GF and Poullier JP. Health spending, access, and outcomes: Trends in industrialized countries. Health Affairs vol 18 no 3. May/June 1999; Office of National Health Statistics, Office of the Actuary. National health expenditures, 1997. Health Care Financing Review vol 20 no 1. HCFA pub no 03412. Washington: Health Care Financing Administration. March 1999; Organization for Economic Cooperation and Development Health Data File: Unpublished data.

Health Care Expenditures

Table 115. Gross domestic product, national health expenditures, Federal and State and local government expenditures, and average annual percent change: United States, selected years 1960–98

[Data are compiled by the Health Care Financing Administration]

Gross domestic product, national health expenditures, and government health expenditures	1960	1965	1970	1975	1980	1985	1990	1995	1996	1997	1998
					Amount in billions						
Gross domestic product (GDP)	$ 527	$ 719	$1,036	$1,631	$2,784	$4,181	$ 5,744	$ 7,270	$ 7,662	$ 8,111	$ 8,511
					Percent						
National health expenditures as percent of GDP	5.1	5.7	7.1	8.0	8.9	10.3	12.2	13.7	13.6	13.4	13.5
Source of funds for national health expenditures					Amount in billions						
National health expenditures	$ 26.9	$ 41.1	$ 73.2	$130.7	$247.3	$428.7	$ 699.4	$ 993.3	$1,039.4	$1,088.2	$1,149.1
Private funds	20.2	30.9	45.5	75.7	142.5	254.5	416.2	537.3	559.0	586.0	626.4
Public funds	6.6	10.3	27.7	55.0	104.8	174.2	283.2	456.0	480.4	502.2	522.7
					Percent distribution						
National health expenditures	100.0	100.0	100.0	100.0	100.0	100.0	100.0	100.0	100.0	100.0	100.0
Private funds	75.2	75.0	62.2	57.9	57.6	59.4	59.5	54.1	53.8	53.8	54.5
Public funds	24.8	25.0	37.8	42.1	42.4	40.6	40.5	45.9	46.2	46.2	45.5
Per capita health expenditures					Amount						
National health expenditures	$ 141	$ 202	$ 341	$ 582	$1,052	$1,734	$ 2,689	$ 3,637	$ 3,772	$ 3,912	$ 4,094
Private health expenditures	106	151	212	337	606	1,030	1,600	1,967	2,028	2,107	2,232
Public health expenditures	35	50	129	245	446	705	1,089	1,669	1,743	1,806	1,862
					Amount in billions						
Federal government expenditures:											
Total	$ 85.8	$116.1	$198.6	$345.4	$576.6	$924.6	$1,228.7	$1,575.7	$1,635.9	$1,676.0	$1,703.8
Health	2.9	4.8	17.8	36.4	72.0	123.2	195.2	326.1	347.3	363.0	376.9
State and local government expenditures:											
Total	$ 38.1	$ 56.8	$107.5	$197.2	$307.8	$447.0	$ 660.8	$ 902.5	$ 939.0	$ 981.5	$1,028.7
Health	3.7	5.5	9.9	18.6	32.8	51.0	88.0	129.8	133.1	139.2	145.8
Health as a percent of total					Percent						
Federal government expenditures	3.4	4.2	9.0	10.5	12.5	13.3	15.9	20.7	21.2	21.7	22.1
State and local government expenditures	9.8	9.6	9.2	9.4	10.7	11.4	13.3	14.4	14.2	14.2	14.2
Growth				Average annual percent change from previous year shown							
Gross domestic product	...	6.4	7.6	9.5	11.3	8.5	6.6	4.8	5.4	5.9	4.9
National health expenditures:											
Total	...	8.9	12.2	12.3	13.6	11.6	10.3	7.3	4.6	4.7	5.6
Per capita	...	7.4	11.1	11.3	12.6	10.5	9.2	6.2	3.7	3.7	4.6
Private health expenditures:											
Total	...	8.8	8.1	10.7	13.5	12.3	10.3	5.2	4.0	4.8	6.9
Per capita	...	7.3	7.0	9.7	12.4	11.2	9.2	4.2	3.1	3.9	5.9
Public health expenditures:											
Total	...	9.1	21.9	14.7	13.7	10.7	10.2	10.0	5.4	4.5	4.1
Per capita	...	7.6	20.7	13.7	12.7	9.6	9.1	8.9	4.4	3.6	3.1
Federal government expenditures:											
Total	...	6.2	11.3	11.7	10.8	9.9	5.9	5.1	3.8	2.5	1.7
Health	...	10.6	29.9	15.4	14.6	11.3	9.6	10.8	6.5	4.5	3.8
State and local government expenditures:											
Total	...	8.3	13.6	12.9	9.3	7.7	8.1	6.4	4.0	4.5	4.8
Health	...	7.9	12.6	13.5	12.0	9.2	11.5	8.1	2.5	4.6	4.7

... Category not applicable.

NOTES: These data include revisions in health expenditures and differ from previous editions of *Health, United States*. They reflect Social Security Administration population revisions as of July 1999. Federal and State and local government total expenditures reflect October 1999 revisions from the Bureau of Economic Analysis.

SOURCE: National Health Statistics Group, Office of the Actuary. National health expenditures, 1998. Health Care Financing Review vol 21 no 2. HCFA pub no 03420. Health Care Financing Administration. Washington: U.S. Government Printing Office, Winter 1999.

Table 116. Consumer Price Index and average annual percent change for all items, selected items, and medical care components: United States, selected years 1960–99

[Data are based on reporting by samples of providers and other retail outlets]

Items and medical care components	1960	1970	1980	1990	1995	1996	1997	1998	1999
	Consumer Price Index (CPI)								
All items	29.6	38.8	82.4	130.7	152.4	156.9	160.5	163.0	166.6
All items excluding medical care	30.2	39.2	82.8	128.8	148.6	152.8	156.3	158.6	162.0
All services	24.1	35.0	77.9	139.2	168.7	174.1	179.4	184.2	188.8
Food	30.0	39.2	86.8	132.4	148.4	153.3	157.3	160.7	164.1
Apparel	45.7	59.2	90.9	124.1	132.0	131.7	132.9	133.0	131.3
Housing	- - -	36.4	81.1	128.5	148.5	152.8	156.8	160.4	163.9
Energy	22.4	25.5	86.0	102.1	105.2	110.1	111.5	102.9	106.6
Medical care	22.3	34.0	74.9	162.8	220.5	228.2	234.6	242.1	250.6
Components of medical care									
Medical care services	19.5	32.3	74.8	162.7	224.2	232.4	239.1	246.8	255.1
Professional services	- - -	37.0	77.9	156.1	201.0	208.3	215.4	222.2	229.2
Physicians' services	21.9	34.5	76.5	160.8	208.8	216.4	222.9	229.5	236.0
Dental services	27.0	39.2	78.9	155.8	206.8	216.5	226.6	236.2	247.2
Eye glasses and eye care[1]	- - -	- - -	- - -	117.3	137.0	139.3	141.5	144.1	145.5
Services by other medical professionals[1]	- - -	- - -	- - -	120.2	143.9	146.6	151.8	155.4	158.7
Hospital and related services	- - -	- - -	69.2	178.0	257.8	269.5	278.4	287.5	299.5
Hospital services[2]	- - -	- - -	- - -	- - -	- - -	- - -	101.7	105.0	109.3
Inpatient hospital services[2]	- - -	- - -	- - -	- - -	- - -	- - -	101.3	104.0	107.9
Outpatient hospital services[1]	- - -	- - -	- - -	138.7	204.6	215.1	224.9	233.2	246.0
Hospital rooms	9.3	23.6	68.0	175.4	251.2	261.0	- - -	- - -	- - -
Other inpatient services[1]	- - -	- - -	- - -	142.7	206.8	216.9	- - -	- - -	- - -
Nursing homes and adult day care	- - -	- - -	- - -	- - -	- - -	- - -	102.3	107.1	111.6
Medical care commodities	46.9	46.5	75.4	163.4	204.5	210.4	215.3	221.8	230.7
Prescription drugs and medical supplies	54.0	47.4	72.5	181.7	235.0	242.9	249.3	258.6	273.4
Nonprescription drugs and medical supplies[1]	- - -	- - -	- - -	120.6	140.5	143.1	145.4	147.7	148.5
Internal and respiratory over-the-counter drugs	- - -	42.3	74.9	145.9	167.0	170.2	173.1	175.4	175.9
Nonprescription medical equipment and supplies	- - -	- - -	79.2	138.0	166.3	169.1	171.5	174.9	176.7
	Average annual percent change from previous year shown								
All items	. . .	4.3	8.9	4.7	3.1	3.0	2.3	1.6	2.2
All items excluding medical care	. . .	4.1	8.8	4.5	2.9	2.8	2.3	1.5	2.1
All services	. . .	5.6	10.2	6.0	3.9	3.2	3.0	2.7	2.5
Food	. . .	4.0	7.7	4.3	2.3	3.3	2.6	2.2	2.1
Apparel	. . .	4.4	4.6	3.2	1.2	-0.2	0.9	0.1	-1.3
Housing	. . .	- - -	9.9	4.7	2.9	2.9	2.6	2.3	2.2
Energy	. . .	2.2	15.4	1.7	0.6	4.7	1.3	-7.7	3.6
Medical care	. . .	6.2	9.5	8.1	6.3	3.5	2.8	3.2	3.5
Components of medical care									
Medical care services	. . .	7.3	9.9	8.1	6.6	3.7	2.9	3.2	3.4
Professional services	. . .	- - -	8.9	7.2	5.2	3.6	3.4	3.2	3.2
Physicians' services	. . .	6.6	9.7	7.7	5.4	3.6	3.0	3.0	2.8
Dental services	. . .	5.3	8.2	7.0	5.8	4.7	4.7	4.2	4.7
Eye glasses and eye care[1]	. . .	- - -	- - -	- - -	3.2	1.7	1.6	1.8	1.0
Services by other medical professionals[1]	. . .	- - -	- - -	- - -	3.7	1.9	3.5	2.4	2.1
Hospital and related services	. . .	- - -	- - -	9.9	7.7	4.5	3.3	3.3	4.2
Hospital services[2]	. . .	- - -	- - -	- - -	- - -	- - -	- - -	3.2	4.1
Inpatient hospital services[2]	. . .	- - -	- - -	- - -	- - -	- - -	- - -	2.7	3.8
Outpatient hospital services[1]	. . .	- - -	- - -	- - -	8.1	5.1	4.6	3.7	5.5
Hospital rooms	. . .	13.9	12.2	9.9	7.4	3.9	- - -	- - -	- - -
Other inpatient services[1]	. . .	- - -	- - -	- - -	7.7	4.9	- - -	- - -	- - -
Nursing homes and adult day care	. . .	- - -	- - -	- - -	- - -	- - -	- - -	4.7	4.2
Medical care commodities	. . .	0.7	7.2	8.0	4.6	2.9	2.3	3.0	4.0
Prescription drugs and medical supplies	. . .	-0.2	7.2	9.6	5.3	3.4	2.6	3.7	5.7
Nonprescription drugs and medical supplies[1]	. . .	- - -	- - -	- - -	3.1	1.9	1.6	1.6	0.5
Internal and respiratory over-the-counter drugs	. . .	1.6	7.7	6.9	2.7	1.9	1.7	1.3	0.3
Nonprescription medical equipment and supplies	. . .	- - -	- - -	5.7	3.8	1.7	1.4	2.0	1.0

- - - Data not available.
. . . Category not applicable.
[1]Dec. 1986 = 100
[2]Dec. 1996 = 100.

NOTES: 1982–84 = 100, except where noted. Data for additional years are available (see Appendix III).

SOURCE: U.S. Department of Labor, Bureau of Labor Statistics. Consumer Price Index. Various releases.

Table 117. Growth in personal health care expenditures and percent distribution of factors affecting growth: United States, 1960–98

[Data are compiled by the Health Care Financing Administration]

Period	Average annual percent increase	Factors affecting growth				
		All factors	Inflation[1]		Population	Intensity[2]
			Economy-wide	Medical		
		Percent distribution				
1960–98	10.4	100	42	16	10	32
1960–61	6.1	100	20	6	27	47
1961–62	7.6	100	17	11	21	51
1962–63	9.3	100	13	7	16	64
1963–64	9.9	100	15	15	14	56
1964–65	8.6	100	23	9	15	53
1965–66	10.4	100	29	21	11	39
1966–67	13.7	100	25	13	8	54
1967–68	12.9	100	35	11	8	46
1968–69	12.8	100	38	10	8	44
1969–70	13.5	100	40	8	8	43
1970–71	9.8	100	54	11	11	24
1971–72	11.4	100	39	–3	9	55
1972–73	11.6	100	50	–15	8	57
1973–74	14.7	100	62	1	6	30
1974–75	14.7	100	66	9	6	19
1975–76	14.0	100	44	21	6	29
1976–77	13.2	100	50	11	7	32
1977–78	11.6	100	64	5	9	22
1978–79	13.7	100	64	4	7	25
1979–80	15.8	100	60	13	7	20
1980–81	16.1	100	60	17	7	16
1981–82	12.4	100	52	35	9	4
1982–83	10.0	100	44	32	11	13
1983–84	9.6	100	39	40	11	10
1984–85	10.2	100	36	36	10	18
1985–86	9.0	100	29	26	11	34
1986–87	9.6	100	33	19	11	37
1987–88	11.0	100	34	24	10	32
1988–89	10.2	100	42	27	11	20
1989–90	11.7	100	38	21	9	31
1990–91	10.6	100	39	16	10	35
1991–92	9.0	100	32	28	12	28
1992–93	6.7	100	39	32	15	14
1993–94	5.5	100	45	25	18	12
1994–95	5.4	100	43	25	17	15
1995–96	5.1	100	38	22	18	23
1996–97	4.8	100	39	7	20	34
1997–98	5.2	100	20	23	18	39

[1]Total inflation is economy-wide and medical inflation is the medical inflation above economy-wide inflation.
[2]The residual percent of growth which cannot be attributed to price increases or population growth represents changes in use or kinds of services and supplies.

NOTE: These data include revisions in health expenditures and in population back to 1990 and differ from previous editions of *Health, United States*.

SOURCE: National Health Statistics Group, Office of the Actuary. National health expenditures, 1998. Health Care Financing Review vol 21 no 2. HCFA pub no 03420. Health Care Financing Administration. Washington: U.S. Government Printing OFfice, Winter 1999.

Table 118 (page 1 of 2). National health expenditures, average annual percent change, and percent distribution, according to type of expenditure: United States, selected years 1960–98

[Data are compiled by the Health Care Financing Administration]

Type of expenditure	1960	1965	1970	1975	1980	1985	1990	1995	1996	1997	1998
						Amount in billions					
All expenditures	$26.9	$41.1	$73.2	$130.7	$247.3	$428.7	$699.4	$993.3	$1,039.4	$1,088.2	$1,149.1
Health services and supplies	25.2	37.7	67.9	122.3	235.6	412.3	674.8	962.5	1,007.5	1,053.5	1,113.7
Personal health care	23.6	35.2	63.8	114.5	217.0	376.4	614.7	879.1	924.0	968.6	1,019.3
Hospital care	9.3	14.0	28.0	52.6	102.7	168.3	256.4	347.0	359.4	370.2	382.8
Physician services	5.3	8.2	13.6	23.9	45.2	83.6	146.3	201.9	208.5	217.8	229.5
Dentist services	2.0	2.8	4.7	8.0	13.3	21.7	31.6	45.0	47.5	51.1	53.8
Nursing home care	0.8	1.5	4.2	8.7	17.6	30.7	50.9	75.5	80.2	84.7	87.8
Other professional services	0.6	0.9	1.4	2.7	6.4	16.6	34.7	53.6	57.4	61.5	66.6
Home health care	0.1	0.1	0.2	0.6	2.4	5.6	13.1	29.1	31.2	30.5	29.3
Drugs and other medical nondurables	4.2	5.9	8.8	13.0	21.6	37.1	59.9	88.6	98.0	108.6	121.9
Vision products and other medical durables	0.6	1.0	1.6	2.5	3.8	6.7	10.5	13.3	14.1	15.1	15.5
Other personal health care	0.7	0.8	1.3	2.5	4.0	6.1	11.2	25.1	27.6	29.2	32.1
Program administration and net cost of health insurance	1.2	1.9	2.7	4.9	11.9	24.3	40.5	53.6	52.1	50.3	57.7
Government public health activities[1]	0.4	0.6	1.3	2.9	6.7	11.6	19.6	29.8	31.3	34.6	36.6
Research and construction	1.7	3.4	5.3	8.4	11.6	16.4	24.5	30.8	32.0	34.8	35.3
Noncommercial research	0.7	1.5	2.0	3.3	5.5	7.8	12.2	16.7	17.2	17.9	19.9
Construction	1.0	1.9	3.4	5.1	6.2	8.5	12.3	14.0	14.8	16.9	15.5
					Average annual percent change from previous year shown						
All expenditures	...	8.9	12.2	12.3	13.6	11.6	10.3	7.3	4.6	4.7	5.6
Health services and supplies	...	8.4	12.5	12.5	14.0	11.8	10.4	7.4	4.7	4.6	5.7
Personal health care	...	8.3	12.7	12.4	13.6	11.6	10.3	7.4	5.1	4.8	5.2
Hospital care	...	8.6	14.8	13.4	14.3	10.4	8.8	6.2	3.6	3.0	3.4
Physician services	...	9.2	10.6	12.0	13.6	13.1	11.8	6.6	3.3	4.5	5.4
Dentist services	...	7.3	10.8	11.2	10.9	10.2	7.8	7.3	5.6	7.6	5.3
Nursing home care	...	11.6	23.4	15.5	15.3	11.7	10.7	8.2	6.3	5.5	3.7
Other professional services	...	7.4	10.2	14.2	18.4	21.2	15.8	9.1	7.1	7.0	8.3
Home health care	...	9.6	19.7	23.2	30.7	18.9	18.4	17.3	7.1	−2.2	−4.0
Drugs and other medical nondurables	...	6.8	8.4	8.1	10.7	11.4	10.1	8.1	10.6	10.8	12.3
Vision products and other medical durables	...	9.1	10.2	9.5	8.1	12.4	9.2	5.0	6.0	6.7	2.7
Other personal health care	...	3.5	9.5	13.8	10.2	8.8	12.9	17.5	9.8	5.9	9.8
Program administration and net cost of health insurance	...	10.6	7.1	12.5	19.3	15.4	10.8	5.7	−2.8	−3.5	14.9
Government public health activities[1]	...	10.8	17.0	16.8	18.1	11.5	11.0	8.7	5.2	10.2	6.0
Research and construction	...	15.1	9.2	9.4	6.8	7.1	8.4	4.6	3.9	8.8	1.6
Noncommercial research	...	17.1	5.1	11.2	10.4	7.5	9.3	6.5	2.6	4.2	11.1
Construction	...	13.7	12.1	8.3	4.1	6.7	7.6	2.7	5.4	14.2	−8.4

See footnotes at end of table.

Table 118 (page 2 of 2). National health expenditures, average annual percent change, and percent distribution, according to type of expenditure: United States, selected years 1960–98

[Data are compiled by the Health Care Financing Administration]

Type of expenditure	1960	1965	1970	1975	1980	1985	1990	1995	1996	1997	1998
					Percent distribution						
All expenditures	100.0	100.0	100.0	100.0	100.0	100.0	100.0	100.0	100.0	100.0	100.0
Health services and supplies	93.7	91.6	92.7	93.6	95.3	96.2	96.5	96.9	96.9	96.8	96.9
Personal health care	88.0	85.5	87.1	87.6	87.8	87.8	87.9	88.5	88.9	89.0	88.7
Hospital care	34.5	34.1	38.2	40.2	41.5	39.3	36.7	34.9	34.6	34.0	33.3
Physician services	19.7	19.9	18.5	18.3	18.3	19.5	20.9	20.3	20.1	20.0	20.0
Dentist services	7.3	6.8	6.4	6.1	5.4	5.0	4.5	4.5	4.6	4.7	4.7
Nursing home care	3.2	3.6	5.8	6.6	7.1	7.2	7.3	7.6	7.7	7.8	7.6
Other professional services	2.3	2.1	1.9	2.1	2.6	3.9	5.0	5.4	5.5	5.6	5.8
Home health care	0.2	0.2	0.3	0.5	1.0	1.3	1.9	2.9	3.0	2.8	2.5
Drugs and other medical nondurables	15.8	14.3	12.0	10.0	8.7	8.6	8.6	8.9	9.4	10.0	10.6
Vision products and other medical durables	2.4	2.4	2.2	2.0	1.5	1.6	1.5	1.3	1.4	1.4	1.3
Other personal health care	2.6	2.0	1.8	1.9	1.6	1.4	1.6	2.5	2.7	2.7	2.8
Program administration and net cost of health insurance	4.3	4.7	3.7	3.8	4.8	5.7	5.8	5.4	5.0	4.6	5.0
Government public health activities[1]	1.4	1.5	1.8	2.2	2.7	2.7	2.8	3.0	3.0	3.2	3.2
Research and construction	6.3	8.4	7.3	6.4	4.7	3.8	3.5	3.1	3.1	3.2	3.1
Noncommercial research	2.6	3.7	2.7	2.5	2.2	1.8	1.7	1.7	1.6	1.6	1.7
Construction	3.7	4.7	4.6	3.9	2.5	2.0	1.8	1.4	1.4	1.6	1.3

. . . Category not applicable.

[1]Includes personal care services delivered by government public health agencies.

NOTE: These data include revisions in health expenditures and differ from previous editions of *Health, United States*.

SOURCE: National Health Statistics Group, Office of the Actuary. National health expenditures, 1998. Health Care Financing Review vol 21 no 2. HCFA pub no 03420. Health Care Financing Administration. Washington: U.S. Government Printing Office, Winter 1999.

[Data are compiled by the Health Care Financing Administration]

Type of personal health care expenditures and source of funds	1960	1965	1970	1975	1980	1985	1990	1995	1996	1997	1998
					Amount in billions						
Total[1]	$ 23.6	$ 35.2	$ 63.8	$114.5	$217.0	$376.4	$614.7	$879.1	$924.0	$968.6	$1,019.3
					Amount						
Per capita	$ 124	$ 172	$ 297	$ 510	$ 923	$1,523	$2,363	$3,219	$3,353	$3,482	$ 3,632
Source of funds					Percent distribution						
All sources	100.0	100.0	100.0	100.0	100.0	100.0	100.0	100.0	100.0	100.0	100.0
Out-of-pocket payments	55.3	52.7	39.0	33.3	27.8	26.7	23.6	19.4	19.3	19.5	19.6
Private health insurance	21.2	24.7	23.2	24.8	28.6	30.3	33.8	32.6	32.3	32.3	33.1
Other private funds	1.8	2.0	2.6	2.4	3.6	3.7	3.4	3.5	3.7	3.7	3.7
Government	21.7	20.6	35.3	39.6	40.1	39.2	39.2	44.5	44.8	44.5	43.6
Federal	9.0	8.4	23.0	27.0	29.2	29.5	28.8	34.0	34.5	34.4	33.7
State and local	12.6	12.2	12.2	12.5	10.9	9.7	10.4	10.5	10.3	10.1	9.9
					Amount in billions						
Hospital care expenditures[2]	$ 9.3	$ 14.0	$ 28.0	$ 52.6	$102.7	$168.3	$256.4	$347.0	$359.4	$370.2	$ 382.8
					Percent distribution						
All sources	100.0	100.0	100.0	100.0	100.0	100.0	100.0	100.0	100.0	100.0	100.0
Out-of-pocket payments	20.7	19.6	9.0	8.3	5.2	5.2	4.3	3.3	3.2	3.3	3.4
Private health insurance	35.6	40.9	32.4	32.9	35.5	35.0	37.3	30.8	30.0	30.0	30.8
Other private funds	1.2	1.9	3.2	2.7	4.9	4.9	4.0	4.2	4.6	4.9	5.0
Government[3]	42.5	37.6	55.4	56.0	54.4	54.8	54.5	61.7	62.2	61.8	60.8
Medicaid	...	...	9.5	10.0	10.3	9.3	11.5	16.3	16.3	15.8	15.9
Medicare	...	...	19.2	22.0	25.7	29.1	26.8	31.4	32.4	33.2	32.4
					Amount in billions						
Nursing home care expenditures[4]	$ 0.8	$ 1.5	$ 4.2	$ 8.7	$ 17.6	$ 30.7	$ 50.9	$ 75.5	$ 80.2	$ 84.7	$ 87.8
					Percent distribution						
All sources	100.0	100.0	100.0	100.0	100.0	100.0	100.0	100.0	100.0	100.0	100.0
Out-of-pocket payments	77.9	60.1	53.5	42.6	41.8	44.3	43.1	35.2	33.6	32.8	32.5
Private health insurance	0.0	0.1	0.4	0.8	1.2	2.7	4.1	4.5	4.7	4.9	5.3
Other private funds	6.3	5.7	4.9	4.8	3.0	1.8	1.8	1.9	1.9	1.8	1.8
Government[3]	15.7	34.1	41.2	51.9	54.0	51.2	51.0	58.5	59.9	60.5	60.4
Medicaid	...	...	22.3	47.1	50.0	47.2	45.4	47.1	47.2	47.1	46.3
Medicare	...	...	3.4	2.5	1.7	1.5	3.4	9.1	10.5	11.3	11.9
					Amount in billions						
Physician services expenditures	$ 5.3	$ 8.2	$ 13.6	$ 23.9	$ 45.2	$ 83.6	$146.3	$201.9	$208.5	$217.8	$ 229.5
					Percent distribution						
All sources	100.0	100.0	100.0	100.0	100.0	100.0	100.0	100.0	100.0	100.0	100.0
Out-of-pocket payments	62.7	60.6	42.2	36.7	32.4	29.2	22.0	15.0	14.9	15.5	15.6
Private health insurance	30.2	32.5	35.2	35.3	37.9	40.1	45.7	51.6	51.2	50.2	50.5
Other private funds	0.1	0.1	0.1	0.2	0.8	1.6	1.8	1.9	2.0	2.1	2.0
Government[3]	7.1	6.8	22.5	27.7	28.9	29.1	30.5	31.5	31.9	32.2	31.9
Medicaid	...	...	4.8	7.5	5.5	4.2	4.8	7.2	7.3	7.1	6.5
Medicare	...	...	12.2	14.1	17.6	19.5	20.0	19.8	20.2	20.9	21.5

See footnotes at end of table.

Table 119 (page 2 of 2). **Personal health care expenditures, according to type of expenditure and source of funds: United States, selected years 1960–98**

[Data are compiled by the Health Care Financing Administration]

Type of personal health care expenditures and source of funds	1960	1965	1970	1975	1980	1985	1990	1995	1996	1997	1998
					Amount in billions						
All other personal health care expenditures[5]	$ 8.2	$ 11.5	$ 18.0	$ 29.4	$ 51.5	$ 93.9	$161.0	$254.8	$275.9	$296.0	$319.2
					Percent distribution						
All sources	100.0	100.0	100.0	100.0	100.0	100.0	100.0	100.0	100.0	100.0	100.0
Out-of-pocket payments	87.4	86.7	79.9	72.4	63.9	57.3	49.6	40.1	39.3	39.0	38.4
Private health insurance	1.5	2.4	5.0	8.7	15.9	22.2	26.9	28.2	28.9	29.7	30.8
Other private funds	3.0	2.9	2.8	2.9	3.6	4.1	4.3	4.4	4.2	4.1	4.0
Government[3]	8.1	8.0	12.3	16.1	16.5	16.4	19.2	27.3	27.6	27.2	26.8
Medicaid	...	...	4.5	6.0	5.5	5.7	7.3	12.0	12.5	13.0	13.5
Medicare	...	...	0.7	1.8	3.2	4.6	5.5	9.9	9.9	9.3	8.4

... Category not applicable.

[1]Includes all expenditures for health services and supplies other than expenses for program administration, net cost of private health insurance, and government public health activities.

[2]Includes expenditures for hospital-based nursing home care and home health agency care.

[3]Includes other government expenditures for these health care services, for example, care funded by the Department of Veterans Affairs and State and locally financed subsidies to hospitals.

[4]Includes expenditures for care in freestanding nursing homes. Expenditures for care in facility-based nursing homes are included with hospital care.

[5]Includes expenditures for dental services, other professional services, home health care, drugs and other medical nondurables, vision products and other medical durables, and other personal health care.

NOTE: These data include revisions in health expenditures and differ from previous editions of *Health, United States*.

SOURCE: National Health Statistics Group, Office of the Actuary. National health expenditures, 1998. Health Care Financing Review vol 21 no 2. HCFA pub no 03420. Health Care Financing Administration. Washington: U.S. Government Printing Office, Winter 1999.

Table 120 (page 1 of 2). Expenditures for health services and supplies and percent distribution, by type of payer: United States, selected calendar years 1965–95

[Data are compiled by the Health Care Financing Administration]

Type of payer	1965	1970	1975	1980	1985	1990	1991	1992	1993	1994	1995
	Amount in billions										
Total[1]	$ 37.7	$ 67.9	$122.3	$235.6	$411.8	$672.9	$736.8	$806.7	$863.1	$906.7	$957.8
Private	29.8	48.9	83.7	158.4	282.2	450.8	483.4	522.4	547.0	569.5	597.4
Private business	5.9	13.6	27.5	61.7	108.6	185.8	200.1	217.9	229.5	239.0	249.4
Employer contribution to private health insurance premiums	4.9	9.7	19.7	45.3	79.1	138.4	148.2	162.4	172.3	177.1	183.8
Private employer contribution to Medicare hospital insurance trust fund[2]	0.0	2.1	5.0	10.5	20.3	29.5	32.7	34.3	36.0	40.2	43.1
Workers compensation and temporary disability insurance	0.8	1.4	2.4	5.1	7.7	15.7	16.7	18.5	18.4	18.6	19.3
Industrial inplant health services	0.2	0.3	0.5	0.9	1.4	2.2	2.4	2.6	2.8	3.1	3.3
Household	23.2	33.8	53.8	89.5	160.5	245.3	261.8	282.2	293.7	306.7	323.3
Employee contribution to private health insurance premiums and individual policy premiums	4.7	5.6	8.2	14.6	30.7	51.3	56.8	62.6	66.4	66.0	68.5
Employee and self-employment contributions and voluntary premiums paid to Medicare hospital insurance trust fund[2]	0.0	2.4	5.7	12.0	24.1	35.5	39.7	41.7	43.8	50.3	55.9
Premiums paid by individuals to Medicare supplementary medical insurance trust fund	0.0	1.0	1.7	2.7	5.2	10.1	10.3	12.1	11.9	14.4	16.3
Out-of-pocket health spending	18.5	24.9	38.1	60.3	100.6	148.4	155.0	165.8	171.6	176.0	182.6
Nonpatient revenues	0.6	1.5	2.4	7.2	13.1	19.8	21.6	22.4	23.8	23.7	24.7
Public	7.9	19.0	38.6	77.3	129.6	222.1	253.3	284.2	316.1	337.3	360.4
Federal Government	3.4	10.4	21.2	42.4	68.4	115.1	135.7	159.1	179.5	189.1	203.4
Employer contributions to private health insurance premiums	0.2	0.3	1.2	2.2	4.3	9.2	9.8	10.7	11.5	11.9	11.3
Medicaid[3]	0.0	2.9	7.6	14.7	23.1	43.4	57.8	69.2	78.2	83.2	88.7
Other[4]	3.2	7.2	12.4	25.5	41.0	62.5	68.1	79.2	89.8	94.0	103.4
State and local government	4.5	8.6	17.4	34.8	61.2	107.0	117.6	125.2	136.6	148.1	157.0
Employer contributions to private health insurance premiums	0.3	0.7	2.2	7.6	18.2	33.5	37.5	41.2	45.2	47.7	47.1
Medicaid[3]	0.0	2.5	6.1	11.7	18.6	33.2	37.9	39.2	43.9	49.8	55.6
Other[5]	4.2	5.4	9.1	15.5	24.4	40.2	42.2	44.8	47.5	50.6	54.3
	Percent distribution										
Total	100.0	100.0	100.0	100.0	100.0	100.0	100.0	100.0	100.0	100.0	100.0
Private	79.0	72.0	68.4	67.2	68.5	67.0	65.6	64.8	63.4	62.8	62.4
Private business	15.6	20.0	22.5	26.2	26.4	27.6	27.2	27.0	26.6	26.4	26.0
Employer contribution to private health insurance premiums	13.0	14.3	16.1	19.2	19.2	20.6	20.1	20.1	20.0	19.5	19.2
Private employer contribution to Medicare hospital insurance trust fund[2]	0.0	3.1	4.1	4.5	4.9	4.4	4.4	4.3	4.2	4.4	4.5
Workers compensation and temporary disability insurance	2.1	2.1	2.0	2.2	1.9	2.3	2.3	2.3	2.1	2.1	2.0
Industrial inplant health services	0.5	0.4	0.4	0.4	0.3	0.3	0.3	0.3	0.3	0.3	0.3
Household	61.5	49.8	44.0	38.0	39.0	36.5	35.5	35.0	34.0	33.8	33.8
Employee contribution to private health insurance premiums and individual policy premiums	12.5	8.2	6.7	6.2	7.5	7.6	7.7	7.8	7.7	7.3	7.2
Employee and self-employment contributions and voluntary premiums paid to Medicare hospital insurance trust fund[2]	0.0	3.5	4.7	5.1	5.9	5.3	5.4	5.2	5.1	5.5	5.8
Premiums paid by individuals to Medicare supplementary medical insurance trust fund	0.0	1.5	1.4	1.1	1.3	1.5	1.4	1.5	1.4	1.6	1.7
Out-of-pocket health spending	49.1	36.7	31.2	25.6	24.4	22.1	21.0	20.6	19.9	19.4	19.1
Nonpatient revenues	1.6	2.2	2.0	3.1	3.2	2.9	2.9	2.8	2.8	2.6	2.6

See footnotes at end of table.

[Data are compiled by the Health Care Financing Administration].

Type of payer	1965	1970	1975	1980	1985	1990	1991	1992	1993	1994	1995
						Percent distribution					
Public	21.0	28.0	31.6	32.8	31.5	33.0	34.4	35.2	36.6	37.2	37.6
Federal Government	9.0	15.3	17.3	18.0	16.6	17.1	18.4	19.7	20.8	20.9	21.2
Employer contributions to private health insurance premiums	0.5	0.4	1.0	0.9	1.0	1.4	1.3	1.3	1.3	1.3	1.2
Medicaid[3]	0.0	4.3	6.2	6.2	5.6	6.4	7.8	8.6	9.1	9.2	9.3
Other[4]	8.5	10.6	10.1	10.8	10.0	9.3	9.2	9.8	10.4	10.4	10.8
State and local government	11.9	12.7	14.2	14.8	14.9	15.9	16.0	15.5	15.8	16.3	16.4
Employer contributions to private health insurance premiums	0.8	1.0	1.8	3.2	4.4	5.0	5.1	5.1	5.2	5.3	4.9
Medicaid[3]	0.0	3.7	5.0	5.0	4.5	4.9	5.1	4.9	5.1	5.5	5.8
Other[5]	11.1	8.0	7.4	6.6	5.9	6.0	5.7	5.6	5.5	5.6	5.7

[1]Excludes research and construction.
[2]Includes one-half of self-employment contribution to Medicare hospital insurance trust fund.
[3]Includes Medicaid buy-in premiums for Medicare.
[4]Includes expenditures for Medicare with adjustments for contributions by employers and individuals and premiums paid to the Medicare insurance trust fund and maternal and child health, vocational rehabilitation, Substance Abuse and Mental Health Services Administration, Indian Health Service, Federal workers' compensation, and other miscellaneous general hospital and medical programs, public health activities, Department of Defense, and Department of Veterans Affairs.
[5]Includes other public and general assistance, maternal and child health, vocational rehabilitation, public health activities, hospital subsidies, and employer contributions to Medicare hospital insurance trust fund.

NOTES: This table disaggregates health expenditures according to four classes of payers: businesses, households (individuals), Federal Government, and State and local governments. Where businesses or households pay dedicated funds into government health programs (for example, Medicare) or employers and employees share in the cost of health premiums, these costs are assigned to businesses or households accordingly. This results in a lower share of expenditures being assigned to the Federal Government than for tabulations of expenditures by source of funds. Estimates of national health expenditure by source of funds aim to track government-sponsored health programs over time and do not delineate the role of business employers in paying for health care. Figures may not sum to totals due to rounding. These data include revisions and differ from previous editions of Health, United States.

SOURCE: Office of National Health Statistics, Office of the Actuary. Business, households, and government: Health spending 1995. Health Care Financing Review vol 18, no 3. Washington: Health Care Financing Administration. Spring 1997.

Table 121. Employers' costs per employee hour worked for total compensation, wages and salaries, and health insurance, according to selected characteristics: United States, selected years 1991–99

[Data are based on surveys of employers]

Characteristic	Total compensation				Wages and salaries			
	1991	1994	1998	1999	1991	1994	1998	1999
	Amount per employee-hour worked							
State and local government............	$22.31	$25.27	$27.28	$28.00	$15.52	$17.57	$19.19	$19.78
Total private industry	15.40	17.08	18.50	19.00	11.14	12.14	13.47	13.87
Industry:								
Goods producing.................	18.48	20.85	22.26	22.86	12.70	13.87	15.35	15.84
Service producing	14.31	15.82	17.31	17.82	10.58	11.56	12.88	13.26
Manufacturing	18.22	20.72	22.29	22.77	12.40	13.69	15.22	15.66
Nonmanufacturing	14.67	16.19	17.66	18.20	10.81	11.76	13.09	13.49
Occupation:								
White collar.....................	18.15	20.26	22.38	23.02	13.40	14.72	16.54	17.02
Blue collar.......................	15.15	16.92	17.56	17.98	10.37	11.31	12.15	12.51
Service...........................	7.82	8.38	9.37	9.58	5.96	6.33	7.25	7.44
Region:								
Northeast	17.56	20.03	20.38	20.94	12.65	14.13	14.70	15.08
Midwest	15.05	16.26	18.15	18.36	10.70	11.34	12.99	13.21
South	13.68	15.05	16.45	16.97	10.03	10.85	12.15	12.55
West	15.97	18.08	19.94	20.74	11.62	13.01	14.75	15.36
Union status:								
Union............................	19.76	23.26	23.59	24.75	13.02	14.76	15.38	16.21
Nonunion........................	14.54	16.04	17.80	18.20	10.78	11.70	13.21	13.54
Establishment employment size:								
1–99 employees	13.38	14.58	15.92	16.27	10.00	10.72	12.01	12.29
100 or more	17.34	19.45	21.20	21.88	12.23	13.48	15.01	15.54
100–499	14.31	15.88	17.52	18.14	10.32	11.37	12.67	13.17
500 or more..................	20.60	23.35	25.56	26.37	14.28	15.79	17.78	18.37

Characteristic	Health insurance				Health insurance as a percent of total compensation			
	1991	1994	1998	1999	1991	1994	1998	1999
	Amount per employee-hour worked							
State and local government............	$1.54	$2.06	$2.05	$2.12	6.9	8.2	7.5	7.6
Total private industry	0.92	1.14	1.00	1.03	6.0	6.7	5.4	5.4
Industry:								
Goods producing.................	1.28	1.70	1.48	1.52	6.9	8.1	6.6	6.6
Service producing	0.79	0.95	0.85	0.88	5.5	6.0	4.9	4.9
Manufacturing	1.37	1.79	1.54	1.58	7.5	8.6	6.9	6.9
Nonmanufacturing	0.80	0.98	0.88	0.91	5.5	6.0	5.0	5.0
Occupation:								
White collar.....................	1.02	1.25	1.11	1.15	5.6	6.2	5.0	5.0
Blue collar.......................	1.06	1.35	1.17	1.20	7.0	8.0	6.7	6.7
Service...........................	0.36	0.45	0.40	0.40	4.6	5.4	4.3	4.2
Region:								
Northeast	1.08	1.37	1.15	1.19	6.2	6.9	5.6	5.7
Midwest	0.95	1.19	1.04	1.07	6.3	7.3	5.7	5.8
South	0.76	0.95	0.87	0.89	5.5	6.3	5.3	5.2
West	0.92	1.10	0.97	1.00	5.8	6.1	4.9	4.8
Union status:								
Union............................	1.63	2.28	1.97	2.02	8.2	9.8	8.4	8.2
Nonunion........................	0.78	0.94	0.86	0.89	5.4	5.9	4.8	4.9
Establishment employment size:								
1–99 employees	0.68	0.84	0.73	0.77	5.1	5.7	4.6	4.7
100 or more	1.14	1.42	1.28	1.30	6.6	7.3	6.0	5.9
100–499	0.90	1.03	1.01	1.01	6.3	6.5	5.8	5.6
500 or more..................	1.40	1.84	1.59	1.64	6.8	7.9	6.2	6.2

NOTES: Costs are calculated from March survey data each year. Data for additional years are available (see Appendix III).

SOURCES: U.S. Department of Labor, Bureau of Labor Statistics: Employment Cost Indexes and Levels, 1975–92. Bulletin 2413, Nov. 1992; U.S. Department of Labor: News pub nos 91–292, 94–290, 96–424, 98–285, and 99–173. June 19, 1991, June 16, 1994, Oct. 10, 1996, July 9, 1998, and June 24, 1999. Washington.

Table 122 (page 1 of 2). Hospital expenses, according to type of ownership and size of hospital: United States, selected years 1975–98

[Data are based on reporting by a census of hospitals]

Type of ownership and size of hospital	1975	1980	1985	1990	1993	1995	1996	1997	1998	1985–93	1993–98
Total expenses				Amount in billions						Average annual percent change	
All hospitals	$48.7	$91.9	$153.3	$234.9	$301.5	$320.3	$330.5	$342.3	$355.5	8.8	3.3
Federal	4.5	7.9	12.3	15.2	19.6	20.2	22.3	22.7	22.6	6.0	2.9
Non-Federal[1]	44.2	84.0	141.0	219.6	281.9	300.0	308.3	319.6	332.9	9.0	3.4
Community[2]	39.0	76.9	130.5	203.7	266.1	285.6	293.8	305.8	318.8	9.3	3.7
Nonprofit	27.9	55.8	96.1	150.7	197.2	209.6	216.0	225.3	238.0	9.4	3.8
For profit	2.6	5.8	11.5	18.8	23.1	26.7	28.4	31.2	31.7	9.1	6.5
State-local government	8.5	15.2	22.9	34.2	45.8	49.3	49.4	49.3	49.1	9.1	1.4
6–24 beds	0.1	0.2	0.3	0.5	0.7	1.1	1.1	1.3	1.4	11.2	14.9
25–49 beds	1.0	1.7	2.6	4.0	5.6	7.2	7.5	8.1	8.8	10.1	9.5
50–99 beds	2.9	5.4	8.6	12.6	15.8	17.8	18.4	19.5	20.0	7.9	4.8
100–199 beds	6.7	12.5	21.4	33.3	44.5	50.7	53.7	54.9	59.4	9.6	5.9
200–299 beds	6.8	13.4	23.3	38.7	50.6	55.8	56.5	57.1	57.1	10.2	2.4
300–399 beds	5.8	11.5	21.8	33.1	43.7	43.3	46.0	48.4	49.6	9.1	2.6
400–499 beds	4.8	10.5	15.7	25.3	30.4	33.7	35.5	35.0	36.4	8.6	3.7
500 beds or more	11.0	21.6	36.8	56.2	74.9	76.1	75.0	81.7	86.0	9.3	2.8
Employee expenses as percent of total expenses[3]				Percent							
Federal	64.5	68.4	68.1	67.1	65.6	65.8	63.0	63.1	65.5	...	...
Non-Federal[1]	54.8	58.1	56.6	54.8	53.7	54.5	53.9	53.2	53.0	...	...
Community[2]	53.0	56.3	55.2	53.6	52.7	53.6	53.0	52.4	52.1	...	...
Nonprofit	53.5	57.2	55.9	54.3	53.4	53.9	53.4	52.7	52.4	...	...
For profit	43.5	45.7	45.2	43.7	45.7	47.9	48.2	47.7	48.5	...	...
State-local government	54.3	57.3	57.1	55.8	53.6	55.2	54.2	54.2	53.3	...	...
6–24 beds	51.3	54.9	55.0	54.4	53.9	54.2	54.1	55.6	54.6	...	...
25–49 beds	50.2	54.0	54.1	53.0	52.8	53.9	53.8	53.0	53.1	...	...
50–99 beds	50.6	53.7	52.9	51.8	52.4	53.7	53.0	53.0	53.2	...	...
100–199 beds	51.0	54.2	52.6	51.7	52.2	52.9	52.9	52.2	52.5	...	...
200–299 beds	52.8	55.6	54.6	53.0	52.6	53.3	52.8	52.0	52.4	...	...
300–399 beds	53.8	56.9	55.7	54.1	53.1	53.4	52.5	52.1	51.4	...	...
400–499 beds	54.2	57.8	56.2	55.1	53.2	54.1	53.9	52.7	51.3	...	...
500 beds or more	54.3	57.9	56.9	54.5	52.9	54.1	53.1	52.6	52.1	...	...
Expenses per inpatient day				Amount							
Community[2]	$151	$245	$460	$687	$881	$968	$1,006	$1,033	$1,067	8.5	3.9
Nonprofit	150	246	463	692	898	994	1,042	1,074	1,111	8.6	4.3
For profit	146	257	500	752	914	947	945	962	968	7.8	1.2
State-local government	157	239	433	634	800	878	903	914	949	8.0	3.5
6–24 beds	121	203	380	526	664	678	757	731	823	7.2	4.4
25–49 beds	111	197	379	489	635	696	749	775	817	6.7	5.2
50–99 beds	115	191	363	493	598	647	664	686	699	6.4	3.2
100–199 beds	134	215	402	585	729	796	827	853	877	7.7	3.8
200–299 beds	146	239	449	665	854	943	993	1,011	1,035	8.4	3.9
300–399 beds	156	248	484	731	956	1,070	1,109	1,129	1,176	8.9	4.2
400–499 beds	159	215	489	756	977	1,135	1,175	1,195	1,256	9.0	5.2
500 beds or more	184	239	527	825	1,087	1,212	1,267	1,304	1,353	9.5	4.5

See footnotes at end of table.

Table 122 (page 2 of 2). Hospital expenses, according to type of ownership and size of hospital: United States, selected years 1975–98

[Data are based on reporting by a census of hospitals]

Type of ownership and size of hospital	1975	1980	1985	1990	1993	1995	1996	1997	1998	1985–93	1993–98
Expenses per inpatient stay					Amount					\multicolumn{2}{c}{Average annual percent change}	
Community[2]	$1,165	$1,851	$3,245	$4,947	$6,132	$6,216	$6,225	$6,262	$6,386	8.3	0.8
Nonprofit	1,178	1,902	3,307	5,001	6,178	6,279	6,344	6,393	6,526	8.1	1.1
For profit	968	1,676	3,033	4,727	5,643	5,425	5,207	5,219	5,262	8.1	−1.4
State-local government	1,197	1,750	3,106	4,838	6,206	6,445	6,419	6,475	6,612	9.0	1.3
6–24 beds	684	1,072	1,876	2,701	3,471	3,578	3,630	3,348	3,757	8.0	1.6
25–49 beds	673	1,138	2,007	2,967	3,687	3,797	3,879	3,989	4,106	7.9	2.2
50–99 beds	785	1,271	2,342	3,461	4,312	4,427	4,474	4,598	4,734	7.9	1.9
100–199 beds	955	1,512	2,683	4,109	4,999	5,103	5,121	5,146	5,219	8.1	0.9
200–299 beds	1,096	1,767	3,044	4,618	5,713	5,851	5,917	5,948	6,012	8.2	1.0
300–399 beds	1,225	1,881	3,394	5,096	6,351	6,512	6,550	6,429	6,642	8.1	0.9
400–499 beds	1,290	2,090	3,571	5,500	6,706	7,164	7,253	7,279	7,431	8.2	2.1
500 beds or more	1,677	2,517	4,254	6,667	8,460	8,531	8,450	8,508	8,670	9.0	0.5

. . . Category not applicable.

[1]The category of non-Federal hospitals is comprised of psychiatric, tuberculosis and other respiratory diseases hospitals, and long-term and short-term hospitals.
[2]Community hospitals are short-term hospitals excluding hospital units in institutions such as prison and college infirmaries, facilities for the mentally retarded, and alcoholism and chemical dependency hospitals.
[3]Includes employee payroll and benefit expenses. Does not include contracted labor services.

NOTE: Data for additional years are available (see Appendix III).

SOURCES: American Hospital Association: Hospital Statistics, 1976, 1981, 1986, 1991–2000 Editions. Chicago, 1976, 1981, 1986, 1991–2000 (Copyrights 1976, 1981, 1986, 1991–2000: Used with the permission of the American Hospital Association); and unpublished data.

Table 123. Nursing home average monthly charges per resident and percent of residents, according to selected facility and resident characteristics: United States, 1973–74, 1977, 1985, 1995, and 1997

[Data are based on reporting by a sample of nursing homes]

Facility and resident characteristic	Average monthly charge[1]					Percent of residents				
	1973–74[2]	1977	1985	1995	1997	1973–74[2]	1977	1985	1995	1997
Facility characteristic										
All facilities....................	$479	$689	$1,456	$3,135	$3,609	100.0	100.0	100.0	100.0	100.0
Ownership:										
Proprietary..................	489	670	1,379	3,047	3,508	69.8	68.2	68.7	63.6	65.5
Nonprofit and government.......	456	732	1,624	3,288	3,792	30.2	31.8	31.3	36.4	34.5
Certification:[3]										
Skilled nursing facility...........	566	880	1,905	- - -	- - -	39.8	20.7	18.5	- - -	- - -
Skilled nursing and intermediate facility.....................	514	762	1,571	- - -	- - -	24.5	40.5	45.2	- - -	- - -
Intermediate facility	376	556	1,179	- - -	- - -	22.4	28.3	24.9	- - -	- - -
Not certified	329	390	875	- - -	- - -	13.3	10.6	11.4	- - -	- - -
Both Medicare and Medicaid......	- - -	- - -	- - -	3,317	3,765	- - -	- - -	- - -	78.4	84.9
Medicare only	- - -	- - -	- - -	4,211	4,221	- - -	- - -	- - -	3.0	2.9
Medicaid only	- - -	- - -	- - -	2,169	2,436	- - -	- - -	- - -	15.8	9.7
Neither......................	- - -	- - -	- - -	2,323	2,422	- -	- - -	- - -	2.8	2.4
Bed size:										
Less than 50 beds.............	397	546	1,036	4,978	3,521	15.2	12.9	8.9	4.5	3.9
50–99 beds..................	448	643	1,335	2,691	3,178	34.1	30.5	27.6	24.9	24.7
100–199 beds................	502	706	1,478	3,028	3,592	35.6	38.8	43.2	51.1	51.9
200 beds or more	576	837	1,759	3,560	4,211	15.1	17.9	20.2	19.5	19.5
Geographic region:										
Northeast	651	918	1,781	3,904	4,589	22.0	22.4	23.6	22.8	23.3
Midwest	433	640	1,399	2,740	3,203	34.6	34.5	32.5	32.3	31.0
South	410	585	1,256	2,752	3,225	26.0	27.2	29.4	32.0	32.6
West	454	653	1,458	3,710	3,791	17.4	15.9	14.5	12.9	13.1
Resident characteristic										
All residents....................	479	689	1,456	3,135	3,609	100.0	100.0	100.0	100.0	100.0
Age:										
Under 65 years	434	585	1,379	3,662	3,760	10.6	13.6	11.6	8.0	8.5
65–74 years	473	669	1,372	3,409	3,877	15.0	16.2	14.2	12.0	12.8
75–84 years	488	710	1,468	3,138	3,595	35.5	35.7	34.1	32.5	32.8
85 years and over	485	719	1,497	2,974	3,521	38.8	34.5	40.0	47.5	45.9
Sex:										
Male........................	466	652	1,438	3,345	3,758	29.1	28.8	28.4	26.6	27.8
Female......................	484	705	1,463	3,059	3,553	70.9	71.2	71.6	73.4	72.2

- - - Data not available.
[1]Includes life-care residents and no-charge residents.
[2]Data exclude residents of personal care homes.
[3]Medicare extended care facilities and Medicaid skilled nursing homes from the 1973–74 survey were considered to be equivalent to Medicare or Medicaid skilled nursing facilities in 1977 and 1985 for the purposes of this comparison. In the 1995 and 1997 surveys the certification categories were based on Medicare and Medicaid certification.

SOURCES: Centers for Disease Control and Prevention: Hing E. Charges for care and sources of payment for residents in nursing homes, United States, National Nursing Home Survey, August 1973–April 1974. National Center for Health Statistics. Vital Health Stat 13(32). 1977; Van Nostrand JF, Zappolo A, Hing E, et al. The National Nursing Home Survey, 1977 summary for the United States. National Center for Health Statistics. Vital Health Stat 13(43). 1979; and Hing E, Sekscenski E, Strahan G. The National Nursing Home Survey: 1985 summary for the United States. National Center for Health Statistics. Vital Health Stat 13(97). 1989; and unpublished data.

Table 124. Nursing home average monthly charges per resident and percent of residents, according to primary source of payments and selected facility characteristics: United States, 1985, 1995, and 1997

[Data are based on reporting by a sample of nursing homes]

Facility characteristic	All sources 1997	Own income or family support[1] 1985	1995	1997	Medicare 1985	1995	1997	Medicaid 1985	1995	1997
					Average monthly charge[2]					
All facilities	$3,609	$1,450	$3,081	$3,643	$ 2,141	$ 5,546	$ 6,037	$1,504	$2,769	$3,081
Ownership										
Proprietary	3,508	1,444	3,190	3,784	2,058	5,668	6,051	1,363	2,560	2,883
Nonprofit and government	3,792	1,462	2,967	3,475	*2,456	5,304	6,008	1,851	3,201	3,516
Certification[3]										
Skilled nursing facility	---	1,797	---	---	2,315	---	---	2,000	---	---
Skilled nursing and intermediate facility	---	1,643	---	---	2,156	---	---	1,509	---	---
Intermediate facility	---	1,222	---	---	...	---	---	1,150	---	---
Not certified	---	999	---	---	...	---	---	...	...	...
Both Medicare and Medicaid	3,765	---	3,365	3,868	---	5,472	6,134	---	2,910	3,179
Medicare only	4,221	---	3,344	4,068	---	*10,074	4,922	---	...	3,451
Medicaid only	2,436	---	2,352	2,485	---	...	2,829	---	2,069	2,409
Neither	2,422	---	2,390	2,482	---	...	2,424	---	...	2,178
Bed size										
Less than 50 beds	3,521	886	3,377	2,972	*1,348	4*17,224	4*10,133	1,335	2,990	2,987
50–99 beds	3,178	1,388	2,849	3,253	1,760	4,929	5,814	1,323	2,335	2,693
100–199 beds	3,592	1,567	3,138	3,788	2,192	4,918	5,877	1,413	2,659	2,975
200 beds or more	4,211	1,701	3,316	4,161	2,767	4,523	6,214	1,919	3,520	3,820
Geographic region										
Northeast	4,589	1,645	4,117	4,884	2,109	4,883	6,542	2,035	3,671	4,039
Midwest	3,203	1,398	2,650	3,231	2,745	5,439	5,546	1,382	2,478	2,732
South	3,225	1,359	2,945	3,320	2,033	4,889	6,173	1,200	2,333	2,642
West	3,791	1,498	3,666	3,916	1,838	8,825	5,630	1,501	2,848	3,240
					Percent of residents					
All facilities	100.0	41.6	27.8	24.5	1.4	9.9	14.4	50.4	60.2	57.9
Ownership										
Proprietary	100.0	40.1	24.1	20.9	1.6	10.4	15.0	52.1	63.8	61.5
Nonprofit and government	100.0	44.9	34.3	31.4	*0.9	9.2	13.2	46.6	54.0	51.0
Certification[3]										
Skilled nursing facility	---	39.1	---	---	2.6	---	---	53.7	---	---
Skilled nursing and intermediate facility	---	36.8	---	---	1.9	---	---	57.8	---	---
Intermediate facility	---	41.4	---	---	...	---	---	55.9	---	---
Not certified	---	65.5	---	---	...	---	---	...	...	...
Both Medicare and Medicaid	100.0	---	23.1	21.9	---	11.6	15.9	---	63.9	59.6
Medicare only	100.0	---	71.2	63.3	---	16.2	23.0	---	...	2.6
Medicaid only	100.0	---	32.1	22.3	---	...	1.1	---	63.0	73.4
Neither	100.0	---	91.0	78.0	---	...	3.9	---	...	4.0
Bed size										
Less than 50 beds	100.0	53.1	35.3	39.1	*1.2	13.1	13.8	33.8	49.9	43.2
50–99 beds	100.0	49.5	34.5	29.4	*1.3	6.2	12.9	42.9	57.6	55.6
100–199 beds	100.0	39.6	26.2	22.9	1.5	10.6	15.4	55.2	61.5	58.8
200 beds or more	100.0	30.1	22.0	19.9	*1.5	12.1	13.6	57.7	62.4	61.3
Geographic region										
Northeast	100.0	34.8	18.2	19.6	1.7	14.0	16.0	52.9	64.9	59.9
Midwest	100.0	49.1	36.3	32.8	*0.8	6.7	11.9	45.9	55.8	52.8
South	100.0	39.4	26.1	20.7	*1.2	10.1	13.9	53.8	62.2	63.3
West	100.0	40.4	27.9	23.3	*2.7	10.5	18.5	49.2	57.9	53.1

* Relative standard error greater than 30 percent.

--- Data not available.

... Category not applicable.

[1]Includes private health insurance.

[2]Includes life-care residents and no-charge residents.

[3]In the 1995 and 1997 surveys the certification categories were based on Medicare and Medicaid certification.

[4]Likely to include a high proportion of patients in subacute units of hospitals.

SOURCES: Centers for Disease Control and Prevention: Hing E, Sekscenski E, Strahan G. The National Nursing Home Survey: 1985 summary for the United States. National Center for Health Statistics. Vital Health Stat 13(97). 1985; and unpublished data.

Table 125. Mental health expenditures, percent distribution, and per capita expenditures, according to type of mental health organization: United States, selected years 1975–94

[Data are based on inventories of mental health organizations]

Type of organization	1975	1979	1983	1986	1988	1990	1992	1994
				Amount in millions				
All organizations	$6,564	$8,764	$14,432	$18,458	$23,028	$28,410	$29,765	$33,136
State and county mental hospitals	3,185	3,757	5,491	6,326	6,978	7,774	7,970	7,825
Private psychiatric hospitals	467	743	1,712	2,629	4,588	6,101	5,302	6,468
Non-Federal general hospitals with separate psychiatric services	621	723	2,176	2,878	3,610	4,662	5,193	5,344
Department of Veterans Affairs medical centers[1]	699	848	1,316	1,338	1,290	1,480	1,530	1,386
Residential treatment centers for emotionally disturbed children	279	436	573	978	1,305	1,969	2,167	2,360
Freestanding psychiatric outpatient clinics	422	589	430	518	657	671	821	878
All other organizations[2]	116	187	2,734	3,792	4,600	5,753	6,782	8,875
				Percent distribution				
All organizations	100.0	100.0	100.0	100.0	100.0	100.0	100.0	100.0
State and county mental hospitals	48.5	42.9	38.0	34.4	30.3	27.4	26.8	23.6
Private psychiatric hospitals	7.1	8.5	11.9	14.2	19.9	21.5	17.8	19.5
Non-Federal general hospitals with separate psychiatric services	9.5	8.2	15.1	15.6	15.7	16.4	17.4	16.1
Department of Veterans Affairs medical centers[1]	10.6	9.7	9.1	7.2	5.6	5.2	5.1	4.2
Residential treatment centers for emotionally disturbed children	4.3	5.0	4.0	5.3	5.7	6.9	7.3	7.1
Freestanding psychiatric outpatient clinics	6.4	6.7	• 3.0	2.8	2.8	2.4	2.8	2.7
All other organizations[2]	1.8	2.1	18.9	20.5	20.0	20.2	22.8	26.8
				Amount per capita[3]				
All organizations	$ 31	$ 40	$ 62	$ 77	$ 95	$ 117	$ 117	$ 128
State and county mental hospitals	15	17	24	26	29	32	31	30
Private psychiatric hospitals	2	3	7	11	19	25	21	25
Non-Federal general hospitals with separate psychiatric services	3	3	9	12	15	19	20	21
Department of Veterans Affairs medical centers[1]	3	4	6	6	5	6	6	5
Residential treatment centers for emotionally disturbed children	1	2	3	4	5	8	9	9
Freestanding psychiatric outpatient clinics	2	3	2	2	3	3	3	3
All other organizations[2]	1	1	12	16	19	24	27	35

[1]Includes Department of Veterans Affairs neuropsychiatric hospitals, general hospital psychiatric services, and psychiatric outpatient clinics.
[2]Includes freestanding outpatient clinics, freestanding day–night organizations, multiservice organizations, and other residential organizations. Multiservice mental health organizations were redefined in 1983; see Appendix I, Substance Abuse and Mental Health Services Administration.
[3]Civilian population.

NOTES: Comparisons of data from 1979 and 1983 with data from other years should be made with caution because changes in reporting procedures may affect the comparability of data. Mental health expenditures include salaries, other operating expenditures, and capital expenditures.

SOURCES: Survey and Analysis Branch, Division of State and Community Systems Development, Center for Mental Health Services. Manderscheid RW, Sonnenschein MA. *Mental health, United States, 1996.* U.S. Government Printing Office, 1996; unpublished data from the 1994 inventory of mental health organizations and general hospital mental health services.

Table 126. Funding for health research and development, according to source of funds: United States, selected fiscal years 1970–97

[Data are compiled by the National Institutes of Health from Federal Government sources]

Source of funds	1970	1980	1985	1990	1993[1]	1994	1995	1996	1997
	Amount in millions								
All funding	$2,847	$7,967	$13,567	$23,095	$31,088	$33,399	$35,816	- - -	- - -
Industry[2]	795	2,459	5,360	10,719	15,711	17,106	18,645	- - -	- - -
Private nonprofit organizations	215	305	538	960	1,215	1,276	1,325	- - -	- - -
State and local governments	170	480	878	1,625	2,054	2,196	2,423	- - -	- - -
Federal government	1,667	4,723	6,791	9,791	12,108	12,821	13,423	- - -	15,081
National Institutes of Health	- - -	- - -	- - -	- - -	9,756	10,329	10,681	11,251	11,993
National Institute on Aging	- - -	- - -	- - -	- - -	382	405	419	441	470
National Institute of Allergy and Infectious Diseases	- - -	- - -	- - -	- - -	1,001	1,060	1,096	1,154	1,230
National Cancer Institute	- - -	- - -	- - -	- - -	1,903	2,015	2,084	2,195	2,340
National Institute of Child Health and Human Development	- - -	- - -	- - -	- - -	497	526	544	573	610
National Institute of Diabetes and Digestive and Kidney Diseases	- - -	- - -	- - -	- - -	637	675	698	735	783
National Institute on Drug Abuse	- - -	- - -	- - -	- - -	396	419	434	457	487
National Institute of General Medical Sciences	- - -	- - -	- - -	- - -	715	757	783	825	879
National Heart, Lung, and Blood Institute	- - -	- - -	- - -	- - -	1,123	1,189	1,229	1,295	1,380
National Institute of Mental Health	- - -	- - -	- - -	- - -	540	572	592	623	664
National Institute of Neurological Disorders and Stroke	- - -	- - -	- - -	- - -	578	613	633	667	711
Other National Institutes of Health[3]	- - -	- - -	- - -	- - -	1,984	2,098	2,169	2,286	2,439
	Average annual percent change from previous year shown								
All funding	. . .	10.8	11.2	11.2	6.3	7.4	7.2	- - -	- - -
Industry[2]	. . .	12.0	16.9	14.9	9.1	8.9	9.0	- - -	- - -
Private nonprofit organizations	. . .	3.6	12.0	12.3	2.7	5.0	9.0	- - -	- - -
State and local governments	. . .	10.9	12.8	13.1	6.3	6.9	10.3	- - -	- - -
Federal government	. . .	11.0	7.5	7.6	3.3	5.9	4.7	- - -	6.0
National Institutes of Health	. . .	. . .	. . .	. . .	. . .	5.9	3.4	5.3	6.6
	Percent distribution of Federal funding								
All Federal agencies	100.0	100.0	100.0	100.0	100.0	100.0	100.0	- - -	100.0
Department of Health and Human Services	70.6	78.2	79.7	85.2	85.0	85.6	85.1	- - -	84.1
National Institutes of Health	52.4	67.4	71.1	72.9	80.7	80.6	79.6	- - -	79.5
Centers for Disease Control and Prevention	- - -	1.8	0.7	1.0	1.3	1.6	2.4	- - -	2.1
Other Public Health Service	16.2	7.9	7.3	10.8	2.4	2.7	2.5	- - -	2.1
Other Department of Health and Human Services	2.0	1.1	0.6	0.5	0.6	0.6	0.6	- - -	0.4
Other departments and agencies	29.4	21.8	20.3	14.8	15.0	14.4	14.9	- - -	15.9
Department of Defense	7.5	4.5	6.5	4.4	5.6	5.3	5.3	- - -	7.3
Department of Energy[4]	6.3	4.5	2.6	2.8	2.6	2.5	2.5	- - -	2.1
Department of Veterans Affairs	3.5	2.8	3.3	2.4	2.0	1.9	1.8	- - -	1.7
Environmental Protection Agency	. . .	1.7	0.8	0.3	0.4	0.3	0.2	- - -	0.8
National Aeronautics and Space Administration	5.2	1.5	1.7	1.5	1.7	1.5	2.6	- - -	1.2
All other departments and agencies	6.9	6.8	5.4	3.4	2.7	2.9	2.5	- - -	2.8

- - - Data not available.
. . . Category not applicable.

[1] In fiscal year 1993 the Alcohol, Drug Abuse, and Mental Health Administration was reorganized and renamed the Substance Abuse and Mental Health Services Administration and its three research institutes were transferred into the National Institutes of Health.
[2] Includes expenditures for drug research. These expenditures are included in the "drugs and sundries" component of the Health Care Financing Administration's National Health Expenditure Series, not under "research."
[3] Includes the National Institutes on Alcohol Abuse and Alcoholism, of Arthritis and Musculoskeletal and Skin Diseases, on Deafness and Other Communication Disorders, of Dental Research, of Environmental Health Sciences, of Nursing Research, and the National Eye Institute, the National Center for Human Genome Research, the National Library of Medicine, the Fogarty International Center, the Division of Research Resources, and the Office of the Director.
[4] Includes Atomic Energy Commission and Energy Research and Development Administration.

NOTES: Data for 1970 and 1975 fiscal years ending June 30; all other data for fiscal year ending September 30. Data on the National Institutes of Health are presented from 1993 onwards since there was frequent reorganization of the Institutes in prior years. Data for additional years are available (see Appendix III).

SOURCE: National Institutes of Health, Office of Reports and Analysis.

Table 127. Federal spending for human immunodeficiency virus (HIV)-related activities, according to agency and type of activity: United States, selected fiscal years 1985–99

[Data are compiled from Federal Government appropriations]

Agency and type of activity	1985	1990	1992	1993	1994	1995	1996	1997	1998	1999[1]
Agency				Amount in millions						
All Federal spending	$205	$3,064	$4,498	$5,328	$6,329	$6,821	$7,522	$8,363	$8,931	$9,988
Department of Health and Human Services, total	197	2,620	3,824	4,426	5,399	4,941	5,598	6,367	6,835	7,708
Department of Health and Human Services discretionary spending, total[2]	109	1,591	1,963	2,081	2,569	2,700	2,898	3,267	3,535	4,108
National Institutes of Health	66	907	1,047	1,073	1,296	1,334	1,411	1,501	1,604	1,799
Substance Abuse and Mental Health Services Administration	–	50	26	26	27	24	54	64	70	93
Centers for Disease Control and Prevention	33	443	480	498	543	590	584	617	625	657
Food and Drug Administration	9	57	72	73	72	73	73	73	73	77
Health Resources and Services Administration	–	113	317	390	608	661	762	1,001	1,155	1,416
Agency for Health Care Policy and Research	–	8	10	10	11	9	6	4	1	2
Office of Public Health and Science[3]	–	8	5	5	5	4	4	4	4	11
Indian Health Service	–	3	3	3	4	4	3	4	4	4
Emergency Fund	...	...	...	...	...	...	...	...	...	50
Other Department of Health and Human Services agencies	–	3	3	3	2	2	2	–	–	1
Health Care Financing Administration	75	780	1,360	1,675	1,990	2,240	2,700	3,100	3,300	3,600
Social Security Administration[4]	13	249	501	670	840	...	...	...	...	...
Social Security Administration[4]	...					940	976	1,001	1,061	1,136
Department of Veterans Affairs	8	220	279	325	312	317	331	332	343	403
Department of Defense	–	125	129	159	129	112	98	100	105	106
Agency for International Development	–	71	94	117	115	120	115	117	121	135
Department of Housing and Urban Development	–	–	107	196	258	171	171	196	204	225
Office of Personnel Management	–	21	58	98	108	212	226	241	253	266
Other departments	–	7	7	7	8	8	7	9	9	9
Activity										
Research	84	1,142	1,311	1,361	1,561	1,589	1,653	1,730	1,831	2,045
Department of Health and Human Services discretionary spending[2]	83	1,093	1,259	1,284	1,508	1,544	1,619	1,702	1,801	2,014
Department of Veterans Affairs	1	15	6	7	6	5	6	6	6	7
Department of Defense	–	34	46	70	47	40	28	22	24	24
Education and prevention	26	486	518	576	619	658	635	685	701	793
Department of Health and Human Services discretionary spending[2]	25	351	378	395	445	492	476	522	534	610
Department of Veterans Affairs	1	31	22	31	31	31	31	31	31	32
Department of Defense	–	28	18	27	22	12	11	12	13	13
Agency for International Development	–	71	94	117	115	120	115	117	121	135
Other	–	5	6	6	6	3	2	3	2	3
Medical care	81	1,187	2,061	2,523	3,051	3,462	4,087	4,752	5,134	5,790
Health Care Financing Administration: Medicaid (Federal share)	70	670	1,080	1,290	1,490	1,640	1,600	1,800	1,900	2,100
Medicare	5	110	280	385	500	600	1,100	1,300	1,400	1,500
Department of Health and Human Services discretionary spending[2]	–	144	323	397	613	664	803	1,044	1,200	1,485
Department of Veterans Affairs	6	174	251	287	275	281	294	295	306	364
Department of Defense	–	63	65	62	60	60	59	66	68	69
Office of Personnel Management	–	21	58	98	108	212	226	241	253	266
Other	–	5	4	4	5	5	5	6	7	6
Cash assistance	13	249	608	866	1,098	1,111	1,147	1,197	1,265	1,361
Social Security Administration: Disability Insurance	10	210	390	505	600	640	696	691	726	776
Supplemental Security Income	3	39	111	165	240	300	280	310	335	360
Department of Housing and Urban Development	–	–	107	196	258	171	171	196	204	225

– Quantity zero.   ... Category not applicable.

[1] Preliminary figures.

[2] Department of Health and Human Services discretionary spending is spending that is not entitlement spending. Medicare and Medicaid are examples of entitlement spending.

[3] The Office of the Assistant Secretary for Health prior to FY 1996.

[4] Prior to 1995 the Social Security Administration was part of the Department of Health and Human Services.

SOURCE: Budget Office, Public Health Service. Unpublished data.

Table 128 (page 1 of 3). **Health care coverage for persons under 65 years of age, according to type of coverage and selected characteristics: United States, selected years 1984–97**

[Data are based on household interviews of a sample of the civilian noninstitutionalized population]

Characteristic	Private insurance						Private insurance obtained through workplace[1]					
	1984	1989	1994[2]	1995	1996	1997[2,3]	1984	1989	1994[2]	1995	1996	1997[2,3]
	Number in millions											
Total[4]	157.5	162.7	160.7	165.0	165.9	165.8	141.8	146.3	146.7	151.4	151.4	152.5
	Percent of population											
Total, age adjusted[4,5]	77.1	76.2	70.7	71.9	71.6	70.9	69.2	68.4	64.5	66.0	65.3	65.1
Total, crude[4]	76.8	75.9	70.3	71.6	71.4	70.7	69.1	68.3	64.2	65.7	65.1	65.0
Age												
Under 18 years	72.6	71.8	63.8	65.7	66.4	66.1	66.5	65.8	59.0	60.9	61.1	61.4
Under 6 years	68.1	67.9	58.3	60.1	61.1	61.3	62.1	62.3	53.9	55.6	56.5	57.3
6–17 years	74.9	74.0	66.8	68.7	69.1	68.5	68.7	67.7	61.8	63.7	63.4	63.4
18–44 years	76.5	75.5	69.8	71.2	70.6	69.4	69.6	68.4	63.9	65.6	64.7	64.4
18–24 years	67.4	64.5	58.3	61.2	60.4	59.3	58.7	55.3	50.7	53.9	52.3	53.8
25–34 years	77.4	75.9	69.4	70.3	69.5	68.1	71.2	69.5	64.1	65.3	64.4	63.6
35–44 years	83.9	82.7	77.1	78.0	77.5	76.4	77.4	76.2	71.6	72.9	72.0	71.2
45–64 years	83.3	82.5	80.3	80.4	79.5	79.0	71.8	71.6	71.8	72.4	71.4	70.8
45–54 years	83.3	83.4	81.3	81.1	80.4	80.4	74.6	74.4	74.6	74.9	74.0	73.6
55–64 years	83.3	81.6	78.8	79.3	78.1	76.9	69.0	68.3	67.9	68.6	67.5	66.6
Sex[5]												
Male	77.7	76.5	71.2	72.3	72.0	71.2	70.1	68.9	65.0	66.5	65.8	65.4
Female	76.5	75.9	70.2	71.6	71.3	70.6	68.4	67.9	64.0	65.4	64.9	64.9
Race[5,6]												
White	80.1	79.3	74.1	74.9	74.6	74.3	72.0	71.2	67.4	68.8	67.9	68.0
Black	59.2	58.7	53.0	55.6	56.2	56.1	53.3	53.6	50.2	51.8	53.0	53.7
Asian or Pacific Islander	70.9	71.6	67.9	68.8	68.3	68.2	64.4	60.2	57.8	60.2	59.4	60.5
Hispanic origin and race[5,6]												
All Hispanic	57.1	53.2	49.4	48.3	48.4	47.9	52.9	48.6	45.1	44.9	44.6	44.5
Mexican	54.9	48.5	46.4	44.7	44.4	43.9	51.7	45.6	44.3	42.7	41.5	41.8
Puerto Rican	51.0	46.8	49.5	49.1	52.5	48.2	48.3	43.4	46.3	45.9	49.9	45.5
Cuban	72.1	70.0	63.7	63.4	65.7	70.7	57.6	56.3	45.7	53.8	54.8	55.9
Other Hispanic	62.0	62.4	53.1	53.1	53.4	51.2	57.7	55.7	47.1	47.9	48.4	47.6
White, non-Hispanic	82.4	82.5	77.7	78.9	78.6	78.0	74.0	74.0	70.7	72.3	71.5	71.4
Black, non-Hispanic	59.4	58.8	53.4	56.1	56.7	56.3	53.4	53.7	50.6	52.3	53.3	53.9
Age and percent of poverty level[7]												
All ages:[5]												
Below 100 percent	33.0	27.5	22.3	22.7	20.7	23.6	23.8	19.7	16.8	17.7	15.8	19.6
100–149 percent	61.8	54.2	46.6	47.7	46.8	42.0	51.1	45.0	40.6	41.7	40.4	36.8
150–199 percent	77.2	70.6	65.2	66.1	67.1	63.6	68.6	61.9	58.3	60.0	60.0	58.1
200 percent or more	91.6	91.0	88.8	89.1	89.3	87.6	85.0	83.9	82.7	83.4	83.0	82.0
Under 18 years:												
Below 100 percent	28.7	22.3	14.9	16.8	16.1	17.5	23.2	17.5	12.4	13.4	13.4	15.4
100–149 percent	66.2	59.6	47.8	48.5	49.5	42.5	58.3	52.5	43.2	43.6	43.7	38.4
150–199 percent	80.9	75.9	69.3	68.5	73.0	66.8	75.8	70.1	64.0	63.0	67.4	63.1
200 percent or more	92.3	92.7	89.7	90.4	90.7	88.9	86.9	86.7	84.5	85.5	84.6	83.7
Geographic region[5]												
Northeast	80.7	82.1	75.3	75.7	75.5	74.3	74.1	75.1	70.0	70.1	69.2	69.7
Midwest	80.9	81.7	77.7	77.8	78.8	77.3	72.1	73.4	71.4	71.6	72.6	71.4
South	74.5	71.7	66.0	67.6	66.7	67.5	66.2	63.8	60.0	62.4	61.0	61.6
West	72.3	71.8	66.0	68.5	67.7	65.8	64.9	64.2	58.8	61.2	60.1	59.4
Location of residence[5]												
Within MSA[8]	77.8	76.8	71.3	72.8	73.0	71.5	71.0	69.8	65.5	67.2	67.0	66.0
Outside MSA[8]	75.5	74.0	68.7	68.3	66.4	68.5	65.3	63.5	60.8	61.0	59.0	61.7

See footnotes at end of table.

[Data are based on household interviews of a sample of the civilian noninstitutionalized population]

Characteristic	Medicaid[9]						Not covered[10]					
	1984	1989	1994[2]	1995	1996	1997[2,3]	1984	1989	1994[2]	1995	1996	1997[2,3]
	Number in millions											
Total[4]	14.0	15.4	24.1	25.3	25.0	22.9	29.8	33.4	40.4	37.4	38.9	41.0
	Percent of population											
Total, age adjusted[4,5]	6.7	7.1	10.3	10.8	10.5	9.6	14.3	15.3	17.4	16.0	16.6	17.4
Total, crude[4]	6.8	7.2	10.6	11.0	10.8	9.7	14.5	15.6	17.7	16.2	16.7	17.5
Age												
Under 18 years	11.9	12.6	20.0	20.6	20.1	18.4	13.9	14.7	15.3	13.6	13.4	14.0
Under 6 years	15.5	15.7	27.2	28.3	27.4	24.7	14.9	15.1	13.7	11.9	11.9	12.5
6–17 years	10.1	10.9	16.2	16.6	16.4	15.2	13.4	14.5	16.2	14.5	14.1	14.7
18–44 years	5.1	5.2	7.3	7.4	7.3	6.6	17.1	18.4	21.9	20.5	21.2	22.4
18–24 years	6.4	6.8	9.6	9.7	9.2	8.8	25.0	27.1	31.1	28.2	29.6	30.1
25–34 years	5.3	5.2	7.7	7.7	7.5	6.8	16.2	18.3	22.1	21.3	22.5	23.8
35–44 years	3.5	4.0	5.4	5.6	6.0	5.2	11.2	12.3	16.0	15.2	15.2	16.7
45–64 years	3.4	4.3	4.5	5.3	5.2	4.6	9.6	10.5	12.0	11.0	12.1	12.4
45–54 years	3.2	3.8	3.8	4.9	4.8	4.0	10.5	11.0	12.6	11.7	12.5	12.8
55–64 years	3.6	4.9	5.5	6.0	5.7	5.6	8.7	10.0	11.2	10.0	11.6	11.8
Sex[5]												
Male	5.2	5.6	8.3	8.9	8.7	8.1	15.0	16.4	18.6	17.3	17.8	18.5
Female	8.0	8.6	12.2	12.6	12.4	11.0	13.6	14.3	16.3	14.8	15.4	16.2
Race[5,6]												
White	4.6	5.1	7.8	8.4	8.4	7.5	13.4	14.2	16.7	15.4	15.9	16.3
Black	18.9	17.8	24.5	24.6	22.2	20.5	20.0	21.4	20.2	18.6	19.8	20.2
Asian or Pacific Islander	9.1	11.3	9.2	10.1	11.3	9.4	18.0	18.5	20.3	18.3	19.1	19.3
Hispanic origin and race[5,6]												
All Hispanic	12.2	12.7	17.8	19.1	17.9	16.0	29.1	32.4	32.3	31.7	32.7	34.3
Mexican	11.1	11.5	16.5	18.0	16.8	15.3	33.2	38.8	36.7	36.5	38.0	39.2
Puerto Rican	28.6	26.9	33.8	30.5	31.1	28.9	18.1	23.3	16.3	18.5	15.1	19.4
Cuban	4.8	7.8	8.4	13.7	12.6	8.2	21.6	20.9	27.5	22.1	18.9	20.5
Other Hispanic	7.4	10.4	14.6	16.5	14.5	13.9	27.5	25.2	31.0	29.9	30.8	32.9
White, non-Hispanic	3.7	4.2	6.3	6.8	6.8	6.2	11.8	11.9	14.5	13.0	13.3	13.7
Black, non-Hispanic	19.1	17.8	24.5	24.3	21.9	20.3	19.7	21.3	19.8	18.5	19.7	20.1
Age and percent of poverty level[7]												
All ages:[5]												
Below 100 percent	30.5	35.3	42.3	44.1	43.9	38.8	34.7	35.8	34.0	32.4	34.4	34.4
100–149 percent	7.5	11.0	15.0	17.2	16.1	17.5	27.0	31.3	35.0	32.1	34.0	36.1
150–199 percent	3.1	5.0	5.5	7.1	7.2	7.4	17.4	21.8	25.8	23.6	23.5	25.9
200 percent or more	0.6	1.1	1.3	1.5	1.5	1.7	5.8	6.8	8.7	8.1	7.8	8.8
Under 18 years:												
Below 100 percent	43.1	47.8	63.6	65.6	65.9	59.7	28.9	31.6	23.3	20.6	21.3	22.4
100–149 percent	9.0	12.3	22.9	26.3	24.8	30.2	22.8	26.1	27.7	25.5	25.2	26.1
150–199 percent	4.4	6.1	8.6	11.7	10.8	12.2	12.7	15.8	19.0	17.7	16.1	19.7
200 percent or more	0.8	1.6	2.2	2.7	2.6	2.9	4.2	4.4	6.8	6.0	5.3	6.1

See footnotes at end of table.

Table 128 (page 3 of 3). Health care coverage for persons under 65 years of age, according to type of coverage and selected characteristics: United States, selected years 1984–97

[Data are based on household interviews of a sample of the civilian noninstitutionalized population]

Characteristic	Medicaid[9]						Not covered[10]					
	1984	1989	1994[2]	1995	1996	1997[2,3]	1984	1989	1994[2]	1995	1996	1997[2,3]
Geographic regions[5]					Percent of population							
Northeast	8.5	6.8	10.8	11.3	11.2	11.2	10.1	10.7	13.7	13.1	13.6	13.4
Midwest	7.2	7.5	9.4	9.8	8.4	8.2	11.1	10.5	12.3	12.2	12.3	13.1
South	5.0	6.4	10.0	10.3	10.7	8.6	17.4	19.4	21.2	19.4	20.1	20.7
West	6.9	8.2	11.4	11.9	12.1	11.4	17.8	18.4	20.6	17.8	18.7	20.4
Location of residence[5]												
Within MSA[8]	7.1	7.0	10.4	10.6	10.0	9.5	13.3	14.9	17.0	15.3	15.8	16.7
Outside MSA[8]	5.9	7.8	10.0	11.6	12.5	9.9	16.4	16.9	19.2	18.8	19.7	19.9

[1]Private insurance originally obtained through a present or former employer or union.
[2]The questionnaire changed compared with previous years. See Appendix II, Health insurance coverage.
[3]Preliminary data.
[4]Includes all other races not shown separately and unknown poverty level.
[5]Estimates are age adjusted to the year 2000 standard using three age groups: Under 18 years, 18–44 years, and 45–64 years. See Appendix II, Age adjustment.
[6]The race groups white, black, and Asian or Pacific Islander include persons of Hispanic and non-Hispanic origin; persons of Hispanic origin may be of any race.
[7]Poverty level is based on family income and family size using Bureau of the Census poverty thresholds. See Appendix II.
[8]Metropolitan statistical area.
[9]Includes other public assistance through 1996. In 1997 includes state-sponsored health plans. In 1997 the age-adjusted percent of the population under 65 years of age covered by Medicaid was 9.5 percent, and 1.2 percent were covered by state-sponsored health plans.
[10]Includes persons not covered by private insurance, Medicaid, public assistance (through 1996), state-sponsored or other government-sponsored health plans (1997), Medicare, or military plans. Estimates of the percentage of persons lacking health care coverage based on the National Health Interview Survey (NHIS) are slightly higher than those based on the March Current Population Survey (CPS) (table 146). See Appendix II, Health insurance coverage.

NOTE: Percents do not add to 100 because the percent with other types of health insurance (for example, Medicare, military) is not shown, and because persons with both private insurance and Medicaid appear in both columns.

SOURCE: Centers for Disease Control and Prevention, National Center for Health Statistics. National Health Interview Survey.

Table 129 (page 1 of 2). Health care coverage for persons 65 years of age and over, according to type of coverage and selected characteristics: United States, selected years 1984–97

[Data are based on household interviews of a sample of the civilian noninstitutionalized population]

Characteristic	Private insurance[1]						Private insurance obtained through workplace[1,2]					
	1984	1989	1994[3]	1995	1996	1997[3,4]	1984	1989	1994[3]	1995	1996	1997[3,4]
	Number in millions											
Total[5]	19.4	22.4	24.0	23.5	22.9	22.3	10.2	11.2	12.5	12.5	12.1	12.0
	Percent of population											
Total, age adjusted[5,6]	72.5	76.1	77.2	74.8	71.9	69.5	37.2	37.3	39.6	39.0	37.6	37.0
Total, crude[5]	73.3	76.5	77.3	74.8	72.0	69.5	38.8	38.4	40.4	39.6	38.1	37.5
Age												
65–74 years	76.5	78.2	78.4	75.3	72.4	69.9	45.1	43.7	45.6	43.3	41.5	42.0
75 years and over	68.1	73.9	75.8	74.2	71.3	69.1	28.6	30.2	33.0	34.3	33.3	31.6
75–84 years	70.8	75.9	77.9	76.0	73.3	70.2	30.8	32.0	35.0	36.1	35.5	33.2
85 years and over	56.8	65.5	67.9	67.8	63.9	64.7	18.9	22.8	25.1	27.5	25.3	25.6
Sex[6]												
Male	73.4	77.4	78.9	76.6	73.8	72.1	42.5	42.1	43.9	43.3	42.0	42.0
Female	71.9	75.4	76.1	73.6	70.7	67.7	33.7	34.0	36.6	36.0	34.5	33.5
Race[6,7]												
White	75.7	79.8	80.9	78.4	75.2	72.7	38.8	38.7	41.2	40.5	38.8	37.9
Black	41.3	42.3	43.6	40.8	42.9	42.5	22.9	23.7	25.3	24.9	28.6	30.8
Hispanic origin and race[6,7]												
All Hispanic	38.2	42.3	50.0	39.9	37.7	30.6	23.1	22.2	20.5	18.4	18.0	17.7
Mexican	39.1	33.5	42.5	31.9	34.4	31.8	23.9	20.2	20.8	15.9	17.3	17.7
White, non-Hispanic	76.9	81.0	82.3	80.5	77.0	74.9	39.4	39.3	42.2	41.7	39.9	39.0
Black, non-Hispanic	41.0	42.4	44.2	40.6	43.5	42.6	22.6	23.7	25.7	24.7	29.2	30.7
Percent of poverty level[6,8]												
Below 100 percent	43.4	46.1	41.6	38.3	34.3	31.9	12.9	11.6	10.7	11.5	10.6	7.2
100–149 percent	67.1	67.7	69.1	68.6	59.0	54.5	27.2	22.2	25.1	25.3	22.2	17.4
150–199 percent	77.9	81.1	81.4	77.8	75.6	69.8	39.7	39.0	37.3	39.5	37.2	33.3
200 percent or more	85.0	85.5	88.5	86.2	84.1	81.8	50.9	49.4	52.4	50.5	48.9	48.5
Geographic region[6]												
Northeast	76.1	76.1	78.0	76.3	72.8	72.7	41.8	42.2	43.9	44.6	41.6	42.3
Midwest	79.0	81.9	84.4	82.4	80.5	78.5	38.9	40.0	42.2	44.8	41.7	40.7
South	66.8	73.0	70.7	71.1	67.3	66.0	33.4	32.0	35.5	33.9	33.6	32.9
West	69.3	74.7	77.9	69.1	68.7	59.9	36.0	37.1	38.0	33.7	35.0	33.6
Location of residence[6]												
Within MSA[9]	73.6	76.6	77.7	75.0	72.1	68.4	40.3	39.9	41.2	41.1	39.6	38.6
Outside MSA[9]	70.7	74.8	75.7	74.0	71.2	73.2	32.0	30.2	35.1	32.2	31.1	31.8

See footnotes at end of table.

Table 129 (page 2 of 2). **Health care coverage for persons 65 years of age and over, according to type of coverage and selected characteristics: United States, selected years 1984–97**

[Data are based on household interviews of a sample of the civilian noninstitutionalized population]

Characteristic	Medicaid[1,10]						Medicare only[11]					
	1984	1989	1994[3]	1995	1996	1997[3,4]	1984	1989	1994[3]	1995	1996	1997[3,4]
	Number in millions											
Total[5]	1.8	2.0	2.5	2.9	2.7	2.5	4.7	4.5	4.1	4.6	5.7	6.7
	Percent of population											
Total, age adjusted[5,6]	7.2	7.2	8.1	9.3	8.6	7.9	18.6	15.7	13.4	14.8	18.1	20.8
Total, crude[5]	7.0	7.0	7.9	9.2	8.5	7.9	17.9	15.4	13.2	14.8	18.1	20.8
Age												
65–74 years	6.0	6.3	6.8	8.3	7.5	7.5	15.2	13.8	12.3	14.4	18.0	20.3
75 years and over	8.5	8.2	9.6	10.4	9.9	8.4	22.3	17.8	14.5	15.2	18.2	21.5
75–84 years.	7.7	7.9	8.4	9.5	9.0	7.9	20.6	16.2	13.3	14.1	16.8	20.5
85 years and over	11.7	9.7	14.2	13.7	13.0	10.2	29.8	24.9	19.0	19.3	23.4	25.2
Sex[6]												
Male.	4.6	5.2	4.9	5.7	5.6	5.1	18.4	14.9	13.0	14.3	16.9	19.6
Female.	8.9	8.6	10.4	11.8	10.7	9.9	18.8	16.2	13.6	15.1	18.8	21.7
Race[6,7]												
White	5.3	5.6	6.3	7.1	6.9	6.5	17.3	13.9	11.9	13.5	16.9	19.3
Black	25.9	21.2	23.0	27.4	22.4	19.7	31.2	34.9	29.2	29.4	30.6	34.8
Hispanic origin and race[6,7]												
All Hispanic.	26.6	26.4	27.9	32.5	29.7	29.0	29.1	22.7	18.5	23.8	28.8	35.1
White, non-Hispanic.	4.6	4.9	5.3	5.8	5.7	5.4	17.0	13.6	11.5	12.9	16.4	18.4
Black, non-Hispanic.	26.2	21.1	22.3	27.5	22.5	19.5	31.3	34.9	29.4	29.5	29.7	34.8
Percent of poverty level[6,8]												
Below 100 percent.	27.6	28.2	37.0	39.9	38.7	40.0	27.9	26.4	22.6	21.8	25.4	27.0
100–149 percent	7.1	9.0	10.6	13.0	12.7	13.9	22.8	20.7	18.5	17.7	26.5	28.3
150–199 percent	3.4	4.7	3.8	5.4	5.1	5.1	16.9	13.6	12.9	15.9	18.9	22.7
200 percent or more	1.9	2.4	2.0	1.9	2.0	2.7	11.6	11.0	8.1	10.1	12.4	14.6
Geographic region[6]												
Northeast	5.4	5.4	7.5	8.9	7.7	6.5	17.8	17.4	14.4	15.3	20.2	19.8
Midwest	4.4	3.7	3.8	5.7	5.0	5.0	15.8	13.8	10.9	11.1	13.3	15.4
South	9.9	9.7	10.9	11.4	10.3	10.0	20.7	16.6	16.2	15.9	19.4	21.6
West	8.3	9.4	9.7	11.1	11.0	9.9	19.5	14.4	10.5	17.3	18.8	28.3
Location of residence[6]												
Within MSA[9]	6.4	6.5	7.5	8.6	7.9	7.5	18.4	15.9	13.2	15.0	18.8	22.3
Outside MSA[9]	8.5	8.8	9.7	11.6	10.9	9.4	18.9	15.5	14.0	14.2	15.7	15.9

[1]Almost all persons 65 years of age and over are covered by Medicare also. In 1997, 92 percent of older persons with private insurance also had Medicare.
[2]Private insurance originally obtained through a present or former employer or union.
[3]The questionnaire changed compared with previous years. See Appendix II, Health insurance coverage.
[4]Preliminary data.
[5]Includes all other races not shown separately and unknown poverty level.
[6]Estimates are age adjusted to the year 2000 standard using two age groups: 65–74 years and 75 years and over. See Appendix II, Age adjustment.
[7]The race groups white and black include persons of Hispanic and non-Hispanic origin; persons of Hispanic origin may be of any race.
[8]Poverty level is based on family income and family size using Bureau of the Census poverty thresholds. See Appendix II.
[9]Metropolitan statistical area.
[10]Includes public assistance through 1996. In 1997 includes state-sponsored health plans. In 1997 the age-adjusted percent of the population 65 years of age and over covered by Medicaid was 7.4 percent, and 0.4 percent were covered by state-sponsored health plans.
[11]Persons covered by Medicare but not covered by private health insurance, Medicaid, public assistance (through 1996), state-sponsored or other government-sponsored health plans (1997), or military plans. See Appendix II, Health insurance coverage.

NOTE: Percents do not add to 100 because persons with both private health insurance and Medicaid appear in more than one column, and because the percent of persons without health insurance (1.1 percent in 1997) is not shown.

SOURCE: Centers for Disease Control and Prevention, National Center for Health Statistics. National Health Interview Survey.

Table 130. Private health insurance by health maintenance organization (HMO) and other types of coverage according to selected characteristics: United States, selected years 1989–97

[Data are based on household interviews of a sample of the civilian noninstitutionalized population]

	Private health insurance									
	Health maintenance organization[1]					Other				
Characteristic	1989	1994	1995	1996	1997[2]	1989	1994	1995	1996	1997[2]
	Number of persons in millions									
Total[3]	45.1	61.2	68.3	76.2	76.5	140.2	123.4	120.1	112.5	111.5
	Percent of population									
Total, age adjusted[3,4]	18.4	23.5	26.0	28.8	29.1	58.0	47.9	46.2	42.9	41.2
Total, crude[3]	18.5	23.6	26.1	28.9	28.7	57.6	47.5	45.9	42.6	41.8
Age										
Under 18 years	20.1	24.0	27.4	30.2	29.9	51.7	39.8	38.3	36.2	36.2
Under 6 years............	20.1	22.7	26.8	28.9	29.8	47.8	35.5	33.2	32.2	31.5
6–17 years.............	20.2	24.6	27.6	30.9	30.0	53.8	42.2	41.0	38.2	38.5
18–44 years.............	20.3	25.6	28.7	31.6	31.4	55.2	44.1	42.5	39.0	38.1
18–24 years	16.6	20.0	22.0	24.6	24.9	47.8	38.2	39.1	35.8	34.4
25–34 years	21.2	26.8	29.3	32.0	32.4	54.7	42.5	41.0	37.5	35.7
35–44 years	21.7	27.8	32.0	35.3	34.1	61.0	49.3	46.0	42.2	42.3
45–64 years.............	17.6	25.5	27.7	31.5	31.3	65.0	54.8	52.6	48.0	47.7
45–54 years	19.6	27.8	29.5	34.3	33.6	63.9	53.4	51.5	46.2	46.9
55–64 years	15.3	22.1	24.9	27.2	27.9	66.4	56.7	54.3	50.9	49.0
65 years or more	10.4	13.1	12.2	12.3	12.5	67.0	64.3	62.6	59.6	57.0
65–74 years	11.4	14.8	13.9	14.0	14.4	67.7	63.6	61.3	58.4	55.5
75 years or more.	8.9	10.6	9.8	10.0	10.0	65.9	65.2	64.4	61.4	59.0
Sex[4]										
Male	18.5	23.4	26.1	28.7	29.0	58.2	48.7	46.7	43.5	41.8
Female	18.3	23.7	25.9	28.8	29.1	57.7	47.3	45.8	42.4	40.7
Race[4,5]										
White	18.1	23.6	26.2	29.1	29.3	61.4	51.3	49.2	45.5	44.7
Black.................	19.7	22.3	24.0	26.5	27.9	37.2	29.5	29.6	28.1	25.8
Asian or Pacific Islander	24.1	30.6	31.8	33.6	35.2	45.0	35.1	33.9	29.9	30.5
Hispanic origin and race[4,5]										
All Hispanic	18.8	23.1	23.2	25.9	25.4	33.3	26.2	23.9	21.1	20.4
Mexican	16.6	23.9	21.6	24.5	23.6	30.3	21.9	21.4	18.6	18.7
Puerto Rican.	16.6	22.5	22.2	23.8	23.9	28.3	26.6	25.6	26.9	20.9
Cuban	25.5	25.0	31.2	34.9	37.7	42.1	37.5	29.5	28.8	28.7
Other Hispanic	22.0	21.1	25.4	28.2	27.4	39.9	32.7	27.1	22.7	21.9
White, non-Hispanic	18.2	23.8	26.7	29.8	30.0	64.3	54.4	52.3	48.7	47.7
Black, non-Hispanic	19.7	22.4	24.2	26.5	27.9	37.3	29.8	29.8	28.5	26.1
Percent of poverty level[4,6]										
Below 100 percent	5.4	6.5	6.8	6.5	8.8	24.5	18.2	17.8	15.9	14.8
100–149 percent	13.4	14.4	16.5	17.2	17.3	42.7	34.9	33.8	31.1	26.0
150–199 percent	17.3	21.7	23.6	26.4	26.2	54.7	45.3	43.9	41.8	38.4
200 percent or more...........	22.5	30.5	33.1	37.3	37.1	68.0	58.2	55.6	51.3	50.0
Geographic region[4]										
Northeast.	20.1	26.3	30.1	31.6	37.7	61.4	49.3	45.6	43.6	36.2
Midwest.....................	20.2	20.8	23.5	27.6	25.6	61.6	57.7	54.9	51.4	51.5
South	11.7	18.3	20.8	23.2	23.6	60.3	48.3	47.1	43.5	43.2
West	25.7	32.0	33.4	36.2	34.9	46.6	35.5	35.2	31.7	29.8
Location of residence[4]										
Within MSA[7]	21.3	27.1	29.2	32.3	32.1	55.6	44.9	43.9	40.6	38.6
Outside MSA[7]	8.1	11.0	13.4	15.6	17.0	66.0	58.5	55.5	51.4	51.5

[1]Persons reporting private health insurance coverage are considered to have health maintenance organization (HMO) coverage if they responded positively to the question "Is this plan an HMO or IPA (individual practice association)?" Does not include Medicaid or Medicare HMO plans.
[2]Preliminary data. The questionnaire changed compared with previous years. See Appendix II, Health insurance coverage.
[3]Includes all other races not shown separately and unknown poverty level.
[4]Estimates are age adjusted to the year 2000 standard using five age groups: Under 18 years, 18–44 years, 45–64 years, 65–74 years, and 75 years and over. See Appendix II, Age adjustment.
[5]The race groups white, black, and Asian or Pacific Islander include persons of Hispanic and non-Hispanic origin; persons of Hispanic origin may be of any race.
[6]Poverty level is based on family income and family size using Bureau of the Census poverty thresholds. See Appendix II.
[7]Metropolitan statistical area.

SOURCE: Centers for Disease Control and Prevention, National Center for Health Statistics. National Health Interview Survey.

Table 131. Health maintenance organizations (HMO's) and enrollment, according to model type, geographic region, and Federal program: United States, selected years 1976–99

[Data are based on a census of health maintenance organizations]

Plans and enrollment	1976	1980	1985[1]	1990	1993	1994[2]	1995[2]	1996[a]	1997[2]	1998[2]	1999[2]
Plans						Number					
All plans	174	235	478	572	551	543	562	630	652	651	643
Model type:[3]											
Individual practice association[4]	41	97	244	360	332	321	332	367	284	317	309
Group[5]	122	138	234	212	150	118	108	122	98	116	123
Mixed	- - -	- - -	- - -	- - -	69	104	122	141	258	212	208
Geographic region:											
Northeast	29	55	81	115	102	101	100	111	110	107	110
Midwest	52	72	157	160	169	159	157	182	184	185	179
South	23	45	141	176	167	173	196	218	236	237	239
West	70	63	99	121	113	110	109	119	121	122	115
Enrollment						Number of persons in millions					
Total	6.0	9.1	21.0	33.0	38.4	45.1	50.9	59.1	66.8	76.6	81.3
Model type:[3]											
Individual practice association[4]	0.4	1.7	6.4	13.7	15.3	17.8	20.1	26.0	26.7	32.6	32.8
Group[5]	5.6	7.4	14.6	19.3	15.4	13.9	13.3	14.1	11.0	13.8	15.9
Mixed	- - -	- - -	- - -	- - -	7.7	13.4	17.6	19.0	29.0	30.1	32.6
Federal program:[6]											
Medicaid[7]	- - -	0.3	0.6	1.2	1.7	2.6	3.5	4.7	5.6	7.8	10.4
Medicare	- - -	0.4	1.1	1.8	2.2	2.5	2.9	3.7	4.8	5.7	6.5
						Percent of HMO enrollees					
Model type:[3]											
Individual practice association[4]	6.6	18.7	30.4	41.6	39.8	39.4	39.4	44.1	39.9	42.6	40.3
Group[5]	93.4	81.3	69.6	58.4	40.1	30.7	26.0	23.7	16.5	18.0	19.6
Mixed	- - -	- - -	- - -	- - -	20.1	29.9	34.5	32.2	43.4	39.2	40.1
Federal program:[6]											
Medicaid[7]	- - -	2.9	2.7	3.5	4.4	5.8	6.9	8.0	8.2	10.2	12.7
Medicare	- - -	4.3	5.1	5.4	5.7	5.5	5.7	6.3	7.2	7.4	8.0
						Percent of population enrolled in HMO's					
Total	2.8	4.0	8.9	13.4	15.1	17.3	19.4	22.3	25.2	28.6	30.1
Geographic region:											
Northeast	2.0	3.1	7.9	14.6	18.0	20.8	24.4	25.9	32.4	37.8	36.7
Midwest	1.5	2.8	9.7	12.6	13.2	15.2	16.4	18.8	19.5	22.7	23.3
South	0.4	0.8	3.8	7.1	8.4	10.2	12.4	15.2	17.9	21.0	23.9
West	9.7	12.2	17.3	23.2	25.1	27.4	28.6	33.2	36.4	39.1	41.4

- - - Data not available.

[1]Increases partly due to changes in reporting methods. See Appendix I, InterStudy.

[2]Open-ended enrollment in HMO plans, amounting to 8.9 million on Jan. 1, 1999, is included from 1994 onwards. See Appendix II, Health maintenance organization.

[3]In 1976, 11 HMO's with 35,000 enrollment did not report model type. In 1997, 11 HMO's with 153,000 enrollment did not report model type. In 1998, 6 HMO's with 109,000 enrollment did not report model type. In 1999, 3 HMO's with 18,000 enrollment did not report model type.

[4]An HMO operating under an individual practice association model contracts with an association of physicians from various settings (a mixture of solo and group practices) to provide health services.

[5]Group includes staff, group, and network model types.

[6]Federal program enrollment in HMO's refers to enrollment by Medicaid or Medicare beneficiaries, where the Medicaid or Medicare program contracts directly with the HMO to pay the appropriate annual premium.

[7]Data for 1990 and later include enrollment in managed care health insuring organizations.

NOTES: Data as of June 30 in 1976–80, December 31 in 1985, and January 1 in 1990–99. Medicaid enrollment in 1990 is as of June 30. HMO's in Guam are included starting in 1994; HMO's in Puerto Rico, starting in 1998. In 1999 HMO enrollment in Guam was 93,000 and in Puerto Rico, 1,354,000. Data for additional years are available (see Appendix III).

SOURCES: Office of Health Maintenance Organizations: Summary of the National HMO census of prepaid plans—June 1976 and National HMO Census 1980. Public Health Service. Washington. U.S. Government Printing Office. DHHS Pub. No. (PHS) 80–50159; InterStudy: National HMO Census: Annual Report on the Growth of HMO's in the U.S., 1984–1985 Editions; The InterStudy Edge, 1990, vol. 2; Competitive Edge, vols. 1–9, 1991–1999; 1986 December Update of Medicare Enrollment in HMO's. 1988 January Update of Medicare Enrollment in HMO's. Excelsior, Minnesota (Copyrights 1983–98: Used with the permission of InterStudy); U.S. Bureau of the Census. Current Population Reports. Series P–25, Nos. 998 and 1058. Washington: U.S. Government Printing Office, Dec. 1986 and Mar. 1990. U.S. Dept. of Commerce. Press release CB 91–100. Mar. 11, 1991; Health Care Financing Administration: Unpublished data.

Table 132 (page 1 of 2). Medical care benefits for employees of private establishments by size of establishment and occupation: United States, selected years 1990–97

[Data are based on a survey of employers]

Size of establishment and type of benefit	All			Professional, technical, and related			Clerical and sales			Blue-collar and service		
	1990	1994	1996	1990	1994	1996	1990	1994	1996	1990	1994	1996
Small private establishments[1]	Percent of all employees											
Participation in medical care benefit:												
Full-time employees..................	69	66	64	82	80	76	75	70	69	60	57	56
Part-time employees	6	7	6	6	11	14	7	9	9	6	5	3
Type of medical care benefit among participating full-time employees	Percent of participating full-time employees											
Fee arrangement	100	100	100	100	100	100	100	100	100	100	100	100
Traditional fee-for-service	74	55	36	69	53	31	77	55	34	73	57	41
Preferred provider organization (PPO)	13	24	35	16	27	41	13	24	36	11	23	32
Health maintenance organization (HMO) ...	14	19	27	15	20	27	10	19	28	15	20	25
Other	0	1	2	0	0	1	0	2	2	0	0	2
Individual coverage:												
Employee contributions not required	58	47	48	56	49	49	53	44	46	62	48	48
Employee contributions required	42	53	52	44	51	51	47	56	54	38	52	51
Family coverage:												
Employee contributions not required	32	19	24	28	17	21	29	15	20	37	23	29
Employee contributions required	68	81	75	72	83	78	71	85	80	63	77	70
Individual coverage:	Average monthly contribution											
Average monthly employee contribution:												
Total	$ 25	$ 41	$ 43	$ 24	$ 47	$ 41	$ 24	$ 41	$ 42	$ 27	$ 38	$ 44
Non-HMO	25	39	43	24	46	40	24	38	43	28	36	45
HMO.............................	25	49	41	24	48	42	27	50	42	25	47	41
Family coverage:												
Average monthly employee contribution:												
Total	109	160	182	112	181	190	106	160	181	111	149	177
Non-HMO	104	151	181	110	173	192	102	155	181	101	137	175
HMO.............................	135	190	182	118	204	183	134	178	183	145	191	182

See footnotes at end of table.

Table 132 (page 2 of 2). **Medical care benefits for employees of private establishments by size of establishment and occupation: United States, selected years 1990–97**

[Data are based on a survey of employers]

Size of establishment and type of benefit	All			Professional, technical, and related			Clerical and sales			Blue-collar and service		
	1991	1995	1997	1991	1995	1997	1991	1995	1997	1991	1995	1997
Medium and large private establishments[2]	Percent of all employees											
Participation in medical care benefit:												
Full-time employees.................	83	77	76	85	80	79	81	76	78	84	75	74
Part-time employees	28	19	21	42	31	29	26	20	20	26	15	19
Type of medical care benefit among participating full-time employees	Percent of participating full-time employees											
Fee arrangement	100	100	100	100	100	100	100	100	100	100	100	100
Traditional fee-for-service	67	37	27	62	29	20	59	30	22	73	45	33
Preferred provider organization (PPO)	16	34	40	19	36	40	21	36	42	12	33	39
Health maintenance organization (HMO) ...	17	27	33	18	33	40	19	32	36	14	21	28
Other	0	1	1	1	1	0	0	2	0	0	1	0
Individual coverage:												
Employee contributions not required	49	33	31	45	21	20	43	24	24	55	44	40
Employee contributions required	51	67	69	55	79	80	57	76	76	45	56	60
Family coverage:												
Employee contributions not required	31	22	20	25	11	10	27	15	14	37	33	29
Employee contributions required	69	78	80	75	89	90	73	85	86	63	67	71
Individual coverage:	Average monthly contribution											
Average monthly employee contribution:												
Total	$ 27	$ 34	$ 39	$ 26	$ 35	$ 37	$ 28	$ 36	$ 39	$ 26	$ 32	$ 40
Non-HMO	26	33	42	26	33	40	27	34	41	25	32	43
HMO.	29	36	34	29	38	33	32	39	36	28	32	34
Family coverage:												
Average monthly employee contribution:												
Total	97	118	130	96	120	125	108	127	135	91	112	131
Non-HMO	92	112	132	93	116	128	104	120	134	84	106	134
HMO.	118	133	126	110	128	120	121	141	138	122	130	124

[1]Less than 100 employees in all private nonfarm industries.
[2]100 or more employees in all private nonfarm industries.

NOTE: In 1992–93, 88 percent of full-time employees in private establishments were offered health care plans by their employers (96 percent in medium and large private establishments and 80 percent in small private establishments\)

SOURCES: U.S. Department of Labor, Bureau of Labor Statistics, Employee benefits in small private establishments, 1990 Bulletin 2388, September 1991, 1994 Bulletin 2475, April 1996, and 1996 Bulletin 2507, April 1999. Employee benefits in medium and large private establishments, 1991 Bulletin 2422, May 1993, 1997 Bulletin 2517, Sept. 1999, and news release USDL 97–246. July 25, 1997. Blostin AP and Pfuntner JN. Employee medical care contributions on the rise. Compensation and Working Conditions, Spring 1998.

Table 133 (page 1 of 2). Medicare enrollees and expenditures and percent distribution, according to type of service: United States and other areas, selected years 1970–98

[Data are compiled by the Health Care Financing Administration]

Type of service	1970	1980	1985	1990	1995	1996	1997	1998[1]
Enrollees				Number in millions				
Total[2]	20.5	28.5	31.1	34.2	37.5	38.1	38.4	38.8
Hospital insurance	20.4	28.1	30.6	33.7	37.1	37.7	38.1	38.4
Supplementary medical insurance	19.6	27.4	30.0	32.6	35.7	36.1	36.5	36.8
Expenditures				Amount in millions				
Total	$7,493	$36,822	$72,294	$110,984	$184,203	$200,337	$213,576	$213,401
Total hospital insurance (HI)	5,281	25,577	48,414	66,997	117,604	129,929	139,452	135,771
HI payments to managed care organizations[3]	- - -	7	768	2,654	6,701	11,777	16,338	18,759
HI payments for fee-for-service utilization	5,281	25,570	47,646	64,343	110,903	118,152	123,114	117,012
Inpatient hospital	4,827	24,109	44,172	56,922	81,984	85,756	88,498	87,029
Skilled nursing facility	246	395	548	2,488	9,236	11,101	12,995	13,487
Home health agency[4]	51	540	1,913	3,661	16,373	17,825	17,680	12,337
Hospice	. . .	. . .	43	325	1,883	1,997	2,082	2,180
Administrative expenses[5]	157	525	970	947	1,428	1,472	1,860	1,980
Total supplementary medical insurance (SMI)	2,212	11,245	23,880	43,987	66,599	70,408	74,124	77,630
SMI payments to managed care organizations[3]	26	203	720	2,827	6,610	9,558	10,962	15,338
SMI payments for fee-for-service utilization[6]	2,186	11,042	23,160	41,160	59,989	60,850	63,162	62,292
Physician/supplies[7]	1,790	8,187	17,312	29,609	- - -	- - -	- - -	- - -
Outpatient hospital[8]	114	1,897	4,319	8,482	- - -	- - -	- - -	- - -
Independent laboratory[9]	11	114	558	1,476	- - -	- - -	- - -	- - -
Physician fee schedule	- - -	- - -	- - -	- - -	31,660	31,631	31,901	32,456
Durable medical equipment	- - -	- - -	- - -	- - -	3,689	3,826	4,237	4,033
Laboratory[10]	- - -	- - -	- - -	- - -	4,255	3,861	3,833	3,564
Other[11]	- - -	- - -	- - -	- - -	9,859	10,770	12,109	12,271
Hospital[12]	- - -	- - -	- - -	- - -	8,663	8,691	9,455	8,844
Home health agency[4]	34	234	38	74	236	262	261	−382
Administrative expenses[5]	237	610	933	1,519	1,627	1,810	1,368	1,505
				Percent distribution of expenditures				
Total hospital insurance (HI)	100.0	100.0	100.0	100.0	100.0	100.0	100.0	100.0
HI payments to managed care organizations[3]	- - -	0.0	1.6	4.0	5.7	9.1	11.7	13.8
HI payments for fee-for-service utilization	100.0	100.0	98.4	96.0	94.3	90.9	88.3	86.2
Inpatient hospital	91.4	94.3	91.2	85.0	69.7	66.0	63.5	64.1
Skilled nursing facility	4.7	1.5	1.1	3.7	7.9	8.5	9.3	9.9
Home health agency[4]	1.0	2.1	4.0	5.5	13.9	13.7	12.7	9.1
Hospice	. . .	. . .	0.1	0.5	1.6	1.5	1.5	1.6
Administrative expenses[5]	3.0	2.1	2.0	1.4	1.2	1.1	1.3	1.5

See footnotes at end of table.

Table 133 (page 2 of 2). Medicare enrollees and expenditures and percent distribution, according to type of service: United States and other areas, selected years 1970–98

[Data are compiled by the Health Care Financing Administration]

Type of service	1970	1980	1985	1990	1995	1996	1997	1998[1]
	Percent distribution of expenditures							
Total supplementary medical insurance (SMI)	100.0	100.0	100.0	100.0	100.0	100.0	100.0	100.0
SMI payments to managed care organizations[3] . . .	1.2	1.8	3.0	6.4	10.0	13.6	14.5	19.8
SMI payments for fee-for-service utilization[6]	98.8	98.2	97.0	93.6	90.0	86.4	85.5	80.2
Physician/supplies[7]	80.9	72.8	72.5	67.3	- - -	- - -	- - -	- - -
Outpatient hospital[8]	5.2	16.9	18.1	19.3	- - -	- - -	- - -	- - -
Independent laboratory[9]	0.5	1.0	2.3	3.4	- - -	- - -	- - -	- - -
Physician fee schedule.	- - -	- - -	- - -	- - -	47.5	44.9	43.0	41.8
Durable medical equipment.	- - -	- - -	- - -	- - -	5.5	5.4	5.7	5.2
Laboratory[10]	- - -	- - -	- - -	- - -	6.4	5.5	5.2	4.6
Other[11]	- - -	- - -	- - -	- - -	14.8	15.3	16.3	15.8
Hospital[12]	- - -	- - -	- - -	- - -	13.0	12.3	12.8	11.4
Home health agency[4]	1.5	2.1	0.2	0.2	0.4	0.4	0.4	−0.5
Administrative expenses[5]	10.7	5.4	3.9	3.5	2.4	2.6	1.8	1.9

- - - Data not available.
. . . Category not applicable.

[1]Preliminary figures; home health agency expenditures for 1998 reflect annual home health SMI to HI transfer amounts.
[2]Number enrolled in the hospital insurance and/or supplementary medical insurance programs on July 1.
[3]Medicare-approved managed care organizations. Prior to 1998 this category was called group practice prepayment.
[4]Reflects annual home health SMI to HI transfer amounts for 1998 and later.
[5]Includes research, costs of experiments and demonstration projects, and peer review activity.
[6]Type of service reporting categories for fee-for-service reimbursement differ before and after 1991.
[7]Includes payment for physicians, practitioners, durable medical equipment and all suppliers other than Independent laboratory, which is shown separately through 1990. Beginning in 1991, those physician services subject to the Physician fee schedule are so broken out. Payments for laboratory services paid under the Laboratory fee schedule and performed in a physician office are included under "Laboratory" beginning in 1991. Payments for durable medical equipment are broken out and so labeled beginning in 1991. The remaining services from the "Physician" category are included in "Other."
[8]Includes payments for hospital outpatient department services, for skilled nursing facility outpatient services, for Part B services received as an inpatient in a hospital or skilled nursing facility setting and for other types of outpatient facilities. Beginning 1991, payments for hospital outpatient department services, except for laboratory services, are listed under "Hospital." Hospital outpatient laboratory services are included in the "Laboratory" line.
[9]Beginning in 1991 most of the independent laboratory services were paid under the Laboratory fee schedule and are included in the "Laboratory" line; the remaining services are included in "Physician fee schedule" and "Other" lines.
[10]Payments for laboratory services paid under the Laboratory fee schedule performed in a physician office, independent lab, or in a hospital outpatient department.
[11]Includes payments for free-standing ambulatory surgical center facility services; ambulance services; supplies; free-standing end-stage renal disease (ESRD) dialysis facility services; rural health clinics; outpatient rehabilitation facilities; psychiatric hospitals; and federally qualified health centers.
[12]Includes the hospital facility costs for Medicare Part B services which are predominantly in the outpatient department, with the exception of hospital outpatient laboratory services, which are included on the "Laboratory" line. The physician reimbursement is included on the "Physician fee schedule" line.

NOTES: Table includes service disbursements as of December 1999 for Medicare enrollees residing in Puerto Rico, Virgin Islands, Guam, other outlying areas, foreign countries, and unknown residence. Some numbers in this table have been revised and differ from previous editions of Health, United States.

SOURCE: Health Care Financing Administration. Medicare and Medicaid Cost Estimates Group, Office of the Actuary and Office of Information Services.

Table 134. Medicare enrollees and program payments among fee-for-service Medicare beneficiaries, according to sex and age: United States and other areas, 1994–97

[Data are compiled by the Health Care Financing Administration]

Sex and age	1994	1995	1996	1997
	Fee-for-service enrollees in thousands			
Total	34,076	34,062	33,704	33,009
Sex				
Male	14,533	14,563	14,440	14,149
Female	19,543	19,499	19,264	18,860
Age				
Under 65 years	4,031	4,239	4,413	4,498
65–74 years	16,713	16,373	15,810	15,099
75–84 years	9,845	9,911	9,915	9,847
85 years and over	3,486	3,540	3,566	3,565
	Fee-for-service program payments in millions			
Total	$146,549	$158,980	$167,063	$175,423
Sex				
Male	63,907	68,758	71,011	75,357
Female	82,642	90,222	95,052	100,066
Age				
Under 65 years	18,835	21,029	24,160	25,798
65–74 years	55,147	58,093	58,737	59,687
75–84 years	50,719	55,256	58,058	61,708
85 years and over	21,847	24,602	26,108	28,231
	Percent distribution of fee-for-service program payments			
Total	100.0	100.0	100.0	100.0
Sex				
Male	43.6	43.2	42.5	43.0
Female	56.4	56.8	56.9	57.0
Age				
Under 65 years	12.9	13.2	14.5	14.7
65–74 years	37.6	36.5	35.2	34.0
75–84 years	34.6	34.8	34.8	35.2
85 years and over	14.9	15.5	15.6	16.1
	Average fee-for-service payment per enrollee			
Total	$ 4,301	$ 4,667	$ 4,957	$ 5,314
Sex				
Male	4,397	4,721	4,918	5,326
Female	4,229	4,627	4,934	5,306
Age				
Under 65 years	4,673	4,960	5,475	5,735
65–74 years	3,300	3,548	3,715	3,953
75–84 years	5,152	5,576	5,856	6,267
85 years and over	6,267	6,950	7,321	7,919

NOTE: Table includes data for Medicare enrollees residing in Puerto Rico, Virgin Islands, Guam, other outlying areas, foreign countries, and unknown residence.

SOURCE: Health Care Financing Administration, Office of Strategic Planning. Health Care Financing Review: Medicare and Medicaid Statistical Supplements for years 1996 to 1999.

Table 135 (page 1 of 2). Medicare beneficiaries by race and ethnicity, according to selected characteristics: United States, selected years 1992–96

[Data are based on household interviews of a sample of current Medicare beneficiaries and Medicare administrative records]

Characteristic	All 1996	White, non-Hispanic 1992	1994	1996	Black, non-Hispanic 1992	1994	1996	Hispanic 1992	1994	1996
		Number of beneficiaries in millions								
All Medicare beneficiaries......	39.4	30.9	31.8	32.5	3.3	3.5	3.5	1.9	2.1	2.4
		Percent distribution of beneficiaries								
All Medicare beneficiaries......	100.0	84.2	83.4	82.4	8.9	9.1	8.9	5.2	5.6	6.2
Medical care use		Percent of beneficiaries with at least one service								
All Medicare beneficiaries:										
Long-term care facility stay ...	9.2	8.0	9.3	9.6	6.2	7.8	7.9	4.2	3.9	4.5
Community only residents:										
Inpatient hospital	18.5	18.1	18.1	18.5	18.4	21.1	20.0	16.6	16.5	17.6
Outpatient hospital	64.6	57.8	61.3	65.1	61.1	59.0	65.7	53.1	59.4	60.2
Physician/supplier[1]	93.6	93.0	94.0	94.3	89.1	88.5	88.7	87.9	89.4	90.7
Dental.................	40.4	43.1	42.5	43.9	23.5	19.4	18.8	29.1	26.6	27.6
Prescription medicine	86.7	85.5	85.7	86.8	83.1	82.0	85.0	84.6	86.1	86.8
Expenditures[2]		Expenditures per beneficiary								
All Medicare beneficiaries:										
Total	$ 9,032	$ 6,718	$ 7,878	$ 8,893	$ 6,912	$ 9,085	$10,670	$ 5,642	$ 7,057	$ 7,798
Long-term care facility	2,263	1,679	2,140	2,373	1,258	1,837	2,005	760	943	1,187
Community only residents:										
Total personal health care	$ 6,635	$ 4,988	$ 5,616	$ 6,492	$ 5,530	$ 6,622	$ 8,058	$ 4,938	$ 5,995	$ 6,328
Inpatient hospital..........	2,410	2,058	2,191	2,358	2,493	2,857	2,895	1,999	2,090	2,243
Outpatient hospital	706	478	547	624	668	657	1,282	511	803	874
Physician/supplier[1]	1,981	1,525	1,639	1,969	1,398	1,679	2,124	1,587	1,838	1,957
Dental	203	153	175	224	70	71	84	97	80	128
Prescription medicine	669	481	546	680	417	506	602	389	508	653
Long-term care facility residents only:										
Long-term care facility.......	29,771	23,177	26,612	29,498	21,272	27,963	28,258	25,026	32,006	34,329
Sex		Percent distribution of beneficiaries								
Both sexes	100.0	100.0	100.0	100.0	100.0	100.0	100.0	100.0	100.0	100.0
Male..................	43.9	42.7	43.0	43.7	42.0	42.1	43.5	46.7	47.7	48.2
Female	56.1	57.3	57.0	56.3	58.0	58.0	56.6	53.3	52.3	51.8
Eligibility criteria and age										
All Medicare beneficiaries......	100.0	100.0	100.0	100.0	100.0	100.0	100.0	100.0	100.0	100.0
Disabled	12.1	8.6	9.2	10.0	19.1	22.2	24.2	16.5	18.5	22.1
Under 45 years..........	4.2	2.9	3.2	3.5	7.6	8.7	9.3	6.9	6.6	5.8
45–64 years	7.9	5.8	6.1	6.5	11.5	13.6	14.9	9.6	11.9	16.3
Aged..................	87.9	91.4	90.8	90.0	81.0	77.7	75.8	83.5	81.7	77.7
65–74 years	46.7	52.0	51.1	46.9	48.0	46.2	42.5	49.4	48.8	47.7
75–84 years	30.6	29.5	29.3	31.9	24.0	23.0	24.4	27.1	24.9	23.1
85 years and over........	10.7	9.9	10.4	11.2	9.0	8.4	8.9	6.9	8.0	6.9
Living arrangement										
All	100.0	100.0	100.0	100.0	100.0	100.0	100.0	100.0	100.0	100.0
Alone	28.8	27.5	27.2	28.9	27.7	27.5	31.3	20.2	20.2	24.0
With spouse..............	49.9	53.3	53.6	52.2	33.3	33.3	32.6	50.4	50.6	46.4
With children	8.3	7.7	7.4	6.8	16.8	16.6	15.3	16.6	16.5	16.5
With others	7.0	6.2	6.1	5.8	18.1	17.9	15.4	10.8	10.8	10.7
Long-term care facility.......	6.0	5.3	5.7	6.3	4.0	4.8	5.4	2.0	1.9	2.5

See footnotes at end of table.

Table 135 (page 2 of 2). Medicare beneficiaries by race and ethnicity, according to selected characteristics: United States, selected years 1992–96

[Data are based on household interviews of a sample of current Medicare beneficiaries and Medicare administrative records]

Characteristic	All	White, non-Hispanic			Black, non-Hispanic			Hispanic		
	1996	1992	1994	1996	1992	1994	1996	1992	1994	1996
Age and limitation of activity[3]	Percent distribution of beneficiaries									
Under 65 years (disabled)	100.0	100.0	100.0	100.0	100.0	100.0	100.0	100.0	100.0	100.0
None.	26.9	21.8	25.3	22.9	26.2	33.0	30.5	21.2	24.5	25.0
IADL only	39.7	38.9	35.1	39.7	35.8	34.0	38.5	46.1	42.5	43.4
1 or 2 ADL.	19.6	21.5	23.9	21.9	21.2	20.0	21.3	20.9	16.9	16.7
3–5 ADL	13.8	17.9	15.7	15.6	16.8	13.0	9.6	11.9	16.2	14.9
65–74 years	100.0	100.0	100.0	100.0	100.0	100.0	100.0	100.0	100.0	100.0
None.	71.8	68.7	70.2	71.7	55.1	54.3	60.7	59.2	63.0	69.8
IADL only	15.4	17.0	16.7	15.5	22.9	22.9	16.5	20.9	21.9	20.1
1 or 2 ADL.	8.1	9.6	8.7	8.3	14.4	13.9	14.9	15.7	10.6	7.4
3–5 ADL	4.7	4.6	4.4	4.5	7.6	8.8	7.9	4.2	4.6	2.7
75–84 years	100.0	100.0	100.0	100.0	100.0	100.0	100.0	100.0	100.0	100.0
None.	52.3	47.5	48.8	54.2	42.0	41.9	47.3	44.3	52.0	47.4
IADL only	21.4	23.6	22.2	20.4	26.7	21.6	18.6	27.8	19.9	24.3
1 or 2 ADL.	14.9	16.8	16.9	14.9	15.3	18.4	19.0	14.9	15.4	14.2
3–5 ADL	11.4	12.2	12.1	10.6	15.9	18.1	15.2	13.0	12.7	14.1
85 years and over	100.0	100.0	100.0	100.0	100.0	100.0	100.0	100.0	100.0	100.0
None.	22.1	20.2	19.3	23.3	19.6	18.7	24.7	19.7	19.5	21.4
IADL only	20.9	20.2	21.7	21.3	22.1	25.0	17.9	24.7	28.7	23.8
1 or 2 ADL.	20.2	23.5	22.3	21.3	24.3	18.3	20.3	23.7	19.6	24.3
3–5 ADL	36.9	36.1	36.7	34.1	34.0	38.0	37.2	31.8	32.1	30.5

[1]Physician/supplier services include medical and osteopathic doctor and health practitioner visits; diagnostic laboratory and radiology services; medical and surgical services; durable medical equipment and nondurable medical supplies.
[2]Total health expenditures by Medicare beneficiaries, including expenses paid by Medicare and all other sources of payment.
[3]See Appendix II for definitions of Limitation of activity, Activities of Daily Living (ADL), and Instrumental Activities of Daily Living (IADL). includes data for both community and long-term care facility residents.

SOURCES: Health Care Financing Administration. Health and Health Care of the Medicare Population: Data from the 1992 Medicare Current Beneficiary Survey; Data from the 1994 Medicare Current Beneficiary Survey. 1996 data from the Medicare Current Beneficiary Survey at http://www.hcfa.gov.

Table 136. Medicaid recipients and medical vendor payments, according to basis of eligibility, and race and ethnicity: United States, selected fiscal years 1972–98

[Data are compiled by the Health Care Financing Administration]

Basis of eligibility and race and ethnicity	1972	1975	1980	1985	1990	1995	1996	1997	1998[1]
Recipients					Number in millions				
All recipients	17.6	22.0	21.6	21.8	25.3	36.3	36.1	34.9	40.6
					Percent of recipients				
Basis of eligibility:[2]									
Aged (65 years and over)	18.8	16.4	15.9	14.0	12.7	11.4	11.9	11.3	9.8
Blind and disabled	9.8	11.2	13.5	13.8	14.7	16.1	17.2	17.6	16.3
Adults in families with dependent children[3]	17.8	20.6	22.6	25.3	23.8	21.0	19.7	19.5	19.5
Children under age 21[4]	44.5	43.6	43.2	44.7	44.4	47.3	46.3	45.3	46.7
Other Title XIX[5]	9.0	8.2	6.9	5.6	3.9	1.7	1.8	6.3	7.8
Race and ethnicity:[6]									
White	---	---	---	---	42.8	45.5	44.8	44.4	41.3
Black	---	---	---	---	25.1	24.7	23.9	23.5	24.2
American Indian or Alaska Native	---	---	---	---	1.0	0.8	0.8	1.0	0.8
Asian or Pacific Islander	---	---	---	---	2.0	2.2	2.1	1.9	2.5
Hispanic	---	---	---	---	15.2	17.2	17.5	14.3	15.6
Unknown	---	---	---	---	14.0	9.6	10.9	14.9	15.5
Vendor payments[7]					Amount in billions				
All payments	$ 6.3	$ 12.2	$ 23.3	$ 37.5	$ 64.9	$120.1	$121.7	$124.4	$ 142.3
					Percent distribution				
Total	100.0	100.0	100.0	100.0	100.0	100.0	100.0	100.0	100.0
Basis of eligibility:									
Aged (65 years and over)	30.6	35.6	37.5	37.6	33.2	30.4	30.4	30.3	28.5
Blind and disabled	22.2	25.7	32.7	35.9	37.6	41.1	42.8	43.5	42.4
Adults in families with dependent children[3]	15.3	16.8	13.9	12.7	13.2	11.2	10.1	9.9	10.4
Children under age 21[4]	18.1	17.9	13.4	11.8	14.0	15.0	14.4	14.1	16.0
Other Title XIX[5]	13.9	4.0	2.6	2.1	1.6	1.2	1.2	2.2	2.6
Race and ethnicity:[6]									
White	---	---	---	---	53.4	54.3	54.1	55.0	54.3
Black	---	---	---	---	18.3	19.2	18.7	18.5	19.6
American Indian or Alaska Native	---	---	---	---	0.6	0.5	0.6	0.6	0.8
Asian or Pacific Islander	---	---	---	---	1.0	1.2	1.1	0.9	1.4
Hispanic	---	---	---	---	5.3	7.3	7.4	6.8	8.2
Unknown	---	---	---	---	21.3	17.6	18.1	18.2	15.7
Vendor payments per recipient[7]					Amount				
All recipients	$ 358	$ 556	$1,079	$1,719	$2,568	$3,311	$3,369	$3,568	$ 3,501
Basis of eligibility:									
Aged (65 years and over)	580	1,206	2,540	4,605	6,717	8,868	8,622	9,538	10,242
Blind and disabled	807	1,276	2,618	4,459	6,564	8,435	8,369	8,832	9,095
Adults in families with dependent children[3]	307	455	662	860	1,429	1,777	1,722	1,809	1,876
Children under age 21[4]	145	228	335	452	811	1,047	1,048	1,111	1,203
Other Title XIX[5]	555	273	398	657	1,062	2,380	2,152	1,242	1,166
Race and ethnicity:[6]									
White	---	---	---	---	3,207	3,953	4,074	4,421	4,609
Black	---	---	---	---	1,878	2,568	2,631	2,798	2,836
American Indian or Alaska Native	---	---	---	---	1,706	2,142	2,298	2,500	3,297
Asian or Pacific Islander	---	---	---	---	1,257	1,713	1,767	1,610	1,924
Hispanic	---	---	---	---	903	1,400	1,428	1,699	1,842
Unknown	---	---	---	---	3,909	6,099	5,603	4,356	3,531

--- Data not available.

[1]Prior to 1998 recipient counts exclude those individuals who only received coverage under prepaid health care and for whom no direct vendor payments were made during the year. Prior to 1998 vendor payments exclude payments to health maintenance organizations and other prepaid health plans ($19.3 billion in 1998 and $18 billion in 1997). The total number of persons who were Medicaid eligible and enrolled was 41.4 million in 1998, 41.6 million in 1997, and 41.2 million in 1996 (HCFA Medicaid Statistics, Program and Financial Statistics FY1996, FY1997, and FY1998. unpublished).
[2]In 1980 and 1985 recipients included in more than one category. In 1990–96, 0.2–2.5 percent of recipients have unknown basis of eligibility. From 1997 onwards, unknowns are included in Other Title XIX.
[3]Includes adults in the Aid to Families with Dependent Children (AFDC) program.
[4]Includes children in the AFDC program. From 1997 onwards includes foster care.
[5]Includes some participants in the Supplemental Security Income program and other people deemed medically needy in participating States. From 1997 onwards excludes foster care and includes unknown eligibility.
[6]Race and ethnicity as determined on initial Medicaid application. Categories are mutually exclusive.
[7]Vendor payments exclude disproportionate share hospital payments ($16 billion in 1997 and $15 billion in 1998).

NOTES: 1972 and 1975 data are for fiscal year ending June 30. All other years are for fiscal year ending September 30. Data for additional years are available (see Appendix III). Some numbers in this table have been revised and differ from the previous edition of Health, United States.

SOURCE: Health Care Financing Administration. Office of Information Services, Enterprise Databases Group, Division of Information Distribution.

Table 137 (page 1 of 2). Medicaid recipients and medical vendor payments, according to type of service: United States, selected fiscal years 1972–98

[Data are compiled by the Health Care Financing Administration]

Type of service	1972	1975	1980	1985	1990	1995	1996	1997	1998[1]
Recipients				Number in millions					
All recipients	17.6	22.0	21.6	21.8	25.3	36.3	36.1	34.9	40.6
				Percent of recipients					
Inpatient general hospitals	16.1	15.6	17.0	15.7	18.2	15.3	14.8	13.6	10.5
Inpatient mental hospitals	0.2	0.3	0.3	0.3	0.4	0.2	0.3	0.3	0.3
Mentally retarded intermediate care facilities	- - -	0.3	0.6	0.7	0.6	0.4	0.4	0.4	0.3
Nursing facilities	- - -	- - -	- - -	- - -	- - -	4.6	4.4	4.6	4.0
Skilled	3.1	2.9	2.8	2.5	2.4	- - -	- - -	- - -	- - -
Intermediate care	- - -	3.1	3.7	3.8	3.4	- - -	- - -	- - -	- - -
Physician	69.8	69.1	63.7	66.0	67.6	65.6	63.3	60.7	45.6
Dental	13.6	17.9	21.5	21.4	18.0	17.6	17.2	17.0	12.2
Other practitioner	9.1	12.1	15.0	15.4	15.3	15.2	14.8	14.7	10.7
Outpatient hospital	29.6	33.8	44.9	46.2	49.0	46.1	44.0	39.1	29.9
Clinic	2.8	4.9	7.1	9.7	11.1	14.7	14.0	13.5	13.0
Laboratory and radiological	20.0	21.5	14.9	29.1	35.5	36.0	34.9	31.8	23.1
Home health	0.6	1.6	1.8	2.5	2.8	4.5	4.8	5.3	3.0
Prescribed drugs	63.3	64.3	63.4	63.8	68.5	65.4	62.5	60.1	47.6
Family planning	. . .	5.5	5.2	7.5	6.9	6.9	6.6	6.0	4.9
Early and periodic screening	. . .	. . .	. . .	8.7	11.7	18.2	18.2	18.5	15.2
Rural health clinic	. . .	. . .	. . .	0.4	0.9	3.4	3.9	4.1	- - -
Prepaid health care	- - -	- - -	- - -	- - -	- - -	- - -	- - -	- - -	49.7
Other care	14.4	13.2	11.9	15.5	20.3	31.5	36.3	35.5	36.0
Vendor payments[2]				Amount in billions					
All payments	$ 6.3	$ 12.2	$ 23.3	$ 37.5	$ 64.9	$120.1	$121.7	$124.4	$142.3
				Percent distribution					
Total	100.0	100.0	100.0	100.0	100.0	100.0	100.0	100.0	100.0
Inpatient general hospitals	40.6	27.6	27.5	25.2	25.7	21.9	20.7	18.6	15.1
Inpatient mental hospitals	1.8	3.3	3.3	3.2	2.6	2.1	1.7	1.6	2.0
Mentally retarded intermediate care facilities	- - -	3.1	8.5	12.6	11.3	8.6	7.9	7.9	6.7
Nursing facilities	- - -	- - -	- ·- -	- - -	- - -	24.2	24.3	24.5	22.4
Skilled	23.3	19.9	15.8	13.5	12.4	- - -	- - -	- - -	- - -
Intermediate care	- - -	15.4	18.0	17.4	14.9	- - -	- - -	- - -	- - -
Physician	12.6	10.0	8.0	6.3	6.2	6.1	5.9	5.7	4.3
Dental	2.7	2.8	2.0	1.2	0.9	0.8	0.8	0.8	0.6
Other practitioner	0.9	1.0	0.8	0.7	0.6	0.8	0.9	0.8	0.4
Outpatient hospital	5.8	3.0	4.7	4.8	5.1	5.5	5.3	5.0	4.0
Clinic	0.7	3.2	1.4	1.9	2.6	3.6	3.5	3.4	2.8
Laboratory and radiological	1.3	1.0	0.5	0.9	1.1	1.0	1.0	0.8	0.7
Home health	0.4	0.6	1.4	3.0	5.2	7.8	8.9	9.8	1.9
Prescribed drugs	8.1	6.7	5.7	6.2	6.8	8.1	8.8	9.6	9.5
Family planning	. . .	0.5	0.3	0.5	0.4	0.4	0.4	0.3	0.3
Early and periodic screening	. . .	. . .	. . .	0.2	0.3	1.0	1.1	1.3	0.9
Rural health clinic	. . .	. . .	. . .	0.0	0.1	0.2	0.2	0.2	- - -
Prepaid health care	- - -	- - -	- - -	- - -	- - -	- - -	- - -	- - -	13.6
Other care	1.8	1.9	1.9	2.5	3.7	7.7	8.4	8.9	13.6

See footnotes at end of table.

Table 137 (page 2 of 2). Medicaid recipients and medical vendor payments, according to type of service: United States, selected fiscal years 1972–98

[Data are compiled by the Health Care Financing Administration]

Type of service	1972	1975	1980	1985	1990	1995	1996	1997	1998[1]
Vendor payments per recipient[2]					Amount				
Total payment per recipient	$ 358	$ 556	$ 1,079	$ 1,719	$ 2,568	$ 3,311	$ 3,369	$ 3,568	$ 3,501
Inpatient general hospitals	903	983	1,742	2,753	3,630	4,735	4,696	4,877	5,031
Inpatient mental hospitals	2,825	6,045	11,742	19,867	18,548	29,847	21,873	22,990	20,701
Mentally retarded intermediate care facilities	- - -	5,507	16,438	32,102	50,048	68,613	68,232	72,033	74,960
Nursing facilities	- - -	- - -	- - -	- - -	- - -	17,424	18,589	19,029	19,379
Skilled	2,665	3,864	6,081	9,274	13,356	- - -	- - -	- - -	- - -
Intermediate care	- - -	2,764	5,326	7,882	11,236	- - -	- - -	- - -	- - -
Physician	65	81	136	163	235	309	317	333	327
Dental	71	86	99	98	130	160	166	175	182
Other practitioner	37	48	61	75	96	178	205	190	135
Outpatient hospital	70	50	113	178	269	397	409	453	474
Clinic	82	358	209	337	602	804	833	902	742
Laboratory and radiological	23	27	38	53	80	90	96	93	100
Home health	229	204	847	2,094	4,733	5,740	6,293	6,575	2,206
Prescribed drugs	46	58	96	166	256	413	474	571	699
Family planning	. . .	55	72	119	151	206	200	200	223
Early and periodic screening	. . .	. . .	. . .	45	67	177	212	251	216
Rural health clinic	. . .	. . .	. . .	81	154	174	215	213	- - -
Prepaid health care	- - -	- - -	- - -	- - -	- - -	- - -	- - -	- - -	955
Other care	44	80	172	274	465	807	782	891	1,331

- - - Data not available.

. . . Category not applicable.

[1]Prior to 1998 recipient counts exclude those individuals who only received coverage under prepaid health care and for whom no direct vendor payments were made during the year. Prior to 1998 vendor payments exclude payments to health maintenance organizations and other prepaid health plans ($19.3 billion in 1998 and $18 billion in 1997). The total number of persons who were Medicaid eligible and enrolled was 41.4 million in 1998, 41.6 million in 1997, and 41.2 million in 1996 (HCFA Medicaid Statistics, Program and Financial Statistics FY1996, FY1997, and FY1998. unpublished).

[2]Payments exclude disproportionate share hospital payments ($16 billion in 1997 and $15 billion in 1998).

NOTES: 1972 and 1975 data are for fiscal year ending June 30. All other years are for fiscal year ending September 30. Data for additional years are available (see Appendix III). Some numbers in this table have been revised and differ from the previous edition of *Health, United States*.

SOURCE: Health Care Financing Administration. Office of Information Services, Enterprise Databases Group, Division of Information Distribution.

Table 138. Department of Veterans Affairs health care expenditures and use, and persons treated according to selected characteristics: United States, selected fiscal years 1970–98

[Data are compiled by Department of Veterans Affairs]

	1970	1980	1990	1993	1994	1995	1996	1997	1998
Health care expenditures					Amount in millions				
All expenditures[1]	$1,689	$ 5,981	$11,500	$14,612	$15,401	$16,126	$16,373	$17,149	$17,441
					Percent distribution				
All services	100.0	100.0	100.0	100.0	100.0	100.0	100.0	100.0	100.0
Inpatient hospital	71.3	64.3	57.5	54.8	53.8	49.0	46.3	43.1	38.3
Outpatient care	14.0	19.1	25.3	28.0	28.4	30.2	33.6	37.1	41.8
Nursing home care	5.5	7.1	9.5	10.4	10.5	10.0	10.1	10.2	10.2
All other[2]	9.1	9.6	7.7	6.8	7.3	10.8	10.0	9.6	9.9
Health care use					Number in thousands				
Inpatient hospital stays[3]	787	1,248	1,029	920	907	879	807	671	617
Outpatient visits	7,312	17,971	22,602	24,236	25,158	27,527	29,295	31,919	34,972
Nursing home stays[4]	47	57	75	78	78	79	79	87	98
Inpatients[5]									
Total	---	---	598	556	547	527	491	417	380
					Percent distribution				
Total	---	---	100.0	100.0	100.0	100.0	100.0	100.0	100.0
Veterans with service-connected disability	---	---	38.9	39.4	39.1	39.3	39.5	39.2	38.2
Veterans without service-connected									
disability	---	---	60.3	59.6	60.0	59.9	59.6	59.7	60.8
Low income	---	---	54.8	55.2	56.6	56.2	55.7	55.5	55.4
Exempt[6]	---	---	2.5	2.4	0.9	0.8	0.8	0.9	0.9
Other[7]	---	---	2.8	1.9	2.4	2.8	3.0	3.2	3.8
Unknown	---	---	0.2	0.1	0.1	0.1	0.1	0.1	0.7
Nonveterans	---	---	0.8	1.0	0.9	0.8	0.8	1.0	1.0
Outpatients[5]					Number in thousands				
Total	---	---	2,564	2,684	2,714	2,790	2,846	2,958	3,235
					Percent distribution				
Total	---	---	100.0	100.0	100.0	100.0	100.0	100.0	100.0
Veterans with service-connected disability	---	---	38.3	37.4	37.4	37.5	37.8	37.9	38.7
Veterans without service-connected									
disability	---	---	49.8	50.6	50.5	50.5	50.2	51.5	52.9
Low income	---	---	41.1	41.5	42.6	42.2	41.9	41.9	41.3
Exempt[6]	---	---	2.9	2.6	1.0	0.9	0.9	0.7	0.5
Other[7]	---	---	3.6	2.9	3.6	4.2	4.7	5.9	8.4
Unknown	---	---	2.2	3.6	3.3	3.2	2.8	3.0	2.7
Nonveterans	---	---	11.8	12.0	12.1	12.0	12.1	10.6	10.4

- - - Data not available.

[1]Health care expenditures exclude construction, medical administration, and miscellaneous operating expenses.

[2]Includes miscellaneous benefits and services, contract hospitals, education and training, subsidies to State veterans hospitals, nursing homes, and domiciliaries, and the Civilian Health and Medical Program of the Department of Veterans Affairs.

[3]One-day dialysis patients were included in fiscal year 1980. Interfacility transfers were included beginning in fiscal year 1990.

[4]Includes Department of Veterans Affairs nursing home and domiciliary stays, and community nursing home stays.

[5]Individuals.

[6]Prisoner of war, exposed to Agent Orange, and so forth. Prior to fiscal year 1994, veterans who reported exposure to Agent Orange were classified as exempt. Beginning in fiscal year 1994 those veterans reporting Agent Orange exposure but not treated for it were means tested and placed in the low income or other group depending on income.

[7]Financial means-tested veterans who receive medical care subject to copayments according to income level

NOTES: Figures may not add to totals due to rounding. In 1970 and 1980, the fiscal year ended June 30; for all other years the fiscal year ends September 30. The veteran population was estimated at 25.2 million in 1998 with 37 percent age 65 or over, compared with 11 percent in 1980. Twenty-five percent had served during World War II, 17 percent during the Korean conflict, 32 percent during the Vietnam era, 8 percent during the Persian Gulf War, and 23 percent during peacetime. Beginning in fiscal year 1995 categories for health care expenditures and health care use were revised. Data for additional years are available (see Appendix III).

SOURCE: Department of Veterans Affairs, Office of Policy and Planning, National Center for Veteran Analysis and Statistics. Unpublished data.

Table 139. Hospital care expenditures by geographic division and State and average annual percent change: United States, selected years 1980–93

[Data are compiled by the Health Care Financing Administration]

Geographic division and State[1]	Amount in millions						Average annual percent change	
	1980	1985	1990	1991	1992	1993	1980–90	1990–93
United States[2]	$101,510	$166,545	$254,239	$279,820	$303,461	$323,919	9.6	8.4
New England	6,467	10,332	15,540	16,773	17,855	19,056	9.2	7.0
Maine	460	735	1,119	1,207	1,280	1,376	9.3	7.1
New Hampshire	313	590	1,056	1,102	1,233	1,388	12.9	9.5
Vermont	174	290	447	494	532	562	9.9	7.9
Massachusetts	3,646	5,628	8,159	8,826	9,380	10,034	8.4	7.1
Rhode Island	481	760	1,095	1,177	1,237	1,314	8.6	6.3
Connecticut	1,396	2,328	3,664	3,967	4,193	4,380	10.1	6.1
Middle Atlantic	18,361	29,462	45,472	49,673	53,779	57,854	9.5	8.4
New York	9,582	14,585	22,739	24,784	26,387	28,001	9.0	7.2
New Jersey	2,763	4,751	7,857	8,586	9,406	10,312	11.0	9.5
Pennsylvania	6,017	10,126	14,876	16,303	17,987	19,540	9.5	9.5
East North Central	19,590	30,093	42,984	47,026	50,835	54,172	8.2	8.0
Ohio	4,808	8,026	11,419	12,359	13,394	14,305	9.0	7.8
Indiana	2,125	3,399	5,288	5,918	6,473	6,998	9.5	9.8
Illinois	6,217	8,998	12,400	13,560	14,744	15,621	7.1	8.0
Michigan	4,482	6,882	9,500	10,309	11,008	11,711	7.8	7.2
Wisconsin	1,959	2,788	4,377	4,880	5,216	5,537	8.4	8.2
West North Central	7,810	12,261	18,012	19,664	21,116	22,252	8.7	7.3
Minnesota	1,740	2,716	4,094	4,473	4,674	4,796	8.9	5.4
Iowa	1,179	1,733	2,634	2,856	2,996	3,111	8.4	5.7
Missouri	2,532	4,172	5,986	6,527	7,077	7,652	9.0	8.5
North Dakota	313	524	717	786	853	903	8.6	8.0
South Dakota	275	450	694	786	863	920	9.7	9.9
Nebraska	681	1,060	1,587	1,749	1,881	2,003	8.8	8.1
Kansas	1,090	1,607	2,300	2,487	2,771	2,868	7.8	7.6
South Atlantic	15,588	26,925	44,077	48,917	52,971	56,711	11.0	8.8
Delaware	259	434	709	777	854	937	10.6	9.7
Maryland	2,034	2,980	4,655	5,097	5,516	5,926	8.6	8.4
District of Columbia	913	1,469	2,133	2,291	2,437	2,612	8.9	7.0
Virginia	2,077	3,530	5,661	6,240	6,618	7,031	10.5	7.5
West Virginia	831	1,219	1,763	1,977	2,190	2,346	7.8	10.0
North Carolina	1,963	3,250	5,901	6,658	7,311	7,801	11.6	9.8
South Carolina	978	1,753	3,108	3,588	3,962	4,221	12.3	10.7
Georgia	2,148	3,885	6,685	7,398	8,092	8,704	12.0	9.2
Florida	4,385	8,404	13,462	14,890	15,992	17,131	11.9	8.4
East South Central	5,713	9,673	15,149	16,955	18,715	19,921	10.2	9.6
Kentucky	1,230	2,157	3,437	3,900	4,268	4,515	10.8	9.5
Tennessee	2,027	3,483	5,511	6,146	6,761	7,208	10.5	9.4
Alabama	1,590	2,606	4,015	4,511	5,028	5,301	9.7	9.7
Mississippi	867	1,427	2,187	2,398	2,658	2,897	9.7	9.8
West South Central	9,210	16,230	25,344	28,335	31,236	33,601	10.7	9.9
Arkansas	746	1,313	2,109	2,336	2,546	2,723	11.0	8.9
Louisiana	1,744	3,155	4,627	5,164	5,575	5,956	10.2	8.8
Oklahoma	1,177	1,896	2,674	2,938	3,182	3,329	8.6	7.6
Texas	5,543	9,866	15,935	17,897	19,932	21,592	11.1	10.7
Mountain	4,255	7,652	11,748	13,092	14,223	15,095	10.7	8.7
Montana	264	438	679	764	841	894	9.9	9.6
Idaho	243	419	665	752	844	900	10.6	10.6
Wyoming	146	248	353	381	396	417	9.2	5.7
Colorado	1,218	2,087	3,101	3,480	3,776	3,932	9.8	8.2
New Mexico	451	873	1,364	1,538	1,703	1,848	11.7	10.7
Arizona	1,093	2,103	3,218	3,532	3,765	3,999	11.4	7.5
Utah	453	816	1,325	1,483	1,631	1,743	11.3	9.6
Nevada	387	667	1,043	1,162	1,267	1,362	10.4	9.3
Pacific	14,515	23,918	35,912	39,384	42,731	45,259	9.5	8.0
Washington	1,396	2,516	3,961	4,546	5,090	5,305	11.0	10.2
Oregon	928	1,486	2,297	2,403	2,714	2,966	9.5	8.9
California	11,632	18,883	27,949	30,554	32,880	34,827	9.2	7.6
Alaska	199	385	557	631	690	701	10.8	8.0
Hawaii	360	648	1,148	1,250	1,358	1,460	12.3	8.3

[1]States where services were provided.
[2]These estimates differ from National Health Expenditures estimates presented elsewhere in *Health, United States*. See Appendix I, Health Care Financing Administration.

NOTE: Figures may not sum to totals due to rounding.

SOURCE: Health Care Financing Administration, Office of the Actuary. Estimates prepared by the Office of National Health Statistics.

Table 140. Physician service expenditures by geographic division and State and average annual percent change: United States, selected years 1980–93

[Data are compiled by the Health Care Financing Administration]

Geographic division and State[1]	Amount in millions						Average annual percent change	
	1980	1985	1990	1991	1992	1993	1980–90	1990–93
United States[2]	$45,245	$83,636	$140,499	$150,318	$161,783	$171,226	12.0	6.8
New England	2,072	4,010	7,656	8,088	8,678	9,250	14.0	6.5
Maine	142	275	480	520	570	601	13.0	7.8
New Hampshire	130	281	491	583	719	780	14.2	16.7
Vermont	68	131	221	229	248	265	12.5	6.2
Massachusetts	978	1,890	3,766	3,892	4,130	4,442	14.4	5.7
Rhode Island	166	304	514	527	543	575	12.0	3.8
Connecticut	589	1,127	2,185	2,336	2,468	2,587	14.0	5.8
Middle Atlantic	6,636	12,255	20,470	22,035	24,044	25,238	11.9	7.2
New York	3,332	5,822	9,697	10,238	11,287	12,003	11.3	7.4
New Jersey	1,353	2,533	4,519	4,771	5,526	5,776	12.8	8.5
Pennsylvania	1,950	3,901	6,254	7,026	7,230	7,460	12.4	6.1
East North Central	8,078	13,646	21,823	23,280	24,837	26,275	10.4	6.4
Ohio	2,130	3,692	6,048	6,486	6,786	7,118	11.0	5.6
Indiana	891	1,607	2,680	2,821	3,061	3,263	11.6	6.8
Illinois	2,118	3,672	5,864	6,191	6,707	6,970	10.7	5.9
Michigan	2,002	3,080	4,668	5,017	5,224	5,562	8.8	6.0
Wisconsin	938	1,595	2,564	2,765	3,059	3,362	10.6	9.5
West North Central	3,286	5,739	9,125	9,594	10,395	10,987	10.8	6.4
Minnesota	944	1,765	2,957	3,202	3,322	3,617	12.1	6.9
Iowa	488	769	1,142	1,178	1,294	1,376	8.9	6.4
Missouri	877	1,537	2,485	2,581	2,879	2,958	11.0	6.0
North Dakota	139	288	368	371	433	445	10.2	6.5
South Dakota	102	173	274	280	319	342	10.4	7.7
Nebraska	276	433	688	700	785	825	9.6	6.2
Kansas	461	774	1,211	1,280	1,362	1,425	10.1	5.6
South Atlantic	7,141	14,169	25,449	26,853	28,588	30,041	13.6	5.7
Delaware	120	214	377	405	439	466	12.1	7.3
Maryland	835	1,702	2,968	3,249	3,498	3,704	13.5	7.7
District of Columbia	237	362	657	662	651	672	10.7	0.8
Virginia	886	1,772	3,172	3,462	3,565	3,769	13.6	5.9
West Virginia	330	642	856	882	973	988	10.0	4.9
North Carolina	866	1,543	3,005	3,213	3,458	3,717	13.2	7.3
South Carolina	399	734	1,325	1,423	1,552	1,685	12.8	8.3
Georgia	987	1,930	3,645	3,957	4,321	4,543	14.0	7.6
Florida	2,482	5,272	9,444	9,600	10,131	10,498	14.3	3.6
East South Central	2,361	4,188	7,379	8,051	8,418	8,913	12.1	6.5
Kentucky	562	955	1,639	1,762	1,950	2,038	11.3	7.5
Tennessee	841	1,499	2,569	2,822	2,988	3,137	11.8	6.9
Alabama	632	1,167	2,247	2,477	2,466	2,631	13.5	5.4
Mississippi	327	568	925	990	1,015	1,107	11.0	6.2
West South Central	4,649	8,666	13,566	14,280	15,334	15,947	11.3	5.5
Arkansas	374	680	1,134	1,228	1,217	1,244	11.7	3.1
Louisiana	743	1,424	2,129	2,282	2,450	2,537	11.1	6.0
Oklahoma	536	972	1,382	1,431	1,558	1,640	9.9	5.9
Texas	2,996	5,590	8,920	9,340	10,108	10,526	11.5	5.7
Mountain	2,211	4,336	7,347	7,731	8,357	8,897	12.8	6.6
Montana	138	205	311	325	350	392	8.5	8.0
Idaho	140	235	374	410	453	486	10.3	9.1
Wyoming	64	118	146	142	152	160	8.6	3.1
Colorado	600	1,230	1,891	2,032	2,242	2,452	12.2	9.0
New Mexico	182	368	574	590	665	716	12.2	7.6
Arizona	635	1,287	2,500	2,559	2,676	2,799	14.7	3.8
Utah	244	472	739	794	832	864	11.7	5.3
Nevada	207	421	812	879	988	1,029	14.6	8.2
Pacific	8,811	16,627	27,682	30,406	33,132	35,677	12.1	8.8
Washington	909	1,667	2,834	3,155	3,413	3,720	12.0	9.5
Oregon	596	990	1,597	1,626	1,798	1,904	10.4	6.0
California	6,959	13,311	22,365	24,654	26,903	28,981	12.4	9.0
Alaska	97	214	258	265	276	301	10.3	5.3
Hawaii	249	444	629	706	742	771	9.7	7.0

[1]States where services were provided.
[2]These estimates differ from National Health Expenditures estimates presented elsewhere in Health, United States. See Appendix I, Health Care Financing Administration.

NOTE: Figures may not sum to totals due to rounding.

SOURCE: Health Care Financing Administration, Office of the Actuary. Estimates prepared by the Office of National Health Statistics.

Table 141. Expenditures for purchases of prescription drugs by geographic division and State and average annual percent change: United States, selected years 1980–93

[Data are compiled by the Health Care Financing Administration]

Geographic division and State[1]	Amount in millions						Average annual percent change	
	1980	1985	1990	1991	1992	1993	1980–90	1990–93
United States	$12,049	$21,405	$38,198	$42,755	$45,730	$48,840	12.2	8.5
New England	625	1,217	2,250	2,463	2,578	2,710	13.7	6.4
Maine	51	93	174	192	202	213	13.1	7.0
New Hampshire	39	77	160	174	185	197	15.2	7.2
Vermont	22	43	86	95	101	108	14.6	7.9
Massachusetts	290	596	1,113	1,214	1,270	1,337	14.4	6.3
Rhode Island	48	96	174	190	198	206	13.7	5.8
Connecticut	174	312	544	597	622	650	12.1	6.1
Middle Atlantic	1,817	3,334	5,911	6,513	6,859	7,219	12.5	6.9
New York	820	1,506	2,665	2,929	3,077	3,232	12.5	6.6
New Jersey	381	723	1,298	1,432	1,515	1,601	13.0	7.2
Pennsylvania	616	1,105	1,948	2,152	2,267	2,386	12.2	7.0
East North Central	2,219	3,850	6,691	7,437	7,895	8,360	11.7	7.7
Ohio	607	1,010	1,684	1,869	1,982	2,095	10.7	7.6
Indiana	305	508	874	974	1,038	1,106	11.1	8.2
Illinois	561	1,006	1,771	1,964	2,084	2,206	12.2	7.6
Michigan	527	939	1,654	1,837	1,947	2,054	12.1	7.5
Wisconsin	218	387	708	791	844	899	12.5	8.3
West North Central	887	1,495	2,557	2,835	3,012	3,195	11.2	7.7
Minnesota	191	324	580	648	691	739	11.7	8.4
Iowa	156	255	419	463	490	516	10.4	7.2
Missouri	274	461	783	868	919	975	11.1	7.6
North Dakota	28	51	86	93	98	103	11.9	6.2
South Dakota	30	50	82	91	97	104	10.6	8.2
Nebraska	80	136	235	261	277	293	11.4	7.6
Kansas	128	218	373	412	439	465	11.3	7.6
South Atlantic	1,997	3,694	7,181	8,120	8,746	9,412	13.7	9.4
Delaware	25	49	98	111	120	129	14.6	9.6
Maryland	226	443	888	998	1,069	1,140	14.7	8.7
District of Columbia	32	57	93	99	101	103	11.3	3.5
Virginia	275	522	1,026	1,154	1,248	1,343	14.1	9.4
West Virginia	116	204	333	369	389	412	11.1	7.4
North Carolina	340	569	1,061	1,199	1,287	1,392	12.1	9.5
South Carolina	154	268	511	580	622	665	12.7	9.2
Georgia	294	540	1,035	1,176	1,283	1,397	13.4	10.5
Florida	536	1,041	2,135	2,435	2,627	2,832	14.8	9.9
East South Central	890	1,537	2,659	2,969	3,175	3,402	11.6	8.6
Kentucky	225	392	667	741	791	846	11.5	8.2
Tennessee	288	500	886	996	1,072	1,153	11.9	9.2
Alabama	235	404	707	790	845	904	11.6	8.5
Mississippi	142	241	399	442	468	499	10.9	7.7
West South Central	1,431	2,440	3,846	4,331	4,671	5,039	10.4	9.4
Arkansas	153	235	382	425	452	484	9.6	8.2
Louisiana	254	440	668	740	788	832	10.2	7.6
Oklahoma	175	299	450	500	535	569	9.9	8.1
Texas	848	1,467	2,346	2,666	2,896	3,153	10.7	10.4
Mountain	489	916	1,738	1,998	2,201	2,436	13.5	11.9
Montana	31	54	90	101	110	120	11.2	10.1
Idaho	44	74	129	149	164	182	11.4	12.2
Wyoming	23	37	49	55	59	64	7.9	9.3
Colorado	127	223	379	434	481	534	11.6	12.1
New Mexico	52	101	190	216	237	259	13.8	10.9
Arizona	123	250	526	600	659	728	15.6	11.4
Utah	54	110	218	249	274	302	15.0	11.5
Nevada	36	67	158	193	218	246	15.9	15.9
Pacific	1,694	2,921	5,365	6,089	6,593	7,067	12.2	9.6
Washington	212	340	618	711	781	853	11.3	11.3
Oregon	125	187	318	364	396	431	9.8	10.7
California	1,296	2,274	4,222	4,776	5,155	5,501	12.5	9.2
Alaska	16	34	58	69	77	85	13.7	13.6
Hawaii	44	87	148	169	184	197	12.9	10.0

[1]State where prescriptions were provided.

NOTES: Prescription drug expenditures are limited to spending for products purchased in retail outlets. The value of drugs and other products provided by hospitals, nursing homes, or other health professionals is included in estimates of spending for these providers' services. Figures may not sum to totals due to rounding.

SOURCE: Health Care Financing Administration, Office of the Actuary. Estimates prepared by the Office of National Health Statistics.

Table 142. State mental health agency per capita expenditures for mental health services and average annual percent change by geographic division and State: United States, selected fiscal years 1981–97

[Data are based on reporting by State mental health agencies]

Geographic division and State	1981	1983	1985	1987	1990[1]	1993[1,2]	1997[1,2]	Average annual percent change 1981–97
	Amount per capita							
United States....................	$ 27	$31	$35	$ 38	$ 48	$ 54	$ 64	5.5
New England:								
Maine............................	25	32	36	42	67	70	88	8.2
New Hampshire.................	35	39	42	36	63	78	99	6.8
Vermont.........................	32	40	44	44	54	74	92	6.8
Massachusetts.................	32	36	46·	62	84	83	90	6.7
Rhode Island...................	36	32	35	41	50	61	63	3.6
Connecticut....................	32	39	44	56	73	82	99	7.4
Middle Atlantic:								
New York........................	67	74	90	99	118	131	113	3.3
New Jersey......................	26	31	36	43	57	68	69	6.2
Pennsylvania...................	41	47	52	50	57	68	68	3.3
East North Central:								
Ohio..............................	25	29	30	34	41	47	52	4.8
Indiana..........................	19	23	27	31	47	39	40	4.8
Illinois...........................	18	21	24	25	34	36	51	6.8
Michigan.........................	33	39	49	61	74	75	87	6.3
Wisconsin.......................	22	27	28	31	37	35	44	4.3
West North·Central:								
Minnesota[3].....................	17	30	32	42	54	69	87	10.8
Iowa.............................	8	10	11	12	17	13	29	8.5
Missouri.........................	24	25	28	32	35	41	56	5.5
North Dakota...................	39	42	36	42	40	43	48	1.4
South Dakota...................	17	21	22	27	25	47	54	7.5
Nebraska........................	17	19	21	21	29	34	39	5.5
Kansas..........................	18	22	27	28	35	48	59	7.9
South Atlantic:								
Delaware........................	44	51	46	41	55	56	73	3.2
Maryland........................	33	37	40	49	61	64	76	5.4
District of Columbia[4].........	- - -	23	28	130	268	315	337	- - -
Virginia..........................	23	29	32	35	45	40	49	4.9
West Virginia....................	20	20	22	23	24	22	23	1.0
North Carolina..................	24	29	38	41	46	50	62	6.2
South Carolina.................	31	33	33	45	51	56	64	4.7
Georgia..........................	25	26	23	32	51	49	47	4.0
Florida...........................	20	23	26	25	37	31	44	5.1
East South Central:								
Kentucky........................	15	17	19	23	23	25	35	5.5
Tennessee......................	18	20	23	24	29	37	23	1.6
Alabama.........................	20	24	28	29	38	43	47	5.5
Mississippi......................	14	16	24	22	34	41	56	9.2
West South Central:								
Arkansas........................	17	20	24	24	26	30	30	3.7
Louisiana........................	19	23	26	25	28	39	43	5.3
Oklahoma.......................	22	33	31	30	36	38	41	3.9
Texas............................	13	16	17·	19·	23	31	39	7.1
Mountain:								
Montana.........................	25	28	29	28	28	34	93	8.7
Idaho............................	13	15	15	17	20	26	29	4.9
Wyoming........................	23	28	31	30	35	42	43	4.0
Colorado........................	24	25	28	30	34	41	57	5.6
New Mexico.....................	24	25	25	24	23	24	31	1.7
Arizona..........................	10	10	12	16	27	60	68	12.7
Utah.............................	13	16	17	19	21	25	28	4.8
Nevada..........................	22	25	26	28	33	32	45	4.6
Pacific:								
Washington.....................	18	24	30	37	43	66	79	9.8
Oregon..........................	21	21	25	28	41	60	68	7.8
California........................	28	29	34	30	42	50	58	4.6
Alaska...........................	38	41	45	50	72	86	79	4.7
Hawaii...........................	19	22	23	26	38	71	85	9.9

- - - Data not available.
[1]Puerto Rico is included in U.S. total.   [2]Guam is included in U.S. total.
[3]Data for 1981 not comparable with 1983–93 data for Minnesota. Average annual percent change is for 1983–97.
[4]Transfer of St. Elizabeths Hospital from the National Institute of Mental Health to the District of Columbia Office of Mental Health took place over the years 1985–93.

NOTE: Expenditures for mental illness, excluding mental retardation and substance abuse.

SOURCES: National Association of State Mental Health Program Directors and the National Association of State Mental Health Program Directors Research Institute, Inc.: Final Report: Funding sources and expenditures of State mental health agencies: Revenue/expenditure study results, fiscal year 1990. Nov. 1992; Supplemental report fiscal year 1993. Mar. 1996; Fiscal year 1997: Final report. July 1999.

Table 143. Medicare enrollees, enrollees in managed care, payments per enrollee, and short-stay hospital utilization by geographic division and State: United States, 1994 and 1997

[Data are compiled by the Health Care Financing Administration]

Geographic division and State	Enrollment in thousands[1] 1997	Percent of enrollees in managed care[2] 1994	Percent of enrollees in managed care[2] 1997	Payments per enrollee[3] 1994	Payments per enrollee[3] 1997	Discharges per 1,000 enrollees[3] 1994	Discharges per 1,000 enrollees[3] 1997	Average length of stay in days[3] 1994	Average length of stay in days[3] 1997
United States	37,657	7.9	14.5	$4,375	$5,416	345	370	7.5	6.3
New England	2,081	4.0	12.2	4,497	5,821	320	334	7.5	6.3
Maine	208	0.1	0.2	3,464	4,325	322	323	7.7	6.2
New Hampshire	160	0.2	4.1	3,414	4,524	281	301	7.6	5.9
Vermont	86	0.1	1.4	3,182	3,771	283	276	7.6	6.1
Massachusetts	949	6.1	19.1	5,147	6,716	350	367	7.6	5.9
Rhode Island	168	7.0	14.2	4,148	5,973	312	355	7.6	6.0
Connecticut	510	2.6	7.8	4,426	5,767	287	299	8.1	6.8
Middle Atlantic	5,917	4.6	15.9	4,917	5,974	354	388	8.1	6.4
New York	2,646	6.2	14.4	4,855	6,117	334	365	9.8	7.9
New Jersey	1,191	2.6	11.4	4,531	5,889	354	369	11.2	9.0
Pennsylvania	2,080	3.3	20.2	5,212	5,831	379	428	10.2	8.2
East North Central	6,274	2.8	6.3	4,045	5,008	345	362	8.0	6.6
Ohio	1,691	2.4	9.9	3,982	4,989	350	374	7.2	6.0
Indiana	827	2.6	3.2	3,945	4,775	345	349	7.1	6.0
Illinois	1,625	5.5	8.9	4,324	5,192	374	385	6.9	5.8
Michigan	1,364	0.7	2.2	4,307	5,442	328	353	7.3	6.1
Wisconsin	766	2.0	3.7	3,246	4,142	310	319	7.6	6.4
West North Central	2,816	6.7	8.5	3,578	4,385	334	353	6.8	5.7
Minnesota	639	19.6	17.2	3,394	4,131	334	346	6.6	5.7
Iowa	477	3.1	3.5	3,080	3,865	322	346	5.7	5.2
Missouri	845	3.4	9.8	4,191	5,038	349	372	6.6	5.6
North Dakota	102	0.6	0.6	3,218	3,650	327	324	7.3	6.1
South Dakota	118	0.1	0.1	2,952	3,737	356	347	6.3	5.6
Nebraska	251	2.2	4.1	2,926	3,938	281	316	6.1	5.5
Kansas	385	3.3	4.8	3,847	4,752	348	363	6.3	5.3
South Atlantic	7,207	6.1	11.5	4,390	5,322	341	359	6.5	5.7
Delaware	108	0.2	8.1	4,712	4,968	326	326	7.4	6.2
Maryland	621	1.4	11.1	4,997	5,561	362	353	8.1	6.5
District of Columbia	77	3.9	11.1	5,655	7,548	376	397	7.5	6.2
Virginia	854	1.5	3.5	3,748	4,587	348	355	10.1	8.1
West Virginia	333	8.3	7.6	3,798	4,896	420	437	7.3	6.4
North Carolina	1,071	0.5	1.4	3,465	4,552	314	349	7.1	6.1
South Carolina	535	0.1	1.0	3,777	4,681	319	346	8.0	6.5
Georgia	876	0.4	2.4	4,402	5,223	378	379	8.3	6.6
Florida	2,732	13.8	23.8	5,027	6,152	326	352	6.9	6.0
East South Central	2,464	0.9	2.9	4,262	5,333	398	416	7.1	6.1
Kentucky	601	2.3	4.1	3,862	4,888	396	404	7.2	5.9
Tennessee	793	0.3	1.5	4,441	5,379	375	384	7.1	6.2
Alabama	661	0.8	5.0	4,454	5,459	413	429	7.0	5.9
Mississippi	408	0.1	0.5	4,189	5,680	423	472	7.4	6.7
West South Central	3,673	2.8	9.8	4,628	6,212	351	386	7.2	6.1
Arkansas	429	0.2	2.1	3,719	4,517	366	383	7.0	6.2
Louisiana	591	0.4	11.0	5,468	6,984	399	449	7.2	6.1
Oklahoma	496	2.5	6.8	4,098	5,557	355	373	7.0	6.1
Texas	2,158	4.1	11.7	4,703	6,531	333	372	7.2	6.1
Mountain	2,067	15.9	23.9	3,806	4,546	290	320	5.9	5.2
Montana	132	0.4	0.4	3,114	3,808	306	312	5.9	5.0
Idaho	158	2.5	4.5	3,045	4,044	274	298	5.2	4.7
Wyoming	62	3.3	2.7	3,537	4,235	315	315	5.6	5.2
Colorado	445	17.2	28.9	3,935	5,021	302	315	6.0	5.2
New Mexico	221	13.6	18.0	3,110	3,939	301	314	6.0	5.4
Arizona	633	24.8	35.4	4,442	4,707	292	358	5.9	5.1
Utah	198	9.4	13.5	3,443	4,334	238	251	5.4	4.9
Nevada	219	19.0	30.2	4,306	5,361	291	341	7.0	5.8
Pacific	5,156	27.2	36.2	4,657	5,740	341	391	6.0	5.4
Washington	709	12.5	23.8	3,401	4,405	269	296	5.3	5.0
Oregon	484	27.7	37.2	3,285	4,274	305	373	5.2	4.6
California	3,768	30.0	38.9	5,219	6,335	366	421	6.1	5.5
Alaska	37	0.6	0.9	3,687	5,487	269	298	6.3	6.0
Hawaii	158	29.8	32.0	3,069	4,043	301	330	9.1	7.8

[1] Total persons enrolled in hospital insurance, supplementary medical insurance, or both, as of July 1. Includes fee-for-service and managed care enrollees.
[2] Includes enrollees in Medicare-approved managed care organizations.
[3] Data are for fee-for-service enrollees only.

NOTES: Figures may not sum to totals due to rounding. Data for additional years are available (see Appendix III).

SOURCE: Health Care Financing Administration, Office of Strategic Planning. Health Care Financing Review: Medicare and Medicaid Statistical Supplements for years 1996 and 1999.

Table 144 (page 1 of 2). **Medicaid recipients, recipients in managed care, payments per recipient, and recipients per 100 persons below the poverty level by geographic division and State: United States, selected fiscal years 1989–98**

[Data are compiled by the Health Care Financing Administration]

Geographic division and State	Recipients in thousands		Percent of recipients in managed care		Payments per recipient			Recipients per 100 persons below the poverty level	
	1996	1998[1]	1996	1998	1990	1996	1998[1]	1989–90	1997–98
United States	36,118	40,649	40	54	$ 2,568	$3,369	$3,501	75	108
New England:									
Maine	167	170	1	11	3,248	4,321	4,383	88	132
New Hampshire	100	94	16	10	5,423	5,496	6,449	53	83
Vermont	102	124	–	48	2,530	2,954	2,834	108	208
Massachusetts[2]	715	908	70	63	4,622	5,285	5,075	103	129
Rhode Island	130	153	63	63	[2]3,778	5,280	6,004	[3]163	116
Connecticut	329	381	61	72	4,829	6,179	6,350	167	98
Middle Atlantic:									
New York	3,281	3,073	23	30	5,099	6,811	7,907	95	103
New Jersey	714	813	43	59	4,054	5,217	5,188	83	94
Pennsylvania	1,168	1,523	53	68	2,449	3,993	3,992	88	95
East North Central:									
Ohio	1,478	1,291	32	28	2,566	3,729	4,742	98	108
Indiana	594	607	31	58	3,859	4,130	4,222	45	106
Illinois	1,454	1,364	13	13	2,271	3,689	4,526	69	107
Michigan	1,172	1,363	73	68	2,094	2,867	3,188	85	119
Wisconsin	434	519	32	49	3,179	4,384	4,255	95	105
West North Central:									
Minnesota	455	538	33	53	3,709	5,342	5,432	70	95
Iowa	308	315	41	92	2,589	3,534	4,092	80	115
Missouri	636	734	35	42	2,002	3,171	3,601	63	110
North Dakota	61	62	55	52	3,955	4,889	5,476	58	67
South Dakota	77	90	65	71	3,368	4,114	3,974	51	85
Nebraska	191	211	27	73	2,595	3,548	3,566	61	111
Kansas	251	242	32	49	2,524	3,425	3,788	71	95
South Atlantic:									
Delaware	82	101	78	77	3,004	3,773	4,138	68	122
Maryland	399	561	64	67	3,300	5,138	4,437	74	123
District of Columbia	143	166	55	45	2,629	4,955	4,402	86	130
Virginia	623	653	68	60	2,596	2,849	3,243	53	86
West Virginia	395	343	30	43	1,443	2,855	3,628	80	117
North Carolina	1,130	1,168	37	69	2,531	3,255	3,437	66	121
South Carolina	503	595	1	4	2,343	3,026	3,393	52	109
Georgia	1,185	1,222	32	76	3,190	2,604	2,465	64	113
Florida	1,638	1,905	64	65	2,273	2,851	2,986	55	88
East South Central:									
Kentucky	641	644	53	63	2,089	3,014	3,763	81	114
Tennessee	1,409	1,844	100	100	1,896	2,049	1,718	67	212
Alabama	546	527	11	71	1,731	2,675	3,609	43	84
Mississippi	510	486	7	40	1,354	2,633	2,969	67	105
West South Central:									
Arkansas	363	425	39	56	2,267	3,375	3,239	55	89
Louisiana	778	721	6	5	2,247	3,154	3,308	58	97
Oklahoma	358	342	19	50	2,516	2,852	3,439	56	72
Texas	2,572	2,325	4	25	1,928	2,672	3,071	47	77
Mountain:									
Montana	101	101	59	98	2,793	3,478	3,585	47	67
Idaho	119	123	37	35	2,973	3,402	3,446	36	68
Wyoming	51	46	1	–	2,036	3,571	4,163	[3]59	81
Colorado	271	345	80	99	2,705	3,815	4,173	45	87
New Mexico	318	329	45	80	2,120	2,757	2,617	39	86
Arizona[4]	528	508	86	85	- - -	- - -	3,238	- - -	65
Utah	152	216	82	91	2,279	2,775	2,867	72	96
Nevada	109	128	41	39	3,161	3,361	3,606	37	61

See footnotes at end of table.

Table 144 (page 2 of 2). Medicaid recipients, recipients in managed care, payments per recipient, and recipients per 100 persons below the poverty level by geographic division and State: United States, selected fiscal years 1989–98

[Data are compiled by the Health Care Financing Administration]

Geographic division and State	Recipients in thousands		Percent of recipients in managed care		Payments per recipient			Recipients per 100 persons below the poverty level	
	1996	1998[1]	1996	1998	1990	1996	1998[1]	1989–90	1997–98
Pacific:									
Washington	621	1413	100	91	2,128	2,242	1,447	98	196
Oregon	450	511	91	89	2,283	2,915	2,695	74	118
California.	5,107	7,082	23	46	1,795	2,178	2,010	88	113
Alaska.	69	75	–	–	3,562	4,027	4,434	70	128
Hawaii.	41	185	80	80	2,252	6,574	2,749	73	133

– Quantity zero.

- - - Data not available.

[1]Prior to 1998 recipient counts exclude those individuals who only received coverage under prepaid health care and for whom no direct vendor payments were made during the year. Prior to 1998 vendor payments exclude payments to health maintenance organizations and other prepaid health plans ($19.3 billion in 1998 and $18 billion in 1997). The total number of persons who were Medicaid eligible and enrolled was 41.4 million in 1998, 41.6 million in 1997, and 41.2 million in 1996 (HCFA Medicaid Statistics, Program and Financial Statistics FY1996, FY1997, and FY1998. unpublished).

[2]Data for categorically eligible blind Medicaid recipients in 1990 are estimated by the Bureau of Data Management and Strategy, HCFA.

[3]Data are estimated by the Bureau of Data Management and Strategy, HCFA.

[4]Arizona has a limited Medicaid program, with care financed largely on a capitated basis.

NOTE: Payments exclude disproportionate share hospital payments ($16 billion in 1997 and $15 billion in 1998).

SOURCES: Health Care Financing Administration. Office of Information Services, Enterprise Databases Group, Division of Information Distribution; Department of Commerce, Bureau of the Census, Housing and Household Economic Statistics Division.

Table 145. Persons enrolled in health maintenance organizations (HMO's) by geographic division and State: United States, selected years 1980–99

[Data are based on a census of health maintenance organizations]

Geographic division and State	Number in thousands 1999	Percent of population								
		1980	1985	1990	1994	1995	1996	1997	1998	1999
United States[1]	81,333	4.0	7.9	13.5	17.3	19.4	22.3	25.2	28.6	30.1
New England:										
Maine	251	0.4	0.3	2.6	5.1	7.0	9.5	15.9	19.1	20.2
New Hampshire	413	1.2	5.6	9.6	14.2	18.5	21.9	23.9	33.8	34.9
Vermont	23	–	–	6.4	11.2	12.5	13.4	–	–	4.0
Massachusetts	3,252	2.9	13.7	26.5	34.5	39.0	39.0	44.6	54.2	52.9
Rhode Island	400	3.7	9.1	20.6	26.6	19.6	23.7	11.8	29.8	40.5
Connecticut	1,272	2.4	7.1	19.9	21.2	21.2	29.8	34.7	42.9	38.8
Middle Atlantic:										
New York	6,940	5.5	8.0	15.1	23.4	26.6	29.2	35.7	37.8	38.2
New Jersey	2,391	2.0	5.6	12.3	11.4	14.7	23.0	27.5	31.3	29.5
Pennsylvania	4,036	1.2	5.0	12.5	18.3	21.5	27.4	29.9	37.1	33.6
East North Central:										
Ohio	2,843	2.2	6.7	13.3	15.2	16.3	18.5	17.6	23.4	25.4
Indiana	777	0.5	3.6	6.1	7.4	8.3	9.9	11.9	14.0	13.2
Illinois	2,506	1.9	7.1	12.6	16.2	17.2	20.0	17.1	20.8	20.8
Michigan	2,648	2.4	9.9	15.2	18.3	20.5	22.2	23.5	25.3	27.0
Wisconsin	1,614	8.5	17.8	21.7	22.4	24.0	27.6	24.9	30.8	30.9
West North Central:										
Minnesota	1,437	9.9	22.2	16.4	25.4	26.5	28.6	32.7	32.4	30.4
Iowa	139	0.2	4.8	10.1	4.6	4.5	4.9	4.6	4.9	4.9
Missouri	1,860	2.3	6.0	8.2	15.0	18.5	24.0	30.2	33.7	34.2
North Dakota	16	0.4	2.5	1.7	0.7	1.2	1.2	1.7	2.2	2.5
South Dakota	45	–	–	3.3	2.9	2.8	2.8	3.5	5.1	6.1
Nebraska	305	1.1	1.8	5.1	6.9	8.6	10.8	15.4	16.9	18.4
Kansas	442	–	3.3	7.9	5.2	4.7	6.3	11.5	14.4	16.8
South Atlantic:										
Delaware	340	–	3.9	17.5	16.6	18.4	29.3	38.8	48.1	45.7
Maryland	2,362	2.0	4.8	14.2	24.5	29.5	30.9	38.0	43.6	46.0
District of Columbia[2]	176	...	...	...	...	...	...	34.1	33.0	33.7
Virginia	1,332	–	1.1	6.1	7.2	7.7	8.7	15.7	16.9	19.6
West Virginia	189	0.7	1.7	3.9	4.1	5.8	7.0	9.4	10.7	10.5
North Carolina	1,416	0.6	1.6	4.8	6.7	8.3	11.1	14.6	17.1	18.8
South Carolina	383	0.2	1.0	1.9	3.6	5.5	9.0	8.4	9.9	10.0
Georgia	1,239	0.1	2.9	4.8	6.7	7.6	9.4	12.7	15.5	16.2
Florida	4,900	1.5	5.6	10.6	15.7	18.8	23.0	29.0	31.5	32.9
East South Central:										
Kentucky	1,281	0.9	1.6	5.7	10.6	16.1	15.3	27.4	35.1	32.5
Tennessee	2,046	–	1.8	3.7	11.0	12.2	13.9	15.3	24.1	37.7
Alabama	437	0.3	0.9	5.3	6.2	7.3	7.9	9.8	10.8	10.0
Mississippi	89	–	–	–	0.1	0.7	1.2	2.4	3.6	3.2
West South Central:										
Arkansas	312	–	0.1	2.2	5.4	3.8	15.2	8.7	10.7	12.3
Louisiana	775	0.6	0.9	5.4	7.5	7.2	11.0	14.7	16.6	17.7
Oklahoma	476	–	2.1	5.5	7.1	7.6	10.3	12.4	13.8	14.2
Texas	3,676	0.6	3.4	6.9	9.1	12.0	12.3	15.3	17.8	18.6
Mountain:										
Montana	58	–	–	1.0	1.6	2.4	2.9	3.1	3.9	6.6
Idaho	79	1.2	–	1.8	1.1	1.4	3.7	4.3	5.7	6.4
Wyoming	6	–	–	–	–	–	–	0.4	0.7	1.2
Colorado	1,563	6.9	10.8	20.0	22.2	23.3	25.8	31.1	36.4	39.4
New Mexico	661	1.4	2.0	12.7	12.7	15.1	15.5	21.0	32.3	38.1
Arizona	1,496	6.0	10.3	16.2	22.5	25.8	29.0	28.8	30.3	32.0
Utah	739	0.6	8.8	13.9	23.4	25.1	30.1	40.7	35.6	35.2
Nevada	410	–	5.8	8.5	11.9	15.9	18.7	20.8	26.8	23.5
Pacific:										
Washington	985	9.4	8.7	14.6	21.0	18.7	23.2	25.1	26.3	17.3
Oregon	1,422	12.0	14.0	24.7	29.6	40.0	44.8	47.2	45.3	43.3
California	17,025	16.8	22.5	30.7	33.7	36.0	40.3	43.8	47.1	52.1
Alaska	–	–	–	–	–	–	–	–	–	–
Hawaii	402	15.3	18.1	21.6	21.1	21.0	21.6	25.0	32.8	33.7

– Quantity zero.　　- - - Data not available.

[1]HMO's in Guam are included starting in 1994; HMO's in Puerto Rico, starting in 1998. In 1999 HMO enrollment in Guam was 93,000 and in Puerto Rico, 1,354,000.
[2]Data for the District of Columbia (DC) were not included for 1980–96 because the data were not adjusted for the high proportion of enrollees of DC-based HMO's living in Maryland and Virginia.

NOTES: Data for 1980–90 are for pure HMO enrollment at midyear. Data for 1994–99 are for pure and open-ended enrollment as of January 1. In 1990 open-ended enrollment accounted for 3 percent of HMO enrollment compared with 11 percent in 1999. See Appendix II, Health maintenance organization.

SOURCE: The InterStudy Edge, Managed care: A decade in review 1980–1990. The InterStudy Competitive Edge, vols 4–9, 1994–1999. St. Paul, Minnesota (Copyrights 1991, 1994–1999: Used with the permission of InterStudy).

Table 146. Persons without health care coverage by geographic division and State: United States, selected years 1987–98

[Data are based on household interviews of a sample of the civilian noninstitutionalized population]

Geographic division and State	Number in thousands 1998	Percent of population								
		1987	1990	1992	1993	1994	1995	1996	1997	1998
United States	44,281	12.9	13.9	15.0	15.3	15.2	15.4	15.6	16.1	16.3
New England:										
Maine	161	8.4	11.2	11.1	11.1	13.1	13.5	12.1	14.9	12.7
New Hampshire	138	10.1	9.9	12.6	12.5	11.9	10.1	9.6	11.8	11.3
Vermont	58	9.8	9.5	9.5	11.9	8.6	13.0	11.0	9.5	9.9
Massachusetts	627	6.3	9.1	10.6	11.7	12.5	11.1	12.4	12.6	10.3
Rhode Island	96	6.8	11.1	9.5	10.3	11.5	12.9	9.9	10.2	10.0
Connecticut	412	6.4	6.9	8.2	10.0	10.4	8.8	11.0	12.0	12.6
Middle Atlantic:										
New York	3,177	11.6	12.1	13.9	13.9	16.0	15.2	17.0	17.5	17.3
New Jersey	1,329	7.9	10.0	13.3	13.7	13.0	14.2	16.8	16.5	16.4
Pennsylvania	1,248	7.2	10.1	8.7	10.8	10.6	10.0	9.5	10.1	10.5
East North Central:										
Ohio	1,169	9.2	10.3	11.0	11.1	11.0	11.9	11.5	11.5	10.4
Indiana	839	13.4	10.7	11.0	11.9	10.5	12.6	10.6	11.4	14.4
Illinois	1,842	9.7	10.9	13.2	12.6	11.4	11.0	11.3	12.4	15.0
Michigan	1,328	8.4	9.4	10.0	11.2	10.8	9.7	8.9	11.6	13.2
Wisconsin	604	6.5	6.7	9.1	8.7	8.9	7.3	8.4	8.0	11.8
West North Central:										
Minnesota	448	6.6	8.9	8.1	10.1	9.5	8.0	10.2	9.2	9.3
Iowa	265	7.3	8.1	10.3	9.2	9.7	11.3	11.6	12.0	9.3
Missouri	570	10.5	12.7	14.4	12.2	12.2	14.6	13.2	12.6	10.5
North Dakota	92	7.7	6.3	8.2	13.4	8.4	8.2	9.8	15.2	14.2
South Dakota	102	13.7	11.6	15.1	13.0	10.0	9.4	9.5	11.8	14.3
Nebraska	155	9.6	8.5	9.4	11.9	10.7	9.0	11.4	10.8	9.0
Kansas	270	10.3	10.8	10.9	12.7	12.9	12.4	11.4	11.7	10.3
South Atlantic:										
Delaware	115	10.5	13.9	11.2	13.4	13.5	15.8	13.3	13.1	14.7
Maryland	837	9.8	12.7	11.3	13.5	12.6	15.3	11.4	13.4	16.6
District of Columbia	87	15.6	19.2	21.7	20.7	16.4	17.3	14.8	16.2	17.0
Virginia	946	10.4	15.7	14.6	13.0	12.0	13.5	12.5	12.6	14.1
West Virginia	302	13.5	13.8	15.4	18.3	16.2	15.3	14.9	17.2	17.2
North Carolina	1,111	13.3	13.8	13.9	14.0	13.3	14.3	16.0	15.5	15.0
South Carolina	594	11.1	16.2	17.2	16.9	14.2	14.6	17.1	16.8	15.4
Georgia	1,341	13.0	15.3	19.1	18.4	16.2	17.9	17.8	17.6	17.5
Florida	2,564	17.4	18.0	19.8	19.6	17.2	18.3	18.9	19.6	17.5
East South Central:										
Kentucky	545	15.2	13.2	14.6	12.5	15.2	14.6	15.4	15.0	14.1
Tennessee	724	14.5	13.7	13.6	13.2	10.2	14.8	15.2	13.6	13.0
Alabama	714	15.8	17.4	16.8	17.2	19.2	13.5	12.8	15.5	17.0
Mississippi	554	17.1	19.9	19.4	17.9	17.8	19.7	18.5	20.1	20.0
West South Central:										
Arkansas	478	20.7	17.4	19.9	19.7	17.4	18.0	21.7	24.4	18.7
Louisiana	817	17.1	19.7	22.3	23.9	19.2	20.5	20.8	14.9	19.0
Oklahoma	599	18.1	18.6	22.0	23.6	17.8	19.2	17.0	17.8	18.3
Texas	4,880	21.1	21.1	23.1	21.8	24.2	24.5	24.3	24.5	24.5
Mountain:										
Montana	181	15.5	14.0	9.4	15.3	13.6	12.7	13.6	19.5	19.6
Idaho	225	15.3	15.2	16.5	14.8	14.0	14.0	16.5	17.7	17.7
Wyoming	82	11.4	12.5	11.7	15.0	15.4	15.9	13.4	15.5	16.9
Colorado	599	13.8	14.7	12.7	12.6	12.4	14.8	16.6	15.1	15.1
New Mexico	386	22.7	22.2	19.8	22.0	23.1	25.6	22.3	22.6	21.1
Arizona	1,187	18.4	15.5	15.5	20.2	20.2	20.4	24.1	24.5	24.2
Utah	293	12.4	9.0	11.8	11.3	11.5	11.8	12.0	13.4	13.9
Nevada	394	15.9	16.5	23.0	18.1	15.7	18.7	15.6	17.5	21.2
Pacific:										
Washington	706	13.0	11.4	10.4	12.6	12.7	12.4	13.5	11.4	12.3
Oregon	481	15.0	12.4	13.6	14.7	13.1	12.5	15.3	13.3	14.3
California	7,373	16.8	19.1	20.0	19.7	21.1	20.6	20.1	21.5	22.1
Alaska	112	16.2	15.4	16.8	13.3	13.3	12.5	13.4	18.1	17.3
Hawaii	121	7.5	7.3	6.1	11.1	9.2	8.9	8.6	7.5	10.0

NOTES: New health insurance questions were introduced for a quarter sample for 1993 data and the full sample for 1994 data. Starting with 1993 data, the collection method changed from paper and pencil to computer-assisted interviewing. 1990 census population controls were implemented starting with 1992 data. Estimates of the percent of persons lacking health care coverage based on the National Health Interview Survey (NHIS) (table 128) are slightly higher than those based on the March Current Population Survey (CPS). See Appendix II, Health insurance coverage.

SOURCES: U.S. Bureau of the Census: Household Economic Studies. Current population reports, series P–60, no 190. Washington: U.S. Government Printing Office. Nov. 1995; press release CB98–172, Sept. 28, 1998; and unpublished data from the Current Population Survey provided by the Income Statistics Branch.

Appendixes

Appendix Contents ....

Sources of Data

Introduction

This report consolidates the most current data on the health of the population of the United States, the availability and use of health resources, and health care expenditures. The information was obtained from the data files and/or published reports of many governmental and nongovernmental agencies and organizations. In each case, the sponsoring agency or organization collected data using its own methods and procedures. Therefore, the data in this report vary considerably with respect to source, method of collection, definitions, and reference period.

Much of the data presented in the detailed tables are from the ongoing data collection systems of the National Center for Health Statistics. For an overview of these systems, see: Kovar MG. Data systems of the National Center for Health Statistics. National Center for Health Statistics. Vital Health Stat 1(23). 1989. However, health care personnel data come primarily from the Bureau of Health Professions, Health Resources and Services Administration, and the American Medical Association. National health expenditures data were compiled by the Office of the Actuary, Health Care Financing Administration.

Although a detailed description and comprehensive evaluation of each data source is beyond the scope of this appendix, users should be aware of the general strengths and weaknesses of the different data collection systems. For example, population-based surveys obtain socioeconomic data, data on family characteristics, and information on the impact of an illness, such as days lost from work or limitation of activity. They are limited by the amount of information a respondent remembers or is willing to report. Detailed medical information, such as precise diagnoses or the types of operations performed, may not be known and so will not be reported. Health care providers, such as physicians and hospitals, usually have good diagnostic information but little or no information about the socioeconomic characteristics of individuals or the impact of illnesses on individuals.

The populations covered by different data collection systems may not be the same, and understanding the differences is critical to interpreting the data. Data on vital statistics and national expenditures cover the entire population. Most data on morbidity and utilization of health resources cover only the civilian noninstitutionalized population. Thus, statistics are not included for military personnel who are usually young; for institutionalized people who may be any age; or for nursing home residents who are usually old.

All data collection systems are subject to error, and records may be incomplete or contain inaccurate information. People may not remember essential information, a question may not mean the same thing to different respondents, and some institutions or individuals may not respond at all. It is not always possible to measure the magnitude of these errors or their impact on the data. Where possible, the tables have notes describing the universe and the method of data collection to enable the user to place his or her own evaluation on the data. In many instances data do not add to totals because of rounding.

Some information is collected in more than one survey and estimates of the same statistic may vary among surveys. For example, cigarette use is measured by the Health Interview Survey, the National Household Survey of Drug Abuse, and the Monitoring the Future Survey. Estimates of cigarette use may differ among surveys because of different survey methodologies, sampling frames, questionnaires, definitions, and tabulation categories.

Overall estimates generally have relatively small sampling errors, but estimates for certain population subgroups may be based on small numbers and have relatively large sampling errors. Numbers of births and deaths from the vital statistics system represent complete counts (except for births in those States where data are based on a 50-percent sample for certain years). Therefore, they are not subject to sampling error. However, when the figures are used for analytical purposes, such as the comparison of rates over a period, the number of events that actually occurred may be considered as one of a large series of possible results that could have arisen under the same circumstances. When the number of events is small and the probability of such an event is small, considerable caution must be observed in interpreting the conditions described by the figures. Estimates that are unreliable because of large sampling errors or small numbers of events are noted with asterisks in selected tables. The criteria used to designate unreliable estimates are indicated as notes to the applicable tables.

The descriptive summaries that follow provide a general overview of study design, methods of data collection, and reliability and validity of the data. More complete and detailed discussions are found in the publications referenced at the end of each summary. The data set or source is listed under the agency or organization that sponsored the data collection.

Department of Health and Human Services

Centers for Disease Control and Prevention

National Center for Health Statistics

National Vital Statistics System

Through the National Vital Statistics System, the National Center for Health Statistics (NCHS) collects and publishes data on births, deaths, marriages, and divorces in the United States. Fetal deaths are classified and tabulated separately from other deaths. The Division of Vital Statistics obtains information on births and deaths from the registration offices of all States, New York City, the District of Columbia, Puerto Rico, the U.S. Virgin Islands, and Guam. Geographic coverage for births and deaths has been complete since 1933. U.S. data shown in detailed tables in this book are for the 50 States and the District of Columbia, unless otherwise specified.

Until 1972 microfilm copies of all death certificates and a 50-percent sample of birth certificates were received from all registration areas and processed by NCHS. In 1972 some States began sending their data to NCHS through the Cooperative Health Statistics System (CHSS). States that participated in the CHSS program processed 100 percent of their death and birth records and sent the entire data file to NCHS on computer tapes. Currently, the data are sent to NCHS through the Vital Statistics Cooperative Program (VSCP), following the same procedures as

CHSS. The number of participating States grew from 6 in 1972 to 46 in 1984. Starting in 1985 all 50 States and the District of Columbia participated in VSCP.

In most areas practically all births and deaths are registered. The most recent test of the completeness of birth registration, conducted on a sample of births from 1964 to 1968, showed that 99.3 percent of all births in the United States during that period were registered. No comparable information is available for deaths, but it is generally believed that death registration in the United States is at least as complete as birth registration.

Demographic information on the birth certificate such as race and ethnicity is provided by the mother at the time of birth. Medical and health information is based on hospital records. Demographic information on the death certificate is provided by the funeral director based on information supplied by an informant. Medical certification of cause of death is provided by a physician, medical examiner, or coroner.

U.S. Standard Certificates—U.S. Standard Live Birth and Death Certificates and Fetal Death Reports are revised periodically, allowing careful evaluation of each item and addition, modification, and deletion of items. Beginning with 1989 revised standard certificates replaced the 1978 versions. The 1989 revision of the birth certificate includes items to identify the Hispanic parentage of newborns and to expand information about maternal and infant health characteristics. The 1989 revision of the death certificate includes items on educational attainment and Hispanic origin of decedents as well as changes to improve the medical certification of cause of death. Standard certificates recommended by NCHS are modified in each registration area to serve the area's needs. However, most certificates conform closely in content and arrangement to the standard certificate, and all certificates contain a minimum data set specified by NCHS. For selected items, reporting areas expanded during the years spanned by this report. For items on the birth certificate, the number of reporting States increased for mother's education, prenatal care, marital status, Hispanic parentage, and tobacco use; and on the death certificate, for educational attainment and Hispanic origin of the decedent.

Appendix I ....

Birth certificate items—

Race—Data on birth rates, birth characteristics, and fetal death rates for 1980 and more recent years for liveborn infants and fetal deaths are presented in this report according to race of mother, unless specified otherwise. Before 1980 data were tabulated by race of newborn and fetus, taking into account the race of both parents. If the parents were of different races and one parent was white, the child was classified according to the race of the other parent. When neither parent was white, the child was classified according to father's race, with one exception: if either parent was Hawaiian, the child was classified Hawaiian. Before 1964, if race was unknown, the birth was classified as white. Beginning in 1964 unknown race was classified according to information on the previous record.

Maternal age—Mother's age was reported on the birth certificate by all States. Data are presented for mothers age 10–49 years through 1996 and 10–54 years starting in 1997, based on mother's date of birth or age as reported on the birth certificate. The age of mother is edited for upper and lower limits. When the age of the mother is computed to be under 10 years or 55 years or over (50 years or over in 1964–96), it is considered not stated and imputed according to the age of the mother from the previous birth record of the same race and total birth order (total of fetal deaths and live births). Before 1963 not stated ages were distributed in proportion to the known ages for each racial group. Beginning in 1997 the birth rate for the maternal age group 45–49 years includes data for mother's age 50–54 years in the numerator and is based on the population of women 45–49 years in the denominator.

Maternal education—Mother's education was reported on the birth certificate by 38 States in 1970. Data were not available from Alabama, Arkansas, California, Connecticut, Delaware, District of Columbia, Georgia, Idaho, Maryland, New Mexico, Pennsylvania, Texas, and Washington. In 1975 these data were available from 4 additional States, Connecticut, Delaware, Georgia, Maryland, and the District of Columbia, increasing the number of States reporting mother's education to 42 and the District of Columbia. Between 1980 and 1988 only three States, California, Texas, and Washington did not report mother's education. In 1988 mother's education was also missing from New York State outside of New York City. In 1989–91 mother's education was missing only from Washington and New York State outside of New York City. Starting in 1992 mother's education was reported by all 50 States and the District of Columbia.

Prenatal care—Prenatal care was reported on the birth certificate by 39 States and the District of Columbia in 1970. Data were not available from Alabama, Alaska, Arkansas, Connecticut, Delaware, Georgia, Idaho, Massachusetts, New Mexico, Pennsylvania, and Virginia. In 1975 these data were available from 3 additional States, Connecticut, Delaware, and Georgia, increasing the number of States reporting prenatal care to 42 and the District of Columbia. Starting in 1980 prenatal care information was available for the entire United States.

Marital status—Mother's marital status was reported on the birth certificate by 39 States and the District of Columbia in 1970, and by 38 States and the District of Columbia in 1975. The incidence of births to unmarried women in States with no direct question on marital status was assumed to be the same as the incidence in reporting States in the same geographic division. Starting in 1980 for States without a direct question, marital status was inferred by comparing the parents' and child's surnames and other information concerning the father. In 1980–96 marital status was reported on the birth certificates of 41–45 States. In 1997, all but four States (Connecticut, Michigan, Nevada, and New York) and, in 1998, all but two States (Michigan and New York) included a direct question about mother's marital status on their birth certificates.

Hispanic origin—In 1980 and 1981 information on births of Hispanic parentage was reported on the birth certificate by the following 22 States: Arizona, Arkansas, California, Colorado, Florida, Georgia, Hawaii, Illinois, Indiana, Kansas, Maine, Mississippi, Nebraska, Nevada, New Jersey, New Mexico, New York, North Dakota, Ohio, Texas, Utah, and Wyoming. In 1982 Tennessee, and in 1983 the District of Columbia began reporting this information. Between 1983 and 1987 information on births of Hispanic parentage was available for 23 States and the District of Columbia. In 1988 this information became available for Alabama, Connecticut, Kentucky, Massachusetts, Montana, North Carolina, and Washington, increasing the number of States reporting information on births of Hispanic parentage to 30 States and the District of Columbia. In 1989 this information became available from an additional 17 States, increasing the number of Hispanic-reporting States to 47 and the District of Columbia. In 1989 only Louisiana, New Hampshire, and Oklahoma did not report Hispanic parentage on the birth certificate. In 1990 Louisiana began reporting Hispanic parentage. Hispanic origin of the mother was reported on the birth certificates of 49 States and the District of Columbia in 1991 and 1992; only New Hampshire did not provide this information. Starting in 1993 Hispanic origin of mother was reported by all 50 States and the District of Columbia. In 1990, 99 percent of birth records included information on mother's origin.

Tobacco use—Information on tobacco use during pregnancy became available for the first time in 1989 with the revision of the U.S. Standard Birth Certificate. In 1989 data on tobacco use were collected by 43 States and the District of Columbia. The following States did not require the reporting of tobacco use in the standard format on the birth certificate: California, Indiana, Louisiana, Nebraska, New York, Oklahoma, and South Dakota. In 1990 information on tobacco use became available from Louisiana and Nebraska, increasing the number of reporting States to 45 and the District of Columbia. In 1991–93

information on tobacco use was available for 46 States and the District of Columbia with the addition of Oklahoma to the reporting area; and in 1994–97, for 46 States, the District of Columbia, and New York City.

Death certificate items—

Education of decedent—Information on educational attainment of decedents became available for the first time in 1989 due to the revision of the U.S. Standard Certificate of Death. Mortality data by educational attainment for 1989 were based on data from 20 States and by 1994–96 increased to 45 States and the District of Columbia. In 1994–96 the following States either did not report educational attainment on the death certificate or the information was more than 20 percent incomplete: Georgia, Kentucky, Oklahoma, Rhode Island, and South Dakota. In 1997 and 1998 information on decedent's education was available from Oklahoma, increasing the reporting area to 46 States and the District of Columbia. Information on the death certificate about the decedent's educational attainment is reported by the funeral director based on information provided by an informant such as next of kin.

Calculation of unbiased death rates by educational attainment based on the National Vital Statistics System requires that the reporting of education on the death certificate be complete and consistent with the reporting of education on the Current Population Survey, the source of population estimates that form the denominators for death rates. Death records with education not stated have not been included in the calculation of rates. Therefore the levels of the rates shown in this report are underestimated by approximately the percent not stated, which ranged from 3 to 5 percent.

The validity of information about the decedent's education was evaluated by comparing self-reported education obtained in the Current Population Survey with education on the death certificate for decedents in the National Longitudinal Mortality Survey (NLMS). (Sorlie

PD, Johnson NJ: Validity of education information on the death certificate, Epidemiology 7(4):437–9, 1996.) Another analysis compared self-reported education collected in the first National Health and Nutrition Examination Survey (NHANES I) with education on the death certificate for decedents in the NHANES I Epidemiologic Followup Study. (Makuc DM, Feldman JJ, Mussolino ME: Validity of education and age as reported on death certificates, American Statistical Association 1996 Proceedings of the Social Statistics Section, 102–6, 1997.) Results of both studies indicated that there is a tendency for some people who did not graduate from high school to be reported as high school graduates on the death certificate. This tendency results in overstating the death rate for high school graduates and understating the death rate for the group with less than 12 years of education. The bias was greater among older than younger decedents and somewhat greater among black than white decedents.

In addition, educational gradients in death rates based on the National Vital Statistics System were compared with those based on the NLMS, a prospective study of persons in the Current Population Survey. Results of these comparisons indicate that educational gradients in death rates based on the National Vital Statistics System were reasonably similar to those based on NLMS for white persons 25–64 years of age and black persons 25–44 years of age. The number of deaths for persons of Hispanic origin in NLMS was too small to permit comparison for this ethnic group

Hispanic origin—In 1985 mortality data by Hispanic origin of decedent were based on deaths to residents of the following 17 States and the District of Columbia whose data on the death certificate were at least 90 percent complete on a place-of-occurrence basis and of comparable format: Arizona, Arkansas, California, Colorado, Georgia, Hawaii, Illinois, Indiana, Kansas, Mississippi, Nebraska, New York, North Dakota, Ohio, Texas, Utah, and Wyoming. In 1986 New

Jersey began reporting Hispanic origin of decedent, increasing the number of reporting States to 18 and the District of Columbia in 1986 and 1987. In 1988 Alabama, Kentucky, Maine, Montana, North Carolina, Oregon, Rhode Island, and Washington were added to the reporting area, increasing the number of States to 26 and the District of Columbia. In 1989 an additional 18 States were added, increasing the Hispanic reporting area to 44 States and the District of Columbia. In 1989 only Connecticut, Louisiana, Maryland, New Hampshire, Oklahoma, and Virginia were not included in the reporting area. Starting with 1990 data in this book, the criterion was changed to include States whose data were at least 80 percent complete. In 1990 Maryland, Virginia, and Connecticut, in 1991 Louisiana, and in 1993 New Hampshire were added, increasing the reporting area for Hispanic origin of decedent to 47 States and the District of Columbia in 1990, 48 States and the District of Columbia in 1991 and 1992, and 49 States and the District of Columbia in 1993–96. Only Oklahoma did not provide this information in 1993–96. Starting in 1997 Hispanic origin of decedent was reported by all 50 States and the District of Columbia. Based on data from the U.S. Bureau of the Census, the 1990 reporting area encompassed 99.6 percent of the U.S. Hispanic population. In 1990 more than 96 percent of death records included information on origin of decedent.

Race and Hispanic origin—Death rates by race and Hispanic origin are based on information from death certificates (numerators of the rates) and on population estimates from the Census Bureau (denominators) (see Appendix I, Bureau of the Census). Race and ethnicity information on the death certificate are reported by the funeral director as provided by an informant, often the surviving next of kin, or, in the absence of an informant, on the basis of observation. Race and ethnicity information from the Census is by self-report. To the extent that race and Hispanic origin are inconsistent between these two data sources, death rates will be biased. Studies have shown that persons self-reported as American Indian, Asian, or Hispanic on census and survey records may sometimes be reported as white or non-Hispanic on the death certificate, resulting in an underestimation of deaths and death rates for the American Indian, Asian, and Hispanic groups. Bias also results from undercounts of some population groups in the census, particularly young black and white males and elderly persons, resulting in an overestimation of death rates. The net effects of misclassification and under coverage result in overstated death rates for the white population and black population estimated to be 1 percent and 5 percent, respectively; and understated death rates for other population groups estimated as follows: American Indians, 21 percent; Asian or Pacific Islanders, 11 percent; and Hispanics, 2 percent. For more information, see Rosenberg HM, Maurer JD, Sorlie PD, Johnson NJ, et al. Quality of death rates by race and Hispanic origin: A summary of current research, 1999. National Center for Health Statistics. Vital Health Stat 2(128). 1999.

Infant and maternal mortality rates are calculated with denominators comprised of number of live births rather than population estimates. Starting with 1980 infant and maternal mortality trends are based on maternal race and ethnicity of the live birth in the denominator. Before 1980 infant and maternal mortality trends were based on child's race in the denominator, which took into account the race of both parents. Infant and maternal mortality trends for Hispanics commenced with 1985 and are based on Hispanic origin of mother.

Vital event rates for the American Indian or Alaska Native population shown in this book are based on the total U.S. resident population of American Indians and Alaska Natives as enumerated by the U.S. Bureau of Census. In contrast the Indian Health Service calculates vital event rates for this population based on U.S. Bureau of Census county data for American Indians and Alaska Natives who reside on or near reservations.

Mortality data in *Health, United States* are presented for four major race groups, white, black, American Indian or Alaska Native, and Asian or Pacific Islander, in accordance with 1977 U.S. Office of Management and Budget (OMB) standards for presenting Federal statistics on race. Over the next several years, major changes will occur in the way Federal agencies collect and tabulate data on race and Hispanic origin in accordance with new guidelines from OMB (see Appendix II, Race). The major difference between the current and new guidelines is the adoption of data-collection procedures in which respondents can identify with more than one race group.

Alaska data—For 1995 the number of deaths occurring in Alaska is in error for selected causes because NCHS did not receive changes resulting from amended records and because of errors in processing the cause-of-death data. Differences are concentrated among selected causes of death, principally Symptoms, signs, and ill-defined conditions (ICD-9 Nos. 780–799) and external causes.

For more information, see: National Center for Health Statistics, Technical Appendix, *Vital Statistics of the United States, 1992*, Vol. I, Natality, DHHS Pub. No. (PHS) 96–1100 and Vol. II, Mortality, Part A, DHHS Pub. No. (PHS) 96–1101, Public Health Service. Washington: U.S. Government Printing Office, 1996; or visit the NCHS home page at www.cdc.gov/nchs/.

National Linked File of Live Births and Infant Deaths

National linked files of live births and infant deaths are data sets for research on infant mortality. To create these data sets, death certificates are linked with corresponding birth certificates for infants who die in the United States before their first birthday. Linked data files include all of the variables on the national natality file, including the more accurate racial and ethnic information, as well as the variables on the national mortality file, including cause of death and age at death. The linkage makes available for the analysis of infant mortality extensive information from

Sources of Data

the birth certificate about the pregnancy, maternal risk factors, and infant characteristics and health items at birth. Each year 97–98 percent of infant death records are linked to their corresponding birth records.

National linked files of live births and infant deaths were first produced for the 1983 birth cohort. Birth cohort linked file data are available for 1983–91 and period linked file data for 1995–97. While birth cohort linked files have methodological advantages, their production incurs substantial delays in data availability, since it is necessary to wait until the close of a second data year to include all infant deaths to the birth cohort. Starting with data year 1995, more timely linked file data are produced in a period data format preceding the release of the corresponding birth cohort format. Other changes to the data set starting with 1995 data include the addition of record weights to correct for the 2.2–2.5 percent of records that could not be linked and the addition of an imputation for not stated birthweight.

For more information, see: Prager K. Infant mortality by birthweight and other characteristics: United States, 1985 birth cohort. National Center for Health Statistics. Vital Health Stat 20(24). 1994; MacDorman MF, Atkinson JO. Infant mortality statistics from the 1997 period linked birth/death data set. Monthly vital statistics report; vol 47 no 23, supp. Hyattsville, MD: National Center for Health Statistics. 1999; or visit the NCHS home page at www.cdc.gov/nchs/.

Compressed Mortality File

The Compressed Mortality File (CMF) used to compute death rates by urbanization level is a county-level national mortality and population database. The mortality data base of CMF is derived from the detailed mortality files of the National Vital Statistics System starting with 1968. The population data base of CMF is derived from intercensal and postcensal population estimates and census counts of the resident population of each U.S. county by age, race, and sex. Counties are categorized according to level of urbanization based on an NCHS-modified version of the 1993 rural-urban continuum codes for metropolitan and nonmetropolitan counties developed by the

Economic Research Service, U.S. Department of Agriculture. See Appendix II, Urbanization. For more information about the CMF, contact: D. Ingram, Analytic Studies Branch, Division of Health and Utilization Analysis, National Center for Health Statistics, 6525 Belcrest Road, Hyattsville, MD 20782.

National Survey of Family Growth

Data from the National Survey of Family Growth (NSFG) are based on samples of women ages 15–44 years in the civilian noninstitutionalized population of the United States. The first and second cycles, conducted in 1973 and 1976, excluded most women who had never been married. The third, fourth, and fifth cycles, conducted in 1982, 1988, and 1995, included all women ages 15–44 years.

The purpose of the survey is to provide national data on factors affecting birth and pregnancy rates, adoption, and maternal and infant health. These factors include sexual activity, marriage, divorce and remarriage, unmarried cohabitation, contraception and sterilization, infertility, breastfeeding, pregnancy loss, low birthweight, and use of medical care for family planning and infertility.

Interviews are conducted in person by professional female interviewers using a standardized questionnaire. In 1973–88 the average interview length was about 1 hour. In 1995 the average interview lasted about 1 hour and 45 minutes. In all cycles black women were sampled at higher rates than white women, so that detailed statistics for black women could be produced.

Interviewing for Cycle 1 of NSFG was conducted from June 1973 to February 1974. Counties and independent cities of the United States were sampled to form a frame of primary sampling units (PSU's), and 101 PSU's were selected. From these 101 PSU's, 10,879 women 15–44 years of age were selected, 9,797 of these were interviewed. Most never-married women were excluded from the 1973 NSFG.

Interviewing for Cycle 2 of NSFG was conducted from January to September 1976. From 79 PSU's, 10,202 eligible women were identified; of these, 8,611 were interviewed. Again, most never-married women were excluded from the sample for the 1976 NSFG.

Interviewing for Cycle 3 of NSFG was conducted from August 1982 to February 1983. The sample design was similar to that in Cycle 2: 31,027 households were selected in 79 PSU'S. Household screener interviews were completed in 29,511 households (95.1 percent). Of the 9,964 eligible women identified, 7,969 were interviewed. For the first time in NSFG, Cycle 3 included women of all marital statuses.

Interviewing for Cycle 4 was conducted between January and August 1988. The sample was obtained from households that had been interviewed in the National Health Interview Survey in the 18 months between October 1, 1985, and March 31, 1987. For the first time, women living in Alaska and Hawaii were included so that the survey covered women from the noninstitutionalized population of the entire United States. The sample was drawn from 156 PSU's; 10,566 eligible women ages 15–44 years were sampled. Interviews were completed with 8,450 women.

Between July and November of 1990, 5,686 women were interviewed by telephone in the first NSFG telephone reinterview. The average length of interview in 1990 was 20 minutes. The response rate for the 1990 telephone reinterview was 68 percent of those responding to the 1988 survey and still eligible for the 1990 survey.

Interviewing for Cycle 5 of NSFG was conducted between January and October of 1995. The sample was obtained from households that had been interviewed in 198 PSU's in the National Health Interview Survey in 1993. Of the 13,795 eligible women in the sample, 10,847 were interviewed. For the first time, Hispanic as well as black women were sampled at a higher rate than other women.

In order to make national estimates from the sample for the millions of women ages 15–44 years in the United States, data for the interviewed sample women were (a) inflated by the reciprocal of the probability of selection at each stage of sampling (for example, if there was a 1 in 5,000 chance that a woman would be selected for the sample, her sampling weight was 5,000), (b) adjusted for nonresponse, and (c) forced to agree with benchmark population values

based on data from the Current Population Survey of the U.S. Bureau of the Census (this last step is called "poststratification").

Quality control procedures for selecting and training interviewers, coding, editing, and processing the data were built into NSFG to minimize nonsampling error.

More information on the methodology of NSFG is available in the following reports: French DK. National Survey of Family Growth, Cycle I: Sample design, estimation procedures, and variance estimation. National Center for Health Statistics. Vital Health Stat 2(76). 1978; Grady WR. National Survey of Family Growth, Cycle II: Sample design, estimation procedures, and variance estimation. National Center for Health Statistics. Vital Health Stat 2(87). 1981; Bachrach CA, Horn MC, Mosher WD, Shimizu I. National Survey of Family Growth, Cycle III: Sample design, weighting, and variance estimation. National Center for Health Statistics. Vital Health Stat 2(98). 1985; Judkins DR, Mosher WD, Botman SL. National Survey of Family Growth: Design, estimation, and inference. National Center for Health Statistics. Vital Health Stat 2(109). 1991; Goksel H, Judkins DR, Mosher WD. Nonresponse adjustments for a telephone followup to a National In-Person Survey. Journal of Official Statistics 8(4):417–32. 1992; Kelly JE, Mosher WD, Duffer AP, Kinsey SH. Plan and operation of the 1995 National Survey of Family Growth. Vital Health Stat 1(36). 1997; Potter FJ, Iannacchione VG, Mosher WD, Mason RE, Kavee JD. Sampling weights, imputation, and variance estimation in the 1995 National Survey of Family Growth. Vital Health Stat 2(124). 1998; or visit the NCHS home page at www.cdc.gov/nchs/.

National Health Interview Survey

The National Health Interview Survey (NHIS) is a continuing nationwide sample survey in which data are collected through personal household interviews. Information is obtained on personal and demographic characteristics including race and ethnicity by self-reporting or as reported by an informant. Information is also obtained on illnesses, injuries, impairments, chronic conditions, utilization of health resources, and other health topics.

The sample design plan of NHIS follows a multistage probability design that permits a continuous sampling of the civilian noninstitutionalized population residing in the United States. The survey is designed in such a way that the sample scheduled for each week is representative of the target population, and the weekly samples are additive over time. The response rate for the ongoing portion of the survey (core) has been between 94 and 98 percent over the years. Response rates for special health topics (supplements) have generally been lower. For example, the response rate was 80 percent for the 1994 Year 2000 Supplement, which included questions about cigarette smoking and use of such preventive services as mammography.

In 1985 NHIS adopted several new sample design features although, conceptually, the sampling plan remained the same as the previous design. Two major changes included reducing the number of primary sampling locations from 376 to 198 for sampling efficiency and oversampling the black population to improve the precision of the statistics. The sample was designed so that a typical NHIS sample for the data collection years 1985–94 consisted of approximately 7,500 segments containing about 59,000 assigned households. Of these households, an expected 10,000 were vacant, demolished, or occupied by persons not in the target population of the survey. The expected sample of 49,000 occupied households yielded a probability sample of about 127,000 persons. In 1994 there was a sample of 116,179 persons.

In 1995 the NHIS sample was redesigned again. Major design changes included increasing the number of primary sampling units from 198 to 358 and oversampling the black and Hispanic populations to improve the precision of the statistics. The sample was designed so that a typical NHIS sample for the data collection years 1995–2004 will consist of approximately 7,000 segments. The expected sample of 44,000 occupied respondent households will yield a probability sample of about 106,000 persons. In 1997 there was a sample of 103,477 persons and in 1998 the sample was comprised of 98,785 persons.

The NHIS questionnaire that was fielded from 1982 to 1996 consisted of two parts: a set of basic health and demographic items known as the Core questionnaire and one or more sets of questions on current health topics (Supplements). Information was collected from responsible family members residing in the household. Proxy responses were acceptable for Core and Supplement questionnaires when family members were not present at the time of interview. Data for children were collected from proxy respondents.

In 1997 the NHIS questionnaire was redesigned and consists of three parts: a basic module, a periodic module, and a topical module. The basic module functions as the new Core questionnaire and is comprised of three components (Family Core, Sample Adult Core, Sample Child Core). For the Family Core, information is obtained about all members of the family by interviewing adult members of the household or from adult proxy respondents. For the Sample Adult Core, one adult in the household is randomly selected to participate; proxy respondents are not used in this component. For families with children under 18 years of age, one child in the household is randomly selected for participation in the Sample Child Core. Data for this component are collected from a knowledgeable adult in the household. Periodic and topical modules will be incorporated into future years of NHIS.

In 1997 the collection methodology changed from paper and pencil questionnaires to computer-assisted personal interviewing (CAPI). The NHIS questionnaire was also revised extensively in 1997. In some instances, basic concepts measured in NHIS changed and in other instances the same concepts were measured in a different way. While some questions remain the same over time, they may be preceded by different questions or topics. For some questions, there was a change in the reference period for reporting an event or condition. Because of the extensive redesign of the questionnaire in 1997 and the introduction of the CAPI method of data collection, data from 1997 and later years may not be comparable with earlier years.

A description of the survey design, the methods used in estimation, and the general qualifications of the data obtained from the survey are presented in: Massey JT, Moore TF, Parsons VL, Tadros W. Design and estimation for the National Health Interview Survey, 1985–94. National Center for Health Statistics. Vital Health Stat 2(110). 1989; Kovar MG, Poe GS. The National Health Interview Survey design, 1973–84, and procedures, 1975–83. National Center for Health Statistics. Vital Health Stat 1(18). 1985; Adams PF, Hendershot G, Marano M. Current estimates from the National Health Interview Survey, 1996. National Center for Health Statistics. Vital Health Stat 10(200). 1999; or visit the NCHS home page at www.cdc.gov/nchs/.

National Immunization Survey

The National Immunization Survey (NIS) is a continuing nationwide telephone sample survey to gather data on children 19–35 months of age. Estimates of vaccine-specific coverage are available for national, State, and 28 urban areas considered to be high risk for undervaccination.

NIS uses a two-phase sample design. First, a random-digit-dialing (RDD) sample of telephone numbers is drawn. When households with age-eligible children are contacted, the interviewer collects information on the vaccinations received by all age-eligible children. In 1998 the overall response rate was 68 percent, yielding data for 32,511 children aged 19–35 months. The interviewer also collects information on the vaccination providers. In the second phase, all vaccination providers are contacted by mail. The vaccination information from providers was obtained for 66 percent of all children who were eligible for provider followup in 1998. Providers' responses are combined with information obtained from the households to provide a more accurate estimate of vaccination coverage levels. Final estimates are adjusted for noncoverage of nontelephone households.

A description of the survey design and the methods used in estimation are presented in: Zell ER, Ezzati-Rice TM, Battaglia PM, Wright RA. National Immunization Survey: The Methodology of a Vaccination Surveillance System. Public Health Reports 2000; 115:65–77; or visit the NCHS home page at www.cdc.gov/nchs/.

National Health and Nutrition Examination Survey

For the first program or cycle of the National Health Examination Survey (NHES I), 1960–62, data were collected on the total prevalence of certain chronic diseases as well as the distributions of various physical and physiological measures, including blood pressure and serum cholesterol levels. For that program, a highly stratified, multistage probability sample of 7,710 adults, of whom 86.5 percent were examined, was selected to represent the 111 million civilian noninstitutionalized adults 18–79 years of age in the United States at that time. The sample areas consisted of 42 primary sampling units (PSU's) from the 1,900 geographic units.

NHES II (1963–65) and NHES III (1966–70) examined probability samples of the nation's noninstitutionalized children between the ages of 6 and 11 years (NHES II) and 12 and 17 years (NHES III) focusing on factors related to growth and development. Both cycles were multistage, stratified probability samples of clusters of households in land-based segments and used the same 40 PSU's. NHES II sampled 7,417 children with a response rate of 96 percent. NHES III sampled 7,514 youth with a response rate of 90 percent.

For more information on NHES I, see: Gordon T, Miller HW. Cycle I of the Health Examination Survey: Sample and response, United States, 1960–62. National Center for Health Statistics. Vital Health Stat 11(1). 1974. For more information on NHES II, see: Plan, operation, and response results of a program of children's examinations. National Center for Health Statistics. Vital Health Stat 1(5). 1967. For more information on NHES III, see: Schaible WL. Quality control in a National Health Examination Survey. National Center for Health Statistics. Vital Health Stat 2(44). 1972.

In 1971 a nutrition surveillance component was added and the survey name was changed to the National Health and Nutrition Examination Survey (NHANES). In NHANES I, conducted from 1971 to

1974, a major purpose was to measure and monitor indicators of the nutrition and health status of the American people through dietary intake data, biochemical tests, physical measurements, and clinical assessments for evidence of nutritional deficiency. Detailed examinations were given by dentists, ophthalmologists, and dermatologists with an assessment of need for treatment. In addition, data were obtained for a subsample of adults on overall health care needs and behavior, and more detailed examination data were collected on cardiovascular, respiratory, arthritic, and hearing conditions.

The NHANES I target population was the civilian noninstitutionalized population 1–74 years of age residing in the coterminous United States, except for people residing on any of the reservation lands set aside for the use of American Indians. The sample design was a multistage, stratified probability sample of clusters of persons in land-based segments. The sample areas consisted of 65 PSU's selected from the 1,900 PSU's in the coterminous United States. A subsample of persons 25–74 years of age was selected to receive the more detailed health examination. Groups at high risk of malnutrition were oversampled at known rates throughout the process. Household interviews were completed for more than 96 percent of the 28,043 persons selected for the NHANES I sample, and about 75 percent (20,749) were examined.

For NHANES II, conducted from 1976 to 1980, the nutrition component was expanded from the one fielded for NHANES I. In the medical area primary emphasis was placed on diabetes, kidney and liver functions, allergy, and speech pathology. The NHANES II target population was the civilian noninstitutionalized population 6 months–74 years of age residing in the United States, including Alaska and Hawaii.

NHANES II utilized a multistage probability design that involved selection of PSU's, segments (clusters of households) within PSU's, households, eligible persons, and finally, sample persons. The sample design provided for oversampling among those persons 6 months–5 years of age, those 60–74 years of age, and those living in poverty areas. A sample of 27,801 persons was selected for NHANES II. Of this

sample 20,322 (73.1 percent) were examined. Race information for NHANES I and NHANES II was determined primarily by interviewer observation.

The estimation procedure used to produce national statistics for NHANES I and NHANES II involved inflation by the reciprocal of the probability of selection, adjustment for nonresponse, and poststratified ratio adjustment to population totals. Sampling errors also were estimated to measure the reliability of the statistics.

For more information on NHANES I, see: Miller HW. Plan and operation of the Health and Nutrition Examination Survey, United States, 1971–73. National Center for Health Statistics. Vital Health Stat 1(10a) and 1(10b). 1977 and 1978; and Engel A, Murphy RS, Maurer K, Collins E. Plan and operation of the NHANES I Augmentation Survey of Adults 25–74 years, United States, 1974–75. National Center for Health Statistics. Vital Health Stat 1(14). 1978.

For more information on NHANES II, see: McDowell A, Engel A, Massey JT, Maurer K. Plan and operation of the second National Health and Nutrition Examination Survey, 1976–80. National Center for Health Statistics. Vital Health Stat 1(15). 1981. For information on nutritional applications of these surveys, see: Yetley E, Johnson C. Nutritional applications of the Health and Nutrition Examination Surveys (HANES). Ann Rev Nutr 7:441–63. 1987.

The Hispanic Health and Nutrition Examination Survey (HHANES), conducted during 1982–84, was similar in content and design to the previous National Health and Nutrition Examination Surveys. The major difference between HHANES and the previous national surveys is that HHANES employed a probability sample of three special subgroups of the population living in selected areas of the United States rather than a national probability sample. The three HHANES universes included approximately 84, 57, and 59 percent of the respective 1980 Mexican-, Cuban-, and Puerto Rican-origin populations in the continental United States. The Hispanic ethnicity of these populations was determined by self-report.

In the HHANES three geographically and ethnically distinct populations were studied: Mexican Americans living in Texas, New Mexico, Arizona,

Colorado, and California; Cuban Americans living in Dade County, Florida; and Puerto Ricans living in parts of New York, New Jersey, and Connecticut. In the Southwest 9,894 persons were selected (75 percent or 7,462 were examined), in Dade County 2,244 persons were selected (60 percent or 1,357 were examined), and in the Northeast 3,786 persons were selected (75 percent or 2,834 were examined).

For more information on HHANES, see: Maurer KR. Plan and operation of the Hispanic Health and Nutrition Examination Survey, 1982–84. National Center for Health Statistics. Vital Health Stat 1(19). 1985.

The third National Health and Nutrition Examination Survey (NHANES III) is a 6-year survey covering the years 1988–94. Over the 6-year period, 39,695 persons were selected for the survey of which 30,818 (77.6 percent) were examined in the mobile examination center.

The NHANES III target population is the civilian noninstitutionalized population 2 months of age and over. The sample design provides for oversampling among children 2–35 months of age, persons 70 years of age and over, black Americans, and Mexican Americans. Race is reported for the household by the respondent.

Although some of the specific health areas have changed from earlier NHANES surveys, the following goals of the NHANES III are similar to those of earlier NHANES surveys:

■　to estimate the national prevalence of selected diseases and risk factors

■　to estimate national population reference distributions of selected health parameters

■　to document and investigate reasons for secular trends in selected diseases and risk factors

Two new additional goals for the NHANES III survey are:

■　to contribute to an understanding of disease etiology

■　to investigate the natural history of selected diseases

For more information on NHANES III, see: Ezzati TM, Massey JT, Waksberg J, et al. Sample design:

Third National Health and Nutrition Examination Survey. National Center for Health Statistics. Vital Health Stat 2(113). 1992; Plan and operation of the Third National Health and Nutrition Examination Survey, 1988–94. National Center for Health Statistics. Vital Health Stat 1(32). 1994; or visit the NCHS home page at www.cdc.gov/nchs/.

National Health Provider Inventory (National Master Facility Inventory)

The National Master Facility Inventories (NMFI's) were a series of surveys of inpatient health facilities in the United States. They included hospitals, nursing and related-care homes, and other custodial care facilities. The last NMFI was conducted in 1982. In 1986 a different inventory was conducted, the Inventory of Long-Term Care Places (ILTCP). This was a survey of nursing and related-care homes and facilities for the mentally retarded. In 1991 the National Health Provider Inventory (NHPI) was conducted. This was a survey of nursing homes, board and care homes, home health agencies, and hospices. The NMFI, ILTCP, and NHPI were used as a basis for sampling frames for other surveys conducted by the National Center for Health Statistics (National Nursing Home Survey and National Home and Hospice Care Survey).

National Home and Hospice Care Survey

The National Home and Hospice Care Survey (NHHCS) is a sample survey of health agencies and hospices. Initiated in 1992, it was also conducted in 1993, 1994, and 1996. The original sampling frame consisted of all home health-care agencies and hospices identified in the 1991 National Health Provider Inventory (NHPI). The 1992 sample contained 1,500 agencies. These agencies were revisited during the 1993 survey (excluding agencies that had been found to be out of scope for the survey). In 1994 in-scope agencies identified in the 1993 survey were revisited, with 100 newly identified agencies added to the sample. For 1996 the universe was again updated, and a new sample of 1,200 agencies was drawn.

The sample design for the 1992–NHHCS was a stratified three-stage probability design. Primary sampling units were selected at the first stage, agencies were selected at the second stage, and current patients and discharges were selected at the third stage. The sample design for the 1996 NHHCS has a two-stage probability design in which agencies were selected at the first stage and current patients and discharges were selected at the second stage. Current patients were on the rolls of the agency as of midnight on the day before the survey. Discharges were selected to estimate the number of discharges from the agency during the year before the survey.

After the samples were selected, a patient questionnaire was completed for each current patient and discharge by interviewing the staff member most familiar with the care provided to the patients. The respondent was requested to refer to the medical records for each patient. For additional information see: Haupt BJ. Development of the National Home and Hospice Care Survey. National Center for Health Statistics. Vital Health Stat 1(33). 1994; or visit the NCHS home page at www.cdc.gov/nchs/.

National Hospital Discharge Survey

The National Hospital Discharge Survey (NHDS) is a continuing nationwide sample survey of short-stay hospitals in the United States. The scope of NHDS encompasses patients discharged from noninstitutional hospitals, exclusive of military and Department of Veterans Affairs hospitals, located in the 50 States and the District of Columbia. Only hospitals having six or more beds for patient use are included in the survey and, before, 1988 those in which the average length of stay for all patients was less than 30 days. In 1988 the scope was altered slightly to include all general and children's general hospitals regardless of the length of stay. Although all discharges of patients from these hospitals are within the scope of the survey, discharges of newborn infants from all hospitals are excluded from this report.

The original sample was selected in 1964 from a frame of short-stay hospitals listed in the National Master Facility Inventory. A two-stage stratified sample design was used, and hospitals were stratified

according to bed size and geographic region. Sample hospitals were selected with probabilities ranging from certainty for the largest hospitals to 1 in 40 for the smallest hospitals. Within each sample hospital, a systematic random sample of discharges was selected from the daily listing sheet. Initially, the within-hospital sampling rates for selecting discharges varied inversely with the probability of hospital selection so that the overall probability of selecting a discharge was approximately the same across the sample. Those rates were adjusted for individual hospitals in subsequent years to control the reporting burden of those hospitals.

In 1985, for the first time, two data collection procedures were used for the survey. The first was the traditional manual system of sample selection and data abstraction. In the manual system, sample selection and transcription of information from the hospital records to abstract forms were performed by either the hospital staff or representatives of NCHS or both. The second was an automated method, used in approximately 17 percent of the sample hospitals in 1985, involving the purchase of data tapes from commercial abstracting services. These tapes were then subjected to the NCHS sampling, editing, and weighting procedures.

In 1988 NHDS was redesigned. The hospitals with the most beds and/or discharges annually were selected with certainty, but the remaining sample was selected using a three-stage stratified design. The first stage is a sample of PSU's used by the National Health Interview Survey. Within PSU's, hospitals were stratified or arrayed by abstracting status (whether subscribing to a commercial abstracting service) and within abstracting status arrayed by type of service and bed size. Within these strata and arrays, a systematic sampling scheme with probability proportional to the annual number of discharges was used to select hospitals. The rates for systematic sampling of discharges within hospitals vary inversely with probability of hospital selection within PSU. Discharge records from hospitals submitting data via commercial abstracting services and selected State data systems (approximately 40 percent of sample hospitals in 1997 and 1998) were arrayed by primary diagnoses, patient sex and age group, and date of discharge before sampling. Otherwise, the procedures for sampling discharges within hospitals are the same as those used in the prior design.

In 1997 the hospital sample was updated by continuing the sampling process among hospitals that were NHDS-eligible for the sampling frame in 1997 but not in 1994. The additional hospitals were added at the end of the list for the strata where they belonged, and the systematic sampling was continued as if the additional hospitals had been present during the initial sample selection. Hospitals that were no longer NHDS-eligible were deleted. A similar updating process occurred in 1991 and 1994.

The basic unit of estimation for NHDS is the sample patient abstract. The estimation procedure involves inflation by the reciprocal of the probability of selection, adjustment for nonresponding hospitals and missing abstracts, and ratio adjustments to fixed totals. In 1997, 513 hospitals were selected, 501 were within scope, 474 participated (95 percent), and 300,000 medical records were abstracted. In 1998, 513 hospitals were selected, 495 were within scope, 478 participated (97 percent), and 307,000 medical records were abstracted.

For more detailed information on the design of NHDS and the magnitude of sampling errors associated with the NHDS estimates, see: Lawrence L, Hall MJ. 1997 Summary: National Hospital Discharge Survey. Advance data from vital and health statistics; no 308. Hyattsville, Maryland: National Center for Health Statistics. 1999; and Haupt BJ, Kozak LJ. Estimates from two survey designs: National Hospital Discharge Survey. National Center for Health Statistics. Vital Health Stat 13(111). 1992; or visit the NCHS home page at www.cdc.gov/nchs/.

National Survey of Ambulatory Surgery

The National Survey of Ambulatory Surgery (NSAS) is a nationwide sample survey of ambulatory surgery patient discharges from short-stay non-Federal hospitals and freestanding surgery centers. NSAS was conducted annually between 1994 and 1996. The sample consisted of eligible hospitals listed in the 1993 SMG Hospital Market Database and the 1993 SMG

Freestanding Outpatient Surgery Center Database or Medicare Provider-of-Service files. Facilities specializing in dentistry, podiatry, abortion, family planning, or birthing were excluded.

A three-State stratified cluster design was used, and facilities were stratified according to primary sampling unit (PSU). The second stage consisted of the selection of facilities from sample PSU's, and the third stage consisted of a systematic random sample of cases from all locations within a facility where ambulatory surgery was performed. Locations within hospitals dedicated exclusively to dentistry, podiatry, pain block, abortion, or small procedures (sometimes referred to as "lump and bump" rooms) were not included. In 1996 of the 751 hospitals and freestanding ambulatory surgery centers selected for the survey, 601 were in-scope and 488 responded for an overall response rate of 81 percent. These facilities provided information for approximately 125,000 ambulatory surgery discharges. Up to six procedures were coded to the *International Classification of Diseases, 9th Revision, Clinical Modification*. Estimates were derived using a multistage estimation procedure: inflation by reciprocals of the probabilities of selection; adjustment for nonresponse; and population weighting ratio adjustments.

For more detailed information on the design of NSAS, see: McLemore T, Lawrence L. Plan and operation of the National Survey of Ambulatory Surgery. National Center for Health Statistics. Vital Health Stat 1(37). 1997; or visit the NCHS home page at www.cdc.gov/nchs/.

National Nursing Home Survey

NCHS conducted five National Nursing Home Surveys, the first survey from August 1973–April 1974; the second survey from May 1977–December 1977; the third from August 1985–January 1986; the fourth from July 1995–December 1995; and the fifth from July 1997–December 1997.

Much of the background information and experience used to develop the first National Nursing Home Survey was obtained from a series of three ad hoc sample surveys of nursing and personal care homes called the Resident Places Surveys (RPS-1, -2,

Appendix I ....

Sources of Data

-3). The three surveys were conducted by the National Center for Health Statistics during April–June 1963, May–June 1964, and June–August 1969. During the first survey, RPS-1, data were collected on nursing homes, chronic disease and geriatric hospitals, nursing home units, and chronic disease wards of general and mental hospitals. RPS-2 concentrated mainly on nursing homes and geriatric hospitals. During the third survey, RPS-3, nursing and personal care homes in the coterminous United States were sampled.

For the initial National Nursing Home Survey (NNHS) conducted in 1973–74, the universe included only those nursing homes that provided some level of nursing care. Homes providing only personal or domiciliary care were excluded. The sample of 2,118 homes was selected from the 17,685 homes that provided some level of nursing care and were listed in the 1971 National Master Facility Inventory (NMFI) or those that opened for business in 1972. Data were obtained from about 20,600 staff and 19,000 residents. Response rates were 97 percent for facilities, 88 percent for expenditures, 98 percent for residents, and 82 percent for staff.

The scope of the 1977 NNHS encompassed all types of nursing homes, including personal care and domiciliary care homes. The sample of about 1,700 facilities was selected from 23,105 nursing homes in the sampling frame, which consisted of all homes listed in the 1973 NMFI and those opening for business between 1973 and December 1976. Data were obtained from about 13,600 staff, 7,000 residents, and 5,100 discharged residents. Response rates were 95 percent for facilities, 85 percent for expenses, 81 percent for staff, 99 percent for residents, and 97 percent for discharges.

The scope of the 1985 NNHS was similar to the 1973–74 survey in that it excluded personal or domiciliary care homes. The sample of 1,220 homes was selected from a sampling frame of 20,479 nursing and related-care homes. The frame consisted of all homes in the 1982 NMFI; homes identified in the 1982 Complement Survey of NMFI as "missing" from the 1982 NMFI; facilities that opened for business between 1982 and June 1984; and hospital-based nursing homes obtained from the Health Care

Financing Administration. Information on the facility was collected through a personal interview with the administrator. Accountants were asked to complete a questionnaire on expenditures or provide a financial statement. Resident data were provided by a nurse familiar with the care provided to the resident. The nurse relied on the medical record and personal knowledge of the resident. In addition to employee data that were collected during the interview with the administrator, a sample of registered nurses completed a self-administered questionnaire. Discharge data were based on information recorded in the medical record. Additional data about the current and discharged residents were obtained in telephone interviews with next of kin. Data were obtained from 1,079 facilities, 2,763 registered nurses, 5,243 current residents, and 6,023 discharges. Response rates were 93 percent for facilities, 68 percent for expenses, 80 percent for registered nurses, 97 percent for residents, 95 percent for discharges, and 90 percent for next of kin.

The scope of the 1995 and 1997 NNHS was similar to the 1985 and the 1973–74 NNHS in that they included only nursing homes that provided some level of nursing care. Homes providing only personal or domiciliary care were excluded. The 1995 sample of 1,500 homes was selected from a sampling frame of 17,500 nursing homes. The frame consisted of an updated version of the 1991 National Health Provider Inventory (NHPI). Data were obtained from about 1,400 nursing homes and 8,000 current residents. Data on current residents were provided by a staff member familiar with the care received by residents and from information contained in resident's medical records.

The 1997 sample of 1,488 nursing homes was the same basic sample used in 1995. Excluded were out-of-scope and out-of-business places identified in the 1995 survey and included were a small number of additions to the sample from a supplemental frame of places not in the 1995 frame. The 1997 NNHS included the discharge component not available in the 1995 survey.

Statistics for all five surveys were derived by a ratio-estimation procedure. Statistics were adjusted for failure of a home to respond, failure to fill out one of the questionnaires, and failure to complete an item on a questionnaire.

For more information on the 1973–74 NNHS, see: Meiners MR. Selected operating and financial characteristics of nursing homes, United States, 1973–74 National Nursing Home Survey. National Center for Health Statistics. Vital Health Stat 13(22). 1975. For more information on the 1977 NNHS, see: Van Nostrand JF, Zappolo A, Hing E, et al. The National Nursing Home Survey, 1977 summary for the United States. National Center for Health Statistics. Vital Health Stat 13(43). 1979. For more information on the 1985 NNHS, see: Hing E, Sekscenski E, Strahan G. The National Nursing Home Survey: 1985 summary for the United States. National Center for Health Statistics. Vital Health Stat 13(97). 1985. For more information on the 1995 NNHS, see: Strahan G. An overview of nursing homes and their current residents: Data from the 1995 National Nursing Home Survey. Advance data from vital and health statistics; no 280. Hyattsville, MD: National Center for Health Statistics. 1997. For more information on the 1997 NNHS, see the Advance Data report available in the summer of 1999; or visit the NCHS home page at www.cdc.gov/nchs/.

National Ambulatory Medical Care Survey

The National Ambulatory Medical Care Survey (NAMCS) is a continuing national probability sample of ambulatory medical encounters. The scope of the survey covers physician-patient encounters in the offices of nonfederally employed physicians classified by the American Medical Association or American Osteopathic Association as "office-based, patient care" physicians. Patient encounters with physicians engaged in prepaid practices (health maintenance organizations (HMO's), independent practice organizations (IPA's), and other prepaid practices) are included in NAMCS. Excluded are visits to hospital-based physicians, visits to specialists in anesthesiology, pathology, and radiology, and visits to physicians who are principally engaged in teaching, research, or administration. Telephone contacts and nonoffice visits are excluded, also.

A multistage probability design is employed. The first-stage sample consists of 84 primary sampling units (PSU's) in 1985 and 112 PSU's in 1992 selected from about 1,900 such units into which the United States has been divided. In each sample PSU, a sample of practicing non-Federal office-based physicians is selected from master files maintained by the American Medical Association and the American Osteopathic Association. The final stage involves systematic random samples of office visits during randomly assigned 7-day reporting periods. In 1985 the survey excluded Alaska and Hawaii. Starting in 1989 the survey included all 50 States.

In the 1998 survey a sample of 2,500 physicians was selected. The response rate was 68 percent, and data were provided on 23,339 records.

The estimation procedure used in NAMCS basically has three components: inflation by the reciprocal of the probability of selection, adjustment for nonresponse, and ratio adjustment to fixed totals.

For more detailed information on NAMCS, see: Woodwell, DA National Ambulatory Medical Care Survey: 1997 summary. Advance data from vital and health statistics; no 305. Hyattsville, MD: National Center for Health Statistics. 1999; or visit the NCHS home page at www.cdc.gov/nchs/.

National Hospital Ambulatory Medical Care Survey

The National Hospital Ambulatory Medical Care Survey (NHAMCS), initiated in 1992, is a continuing annual national probability sample of visits by patients to emergency departments (ED's) and outpatient departments (OPD's) of non-Federal, short-stay or general hospitals. Telephone contacts are excluded.

A four-stage probability sample design is used in NHAMCS, involving samples of primary sampling units (PSU's), hospitals with ED's and/or OPD's within PSU's, ED's within hospitals and/or clinics within OPD's, and patient visits within ED's and/or clinics. In 1997 and 1998 the hospital response rate for NHAMCS was 96 percent for ED's and 88–90 percent for OPD's. Hospital staff were asked to complete Patient Record Forms (PRF) for a systematic random sample of patient visits occurring during a randomly assigned 4-week reporting period. On the PRF, up to three physicians' diagnoses were collected and coded by NCHS to the *International Classification of Diseases, Clinical Modification* (ICD–9–CM).

Sources of Data

Additionally, if the cause-of-injury check box was marked on the PRF, up to three external causes of injury were coded by NCHS to the ICD–9–CM Supplementary Classification of External Causes of Injury and Poisoning. In 1997 the number of PRF's completed for ED's was 22,209 and for OPD's was 30,107. In 1998 the number of PRF's completed for ED's was 24,175 and for OPD's 29,402.

For more detailed information on NHAMCS, see: McCaig LF, McLemore T. Plan and operation of the National Hospital Ambulatory Medical Care Survey. National Center for Health Statistics. Vital Health Stat 1(34). 1994; or visit the NCHS home page at www.cdc.gov/nchs/.

National Center for HIV, STD, and TB Prevention

AIDS Surveillance

Acquired immunodeficiency syndrome (AIDS) surveillance is conducted by health departments in each State, territory, and the District of Columbia. Although surveillance activities range from passive to active, most areas employ multifaceted active surveillance programs, which include four major reporting sources of AIDS information: hospitals and hospital-based physicians, physicians in nonhospital practice, public and private clinics, and medical record systems (death certificates, tumor registries, hospital discharge abstracts, and communicable disease reports). Using a standard confidential case report form, the health departments collect information that is then transmitted electronically to CDC without personal identifiers.

AIDS surveillance data are used to detect epidemiologic trends, to identify unusual cases requiring followup, and for semiannual publication in the *HIV/AIDS Surveillance Report*. Studies to determine the completeness of reporting of AIDS cases meeting the national surveillance definition suggest reporting at greater than or equal to 90 percent.

Decreases in the AIDS incidence and in the number of AIDS deaths, first noted in 1996, have been ascribed to the effect of new treatments, which prevent or delay the onset of AIDS and premature death among HIV-infected persons, and result in an increase in the number of persons living with HIV and AIDS. A growing number of States require confidential reporting of persons with HIV infection and participate in CDC's integrated HIV/AIDS surveillance system that compiles information on the population of persons newly diagnosed with and living with HIV infection.

For more information on AIDS surveillance, see: Centers for Disease Control and Prevention. *HIV/AIDS Surveillance Report*, published semiannually; or contact: Chief, Surveillance Branch, Division of HIV/AIDS Prevention Surveillance and Epidemiology, National Center for HIV, STD, and TB Prevention (NCHSTP), Centers for Disease Control and Prevention, Atlanta, GA 30333; or visit the NCHSTP home page at www.cdc.gov/nchstp/od/nchstp.html.

Epidemiology Program Office

National Notifiable Diseases Surveillance System

The Epidemiology Program Office (EPO) of CDC, in partnership with the Council of State and Territorial Epidemiologists (CSTE), operates the National Notifiable Diseases Surveillance System. The purpose of this system is primarily to provide weekly provisional information on the occurrence of diseases defined as notifiable by CSTE. In addition, the system also provides summary data on an annual basis. State epidemiologists report cases of notifiable diseases to EPO, and EPO tabulates and publishes these data in the *Morbidity and Mortality Weekly Report* (MMWR) and the *Summary of Notifiable Diseases, United States* (entitled *Annual Summary* before 1985). Notifiable disease surveillance is conducted by public health practitioners at local, State, and national levels to support disease prevention and control activities.

Notifiable disease reports are received from 52 areas in the United States and 5 territories. To calculate U.S. rates, data reported by 50 States, New York City, and the District of Columbia are used. (New York State is reported as Upstate New York, which excludes New York City.)

CSTE and CDC annually review the status of national infectious disease surveillance and recommend additions or deletions to the list of nationally notifiable diseases based on the need to respond to emerging priorities. For example, genital chlamydial infections became nationally notifiable in 1995. However, reporting nationally notifiable diseases to CDC by States is voluntary. Reporting is currently mandated by law or regulation only at the State level. Therefore, the list of diseases that are considered notifiable varies slightly by State. For example, reporting of mumps to CDC is not done by some States in which this disease is not notifiable to local or State authorities.

Completeness of reporting varies because not all cases receive medical care and not all treated conditions are reported. Estimates of underreporting of some diseases have been made. For example, it is estimated that only 22 percent of cases of congenital rubella syndrome are reported. Only 10–15 percent of all measles cases were reported before the institution of the Measles Elimination Program in 1978. Recent investigations suggest that fewer than 50 percent of measles cases were reported following an outbreak in an inner city and that 40 percent of hospitalized measles cases are currently reported. Data from a study of pertussis suggest that only one-third of severe cases causing hospitalization or death are reported. Data from a study of tetanus deaths suggest that only 40 percent of tetanus cases are reported to CDC.

For more information, see: Centers for Disease Control and Prevention, Summary of Notifiable Diseases, United States, 1998 *Morbidity and Mortality Weekly Report*, 47(53) Public Health Service, DHHS, Atlanta, GA, 1998; or write: Chief, Surveillance Systems Branch, Division of Public Health Surveillance and Informatics. Epidemiology Program Office, Centers for Disease Control and Prevention, 4770 Buford Highway, MS K74, Atlanta, GA, 30341–3717; or visit the EPO home page at www.cdc.gov/epo/phs.htm.

National Center for Chronic Disease Prevention and Health Promotion

Abortion Surveillance

In 1969 CDC began abortion surveillance to document the number and characteristics of women obtaining legal induced abortions, monitor unintended pregnancy, and assist efforts to identify and reduce preventable causes of morbidity and mortality associated with abortions. For each year since 1969 abortion data have been available from 52 reporting areas: 50 States, the District of Columbia, and New York City. The total number of legal induced abortions is available from all reporting areas; however, not all areas collect information regarding the characteristics of women who obtain abortions. Furthermore the number of States reporting each characteristic and the number of States with complete data for each characteristic vary from year to year. State data with more than 15 percent unknown for a given characteristic are excluded from the analysis of that characteristic.

For 48 reporting areas, data concerning the number and characteristics of women who obtain legal induced abortions are provided by central health agencies such as State health departments and the health departments of New York City and the District of Columbia. For the other four areas, data concerning the number of abortions are provided by hospitals and other medical facilities. In general the procedures are reported by the State in which the procedure is performed. However, two reporting areas (the District of Columbia and Wisconsin) report abortions by State of residence; occurrence data are unavailable for these areas.

The total number of abortions reported to CDC is about 10 percent less than the total estimated independently by the Alan Guttmacher Institute, a not-for-profit organization for reproductive health research, policy analysis, and public education.

For more information, see: Centers for Disease Control and Prevention, CDC Surveillance Summaries, July 30, 1999. *Morbidity and Mortality Weekly Report* 1999; 48 (NoSS-4), Abortion Surveillance-United States, 1996; or contact: Director, Division of Reproductive Health, National Center for Chronic Disease Prevention and Health Promotion (NCCDPHP), Centers for Disease Control and Prevention, Atlanta, GA 30341; or visit the NCCDPHP home page at www.cdc.gov/nccdphp.

Appendix I

Health Resources and Services Administration

Bureau of Health Professions

Nurse Supply Estimates

Nursing estimates in this report are based on a model developed by the Bureau of Health Professions to meet the requirements of Section 951, P.L. 94–63. The model estimates the following for each State: (a) population of nurses currently licensed to practice; (b) supply of full- and part-time practicing nurses (or available to practice); and (c) full-time equivalent supply of nurses practicing full time plus one-half of those practicing part time (or available on that basis).

The three estimates are divided into three levels of highest educational preparation: associate degree or diploma, baccalaureate, and master's and doctorate.

Among the factors considered are new graduates, changes in educational status, nursing employment rates, age, migration patterns, death rates, and licensure phenomena. The base data for the model are derived from the National Sample Surveys of Registered Nurses, conducted by the Division of Nursing, Bureau of Health Professions, HRSA. Other data sources include National League for Nursing for data on nursing education and National Council of State Boards of Nursing for data on licensure.

Substance Abuse and Mental Health Services Administration

Office of Applied Studies

National Household Surveys on Drug Abuse

Data on trends in use of marijuana, cigarettes, alcohol, and cocaine among persons 12 years of age and over are from the National Household Survey on Drug Abuse (NHSDA). The 1998 survey is the 18th in a series that began in 1971 under the auspices of the National Commission on Marijuana and Drug Abuse. From 1974 to September 1992, the survey was sponsored by the National Institute on Drug Abuse. Since October 1992, the survey has been sponsored by the Substance Abuse and Mental Health Services Administration (SAMHSA).

Since 1991 the National Household Survey on Drug Abuse has covered the civilian noninstitutionalized population 12 years of age and over in the United States. This includes civilians living on military bases and persons living in noninstitutionalized group quarters, such as college dormitories, rooming houses, and shelters. Hawaii and Alaska were included for the first time in 1991.

In 1994 the survey underwent major changes that affect the reporting of substance abuse prevalence rates. New questionnaire and data-editing procedures were implemented to improve the measurement of trends in prevalence and to enhance the timeliness and quality of the data. Because it was anticipated that the new methodology would affect the estimates of prevalence, the 1994 NHSDA was designed to generate two sets of estimates. The first set, called the 1994-A estimates, was based on the same questionnaire and editing method that was used in 1993. The second set, called the 1994-B estimates, was based on the new questionnaire and editing methodology. A description of this new methodology can be found in Advance Report 10, available from SAMHSA. Because of the 1994 changes, many of the estimates from the 1994-A and earlier NHSDA's are not comparable with estimates from the 1994-B and later NHSDA's. To be able to describe long-term trends in drug use accurately, an adjustment procedure was developed and applied to the pre-1994 estimates. This adjustment uses the 1994 split sample design to estimate the magnitude of the impact of the new methodology for each drug category. The adjusted estimates are presented in this volume of *Health, United States*. A description of the adjustment method can be found in the 1998 NHSDA Main Findings, NHSDA Series H-11, Appendix E, available from SAMHSA.

The 1998 survey employed a multistage probability sample design. Young people (age 12–34 years), black Americans, Hispanics, and residents of Arizona and California were oversampled. The sample included 25,500 respondents. The screening and interview response rates were 93.0 percent and 77.0 percent, respectively.

For more information on the National Household Survey on Drug Abuse (NHSDA), see: NHSDA Series:

H-9 National Household Survey on Drug Abuse: Population Estimates 1998, H-10 Summary of Findings from the 1998 National Household Survey on Drug Abuse, and H-11 National Household Survey on Drug Abuse Main Findings 1998; or write: Office of Applied Studies, Substance Abuse and Mental Health Services Administration, Room 16C-06, 5600 Fishers Lane, Rockville, MD 20857; or visit the SAMHSA Web site at www.samhsa.gov.

Drug Abuse Warning Network

The Drug Abuse Warning Network (DAWN) is a large-scale, ongoing drug abuse data collection system based on information from hospital emergency departments and from medical examiner facilities. The major objectives of the DAWN data system include the monitoring of drug abuse patterns and trends, the identification of substances associated with drug abuse episodes, and the assessment of drug-related consequences and other health hazards. Estimates reported in this publication are from the hospital emergency department (ED) component of DAWN.

Hospitals eligible for DAWN are non-Federal, short-stay general hospitals that have a 24-hour emergency department. Since 1988 the DAWN emergency department data have been collected from a representative sample of these hospitals located throughout the coterminous United States, including 21 oversampled metropolitan areas. Within each facility, a designated DAWN reporter is responsible for identifying eligible drug-abuse episodes by reviewing emergency department records and abstracting and submitting data on each reportable case. To be included in DAWN, the patient presenting to the ED must meet all of the following four criteria: (a) The patient was between the ages of 6 and 97 and was treated in the hospital's ED. (b) The patient's presenting problem(s)—the reason for the ED visit—was induced by or related to drug use, regardless of when the drug use occurred. (c) The episode involved the use of an illegal drug or the use of a legal drug or other chemical substance contrary to directions. (d) The patient's reason for using the substance(s) was dependence, suicide attempt or gesture, and/or psychic effect.

The data from the DAWN sample are used to generate estimates of the total number of emergency department drug abuse episodes and drug mentions in all eligible hospitals in the coterminous United States and in the 21 metropolitan areas. Overall, a response rate of 77 percent of sample hospitals was obtained in the 1997 survey.

For further information, see Drug Abuse Warning Network (DAWN) Series D-9, Drug Abuse Warning Network Annual Emergency Department Data, 1997; DAWN Series: D-10, Mid-Year 1998 Preliminary Emergency Department Data from the Drug Abuse Warning Network; DAWN Series D-4, Drug Abuse Warning Network Annual Medical Examiner Data 1996; or write: Office of Applied Studies, Substance Abuse and Mental Health Services Administration, Room 16-105, 5600 Fishers Lane, Rockville, MD 20857; or visit the SAMHSA home page at www.samhsa.gov.

Uniform Facility Data Set

The Uniform Facility Data Set (UFDS), is part of the Drug and Alcohol Services Information System (DASIS) maintained by the Substance Abuse and Mental Health Services Administration. UFDS is a census of all substance abuse treatment and prevention facilities that are licensed, certified, or otherwise recognized by the individual State substance abuse agencies, and an additional group of substance abuse treatment facilities identified from other sources. It seeks information from all specialized facilities that treat substance abuse. These include facilities that only treat substance abuse, as well as specialty substance abuse units operating within larger mental health (for example, community mental health centers), general health (for example, hospitals), social service (for example, family assistance centers), and criminal justice (for example, probation departments) agencies. UFDS solicits data concerning facility and client characteristics for a specific reference day (on or about October 1) including number of individuals in treatment, substance of abuse (alcohol, drugs, or both), types of services, and source of revenue. Public and private facilities are included.

Sources of Data

Treatment facilities contacted through UFDS are identified from the National Master Facility Inventory (NMFI), which lists all State-sanctioned substance abuse treatment and prevention facilities and additional treatment facilities identified through business directories and other sources. In 1996 only State-sanctioned facilities were included in the published tables. The 1997 and 1998 data include the facilities identified through business directories and other sources. Response rates to the surveys were 86, 88, and 91 percent in 1996, 1997, and 1998, respectively.

For further information on UFDS, contact: Office of Applied Studies, Substance Abuse and Mental Health Services Administration, Room 16–105, 5600 Fishers Lane, Rockville, MD 20857; or visit the OAS statistical information section of the SAMHSA home page: www.samhsa.gov.

Center for Mental Health Services

Surveys of Mental Health Organizations

The Survey and Analysis Branch of the Division of State and Community Systems Development conducts a biennial inventory of mental health organizations (IMHO's) and general hospital mental health services (GHMHS). One version is designed for specialty mental health organizations and another for non-Federal general hospitals with separate psychiatric services. The response rate to most of the items on these inventories is relatively high (90 percent or better) as is the rate for data presented in this report. However, for some inventory items, the response rate may be somewhat lower.

IMHO and GHMHS are the primary sources for Center for Mental Health Services data included in this report. This data system is based on questionnaires mailed every other year to mental health organizations in the United States, including psychiatric hospitals, non-Federal general hospitals with psychiatric services, Department of Veterans Affairs psychiatric services, residential treatment centers for emotionally disturbed children, freestanding outpatient psychiatric clinics, partial care organizations, freestanding day-night

organizations, and multiservice mental health organizations, not elsewhere classified.

Federally funded community mental health centers (CMHC's) were included separately through 1980. In 1981, with the advent of block grants, the changes in definition of CMHC's and the discontinuation of CMHC monitoring by the Center for Mental Health Services, organizations formerly classified as CMHC's, have been reclassified as other organization types, primarily "multiservice mental health organizations, not elsewhere classified," and "freestanding psychiatric outpatient clinics."

Beginning in 1983 any organization that provides services in any combination of two or more services (for example, outpatient plus partial care, residential treatment plus outpatient plus partial care) and is neither a hospital nor a residential treatment center for emotionally disturbed children is classified as a multiservice mental health organization.

Other surveys conducted by the Survey and Analysis Branch encompass samples of patients admitted to State and county mental hospitals, private mental hospitals, multiservice mental health organizations, the psychiatric services of non-Federal general hospitals and Department of Veterans Affairs medical centers, residential treatment centers for emotionally disturbed children, and freestanding outpatient and partial care programs. The purpose of these surveys is to determine the sociodemographic, clinical, and treatment characteristics of patients served by these facilities.

For more information, write: Survey and Analysis Banc, Division of State and Community Systems Development, Center for Mental Health Services, Room 15C-O4, 5600 Fishers Lane, Rockville, MD 20857. For further information on mental health, see: Center for Mental Health Services, *Mental Health, United States, 1998.* Manderscheid R, Henderson MJ, eds. DHHS Pub. No. (SMA) 99–3285. Washington: Superintendent of Documents, U.S. Government Printing Office. 1998; or visit the Center for Mental Health Services home page at www.samhsa.gov/cmhs/cmhs.htm.

National Institutes of Health

National Cancer Institute

Surveillance, Epidemiology, and End Results Program

In the Surveillance, Epidemiology, and End Results (SEER) Program the National Cancer Institute (NCI) contracts with 11 population-based registries throughout the United States to provide data on all residents diagnosed with cancer during the year and to provide current followup information on all previously diagnosed patients.

This report covers residents of one of the following geographic areas at the time of the initial diagnosis of cancer: Atlanta, Georgia; Detroit, Michigan; Seattle-Puget Sound, Washington; San Francisco-Oakland, California; Connecticut; Iowa; New Mexico; Utah; and Hawaii.

Population estimates used to calculate incidence rates are obtained from the U.S. Bureau of the Census. NCI uses estimation procedures as needed to obtain estimates for years and races not included in the data provided by the U.S. Bureau of the Census. Rates presented in this report may differ somewhat from previous reports due to revised population estimates and the addition and deletion of small numbers of incidence cases.

Life tables used to determine normal life expectancy when calculating relative survival rates were obtained from NCHS and in-house calculations. Separate life tables are used for each race-sex-specific group included in the SEER Program.

For further information, see: National Cancer Institute, *Cancer Statistics Review 1973–96* by L.A.G. Ries, et al. Public Health Service. Bethesda, MD, 1999; or visit the SEER home page: www.seer.ims.nci.nih.gov.

National Institute on Drug Abuse

Monitoring the Future Study (High School Senior Survey)

Monitoring the Future Study (MTF) is a large-scale epidemiological survey of drug use and related attitudes. It was initiated by the National Institute on Drug Abuse (NIDA) in 1975 and is conducted annually through a NIDA grant awarded to the University of Michigan's Institute for Social Research. MTF is composed of three substudies: (a) annual survey of high school seniors initiated in 1975; (b) ongoing panel studies of representative samples from each graduating class that have been conducted by mail since 1976; and (c) annual surveys of 8th and 10th graders initiated in 1991.

The survey design is a multistage random sample with stage one being the selection of particular geographic areas, stage two the selection of one or more schools in each area, and stage three the selection of students within each school. Data are collected using self-administered questionnaires administered in the classroom by representatives of the Institute for Social Research. Dropouts and students who are absent on the day of the survey are excluded. Recognizing that the dropout population is at higher risk for drug use, this survey was expanded to include similar nationally representative samples of 8th and 10th graders in 1991. Statistics that are published in the *Dropout Rates in the United States: 1997* (published by the National Center for Educational Statistics, Pub. No. 1999–082) stated that among persons 15–16 years of age, 2.7 percent have dropped out of school. Among persons 17 years of age, 2.4 percent have dropped out of school, while the dropout percent increases to 5.9 percent of persons 18 years of age, and to 10.2 percent for persons 19 years of age. Therefore, surveying eighth graders (where drop out rates are much lower than for high school seniors) should be effective for picking up students at higher risk for drug use.

Approximately 45,300 8th, 10th, and 12th graders in 433 schools were surveyed in 1999. In 1999 the annual senior samples were comprised of roughly 14,100 seniors in 143 public and private high schools nationwide, selected to be representative of all seniors in the continental United States. The 10th grade samples involve about 13,900 students in 140 schools in 1999, and the 1999 eighth grade samples have approximately 17,300 students in 150 schools.

For further information on Monitoring the Future Study, see: National Institute on Drug Abuse, National

Survey Results on Drug Use from the Monitoring the
Future Study, 1975–1998, Vol. I, Secondary School
Students, NIH Pub. No. 99–4660, Bethesda, MD:
Public Health Service, printed September 1999; or visit
the NIDA home page at www.nida.nih.gov or the
Monitoring the Future home page at
monitoringthefuture.org/.

Health Care Financing Administration

Office of the Actuary

Estimates of National Health Expenditures

Estimates of expenditures for health (National
Health Accounts) are compiled annually by type of
expenditure and source of funds.

Estimates of expenditures for health services come
from an array of sources. The American Hospital
Association (AHA) data on hospital finances are the
primary source for estimates relating to hospital care.
The salaries of physicians and dentists on the staffs of
hospitals, hospital outpatient clinics, hospital-based
home health agencies, and nursing home care provided
in the hospital setting are considered to be components
of hospital care. Expenditures for home health care and
for services of health professionals (for example,
doctors, chiropractors, private duty nurses, therapists,
and podiatrists) are estimated primarily using a
combination of data from the U.S. Bureau of the
Census' Service Annual Survey and the quinquennial
Census of Service Industries.

The estimates of retail spending for prescription
drugs are based on results of HCFA-sponsored study
conducted by the Actuarial Research Corporation and
on industry data on prescription drug transactions.
Expenditures for other medical nondurables and vision
products and other medical durables purchased in retail
outlets are based on estimates of personal consumption
expenditures prepared by the U.S. Department of
Commerce's Bureau of Economic Analysis, U.S.
Bureau of Labor Statistics/Consumer Expenditure
Survey, and the 1987 National Medical Expenditure
Survey conducted by the Agency for Health Care
Policy and Research. Those durable and nondurable
products provided to inpatients in hospitals or nursing

homes, and those provided by licensed professionals or
through home health agencies are excluded here, but
are included with the expenditure estimates of the
provider service category.

Nursing home expenditures cover care rendered in
establishments providing inpatient nursing and
health-related personal care through active treatment
programs for medical and health-related conditions.
These establishments cover skilled nursing and
intermediate care facilities, including those for the
mentally retarded. Spending estimates are based upon
data from the U.S. Bureau of the Census Services
Annual Survey, and the quinequennial Census of
Service Industries.

Expenditures for construction include those spent
on the erection or renovation of hospitals, nursing
homes, medical clinics, and medical research facilities,
but not for private office buildings providing office
space for private practitioners. Expenditures for
noncommercial research (the cost of commercial
research by drug companies is assumed to be
imbedded in the price charged for the product; to
include this item again would result in double
counting) are developed from information gathered by
the National Institutes of Health.

Source of funding estimates likewise come from a
multiplicity of sources. Data on the Federal health
programs are taken from administrative records
maintained by the servicing agencies. Among the
sources used to estimate State and local government
spending for health are the U.S. Bureau of the Census'
Government Finances and Social Security
Administration reports on State-operated Workers'
Compensation programs. Federal and State-local
expenditures for education and training of medical
personnel are excluded from these measures where
they are separable. For the private financing of health
care, data on the financial experience of health
insurance organizations come from special Health Care
Financing Administration analyses of private health
insurers, and from the Bureau of Labor Statistics'
survey on the cost of employer-sponsored health
insurance and on consumer expenditures. Information
on out-of-pocket spending from the U.S. Bureau of the
Census' Services Annual Survey, U.S. Bureau of Labor

Statistics' Consumer Expenditure Survey, the 1987 National Medical Expenditure Survey conducted by the Agency for Health Care Policy and Research, and from private surveys conducted by the American Hospital Association, American Medical Association, and the American Dental Association are used to develop estimates of direct spending by customers.

For more specific information on definitions, sources, and methods used in the National health accounts, see: National Health Accounts: Lessons from the U.S. experience, by Lazenby HC, Levit KR, Waldo DR, et al. Health Care Financing Review, vol 14 no 4. Health Care Financing Administration. Washington: Public Health Service. 1992 and National Health Expenditures, 1994, Levit KR, Lazenby HC, Sivarajan L, et al. Health Care Financing Review, vol 17 no 3. Health Care Financing Administration. Washington: Public Health Service. 1996; or visit the Health Care Financing Administration home page at www.hcfa.gov.

Estimates of State Health Expenditures

Estimates of spending by State are created using the same definitions of health care sectors used in producing the National Health Expenditures (NHE). The same data sources used in creating NHE are also used to create State estimates whenever possible. Frequently, however, surveys that are used to create valid national estimates lack sufficient size to create valid State-level estimates. In these cases, alternative data sources that best represent the State-by-State distribution of spending are substituted, and the U.S. aggregate expenditures for the specific type of service or source of funds are used to control the level of State-by-State distributions. This procedure implicitly assumes that national spending estimates can be created more accurately than State-specific expenditures.

Despite definitional correspondence, NHE differ from the sum of State estimates. NHE include expenditures for persons living in U.S. territories and for military and Federal civilian employees and their families stationed overseas. The sum of the State level expenditures exclude health spending for those groups. For hospital care, exclusion of purchases of services in

non-U.S. areas accounts for a 0.9 percent reduction in hospital expenditures from those measured as part of NHE.

For more information, contact: Office of the Actuary, Health Care Financing Administration, 7500 Security Blvd., Baltimore, MD 21244–1850; or visit the Health Care Financing Administration home page at www.hcfa.gov.

Medicare National Claims History Files

The Medicare Common Working File (CWF) is a Medicare Part A and Part B benefit coordination and claims validation system. There are two National Claims History (NCH) files, the NCH 100 percent-Nearline File, and the NCH Beneficiary Program Liability (BPL) File. The NCH files contain claims records and Medicare beneficiary information. The NCH 100 percent Nearline File contains all institutional and physician/supplier claims from the CWF. It provides records of every claim submitted, including all adjustment claims. The NCH BPL file contains Medicare Part A and Part B beneficiary liability information (such as deductible and coinsurance amounts remaining). The records include all Part A and Part B utilization and entitlement data. Records for 1998 were maintained on more than 38 million enrollees and 49,290 institutional providers including 6,176 hospitals, 15,022 skilled nursing facilities, 9,662 home health agencies, 2,290 hospices, 2,905 outpatient physical therapy facilities, 582 comprehensive outpatient rehabilitation facilities, 3,512 end-state renal dialysis facilities, 3,560 rural health clinics, 1,100 community mental health centers, 2,623 ambulatory surgical centers, and 1,858 federally qualified health centers. About 860 million claims were processed in fiscal year 1998.

Data from the NCH files provide information about enrollee use of benefits for a point in time or over an extended period. Statistical reports are produced on enrollment, characteristics of participating providers, reimbursement, and services used.

For further information on the NCH files see: Health Care Financing Administration, Office of Information Services, Enterprise Data Base Group,

Division of Information Distribution, Data Users Reference Guide or call the Medicare Hotline at 410 786-3689.

For further information on Medicare, visit the HCFA home page at www.hcfa.gov.

Medicare Current Beneficiary Survey

The Medicare Current Beneficiary Survey (MCBS) is a continuous survey of a nationally representative sample of about 18,000 aged and disabled Medicare beneficiaries enrolled in Medicare Part A (hospital insurance), or Part B (medical insurance), or both, and residing in households or long-term care facilities. The survey provides comprehensive time-series data on utilization of health services, health and functional status, health care expenditures, and health insurance, and beneficiary information such as income, assets, living arrangement, family assistance, and quality of life. The longitudinal design of the survey allows each sample person to be interviewed three times a year for 4 years, whether he or she resides in the community or a facility or moves between the two settings, using the version of the questionnaire appropriate to the setting. Sample persons in the community are interviewed using computer-assisted personal interviewing (CAPI) survey instruments. Because long-term care facility residents often are in poor health, information about institutionalized patients is collected from proxy respondents such as nurses and other primary care givers affiliated with the facility. The sample is selected from the Medicare enrollment files with oversampling among disabled persons under age 65 and among persons 80 years of age and over.

Medicare claims are linked to survey-reported events to produce the Cost and Use file that provides complete expenditure and source of payment data on all health care services, including those not covered by Medicare.

For a description of the MCBS, see: A profile of the Medicare Current Beneficiary Survey, by GS Adler. Health Care Financing Review, vol 15 no 4. Health Care Financing Administration. Washington: Public Health Service. 1994. For further information on the MCBS visit the HCFA home page at www.hcfa.gov.

Medicaid Data System

Many State Medicaid agencies continue to submit data annually to the Health Care Financing Administration (HCFA) using the Form HCFA-2082, *Statistical Report on Medical Care: Eligibles, Recipients, Payments, and Services*. However, the majority of Medicaid data are derived from the Medicaid Statistical Information System (MSIS). States participating in MSIS provide HCFA with a larger data base through the submission of computer tapes. HCFA then extracts comparable data to produce a mirror copy of the HCFA-2082 report. The Federal reporting period is between October 1 and September 30 of the fiscal year.

The following information may help when using the Medicaid data:

■ HCFA performs many statistical edits to ensure consistency and identification of aberrant and missing data. HCFA may substitute cell values only when necessary in order to maintain consistency.

■ Medical Vendor Payments exclude lump sum adjustments (such as payments to disproportionate share (DSH) hospitals). States must adjust payments to qualified hospitals that provide inpatient services to a disproportionate number of Medicaid recipients and/or other low income persons.

■ The number of recipients and eligibles reported on the HCFA-2082 are referred to as "Unduplicated," which simply means that each person is counted once based on their eligibility grouping (for example, Aged or Blind or Disabled) when they first receive medical services.

■ The Medicaid data presented in *Health, United States* are contained in the Medicaid statistical system (HCFA-2082 Report and the MSIS tapes). Data reported on the quarterly Medicaid financial report (HCFA-64) submitted to HCFA by States for reimbursement may differ from the Medicaid statistical report primarily because the HCFA-64 includes disproportionate share hospital payments, payments to health maintenance organizations and Medicare, and quarterly payment adjustments.

For further information on Medicaid data, see *Medicaid Statistics, Program and Financial Statistics, Fiscal Year 1997*, HCFA Pub. No. 10129, Health Care Financing Administration, Baltimore, MD. U.S. Government Printing Office, May 1999; or call the Medicaid Hotline at 410-786-0165. For additional information and data visit the HCFA Web site at www.hcfa.gov.

Online Survey Certification and Reporting Database

The Online Survey Certification and Reporting (OSCAR) database has been maintained by the Health Care Financing Administration (HCFA) since 1992. OSCAR is an updated version of the Medicare and Medicaid Automated Certification System that has been in existence since 1972. OSCAR is an administrative database containing detailed information on all Medicare and Medicaid health care providers in addition to all currently certified Medicare and Medicaid nursing home facilities in the United States and Territories. (Data for the territories are not shown in this report.) The purpose of the nursing home facility survey certification process is to ensure that nursing facilities meet the current HCFA long-term care requirements and thus can participate in serving Medicare and Medicaid beneficiaries. Included in the OSCAR database are all certified nursing facilities, certified hospital-based nursing homes, and certified units for other types of nursing home facilities (for example, life-care communities or board and care homes). Facilities not included in OSCAR are all noncertified facilities (that is, facilities that are only licensed by the State and are limited to private payment sources) and nursing homes that are part of the Department of Veterans Affairs. Also excluded are nursing homes that are intermediate care facilities for the mentally retarded.

Information on the number of beds, residents, and resident characteristics is collected during an inspection of all certified facilities. The information present on OSCAR is based on each facility's own administrative record system in addition to interviews with key administrative staff members.

All certified nursing homes are inspected by representatives of the State survey agency (generally the Department of Health) at least once every 15 months. Therefore a complete census must be based on a 15-month reporting cycle rather than a 12-month cycle. The 1995 data shown in *Health, United States, 2000*, come from a 15-month cycle ending on July 31, 1995. The 1996 data are based on a cycle ending on January 24, 1997, and the 1997 and 1998 data from cycles ending December 29, 1997, and December 13, 1998, respectively. Some nursing homes are inspected twice or more often during any given reporting cycle. In order to avoid overcounting, the data must be edited and duplicates removed. The editing and compilation of the data were performed by Cowles Research Group and published in the group's *Nursing Home Statistical Yearbook* series.

For more information, see: Cowles CM, 1995 Nursing Home Statistical Yearbook. 1996 Nursing Home Statistical Yearbook. 1997 Nursing Home Statistical Yearbook. Anacortes, WA: Cowles Research Group (CRG), 1995; 1997; 1998; Cowles CM, 1998 Nursing Home Statistical Yearbook. Washington, DC: American Association of Homes and Services for the Aging (AAHSA), 1999; HCFA: OSCAR Data Users Reference Guide, 1995, available from HCFA, Health Standards and Quality Bureau, HCFA/HSQB S2 11-07, 7500 Security Boulevard, Baltimore, MD 21244; or visit the HCFA home page at www.hcfa.gov or the CRG Web page at www.LongTermCareInfo.com/CRG. The e-mail contact for CRG is MickCowles@aol.com and for AAHSA is akerman@aahsa.org.

Department of Commerce

Bureau of the Census

Census of Population

The census of population has been taken in the United States every 10 years since 1790. In the 1990 census data were collected on sex, race, age, and marital status from 100 percent of the enumerated population. More detailed information such as income, education, housing, occupation, and industry were collected from a representative sample of the population. For most of the country, one out of six households (about 17 percent) received the more detailed questionnaire. In places of residence estimated to have less than 2,500 population, 50 percent of households received the long form.

For more information on the 1990 census, see: U.S. Bureau of the Census, *1990 Census of Population, General Population Characteristics*, Series 1990, CP-1; or visit the Census Bureau home page at www.census.gov.

Current Population Survey

The Current Population Survey (CPS) is a household sample survey of the civilian noninstitutionalized population conducted monthly by the U.S. Bureau of the Census. CPS provides estimates of employment, unemployment, and other characteristics of the general labor force, the population as a whole, and various other subgroups of the population.

The 1999 CPS sample is located in 754 sample areas, with coverage in every State and the District of Columbia. In an average month during 1999, the number of housing units or living quarters eligible for interview was about 50,000; of these about 7 percent were, for various reasons, unavailable for interview. In 1994 major changes were introduced, which included a complete redesign of the questionnaire and the introduction of computer-assisted interviewing for the entire survey. In addition, there were revisions to some of the labor force concepts and definitions.

The estimation procedure used involves inflation by the reciprocal of the probability of selection, adjustment for nonresponse, and ratio adjustment. Beginning in 1994 new population controls based on the 1990 census adjusted for the estimated population undercount were utilized.

For more information, see: U.S. Bureau of the Census, *The Current Population Survey, Design, and Methodology*, Technical Paper 40, Washington: U.S. Government Printing Office, Jan. 1978; U.S. Department of Labor, Bureau of Labor Statistics, Employment and Earnings, Feb. 1994, vol 41 no 2 and Feb. 1995, vol 42 no 2, Washington: U.S. Government Printing Office, Feb. 1994 and Feb. 1995; or visit the CPS home page at www.bls.gov.

Population Estimates

National population estimates are derived by using decennial census data as benchmarks and data available from various agencies as follows: births and deaths (National Center for Health Statistics); immigrants (Immigration and Naturalization Service); Armed Forces (Department of Defense); net movement between Puerto Rico and the U.S. mainland (Puerto Rico Planning Board); and Federal employees abroad (Office of Personnel Management and Department of Defense). State estimates are based on similar data and also on a variety of data series, including school statistics from State departments of education and parochial school systems. Current estimates are consistent with official decennial census figures and do not reflect estimated decennial census underenumeration.

After decennial population censuses, intercensal population estimates for the preceding decade are prepared to replace postcensal estimates. Intercensal population estimates are more accurate than postcensal estimates because they take into account the census of population at the beginning and end of the decade. Intercensal estimates have been prepared for the 1960's, 1970's, and 1980's to correct the "error of closure" or difference between the estimated population at the end of the decade and the census count for that date. The "error of closure" at the national level was quite small during the 1960's (379,000). However, for the 1970's it amounted to almost 5 million and for the 1980's, 1.5 million.

For more information, see: U.S. Bureau of the Census, U.S. population estimated by age, sex, race, and Hispanic origin: 1990–96, release PPL-57, March 1997; or visit the Census Bureau home page: www.census.gov.

Department of Labor

Bureau of Labor Statistics

Annual Survey of Occupational Injuries and Illnesses

Since 1971 the Bureau of Labor Statistics (BLS) has conducted an annual survey of establishments in the private sector to collect statistics on occupational injuries and illnesses. The Survey of Occupational Injuries and Illnesses is a Federal/State program in which employer reports are collected from about 169,000 private industry establishments and processed by State agencies cooperating with BLS. Data for the mining industry and for railroad activities are provided by Department of Labor's Mine Safety and Health Administration and Department of Transportation's Federal Railroad Administration. Excluded from the survey are self-employed individuals; farmers with fewer than 11 employees; private households; Federal Government agencies; and employees in State and local government agencies. Establishments are classified in industry categories based on the 1987 Standard Industrial Classification (SIC) Manual, as defined by the Office of Management and Budget.

Survey estimates of occupational injuries and illnesses are based on a scientifically selected probability sample, rather than a census of the entire population. An independent sample is selected for each State and the District of Columbia that represents industries in that jurisdiction. BLS includes all the State samples in the national sample.

Establishments included in the survey are instructed in a mailed questionnaire to provide summary totals of all entries for the previous calendar year to its Log and Summary of Occupational Injuries and Illnesses (OSHA No. 200 form). Additionally, from the selected establishments, approximately 550,000 injuries and illnesses with days away from work are sampled in order to obtain demographic and detailed case characteristic information. An occupational injury is any injury, such as a cut, fracture, sprain, or amputation, that results from a work-related event or from a single instantaneous exposure in the work environment. An occupational illness is any abnormal condition or disorder, other than one resulting from an occupational injury, caused by exposure to factors associated with employment. It includes acute and chronic illnesses or diseases that may be caused by inhalation, absorption, ingestion, or direct contact. Lost workday cases are cases that involve days away from work, or days of restricted work activity, or both. The response rate is about 92 percent.

The number of injuries and illnesses reported in any given year can be influenced by the level of economic activity, working conditions and work practices, worker experience and training, and the number of hours worked. Long-term latent illnesses caused by exposure to carcinogens are believed to be understated in the survey's illness measures. In contrast, new illnesses such as contact dermatitis and carpal tunnel syndrome are easier to relate directly to workplace activity.

For more information, see: Bureau of Labor Statistics, Occupational Injuries and Illnesses in 1998, Washington: U.S. Department of Labor, December 1999; or visit the BLS Internet site at stats.bls.gov/oshhome.htm.

Census of Fatal Occupational Injuries

The Census of Fatal Occupational Injuries (CFOI), administered by the Bureau of Labor Statistics (BLS) in conjunction with participating State agencies, compiles comprehensive and timely information on fatal work injuries occurring in the 50 States and the District of Columbia. To compile counts that are as complete as possible, the BLS census uses diverse sources to identify, verify, and profile fatal work injuries. Key information about each workplace fatality (occupation and other worker characteristics, equipment or machinery involved, and circumstances of the event) is obtained by cross-referencing the source records. Work relationship is verified for each work injury fatality by using at least two independent source documents. For a fatality to be included in the census, the decedent must have been employed (that is, working for pay, compensation, or profit) at the time of the event, engaged in a legal work activity, or present at the site of the incident as a requirement of his or her job. These criteria are generally broader than those used by Federal and State agencies administering specific laws and regulations. Fatalities that occur during a person's commute to or from work are excluded from the census counts.

Data for the CFOI are compiled from various Federal, State, and local administrative sources—including death certificates, workers' compensation reports and claims, reports to various regulatory agencies, medical examiner reports, and police reports—as well as news reports. Diverse sources are used because studies have shown that no single source captures all job-related fatalities. Source documents are matched so that each fatality is counted only once. To ensure that a fatality occurred while the decedent was at work, information is verified from two or more independent source documents or from a source document and a follow-up questionnaire.

States may identify additional fatal work injuries after data collection closeout for a reference year. In addition, other fatalities excluded from the published count because of insufficient information to determine work relationship may subsequently be verified as work related. States have up to one year to update their initial published State counts. Occupational fatalities and rates shown in this report are revised, except for the most recent year, and may differ from original data published by CFOI. Increases in the published counts based on additional information have averaged less than 100 fatalities per year or less than 1.5 percent of the total.

For more information, see: Bureau of Labor Statistics, *Fatal Workplace Injuries in 1997: A Collection of Data and Analysis. Report 934*, Washington: U.S. Department of Labor, July 1999; or visit the CFOI Internet site at www.bls.gov/oshfat1.htm.

Consumer Price Index

The Consumer Price Index (CPI) is a monthly measure of the average change in the prices paid by urban consumers for a fixed market basket of goods and services. The all-urban index (CPI-U) introduced in 1978 covers residents of metropolitan areas as well as residents of urban parts of nonmetropolitan areas (about 87 percent of the U. S. population in 1990).

In calculating the index, price changes for the various items in each location were averaged together with weights that represent their importance in the spending of all urban consumers. Local data were then combined to obtain a U.S. city average.

The index measures price changes from a designated reference date, 1982–84, which equals 100. An increase of 22 percent, for example, is shown as

122. This change can also be expressed in dollars as follows: the price of a base period "market basket" of goods and services bought by all urban consumers has risen from $10 in 1982–84 to $16.30 in 1998.

The current revision of CPI, projected to be completed in 2000, reflects spending patterns based on the Survey of Consumer Expenditures from 1993 to 1995, the 1990 Census of Population, and the ongoing Point-of-Purchase Survey. Using an improved sample design, prices for the goods and services required to calculate the index are collected in urban areas throughout the country and from retail and service establishments. Data on rents are collected from tenants of rented housing and residents of owner-occupied housing units. Food, fuels, and other goods and services are priced monthly in urban locations. Price information is obtained through visits or calls by trained BLS field representatives using computer-assisted telephone interviews.

The earlier 1987 revision changed the treatment of health insurance in the cost-weight definitions for medical care items. This change has no effect on the final index result but provides a clearer picture of the role of health insurance in the CPI. As part of the revision, three new indexes have been created by separating previously combined items, for example, eye care from other professional services and inpatient and outpatient treatment from other hospital and medical care services.

Effective January 1997 the hospital index was restructured by combining the three categories—room, inpatient services and outpatient services—into one category, hospital services. Differentiation between inpatient and outpatient and among service types are under this broad category. In addition new procedures for hospital data collection identify a payor, diagnosis, and the payor's reimbursement arrangement from selected hospital bills.

A new geographic sample and item structure were introduced in January 1998 and expenditure weights were updated to 1993–95. Pricing of a new housing sample using computer-assisted data collection started in June 1998. In January 1999 the index will be rebased from the 1982–84 time period to 1993–95.

For more information, see: Bureau of Labor Statistics, *Handbook of Methods*, BLS Bulletin 2490, U.S. Department of Labor, Washington, Apr. 1997; IK Ford and P Sturm. CPI revision provides more accuracy in the medical care services component, *Monthly Labor Review*, U.S. Department of Labor, Bureau of Labor Statistics, Washington, Apr. 1988; or visit the BLS home page at www.bls.gov.

Employment and Earnings

The Division of Monthly Industry Employment Statistics and the Division of Employment and Unemployment Analysis of the Bureau of Labor Statistics publish data on employment and earnings. The data are collected by the U.S. Bureau of the Census, State Employment Security Agencies, and State Departments of Labor in cooperation with BLS.

The major data source is the Current Population Survey (CPS), a household interview survey conducted monthly by the U.S. Bureau of the Census to collect labor force data for BLS. CPS is described separately in this appendix. Data based on establishment records are also compiled each month from mail questionnaires by BLS, in cooperation with State agencies.

For more information, see: U.S. Department of Labor, Bureau of Labor Statistics, *Employment and Earnings*, Jan. 2000, vol 47 no 1, Washington: U.S. Government Printing Office. Jan. 2000.

Employer Costs for Employee Compensation

Employer costs for employee compensation cover all occupations in private industry, excluding farms and households and State and local governments. These cost levels are published once a year with the payroll period including March 12th as the reference period.

The cost levels are based on compensation cost data collected for the Bureau of Labor Statistics Employment Cost Index (ECI), released quarterly. Employee Benefits Survey (EBS) data are jointly collected with the ECI data. Cost data were collected from the ECI's March 1993 sample that consisted of about 23,000 occupations within 4,500 sample establishments in private industry and 7,000 occupations within 1,000 establishments in State and local governments. The sample establishments are

classified industry categories based on the 1987 Standard Industrial Classification (SIC) system, as defined by the U.S. Office of Management and Budget. Within an establishment, specific job categories are selected to represent broader major occupational groups such as professional specialty and technical occupations. The cost levels are calculated with current employment weights each year.

For more information, see: U.S. Department of Labor, Bureau of Labor Statistics, *Employment Cost Indexes and Levels, 1975–95*, Bulletin 2466, Oct. 1995.

Department of Veterans Affairs

Data are obtained from the Department of Veterans Affairs (VA) administrative data systems. These include budget, patient treatment, patient census, and patient outpatient-clinic information. Data from the three patient files are collected locally at each VA medical center and are transmitted to the national databank at the VA Austin Automated Center where they are stored and used to provide nationwide statistics, reports, and comparisons.

The Patient Treatment File

The patient treatment file (PTF) collects data, at the time of the patient's discharge, on each episode of inpatient care provided to patients at VA hospitals, VA nursing homes, VA domiciliaries, community nursing homes, and other non-VA facilities. The PTF record contains the scrambled social security number, dates of inpatient treatment, date of birth, State and county of residence, type of disposition, place of disposition after discharge, as well as the ICD–9–CM diagnostic and procedure or operative codes for each episode of care.

The Patient Census File

The patient census file collects data on each patient remaining in a VA medical facility at midnight on a selected date of each year, normally September 30. This file includes patients admitted to VA hospitals, VA nursing homes, and VA domiciliaries. The census record includes information similar to that reported in the patient treatment file record.

Sources of Data

The Outpatient Clinic File

The outpatient clinic file (OPC) collects data on each instance of medical treatment provided to a veteran in an outpatient setting. The OPC record includes the age, scrambled social security number, State and county of residence, VA eligibility code, clinic(s) visited, purpose of visit, and the date of visit for each episode of care.

For more information, write: Department of Veterans Affairs, National Center for Veteran Analysis and Statistics, Biometrics Division 008C12, 810 Vermont Ave., NW, Washington, DC 20420; or visit the VA home page at www.va.gov.

Environmental Protection Agency

Aerometric Information Retrieval System

The Environmental Protection Agency's Aerometric Information Retrieval System (AIRS) compiles data on ambient air levels of particulate matter smaller than 10 microns (PM-10), lead, carbon monoxide, sulphur dioxide, nitrogen dioxide, and tropospheric ozone. These pollutants were identified in the Clean Air Act of 1970 and in its 1977 and 1990 amendments because they pose significant threats to public health. The National Ambient Air Quality Standards (NAAQS) define for each pollutant the maximum concentration level (micrograms per cubic meter) that cannot be exceeded during specific time intervals. Data shown in this publication reflect attainment of NAAQS during a 12-month period based on analysis using county level air-monitoring data from AIRS and population data from the Bureau of the Census.

Data are collected at State and local air pollution monitoring sites. Each site provides data for one or more of the six pollutants. The number of sites has varied, but generally increased over the years. In 1993 there were 4,469 sites, 4,668 sites in 1994, and 4,800 sites in 1995. The monitoring sites are located primarily in heavily populated urban areas. Air quality for less populated areas is assessed through a combination of data from supplemental monitors and air pollution models.

For more information, see: Environmental Protection Agency, *National Air Quality and Emissions Trend Report, 1994*, EPA-454/R-95-014, Research Triangle Park, NC, Oct. 1995, or write: Office of Air Quality Planning and Standards, Environmental Protection Agency, Research Triangle Park, NC 27711. For additional information on this measure and similar measures used to track the Healthy People 2000 Objectives and Health Status Indicators, see: National Center for Health Statistics, *Monitoring Air Quality in Healthy People 2000*, Statistical Notes, No. 9. Hyattsville, MD: 1995; or visit the EPA AIRS home page at www.epa.gov/airs/.

United Nations

Demographic Yearbook

The Statistical Office of the United Nations prepares the *Demographic Yearbook*, a comprehensive collection of international demographic statistics.

Questionnaires are sent annually and monthly to more than 220 national statistical services and other appropriate government offices. Data forwarded on these questionnaires are supplemented, to the extent possible, by data taken from official national publications and by correspondence with the national statistical services. To ensure comparability, rates, ratios, and percents have been calculated in the statistical office of the United Nations.

Lack of international comparability between estimates arises from differences in concepts, definitions, and time of data collection. The comparability of population data is affected by several factors, including (a) the definitions of the total population, (b) the definitions used to classify the population into its urban and rural components, (c) the difficulties relating to age reporting, (d) the extent of over- or underenumeration, and (e) the quality of population estimates. The completeness and accuracy of vital statistics data also vary from one country to another. Differences in statistical definitions of vital events may also influence comparability.

International demographic trend data are available from the United Nations on a CD-ROM entitled United Nations Demographic Yearbook: Historical

Supplement, 1948–97. First Issue DYB-CD, in press. United Nations publication sales number E/F.99.XIII.12.

For more information, see: United Nations, *Demographic Yearbook 1996*, United Nations, New York, 1998; or visit the United Nations home page at www.un.org or their Web site locator at www.unsystem.org.

World Health Statistics Annual

The World Health Organization (WHO) prepares the *World Health Statistics Annual*, an annual volume of information on vital statistics and causes of death designed for use by the medical and public health professions. Each volume is the result of a joint effort by the national health and statistical administrations of many countries, the United Nations, and WHO. United Nations estimates of vital rates and population size and composition, where available, are reprinted directly in the *Statistics Annual*. For those countries for which the United Nations does not prepare demographic estimates, primarily smaller populations, the latest available data reported to the United Nations and based on reasonably complete coverage of events are used.

Information published on late fetal and infant mortality is based entirely on official national data either reported directly or made available to WHO.

Selected life table functions are calculated from the application of a uniform methodology to national mortality data provided to WHO, in order to enhance their value for international comparisons. The life table procedure used by WHO may often lead to discrepancies with national figures published by countries, due to differences in methodology or degree of age detail maintained in calculations.

The international comparability of estimates published in the *World Health Statistics Annual* is affected by the same problems discussed above for the *Demographic Yearbook*. Cross-national differences in statistical definitions of vital events, in the completeness and accuracy of vital statistics data, and in the comparability of population data are the primary factors affecting comparability.

For more information, see: World Health Organization, *World Health Statistics Annual 1996*, World Health Organization, Geneva, 1998; or visit the WHO home page at www.who.org.

Alan Guttmacher Institute

Abortion Survey

The Alan Guttmacher Institute (AGI) conducts an annual survey of abortion providers. Data are collected from hospitals, nonhospital clinics, and physicians identified as providers of abortion services. A universal survey of 3,092 hospitals, nonhospital clinics, and individual physicians was compiled. To assess the completeness of the provider and abortion counts, supplemental surveys were conducted of a sample of obstetrician-gynecologists and a sample of hospitals (not in original universe) that were identified as providing abortion services through the American Hospital Association Survey.

The number of abortions estimated by AGI through the mid to late 1980's was about 20 percent more than the number reported to the Centers for Disease Control and Prevention (CDC). Since 1989 the AGI estimates have been about 12 percent higher than those reported by CDC.

For more information, write: The Alan Guttmacher Institute, 120 Wall Street, New York, NY 10005; or visit AGI's home page at www.agi-usa.org.

American Association of Colleges of Osteopathic Medicine

The American Association of Colleges of Osteopathic Medicine (AACOM) compiles data on various aspects of osteopathic medical education for distribution to the profession, the government, and the public. Questionnaires are sent annually to all schools of osteopathic medicine requesting information on characteristics of applicants and students, curricula, faculty, grants, contracts, revenues, and expenditures. The response rate is 100 percent.

For more information, see: *Annual Statistical Report, 1998*, American Association of Colleges of Osteopathic Medicine: Rockville, MD, 1998; or visit the AACOM home page at www.aacom.org.

American Association of Colleges of Pharmacy

The American Association of Colleges of Pharmacy (AACP) compiles data on the Colleges of Pharmacy, including information on student enrollment and types of degrees conferred. Data are collected through an annual survey; the response rate is 100 percent.

For further information, see: *Profile of Pharmacy Students*. The American Association of Colleges of Pharmacy, 1426 Prince Street, Alexandria, VA; or visit the AACP home page at www.aacp.org.

American Association of Colleges of Podiatric Medicine

The American Association of Colleges of Podiatric Medicine (AACPM) compiles data on the Colleges of Podiatric Medicine, including information on the schools and enrollment. Data are collected annually through written questionnaires. The response rate is 100 percent.

For further information, write: The American Association of Colleges of Podiatric Medicine, 1350 Piccard Drive, Suite 322, Rockville, MD 20850–4307; or visit the AACPM home page at www.aacpm.org.

American Dental Association

The Division of Educational Measurement of the American Dental Association (ADA) conducts annual surveys of predoctoral dental educational institutions. The questionnaire, mailed to all dental schools, collects information on student characteristics, financial management, and curricula.

For more information, see: American Dental Association, *1997–98 Survey of Predoctoral Dental Educational Institutions*. Chicago, 1998; or visit the ADA home page at www.ada.org.

American Hospital Association

Annual Survey of Hospitals

Data from the American Hospital Association (AHA) annual survey are based on questionnaires sent to all hospitals, AHA-registered and nonregistered, in the United States and its associated areas. U.S. government hospitals located outside the United States were excluded. Questionnaires were mailed to all hospitals on AHA files. For nonreporting hospitals and for the survey questionnaires of reporting hospitals on which some information was missing, estimates were made for all data except those on beds, bassinets, and facilities. Data for beds and bassinets of nonreporting hospitals were based on the most recent information available from those hospitals. Facilities and services and inpatient-service area data include only reporting hospitals and, therefore, do not include estimates.

Estimates of other types of missing data were based on data reported the previous year, if available. When unavailable, the estimates were based on data furnished by reporting hospitals similar in size, control, major service provided, length of stay, and geographic and demographic characteristics.

For more information on the AHA Annual Survey of Hospitals, see: American Hospital Association, (Health Forum), *Hospital Statistics, 2000 ed.* Chicago, 1999; or visit an AHA page at www.aha.org.

American Medical Association

Physician Masterfile

A masterfile of physicians has been maintained by the American Medical Association (AMA) since 1906. The Physician Masterfile contains data on almost every physician in the United States, members and nonmembers of AMA, and on those graduates of American medical schools temporarily practicing overseas. The file also includes graduates of international medical schools who are in the United States and meet education standards for primary recognition as physicians.

A file is initiated on each individual upon entry into medical school or, in the case of international graduates, upon entry into the United States. Between 1969–85 a mail questionnaire survey was conducted every 4 years to update the file information on professional activities, self-designated area of specialization, and present employment status. Since 1985 approximately one-third of all physicians are surveyed each year.

For more information on the AMA Physician Masterfile, see: Division of Survey and Data Resources, American Medical Association, *Physician Characteristics and Distribution in the U.S.*, 2000–2001 ed. Chicago, 1999; or visit the AMA home page at www.ama-assn.org.

Annual Census of Hospitals

From 1920 to 1953 the Council on Medical Education and Hospitals of the AMA conducted annual censuses of all hospitals registered by AMA.

In each annual census, questionnaires were sent to hospitals asking for the number of beds, bassinets, births, patients admitted, average census of patients, lists of staff doctors and interns, and other information of importance at the particular time. Response rates were always nearly 100 percent.

The community hospital data from 1940 and 1950 presented in this report were calculated using published figures from the AMA Annual Census of Hospitals. Although the hospital classification scheme used by AMA in published reports is not strictly comparable with the definition of community hospitals, methods were employed to achieve the greatest comparability possible.

For more information on the AMA Annual Census of Hospitals, see: American Medical Association, Hospital service in the United States, Journal of the American Medical Association, 16(11):1055–1144. 1941; or visit the AMA home page at www.ama-assn.org.

Association of American Medical Colleges

The Association of American Medical Colleges (AAMC) collects information on student enrollment in medical schools through the annual Liaison Committee on Medical Education questionnaire, the fall enrollment questionnaire, and the American Medical College Application Service (AMCAS) data system. Other data sources are the institutional profile system, the premedical students questionnaire, the minority

student opportunities in medicine questionnaire, the faculty roster system, data from the Medical College Admission Test, and one-time surveys developed for special projects.

For more information, see: Association of American Medical Colleges, *Statistical Information Related to Medical Education*, Washington. 1999, or visit the AAMC home page at www.aamc.org.

Association of Schools and Colleges of Optometry

The Association of Schools and Colleges of Optometry (ASCO) compiles data on the various aspects of optometric education including data on schools and enrollment. Questionnaires are sent annually to all the schools and colleges of optometry. The response rate is 100 percent.

For further information, write: Annual Survey of Optometric Educational Institutions, Association of Schools and Colleges of Optometry, 6110 Executive Blvd., Suite 690, Rockville, MD 20852; or visit the ASCO home page at www.opted.org.

Association of Schools of Public Health

The Association of Schools of Public Health (ASPH) compiles data on the 29 schools of public health in the United States and Puerto Rico. Questionnaires are sent annually to all member schools, and the response rate is 100 percent.

Unlike health professional schools that emphasize specific clinical occupations, schools of public health offer study in specialty areas such as biostatistics, epidemiology, environmental and occupational health, health administration, health planning, nutrition, maternal and child health, social and behavioral sciences, and other population-based sciences.

For further information, write: Association of Schools of Public Health, 1660 L Street, NW, Suite 204, Washington, D.C. 20036–5603; or visit the ASPH home page at www.asph.org.

Appendix I

InterStudy

National Health Maintenance Organization Census

From 1976 to 1980 the Office of Health Maintenance Organizations conducted a census of health maintenance organizations (HMO's). Since 1981 InterStudy has conducted the census. A questionnaire is sent to all HMO's in the United States asking for updated enrollment, profit status, and Federal qualification status. New HMO's are also asked to provide information on model type. When necessary, information is obtained, supplemented, or clarified by telephone. For nonresponding HMO's State-supplied information or the most current available data are used.

In 1985 a large increase in the number of HMO's and enrollment was partly attributable to a change in the categories of HMO's included in the census: Medicaid-only and Medicare-only HMO's have been added. Also component HMO's, which have their own discrete management, can be listed separately; whereas, previously the oldest HMO reported for all of its component or expansion sites, even when the components had different operational dates or were different model types.

For further information, see: *The InterStudy Competitive Edge,*. InterStudy Publications, St. Paul, MN, 1999; or visit the InterStudy home page at www.hmodata.com.

National League for Nursing

The division of research of the National League for Nursing (NLN) conducts The Annual Survey of Schools of Nursing in October of each year. Questionnaires are sent to all graduate nursing programs (master's and doctoral), baccalaureate programs designed exclusively for registered nurses, basic registered nursing programs (baccalaureate, associate degree, and diploma), and licensed practical nursing programs. Data on enrollments, first-time admissions, and graduates are completed for all nursing education programs. Response rates of approximately 80 percent are achieved for other areas of inquiry.

For more information, see: National League for Nursing, *Nursing Data Review*, New York, 1998; or visit the NLN home page at www.nln.org.

The glossary is an alphabetical listing of terms used in *Health, United States*. It includes cross references to related terms and synonyms. It also contains the standard populations used for age adjustment and *International Classification of Diseases* (ICD) codes for cause of death and diagnostic and procedure categories. New standards for presenting Federal data on race and ethnicity are described under Race.

Abortion—The Centers for Disease Control and Prevention's (CDC) surveillance system counts legal induced abortions only. For surveillance purposes, legal abortion is defined as a procedure performed by a licensed physician or someone acting under the supervision of a licensed physician to induce the termination of a pregnancy.

Acquired immunodeficiency syndrome (AIDS)—All 50 States and the District of Columbia report AIDS cases to CDC using a uniform surveillance case definition and case report form. The case reporting definitions were expanded in 1985 (*MMWR* 1985; 34:373–5); 1987 (*MMWR* 1987; 36 (supp. no. 1S): 1S-15S); 1993 for adults and adolescents (*MMWR* 1992; 41 (no. RR-17): 1–19); and 1994 for pediatric cases (*MMWR* 1994; 43 (no. RR-12): 1–19). The revisions incorporated a broader range of AIDS-indicator diseases and conditions and used HIV diagnostic tests to improve the sensitivity and specificity of the definition. The 1993 expansion of the case definition caused a temporary distortion of AIDS incidence trends. In 1995 new treatments for HIV and AIDS (protease inhibitors) were approved. These therapies have prevented or delayed the onset of AIDS and premature death among many HIV-infected persons. AIDS incidence data are published semiannually by CDC in HIV/AIDS Surveillance Report. See related *Human immunodeficiency virus (HIV) infection.*

Active physician—See *Physician*.

Activities of daily living (ADL)—Activities of daily living are activities related to personal care and include bathing or showering, dressing, getting in or out of bed or a chair, using the toilet, and eating. If a sample person from the Medicare Current Beneficiary Survey had any difficulty performing an activity by himself or herself and without special equipment, or did not perform the activity at all because of health problems, the person was categorized as having a limitation in that activity. The limitation may have been temporary or chronic at the time of the interview. Sample persons who were administered a community interview answered health status and functioning questions themselves if able to do so. A proxy, such as a nurse, answered questions about the sample person's health status and functioning for long-term care facility interview. In the National Health Interview Survey respondents were asked about needing the help of another person with personal care needs because of a physical, mental, or emotional problem. Persons are considered to have an ADL limitation if the causal condition for the ADL limitation is chronic. See related *Instrumental activities of daily living (IADL); Limitation of activity.*

Addition—An addition to a psychiatric organization is defined by the Center for Mental Health Services as a new admission, a readmission, a return from long-term leave, or a transfer from another service of the same organization or another organization. See related *Mental health disorder; Mental health organization; Mental health service type.*

Admission—The American Hospital Association defines admissions as patients, excluding newborns, accepted for inpatient services during the survey reporting period. See related *Days of care; Discharge; Patient.*

Age—Age is reported as age at last birthday, that is, age in completed years, often calculated by subtracting date of birth from the reference date, with the reference date being the date of the examination, interview, or other contact with an individual.

Age adjustment—Age adjustment, using the direct method, is the application of age-specific rates in a population of interest to a standardized age distribution in order to eliminate differences in observed rates that result from age differences in population composition. This adjustment is usually done when comparing two or more populations at one point in time or one population at two or more points in time.

Age-adjusted rates are calculated by the direct method as follows:

$$\sum_{i=1}^{n} r_i \times (p_i/P)$$

where r_i = age-specific rates for the population of interest

p_i = standard population in age group i

$P = \sum_{i=1}^{n} p_i$ for the age groups that comprise the age range of the rate being age adjusted

n = total number of age groups over the age range of the age-adjusted rate

Age adjustment by the direct method requires use of a standard age distribution. Historically, NCHS and the States used a standard distribution for mortality statistics based on the 1940 U.S. population. Morbidity statistics were age adjusted to different standards including 1970 and 1980. Findings from a Department of Health and Human Services workshop on age adjustment recommended that a new standard based on the year 2000 projected resident population be implemented beginning with data year 1999 for mortality statistics (Anderson RN, Rosenberg HM. Age Standardization of Death Rates: Implementation of the Year 2000 Standard. National vital statistics reports; vol 47 no 3. Hyattsville, Maryland: National Center for Health Statistics. 1998. This report is available through the NCHS homepage at: www.cdc.gov/nchs. The year 2000 projected resident population is available through the Bureau of the Census homepage at: www.census.gov/prod/1/pop/p25-1130/.) In *Health, United States* the new standard will be used for all data systems and implementation will be phased in by data system. In this edition of *Health, United States,* estimates from the National Health Interview Survey, the National Ambulatory Medical Care Survey, the National Hospital Ambulatory Medical Care Survey, the National Nursing Home Survey (resident rates

Table I. Standard million age distribution used to adjust death rates to the U.S. population in 1940

Age	Standard million
All ages	1,000,000
Under 1 year	15,343
1–4 years	64,718
5–14 years	170,355
15–24 years	181,677
25–34 years	162,066
35–44 years	139,237
45–54 years	117,811
55–64 years	80,294
65–74 years	48,426
75–84 years	17,303
85 years and over	2,770

table), and the National Home and Hospice Care Survey are age adjusted to the year 2000 standard.

Mortality data—Death rates are age adjusted to the U.S. standard million population (relative age distribution of 1940 enumerated population of the United States totaling 1,000,000) (table I). Age-adjusted rates are calculated using age-specific death rates per 100,000 population rounded to 1 decimal place. Adjustment is based on 11 age groups with 2 exceptions. First, age-adjusted death rates for black males and black females in 1950 are based on nine age groups, with under 1 year and 1–4 years of age combined as one group and 75–84 years and 85 years of age and over combined as one group. Second, age-adjusted death rates by educational attainment for the age group 25–64 years are based on four 10-year age groups (25–34 years, 35–44 years, 45–54 years, and 55–64 years).

The rate for years of potential life lost (YPLL) before age 75 years is age adjusted to the U.S. standard million population (table I) and is based on eight age groups (under 1 year, 1–14 years, 15–24 years, and 10-year age groups through 65–74 years).

Maternal mortality rates for Complications of pregnancy, childbirth, and the puerperium, ICD-9 codes 630–676, are calculated as the number of deaths per 100,000 live births. These rates are age adjusted to the 1970 distribution of live births by mother's age in the United States as shown in table II. See related *Rate: Death and related rates; Years of potential life lost.*

Table II. Numbers of live births and mother's age groups used to adjust maternal mortality rates to live births in the United States in 1970

Mother's age	Number
All ages	3,731,386
Under 20 years	656,460
20–24 years	1,418,874
25–29 years	994,904
30–34 years	427,806
35 years and over	233,342

SOURCE: U.S. Bureau of the Census: Population estimates and projections. *Current Population Reports.* Series P-25, No. 499. Washington. U.S. Government Printing Office, May 1973.

National Health Interview Survey—Beginning with *Health, United States 2000* data from the National Health Interview Survey (NHIS) are age adjusted to the year 2000 projected resident population (table III). Information on the age groups utilized in the age adjustment procedure is contained in the footnotes on the relevant tables. In editions before *Health, United States 2000* data from NHIS were age adjusted to the 1970 civilian noninstitutionalized population. The 1970 civilian noninstitutionalized population was derived as follows: Civilian noninstitutionalized population = civilian population on July 1, 1970 - institutionalized population. Institutionalized population = (1 - proportion of total population not institutionalized on April 1, 1970) x total population on July 1, 1970.

Health Care Surveys—Data from the National Hospital Discharge Survey (NHDS) and the National Survey of Ambulatory Surgery (NSAS) are age adjusted to the 1970 civilian noninstitutionalized population using five age groups: under 15 years, 15–44 years, 45–64 years, 65–74 years, and 75 years and over (table III). Data from the National Ambulatory Medical Care Survey (NAMCS), the National Hospital Ambulatory Medical Care Survey (NHAMCS), the National Nursing Home Survey (NNHS) (resident rates table), and the National Home and Hospice Care Survey (NHHCS) are age adjusted to the year 2000 standard. Information on the age groups utilized in the age adjustment procedure is contained in the footnotes on the relevant tables.

National Health and Nutrition Examination Survey—Data from the National Health Examination

Table III. Populations and age groups used to age adjust NCHS survey data

Population, survey, and age	Number in thousands
U.S. civilian noninstitutionalized population in 1970 NHDS and NSAS	
All ages	199,584
Under 15 years	57,745
15–44 years	81,189
45–64 years	41,537
65 years and over	19,113
65–74 years	12,224
75 years and over	6,889
U.S. resident population in 1980 NHES and NHANES	
6–11 years	20,834
6–8 years	9,777
9–11 years	11,057
12–17 years	23,410
12–14 years	10,945
15–17 years	12,465
20–74 years	144,120
20–34 years	58,401
35–44 years	25,635
45–54 years	22,800
55–64 years	21,703
65–74 years	15,581
U.S. resident population projected in 2000 NHIS, NAMCS, NHAMCS, NHHCS, and NNHS	
All ages	274,634
18 years and over	203,851
25 years and over	117,593
65 years and over	34,710
Under 18 years	70,783
2–17 years	63,229
18–44 years	108,150
25–34 years	37,233
35–44 years	44,659
45–64 years	60,991
45–54 years	37,030
55–64 years	23,961
65–74 years	18,136
75 years and over	16,574

SOURCES: U.S. Bureau of Census: *Current Population Reports.* P25-721, Estimates of the Population of the United States by Age, Sex, and Race: 1970 to 1977; P25-1095, U.S. Population Estimates by Age, Sex, Race, Hispanic Origin: 1980 to 1991, table 1; P25-1130, Population Projections of the United States by Age, Sex, Race, and Hispanic Origin, table 2. U.S. Government Printing Office, Washington, DC, 1978; 1993; 1996.

Survey (NHES) and the National Health and Nutrition Examination Survey (NHANES) are age adjusted to the 1980 U.S. resident population using five age groups for adults: 20–34 years, 35–44 years, 45–54 years, 55–64 years, and 65–74 years (table III). Data for children aged 6–11 years and 12–17 years are age adjusted within each group using two subgroups: 6–8 years and 9–11 years; and 12–14 years and 15–17 years (table III).

AIDS—See *Acquired immunodeficiency syndrome*.

Air quality standards—See *National ambient air quality standards*.

Air pollution—See *Pollutant*.

Alcohol abuse treatment clients—See *Substance abuse treatment clients*.

Ambulatory care—Health care provided to persons without their admission to a health facility.

Ambulatory surgery—According to the National Survey of Ambulatory Surgery (NSAS), ambulatory surgery refers to previously scheduled surgical and nonsurgical procedures performed on an outpatient basis in a hospital or freestanding ambulatory surgery center's general or main operating rooms, satellite operating rooms, cystoscopy rooms, endoscopy rooms, cardiac catheterization labs, and laser procedure rooms. Procedures performed in locations dedicated exclusively to dentistry, podiatry, abortion, pain block, or small procedures were not included. In NSAS, data on up to six surgical and nonsurgical procedures are collected and coded. See related *Outpatient surgery; Procedure*.

Average annual rate of change (percent change)—In this report average annual rates of change or growth rates are calculated as follows:

$$[(P_n/P_o)^{1/N} - 1] \times 100$$

where P_n = later time period
P_o = earlier time period
N = number of years in interval.

This geometric rate of change assumes that a variable increases or decreases at the same rate during each year between the two time periods.

Average length of stay—In the National Health Interview Survey, the average length of stay per discharged patient is computed by dividing the total number of hospital days for a specified group by the total number of discharges for that group. Similarly, in the National Hospital Discharge Survey, the average length of stay is computed by dividing the total number of days of care, counting the date of admission but not the date of discharge, by the number of patients discharged. The American Hospital Association computes the average length of stay by dividing the number of inpatient days by the number of admissions. See related *Days of care; Discharge; Patient*.

Bed—Any bed that is set up and staffed for use by inpatients is counted as a bed in a facility. For the American Hospital Association the count is the average number of beds, cribs, and pediatric bassinets during the entire reporting period. In the Health Care Financing Administration's Online Survey Certification and Reporting database, all beds in certified facilities are counted on the day of certification inspection. The World Health Organization defines a hospital bed as one regularly maintained and staffed for the accommodation and full-time care of a succession of inpatients and situated in a part of the hospital where continuous medical care for inpatients is provided. The Center for Mental Health Services counts the number of beds set up and staffed for use in inpatient and residential treatment services on the last day of the survey reporting period. See related *Hospital; Mental health organization; Mental health service type; Occupancy rate*.

Birth cohort—A birth cohort consists of all persons born within a given period of time, such as a calendar year.

Birth rate—See *Rate: Birth and related rates*.

Birthweight—The first weight of the newborn obtained after birth. Low birthweight is defined as less than 2,500 grams or 5 pounds 8 ounces. Very low birthweight is defined as less than 1,500 grams or 3 pounds 4 ounces. Before 1979 low birthweight was defined as 2,500 grams or less and very low birthweight as 1,500 grams or less.

Body mass index (BMI)—BMI is a measure that adjusts body weight for height. It is calculated as weight in kilograms divided by height in meters squared. Sex- and age- specific cut points of BMI are used in this book in the definition of overweight for children and adolescents. Healthy weight for adults is defined as a BMI of 19 to less than 25; overweight, as greater than or equal to a BMI of 25; and obesity, as greater than or equal to a BMI of 30. BMI cut points are defined in the Report of the Dietary Guidelines. Advisory Committee on the Dietary Guidelines for Americans, 1995. U.S. Department of Agriculture, Agricultural Research Service, Dietary Guidelines Advisory Committee. 1995. pp.23–4; NHLBI Obesity Education Initiative Expert Panel on the Identification, Evaluation, and Treatment of Overweight and Obesity in Adults. Clinical Guidelines on the Identification, Evaluation, and Treatment of Overweight and Obesity in Adults—The Evidence Report. Obes Res 1998;6:51S–209S or access on the internet at www.nhlbi.nih.gov/guidelines/obesity/ob_gdlns.htm; and in the Healthy People 2010 Objectives: Draft for Public Comment. September 15, 1998. Objectives 2.1, 2.2, and 2.3.

Cause of death—For the purpose of national mortality statistics, every death is attributed to one underlying condition, based on information reported on the death certificate and utilizing the international rules for selecting the underlying cause of death from the reported conditions. Beginning with 1979 the *International Classification of Diseases, Ninth Revision* (ICD-9) has been used for coding cause of death. Data from earlier time periods were coded using the appropriate revision of the ICD for that time period. (See tables IV and V.) Changes in classification of causes of death in successive revisions of the ICD may introduce discontinuities in cause-of-death statistics over time. For further discussion, see Technical Appendix in National Center for Health Statistics: *Vital Statistics of the United States, 1995, Volume II, Mortality, Part A* available on the NCHS web site at www.cdc.gov/nchs/about/major/dvs/mortdata.htm. See related *Human immunodeficiency virus infection; International Classification of Diseases, Ninth Revision.*

Cause-of-death ranking—Cause-of-death ranking for infants is based on the List of 61 Selected Causes of Infant Death and HIV infection (ICD-9 Nos. *042-*044). Cause-of-death ranking for other ages is based on the List of 72 Selected Causes of Death, HIV infection, and Alzheimer's disease. The List of 72 Selected Causes of Death was adapted from one of the special lists for mortality tabulations recommended by the World Health Organization for use with the *Ninth Revision of the International Classification of Diseases.* Two group titles—Certain conditions originating in the perinatal period and Symptoms, signs, and ill-defined conditions—are not ranked from the List of 61 Selected Causes of Infant Death; and two group titles—Major cardiovascular diseases and Symptoms, signs, and ill-defined conditions— are not ranked from the List of 72 Selected Causes. In addition, category titles that begin with the words "Other" and "All other" are not ranked. The remaining category titles are ranked according to number of deaths to determine the leading causes of death. When one of the titles that represent a subtotal is ranked (for example, unintentional injuries), its component parts are not ranked (in this case, motor vehicle-related injuries and all other unintentional injuries). See related *International Classification of Diseases, Ninth Revision.*

Civilian noninstitutionalized population; Civilian population—See *Population.*

Cocaine-related emergency department episodes—The Drug Abuse Warning Network monitors selected adverse medical consequences of cocaine and other drug abuse episodes by measuring contacts with hospital emergency departments. Contacts may be for drug overdose, unexpected drug reactions, chronic

Table IV. Revision of the *International Classification of Diseases,* according to year of conference by which adopted and years in use in the United States

Revision of the International Classification of Diseases	Year of conference by which adopted	Years in use in United States
First.	1900	1900–1909
Second.	1909	1910–1920
Third	1920	1921–1929
Fourth	1929	1930–1938
Fifth.	1938	1939–1948
Sixth	1948	1949–1957
Seventh	1955	1958–1967
Eighth.	1965	1968–1978
Ninth	1975	1979–1998

Table V. Cause-of-death codes, according to applicable revision of *International Classification of Diseases*

	Code numbers			
Cause of death	Sixth Revision	Seventh Revision	Eighth Revision	Ninth Revision
Natural causes.	. . .	. . .	. . .	001–799
Communicable diseases.	. . .	. . .	. . .	001–139, 460–466, 480–487
Chronic and other noncommunicable diseases.	. . .	. . .	. . .	140–459, 467–479, 488–799
Injury and adverse effects/External causes . . .	. . .	. . .	. . .	E800–E999
Meningococcal infection	. . .	. . .	. . .	036
Septicemia	. . .	. . .	. . .	038
Human immunodeficiency virus infection[1] . . .	. . .	. . .	. . .	*042–*044
Malignant neoplasms.	140–205	140–205	140–209	140–208
Colorectal	153–154	153–154	153–154	153, 154
Peritoneum and pleura	. . .	. . .	158, 163.0	158, 163
Respiratory system	160–164	160–164	160–163	160–165
Trachea, bronchus and lung	. . .	. . .	. . .	162
Breast	170	170	174	174–175
Prostate	177	177	185	185
Benign neoplasms	. . .	. . .	. . .	210–239
Diabetes mellitus	260	260	250	250
Anemias	. . .	. . .	. . .	280–285
Meningitis.	. . .	. . .	. . .	320–322
Alzheimer's disease				331.0
Diseases of heart	410–443	400–402, 410–443	390–398, 402, 404, 410–429	390–398, 402, 404–429
Ischemic heart disease	. . .	. . .		410–414
Cerebrovascular diseases.	330–334	330–334	430–438	430–438
Atherosclerosis	. . .	. . .		440
Pneumonia and influenza	480–483, 490–493	480–483, 490–493	470–474, 480–486	480–487
Chronic obstructive pulmonary diseases	241, 501, 502, 527.1	241, 501, 502, 527.1	490–493, 519.3	490–496
Coalworkers' pneumoconiosis	. . .	. . .	515.1	500
Asbestosis	. . .	. . .	515.2	501
Silicosis	. . .	. . .	515.0	502
Chronic liver disease and cirrhosis	581	581	571	571
Nephritis, nephrotic syndrome, and nephrosis	. . .	. . .	. . .	580–589
Complications of pregnancy, childbirth, and the puerperium.	640–689	640–689	630–678	630–676
Congenital anomalies	. . .	. . .	. . .	740–759
Certain conditions originating in the perinatal period	. . .	. . .	. . .	760–779
Newborn affected by maternal complications of pregnancy	. . .	. . .		761
Newborn affected by complications of placenta, cord, and membranes	. . .	. . .		762
Disorders relating to short gestation and unspecified low birthweight	. . .		. . .	765
Birth trauma	. . .	. . .	. . .	767
Intrauterine hypoxia and birth asphyxia . . .	. . .	. . .	. . .	768
Respiratory distress syndrome	. . .	. . .	. . .	769
Infections specific to the perinatal period . .	. . .	. . .	. . .	771
Sudden infant death syndrome.		. . .	. . .	798.0
Unintentional injuries[2]	E800–E962	E800–E962	E800–E949	E800–E949
Motor vehicle-related injuries[2]	E810–E835	E810–E835	E810–E823	E810–E825
Suicide	E963, E970–E979	E963, E970–E979	E950–E959	E950–E959
Homicide and legal intervention	E964, E980–E985	E964, E980–E985	E960–E978	E960–E978
Firearm-related injuries	. . .	. . .	E922, E955, E965, E970, E985	E922, E955.0–E955.4, E965.0–E965.4, E970, E985.0–E985.4

. . . Cause-of-death code numbers are not provided for causes not shown in *Health, United States*.

[1]Categories for coding human immunodeficiency virus infection were introduced in 1987. The * indicates codes are not part of the Ninth Revision.

[2]In the public health community, the term "unintentional injuries" is preferred to "accidents and adverse effects" and "motor vehicle-related injuries" to "motor vehicle accidents."

abuse, detoxification, or other reasons in which drug use is known to have occurred.

Cohort fertility—Cohort fertility refers to the fertility of the same women at successive ages. Women born during a 12-month period comprise a birth cohort. Cohort fertility for birth cohorts of women is measured by central birth rates, which represent the number of births occurring to women of an exact age divided by the number of women of that exact age. Cumulative birth rates by a given exact age represent the total childbearing experience of women in a cohort up to that age. Cumulative birth rates are sums of central birth rates for specified cohorts and show the number of children ever born up to the indicated age. For example, the cumulative birth rate for women exactly 30 years of age as of January 1, 1960, is the sum of the central birth rates for the 1930 birth cohort for the years 1944 (when its members were age 14) through 1959 (when they were age 29). Cumulative birth rates are also calculated for specific birth orders at each exact age of woman. The percent of women who have not had at least one live birth by a certain age is found by subtracting the cumulative first birth rate for women of that age from 1,000 and dividing by 10. For method of calculation, see Heuser RL. *Fertility tables for birth cohorts by color: United States, 1917–73.* Rockville, Maryland. NCHS. 1976. See related *Rate: Birth and related rates.*

Community hospitals—See *Hospital.*

Compensation—See *Employer costs for employee compensation.*

Condition—A health condition is a departure from a state of physical or mental well-being. An impairment is a health condition that includes chronic or permanent health defects resulting from disease, injury, or congenital malformations. All health conditions, except impairments, are coded according to the *International Classification of Diseases, Ninth Revision, Clinical Modification (ICD–9–CM).*

Based on duration, there are two categories of conditions, acute and chronic. In the National Health Interview Survey, an *acute condition* is a condition that has lasted less than 3 months and has involved either a physician visit (medical attention) or restricted activity. A *chronic condition* refers to any condition lasting 3 months or more or is a condition classified as chronic regardless of its time of onset (for example, diabetes, heart conditions, emphysema, and arthritis). The National Nursing Home Survey uses a specific list of chronic conditions, also disregarding time of onset. See related *International Classification of Diseases, Ninth Revision, Clinical Modification.*

Consumer Price Index (CPI)—CPI is prepared by the U.S. Bureau of Labor Statistics. It is a monthly measure of the average change in the prices paid by urban consumers for a fixed market basket of goods and services. The medical care component of CPI shows trends in medical care prices based on specific indicators of hospital, medical, dental, and drug prices. A revision of the definition of CPI has been in use since January 1988. See related *Gross domestic product; Health expenditures, national.*

Crude birth rate; Crude death rate—See *Rate: Birth and related rates; Rate: Death and related rates.*

Current drinker—Starting with 1997 the National Health Interview Survey is collecting information on alcohol consumption in the sample adult questionnaire. Adult respondents are asked two screening questions about lifetime alcohol consumption: "In any one year, have you had at least 12 drinks of any type of alcoholic beverage? In your entire life, have you had at least 12 drinks of any type of alcoholic beverage?" Persons who report at least 12 drinks in a lifetime are then asked a series of questions about alcohol consumption in the past year: "In the past year, how often did you drink any type of alcoholic beverage? In the past year, on those days that you drank alcoholic beverages, on the average, how many drinks did you have? In the past year, on how many days did you have 5 or more drinks of any alcoholic beverage?"

Current smoker— Before 1992 a current smoker was defined by the following questions from the National Health Interview Survey (NHIS) "Have you ever smoked 100 cigarettes in your lifetime?" and "Do you smoke now?" (traditional definition). In 1992 the

Appendix II

definition of current smoker in the NHIS was modified to specifically include persons who smoked on "some days." In 1992 cigarette smoking data were collected for a half-sample with half the respondents (one-quarter sample) using the traditional smoking questions and for the other half of respondents (one-quarter sample) using a revised smoking question ("Do you smoke every day, some days, or not at all?"). An unpublished analysis of the 1992 traditional smoking measure revealed that the crude percent of current smokers 18 years of age and over remained the same as 1991. The statistics for 1992 combine data collected using the traditional and the revised questions. For further information on survey methodology and sample sizes pertaining to the NHIS cigarette data for data years 1965–92 and other sources of cigarette smoking data available from the National Center for Health Statistics, see: National Center for Health Statistics, *Bibliographies and Data Sources, Smoking Data Guide,* No. 1, DHHS Pub. No. (PHS) 91–1308–1, Public Health Service. Washington. U.S. Government Printing Office. 1991.

Starting with 1993 data estimates of cigarette smoking prevalence were based on the revised definition that is considered a more complete estimate of smoking prevalence. In 1993–95 estimates of cigarette smoking prevalence were based on a half-sample. Smoking data were not collected in 1996. Starting in 1997 smoking data were collected in the sample adult questionnaire.

Days of care—According to the American Hospital Association, days, hospital days, or inpatient days are the number of adult and pediatric days of care rendered during the entire reporting period. Days of care for newborns are excluded.

In the National Health Interview Survey, hospital days during the year refer to the total number of hospital days occurring in the 12-month period before the interview week. A hospital day is a night spent in the hospital for persons admitted as inpatients.

In the National Hospital Discharge Survey, days of care refers to the total number of patient days accumulated by patients at the time of discharge from non-Federal short-stay hospitals during a reporting period. All days from and including the date of admission but not including the date of discharge are counted. See related *Admission; Average length of stay; Discharge; Hospital; Patient.*

Death rate—See *Rate: Death and related rates.*

Dental visit—In the National Health Interview Survey respondents are asked "About how long has it been since you last saw or talked to a dentist? Include all types of dentists, such as orthodontists, oral surgeons, and all other dental specialists as well as hygienists."

Diagnosis—See *First-listed diagnosis.*

Diagnostic and other nonsurgical procedures—See *Procedure.*

Discharge—The National Health Interview Survey defines a hospital discharge as the completion of any continuous period of stay of one night or more in a hospital as an inpatient. According to the National Hospital Discharge Survey and the American Hospital Association, discharge is the formal release of an inpatient by a hospital (excluding newborn infants), that is, the termination of a period of hospitalization (including stays of 0 nights) by death or by disposition to a place of residence, nursing home, or another hospital. See related *Admission; Average length of stay; Days of care; Patient.*

Domiciliary care homes—See *Nursing home.*

Drug abuse treatment clients—See *Substance abuse treatment clients.*

Education—Two approaches to defining educational categories are used in this report. The more recent approach used to collect and present survey data defines education categories based on information about educational credentials, such as diplomas and degrees. The older approach defines education categories based on years of education completed. Educational attainment is used to present vital statistics data and National Health Interview Survey (NHIS) data prior to 1997. In the older approach, the education variable in NHIS was measured by asking, "What is the highest grade or year of regular school ___ has ever attended?" and "Did___ finish the grade/year?" Responses were used to categorize individuals according to years of education completed (for example, less than 12 years, 12 years, 13–15 years, 16 or more years).

Beginning in 1997 the NHIS questionnaire was changed to ask "What is the highest level of school ___ has completed or the highest degree received?" Responses were used to categorize individuals according to educational credentials (for example, no high school diploma or general equivalency diploma (GED); high school diploma or GED; some college, no bachelor's degree; bachelor's degree or higher).

Data from the 1996 and 1997 NHIS were used to compare distributions of educational attainment for adults 25 years of age and over using categories based on educational credentials (1997) with categories based on years of education completed (1996). A larger percent of persons reported "some college" than "13–15 years" of education and a correspondingly smaller percent reported "high school diploma or GED" than "12 years of education." In 1997, 19 percent of adults reported no high school diploma, 31 percent high school diploma or GED, 26 percent some college, and 24 percent bachelor's degree or higher. In 1996, 18 percent of adults reported less than 12 years of education, 37 percent 12 years of education, 20 percent 13–15 years, and 25 percent 16 or more years of education.

See related Appendix I, *National Vital Statistics System.* For further information on measurement of education see Kominski R and Siegel PM. Measuring education in the Current Population Survey. *Monthly Labor Review*, Sept. 1993: 34–38.

Emergency department—According to the National Hospital Ambulatory Medical Care Survey (NHAMCS), an emergency department is a hospital facility for the provision of unscheduled outpatient services to patients whose conditions require immediate care and is staffed 24 hours a day. Off-site emergency departments open less than 24 hours are included if staffed by the hospital's emergency department. See related *Emergency department visit; Outpatient department.*

Emergency department visit—Starting with the 1997 National Health Interview Survey, respondents to the sample adult and sample child questionnaires are asked about the number of visits to hospital emergency rooms during the past 12 months. Visits resulting in a hospital admission are included. In the National Hospital Ambulatory Medical Care Survey an emergency department visit is a direct personal exchange between a patient and a physician or other health care providers working under the physician's supervision, for the purpose of seeking care and receiving personal health services. Visits resulting in a hospital admission are excluded. See related *Emergency department; Injury-related visit.*

Employer costs for employee compensation—A measure of the average cost per employee hour worked to employers for wages and salaries and benefits. Wages and salaries are defined as the hourly straight-time wage rate, or for workers not paid on an hourly basis, straight-time earnings divided by the corresponding hours. Straight-time wage and salary rates are total earnings before payroll deductions, excluding premium pay for overtime and for work on weekends and holidays, shift differentials, nonproduction bonuses, and lump-sum payments provided in lieu of wage increases. Production bonuses, incentive earnings, commission payments, and cost-of-living adjustments are included in straight-time wage and salary rates. Benefits covered are paid leave—paid vacations, holidays, sick leave, and other leave; supplemental pay— premium pay for overtime and work on weekends and holidays, shift differentials, nonproduction bonuses, and lump-sum payments provided in lieu of wage increases; insurance benefits—life, health, and sickness and accident insurance; retirement and savings benefits—pension and other retirement plans and savings and thrift plans; legally required benefits—social security, railroad retirement and supplemental retirement, railroad unemployment insurance, Federal and State unemployment insurance, workers' compensation, and other benefits required by law, such as State temporary disability insurance; and other benefits—severance pay and supplemental unemployment plans.

Expenditures—See *Health expenditures, national.*

Family income—For purposes of the National Health Interview Survey and National Health and Nutrition Examination Survey, all people within a household related to each other by blood, marriage, or adoption constitute a family. Each member of a family is classified according to the total income of the family. Unrelated individuals are classified according to their own income. In the National Health and Nutrition Examination Survey and the National Health Interview Survey (in years prior to 1997) family income is the total income received by members of a family (or by an unrelated individual) in the 12 months before the interview. Starting in 1997 the National Health Interview Survey collected family income data on the calendar year prior to the interview. (For example, 1997 family income data are based on 1996 calendar year information). Family income includes wages, salaries, rents from property, interest, dividends, profits and fees from their own businesses, pensions, and help from relatives. In the National Health Interview Survey, family income data are used in the computation of poverty level. For data years 1990–96, about 16–18 percent of persons had missing data on poverty level. Missing values were imputed for family income using a sequential hot deck within matrix cells imputation approach. A detailed description of the imputation procedure as well as data files with imputed annual family income for 1990–96 are available from NCHS on CD-ROM NHIS Imputed Annual Family Income 1990–96, Series 10, Number 9A. See related *Poverty level.*

Federal hospitals—See *Hospital.*

Federal physicians—See *Physician.*

Fee-for-service health insurance—This is private (commercial) health insurance that reimburses health care providers on the basis of a fee for each health service provided to the insured person. Also known as indemnity health insurance. See related *Health insurance coverage.*

Fertility rate—See *Rate: Birth and related rates.*

Fetal death—In the World Health Organization's definition, also adopted by the United Nations and the National Center for Health Statistics, a fetal death is death before the complete expulsion or extraction from its mother of a product of conception, irrespective of the duration of pregnancy; the death is indicated by the fact that after such separation, the fetus does not breathe or show any other evidence of life, such as beating of the heart, pulsation of the umbilical cord, or definite movement of voluntary muscles. For statistical purposes, fetal deaths are classified according to gestational age. In this report tabulations are shown for fetal deaths with stated or presumed gestation of 20 weeks or more and of 28 weeks or more, the latter gestational age group also known as late fetal deaths. See related *Gestation; Live birth; Rate: Death and related rates.*

First-listed diagnosis—In the National Hospital Discharge Survey this is the first recorded final diagnosis on the medical record face sheet (summary sheet).

First-listed external cause of injury—In the National Hospital Ambulatory Medical Care Survey this is the first-listed external cause of injury coded from the Patient Record Form (PRF). Up to three causes of injury can be reported on the PRF. Injuries are coded by NCHS to the *International Classification of Diseases, Ninth Revision, Clinical Modification* Supplementary Classification of External Causes of

Table VI. Codes for first-listed external causes of injury from the *International Classification of Diseases, Ninth Revision, Clinical Modification*

External cause of injury category	E-Code numbers
Unintentional	E800–E869, E880–E929
Motor vehicle traffic	E810–E819
Falls	E880–E886, E888
Struck by or against objects or persons	E916–E917
Caused by cutting and piercing instruments or objects	E920
Intentional (suicide and homicide)	E950–E969

Injury and Poisoning. See table VI for listing of injury categories and codes. See related *Injury-related visit*.

General hospitals—See *Hospital*.

General hospitals providing separate psychiatric services—See *Mental health organization*

Geographic region and division—The 50 States and the District of Columbia are grouped for statistical purposes by the U.S. Bureau of the Census into 4 geographic regions and 9 divisions. The groupings are as follows:

■ Northeast

New England

Maine, New Hampshire, Vermont, Massachusetts, Rhode Island, Connecticut

Middle Atlantic

New York, New Jersey, Pennsylvania

■ Midwest

East North Central

Ohio, Indiana, Illinois, Michigan, Wisconsin

West North Central

Minnesota, Iowa, Missouri, North Dakota, South Dakota, Nebraska, Kansas

■ South

South Atlantic

Delaware, Maryland, District of Columbia, Virginia, West Virginia, North Carolina, South Carolina, Georgia, Florida

East South Central

Kentucky, Tennessee, Alabama, Mississippi

West South Central

Arkansas, Louisiana, Oklahoma, Texas

■ West

Mountain

Montana, Idaho, Wyoming, Colorado, New Mexico, Arizona, Utah, Nevada

Pacific

Washington, Oregon, California, Alaska, Hawaii

Gestation—For the National Vital Statistics System and the Centers for Disease Control and Prevention's Abortion Surveillance, the period of gestation is defined as beginning with the first day of the last normal menstrual period and ending with the day of birth or day of termination of pregnancy. See related *Abortion; Fetal death; Live birth*.

Gross domestic product (GDP)—GDP is the market value of the goods and services produced by labor and property located in the United States. As long as the labor and property are located in the United States, the suppliers (that is, the workers and, for property, the owners) may be either U.S. residents or residents of the rest of the world. See related *Consumer Price Index; Health expenditures, national*.

Health care contact—Starting with 1997 the National Health Interview Survey is collecting information on health care contacts with doctors and other health care professionals. This information is collected in a detailed section pertaining to all types of health care contacts. Analyses of interval since last health care contact are based upon the following question: "About how long has it been since you last saw or talked to a doctor or other health care professional about your own health? Include doctors seen while a patient in a hospital." Analyses of the percent of children without a health care visit are based upon the following question: "During the past 12 months, how many times has ___ seen a doctor or other health care professional about (his/her) health at a doctor's office, a clinic or some other place? Do not include times ____ was hospitalized overnight, visits to hospital emergency rooms, home visits or telephone calls." Analyses of the distribution of health care visits are based on a summary measure combining information about visits to doctor's offices or clinics, emergency departments, and home visits. See related *Emergency department visit; Home visit*.

Health expenditures, national—See related *Consumer Price Index; Gross domestic product*.

Health services and supplies expenditures—These are outlays for goods and services relating directly to patient care plus expenses for administering health insurance programs and government public health activities. This category is equivalent to total national health expenditures minus expenditures for research and construction.

National health expenditures—This measure estimates the amount spent for all health services and supplies and health-related research and construction activities consumed in the United States during the calendar year. Detailed estimates are available by source of expenditures (for example, out-of-pocket payments, private health insurance, and government programs), type of expenditures (for example, hospital care, physician services, and drugs), and are in current dollars for the year of report. Data are compiled from a variety of sources.

Nursing home expenditures—These cover care rendered in skilled nursing and intermediate care facilities, including those for the mentally retarded. The costs of long-term care provided by hospitals are excluded.

Personal health care expenditures—These are outlays for goods and services relating directly to patient care. The expenditures in this category are total national health expenditures minus expenditures for research and construction, expenses for administering health insurance programs, and government public health activities.

Private expenditures—These are outlays for services provided or paid for by nongovernmental sources—consumers, insurance companies, private industry, philanthropic, and other nonpatient care sources.

Public expenditures—These are outlays for services provided or paid for by Federal, State, and local government agencies or expenditures required by governmental mandate (such as, workmen's compensation insurance payments).

Health insurance coverage—National Health Interview Survey (NHIS) respondents were asked about their health insurance coverage at the time of the interview in 1984, 1989, and 1997 and in the previous month in 1993–96. Questions on health insurance coverage were expanded starting in 1993 compared with previous years. In 1997 the entire questionnaire was redesigned and data were collected using a computer assisted personal interview (CAPI).

Respondents are covered by private health insurance if they indicate private health insurance or if they are covered by a single service hospital plan, except in 1997 when no information on single service plans was obtained. Private health insurance includes managed care such as health maintenance organizations (HMO's).

Until 1996 persons were defined as having Medicaid or other public assistance coverage if they indicated that they had either Medicaid or other public assistance, or if they reported receiving Aid to Families with Dependent Children (AFDC) or Supplementary Security Income (SSI). After welfare reform in late 1996, Medicaid was delinked from AFDC and SSI. In 1997 persons were considered to be covered by Medicaid if they reported Medicaid or a State-sponsored health program.

Medicare or military health plan coverage is also determined in the interview, and in 1997 other government-sponsored program was determined.

If respondents do not report coverage under one of the above types of plans and they have unknown coverage on either private health insurance or Medicaid then they are considered to have unknown coverage.

The remaining respondents are considered uninsured. The uninsured are persons who do not have coverage under private health insurance, Medicare, Medicaid, public assistance, a State-sponsored health plan, other government-sponsored programs, or a military health plan. Persons with only Indian Health Service coverage are considered uninsured. Estimates of the percent of persons who are uninsured based on the NHIS (table 128) are slightly higher than those based on the March Current Population Survey (CPS) (table 146). The NHIS asks about coverage at the time of the survey (or in some survey years, coverage during the previous month), whereas the CPS asks about coverage over the previous calendar year. This may result in higher estimates of Medicaid and other health insurance coverage and correspondingly lower estimates of persons without health care coverage in the CPS compared with the NHIS. In addition, the CPS estimate is for persons of all ages whereas the NHIS estimate is for persons under age 65. See related

Fee-for-service health insurance; Health maintenance organization; Managed care; Medicaid; Medicare.

Health maintenance organization (HMO)—An HMO is a prepaid health plan delivering comprehensive care to members through designated providers, having a fixed monthly payment for health care services, and requiring members to be in a plan for a specified period of time (usually 1 year). Pure HMO enrollees use only the prepaid capitated health services of the HMO's panel of medical care providers. Open-ended HMO enrollees use the prepaid HMO health services but in addition may receive medical care from providers who are not part of the HMO's panel. There is usually a substantial deductible, copayment, or coinsurance associated with the use of nonpanel providers. These open-ended products are governed by State HMO regulations. HMO model types are:

Group—An HMO that delivers health services through a physician group that is controlled by the HMO unit or an HMO that contracts with one or more independent group practices to provide health services.

Individual practice association (IPA)—An HMO that contracts directly with physicians in independent practice, and/or contracts with one or more associations of physicians in independent practice, and/or contracts with one or more multispecialty group practices. The plan is predominantly organized around solo-single-specialty practices.

Mixed—An HMO that combines features of group and IPA. This category was introduced in mid-1990 because HMO's are continually changing and many now combine features of group and IPA plans in a single plan.
See related *Managed care.*

Health services and supplies expenditures—See *Health expenditures, national.*

Health status, respondent-assessed—Health status was measured in the National Health Interview Survey by asking the respondent, "Would you say _____'s health is excellent, very good, good, fair, or poor?"

Hispanic origin—Hispanic origin includes persons of Mexican, Puerto Rican, Cuban, Central and South American, and other or unknown Latin American or Spanish origins. Persons of Hispanic origin may be of any race. See related *Race.*

HIV—See *Human immunodeficiency virus infection.*

Home health care—Home health care as defined by the National Home and Hospice Care Survey is care provided to individuals and families in their place of residence for promoting, maintaining, or restoring health; or for minimizing the effects of disability and illness including terminal illness.

Home visits—Starting with 1997 the National Health Interview Survey is collecting information on home visits received during the past 12 months. Respondents are asked: "During the past 12 months, did you receive care at home from a nurse or other health care professional? What was the total number of home visits received?" These data are combined with data on visits to doctor's offices, clinics, and emergency departments to provide a summary measure of health care visits. See related *Emergency department visit; Health care contact.*

Hospice care—Hospice care as defined by the National Home and Hospice Care Survey is a program of palliative and supportive care services providing physical, psychological, social, and spiritual care for dying persons, their families, and other loved ones. Hospice services are available in home and inpatient settings.

Hospital—According to the American Hospital Association, hospitals are licensed institutions with at least six beds whose primary function is to provide diagnostic and therapeutic patient services for medical conditions by an organized physician staff, and have continuous nursing services under the supervision of registered nurses. The World Health Organization considers an establishment to be a hospital if it is permanently staffed by at least one physician, can offer inpatient accommodation, and can provide active medical and nursing care. Hospitals may be classified by type of service, ownership, size in terms of number of beds, and length of stay. In the National Hospital Ambulatory Medical Care Survey (NHAMCS) hospitals include all those with an average length of stay for all patients of less than 30 days (short-stay) or hospitals whose specialty is general (medical or surgical) or children's general. Federal hospitals and hospital units of institutions and hospitals with fewer than six beds staffed for patient use are excluded. See related *Average length of stay; Bed; Days of care; Emergency department; Outpatient department; Patient.*

Community hospitals traditionally included all non-Federal short-stay hospitals except facilities for the mentally retarded. In the revised definition the following additional sites are excluded: hospital units of institutions, and alcoholism and chemical dependency facilities.

Federal hospitals are operated by the Federal Government.

For profit hospitals are operated for profit by individuals, partnerships, or corporations.

General hospitals provide diagnostic, treatment, and surgical services for patients with a variety of medical conditions. According to the World Health Organization, these hospitals provide medical and nursing care for more than one category of medical discipline (for example, general medicine, specialized medicine, general surgery, specialized surgery, and obstetrics). Excluded are hospitals, usually in rural areas, that provide a more limited range of care.

Nonprofit hospitals are operated by a church or other nonprofit organization.

Psychiatric hospitals are ones whose major type of service is psychiatric care. See *Mental health organization.*

Registered hospitals are hospitals registered with the American Hospital Association. About 98 percent of hospitals are registered.

Short-stay hospitals in the National Hospital Discharge Survey are those in which the average length of stay is less than 30 days. The National Health Interview Survey defines short-stay hospitals as any hospital or hospital department in which the type of service provided is general; maternity; eye, ear, nose, and throat; children's; or osteopathic.

Specialty hospitals, such as psychiatric, tuberculosis, chronic disease, rehabilitation, maternity, and alcoholic or narcotic, provide a particular type of service to the majority of their patients.

Hospital-based physician—See *Physician.*

Hospital days—See *Days of care.*

Human immunodeficiency virus (HIV) infection—Mortality coding: Beginning with data for 1987, NCHS introduced category numbers *042-*044 for classifying and coding HIV infection as a cause of death. HIV infection was formerly referred to as human T-cell lymphotropic virus-III/lymphadenopathy-associated virus (HTLV-III/LAV) infection. The asterisk before the category numbers indicates that these codes are not part of the *Ninth Revision of the International Classification of Diseases* (ICD-9). Before 1987 deaths involving HIV infection were classified to Deficiency of cell-mediated immunity (ICD-9 279.1) contained in the title All other diseases; to Pneumocystosis (ICD-9 136.3) contained in the title All other infectious and parasitic diseases; to Malignant neoplasms, including neoplasms of lymphatic and hematopoietic tissues; and to a number of other causes. Therefore, before 1987, death statistics for HIV infection are not strictly comparable with data for 1987 and later years, and are not shown in this report.

Morbidity coding: The National Hospital Discharge Survey codes diagnosis data using the *International Classification of Diseases, Ninth Revision, Clinical Modification* (ICD–9–CM). Discharges with diagnosis of HIV as shown in *Health, United States*, have at least one HIV diagnosis listed on the face sheet of the medical record and are not limited to the first-listed diagnosis. During 1984 and 1985 only data for AIDS (ICD–9–CM 279.19) were included. In 1986–94, discharges with the following diagnoses were included: acquired immunodeficiency syndrome (AIDS), human immunodeficiency virus (HIV) infection and associated conditions, and positive serological or viral culture findings for HIV (ICD–9–CM 042- 044, 279.19, and 795.8). Beginning in 1995 discharges with the following diagnoses were included: human immunodeficiency virus (HIV) disease and asymptomatic human immunodeficiency virus (HIV) infection status (ICD–9–CM 042 and V08). See related *Acquired immunodeficiency syndrome; Cause of death; International Classification of Diseases, Ninth Revision; International Classification of Diseases, Ninth Revision, Clinical Modification.*

ICD; ICD codes—See *Cause of death; International Classification of Diseases, Ninth Revision.*

Incidence—Incidence is the number of cases of disease having their onset during a prescribed period of time. It is often expressed as a rate (for example, the incidence of measles per 1,000 children 5–15 years of age during a specified year). Incidence is a measure of morbidity or other events that occur within a specified period of time. See related *Prevalence.*

Individual practice association (IPA)—See *Health maintenance organization (HMO).*

Industry of employment—Industries are classified according to the *Standard Industrial*

Table VII. Codes for industries, according to the *Standard Industrial Classification (SIC) Manual*

Industry	Code numbers
Agriculture, forestry, and fishing.	01–09
Mining	10–14
Construction.	15–17
Manufacturing.	20–39
Transportation and public utilities	40–49
Wholesale trade	50–51
Retail trade	52–59
Finance, insurance, and real estate	60–67
Services	70–89
Public administration.	91–97

Classification (SIC) Manual of the Office of Management and Budget. Two editions of the SIC are used for coding industry data in *Health, United States*: the 1977 supplement to the 1972 edition and the 1987 edition. The changes between versions include a few detailed titles created to correct or clarify industries or to recognize changes within the industry. Codes for major industry divisions (table VII) were not changed between versions.

Establishments engaged in the same kind of economic activity are classified by the same industry code, regardless of the type of ownership—corporations, sole proprietorships, and government agencies. Data from the Census of Fatal Occupational Injuries are therefore further broken out by private sector and government. Data from the Survey of Occupational Injuries and Illnesses are provided for the private sector only and exclude the self-employed.

The category "Private sector" includes all industry divisions except public administration and military. The category "Not classified" is used for fatalities for which there was insufficient information to determine a specific industry classification.

Infant death—An infant death is the death of a live-born child before his or her first birthday. Deaths in the first year of life may be further classified according to age as neonatal and postneonatal. Neonatal deaths are those that occur before the 28th day of life; postneonatal deaths are those that occur between 28 and 365 days of age. See related *Live birth; Rate: Death and related rates.*

Injury-related visit—In the National Hospital Ambulatory Medical Care Survey an emergency department visit was considered injury-related if, on the Patient Record Form (PRF), the checkbox for injury was indicated. In addition, injury visits were identified if the physician's diagnosis or the patient's reason for visit code was injury related. See related *Emergency department visit; First-listed external cause of injury.*

Inpatient care—See *Mental health service type.*

Inpatient days—See *Days of care.*

Instrumental activities of daily living (IADL)—Instrumental activities of daily living are activities related to independent living and include preparing meals, managing money, shopping for groceries or personal items, performing light or heavy housework and using a telephone. If a sample person from the Medicare Current Beneficiary Survey had any difficulty performing an activity by himself or herself and without special equipment, or did not perform the activity at all because of health problems, the person was categorized as having a limitation in that activity. The limitation may have been temporary or chronic at the time of the interview. Sample persons who were administered a community interview answered health status and functioning questions themselves if able to do so. A proxy, such as a nurse, answered questions about the sample person's health status and functioning for long-term care facility interview. In the National Health Interview Survey respondents are asked about needing the help of another person for handling routine IADL needs due to a physical, mental, or emotional problem. Persons are considered to have an IADL

limitation if the causal condition for the IADL limitation is chronic. See related *Activities of daily living (ADL); Limitation of activity.*

Insured—See *Health insurance coverage.*

Intermediate care facilities—See *Nursing home.*

International Classification of Diseases, Ninth Revision (ICD–9)—The *International Classification of Diseases* (ICD) classifies mortality information for statistical purposes. The ICD was first used in 1900 and has been revised about every 10 years since then. The ICD-9, published in 1977, is used to code U.S. mortality data beginning with data year 1979. (See tables IV and V.) See related *Cause of death; International Classification of Diseases, Ninth Revision, Clinical Modification.*

International Classification of Diseases, Ninth Revision, Clinical Modification (ICD–9–CM)—The ICD–9–CM is based on and is completely compatible with the *International Classification of Diseases, Ninth Revision.* The ICD–9–CM is used to code morbidity

Table VIII. Codes for diagnostic categories from the *International Classification of Diseases, Ninth Revision, Clinical Modification*

Diagnostic category	Code numbers
Females with delivery	V27
Human immunodeficiency virus (HIV) (1984–85)	279.19
(1986–94)	042–044, 279.19, 795.8
(Beginning in 1995)	042, V08
Malignant neoplasms	140–208
Large intestine and rectum	153–154, 197.5
Trachea, bronchus, and lung	162, 197.0, 197.3
Breast	174–175, 198.81
Prostate	185
Diabetes	250
Psychoses (excluding alcoholic and drug psychoses)	293–299
Diseases of the nervous system and sense organs	320–389
Diseases of the circulatory system	390–459
Diseases of heart	391–392.0, 393–398, 402, 404, 410–416, 420–429
Ischemic heart disease	410–414
Acute myocardial infarction	410
Congestive heart failure	428.0
Cerebrovascular diseases	430–438
Diseases of the respiratory system	460–519
Bronchitis	466.0, 490–491
Pneumonia	466.1, 480–487.0
Asthma	493
Hyperplasia of prostate	600
Decubitus ulcers	707.0
Diseases of the musculoskeletal system and connective tissue	710–739
Osteoarthritis	715
Intervertebral disc disorders	722
Injuries and poisoning	800–999
Fracture, all sites	800–829
Fracture of neck of femur (hip)	820

Table IX. Codes for procedure categories from the *International Classification of Diseases, Ninth Revision, Clinical Modification*

Procedure category	Code numbers
Extraction of lens.	13.1–13.6
Insertion of prosthetic lens (pseudophakos)	13.7
Myringotomy with insertion of tube	20.01
Tonsillectomy, with or without adenoidectomy	28.2–28.3
Coronary angioplasty (Prior to 1997).	36.0
(Beginning in 1997)	36.01–36.05, 36.09
Coronary artery bypass graft.	36.1
Cardiac catheterization	37.21–37.23
Pacemaker insertion or replacement.	37.7–37.8
Carotid endarterectomy	38.12
Endoscopy of large or small intestine with or without biopsy	45.11–45.14, 45.16, 45.21–45.25
Cholecystectomy.	51.2
Prostatectomy.	60.2–60.6
Bilateral destruction or occlusion of fallopian tubes	66.2–66.3
Hysterectomy.	68.3–68.7, 68.9
Cesarean sectioh.	74.0–74.2, 74.4, 74.99
Repair of current obstetrical laceration.	75.5–75.6
Reduction of fracture.	76.7, 79.0–79.3
Arthroscopy of knee.	80.26
Excision or destruction of intervertebral disc.	80.5
Total hip replacement.	81.51
Lumpectomy.	85.21
Mastectomy.	85.4
Angiocardiography with contrast material.	88.5

data and the ICD-9 is used to code mortality data. Diagnostic groupings and code number inclusions for ICD–9–CM are shown in table VIII; procedures and code number inclusions are shown in table IX.

ICD-9 and ICD–9–CM are arranged in 17 main chapters. Most of the diseases are arranged according to their principal anatomical site, with special chapters for infective and parasitic diseases; neoplasms; endocrine, metabolic, and nutritional diseases; mental diseases; complications of pregnancy and childbirth; certain diseases peculiar to the perinatal period; and ill-defined conditions. In addition, two supplemental classifications are provided: the classification of factors influencing health status and contact with health service and the classification of external causes of injury and poisoning. See related *Condition; International Classification of Diseases, Ninth Revision; Mental health disorder.*

Late fetal death rate—See *Rate: Death and related rates.*

Leading causes of death—See *Cause-of-death ranking.*

Length of stay—See *Average length of stay.*

Life expectancy—Life expectancy is the average number of years of life remaining to a person at a particular age and is based on a given set of age-specific death rates, generally the mortality conditions existing in the period mentioned. Life expectancy may be determined by race, sex, or other characteristics using age-specific death rates for the population with that characteristic. See related *Rate: Death and related rates.*

Limitation of activity—In the National Health Interview Survey limitation of activity refers to a long-term reduction in a person's capacity to perform the usual kind or amount of activities associated with his or her age group due to a chronic condition. Limitation of activity is assessed by asking respondents a series of questions about limitations in their ability to perform activities usual for their age group because of a physical, mental, or emotional problem. Respondents are asked about limitations in activities of daily living, instrumental activities of daily living, play, school, work, and difficulty in walking or remembering. For reported limitations the condition causing the limitation is determined and respondents are considered limited if the causal conditions are chronic in nature.

Sample persons from the Medicare Current Beneficiary Survey who reported no limitations in the activities of daily living (ADL) or instrumental activities of daily living (IADL) due to health problems were included in the category "none". Sample persons with limitations in at least one IADL, but no ADL, were included in the category "IADL" only. Sample persons with ADL limitations were categorized by the number of limitations (1 to 2, 3 to 5) regardless of the number of IADL limitations. See related *Activities of daily living; Condition; Instrumental activities of daily living.*

Live birth—In the World Health Organization's definition, also adopted by the United Nations and the National Center for Health Statistics, a live birth is the complete expulsion or extraction from its mother of a product of conception, irrespective of the duration of the pregnancy, which, after such separation, breathes or shows any other evidence of life such as heartbeat, umbilical cord pulsation, or definite movement of voluntary muscles, whether the umbilical cord has been cut or the placenta is attached. Each product of such a birth is considered live born. See related *Gestation; Rate: Birth and related rates.*

Live-birth order—In the National Vital Statistics System this item from the birth certificate refers to the total number of live births the mother has had, including the present birth as recorded on the birth certificate. Fetal deaths are excluded. See related *Live birth.*

Low birthweight—See *Birthweight.*

Managed care—Managed care is a health care plan that integrates the financing and delivery of health care services by using arrangements with selected health care providers to provide services for covered individuals. Plans are generally financed using capitation fees. There are signifcant financial incentives for members of the plan to use the health care providers associated with the plan. The plan includes formal programs for quality assurance and utilization review. Health maintenance organizations (HMO's), preferred provider organizations (PPO's), and point of service (POS) plans are examples of managed care.

See related *Health maintenance organization; Preferred provider organization.*

Marital status—Marital status is classified through self-reporting into the categories married and unmarried. The term married encompasses all married people including those separated from their spouses. Unmarried includes those who are single (never married), divorced, or widowed. The Abortion Surveillance Reports of the Centers for Disease Control and Prevention classified separated people as unmarried before 1978.

Maternal mortality rate—See *Rate: Death and related rates.*

Medicaid—This program is State operated and administered but has Federal financial participation. Within certain broad federally determined guidelines, States decide who is eligible; the amount, duration, and scope of services covered; rates of payment for providers; and methods of administering the program. Medicaid provides health care services for certain low-income persons. Medicaid does not provide health services to all poor people in every State. It categorically covers participants in the Aid to Families with Dependent Children program and in the Supplemental Security Income program. In most States it also covers certain other people deemed to be medically needy. The program was authorized in 1965 by Title XIX of the Social Security Act. See related *Health expenditures, national; Health maintenance organization; Medicare.*

Medical specialties—See *Physician specialty.*

Medical vendor payments—Under the Medicaid program, medical vendor payments are payments (expenditures) to medical vendors from the State through a fiscal agent or to a health insurance plan. Adjustments are made for Indian Health Service payments to Medicaid, cost settlements, third party recoupments, refunds, voided checks, and other financial settlements that cannot be related to specific provided claims. Excluded are payments made for medical care under the emergency assistance provisions, payments made from State medical assistance funds that are not federally matchable,

Table X. Mental health codes, according to applicable revision of the *Diagnostic and Statistical Manual of Mental Disorders* and *International Classification of Diseases*

Diagnostic category	DSM-II/ICDA-8	DSM-IIIR/ICD-9-CM
Alcohol related	291, 303, 309.13	291, 303, 305.0
Drug related	294.3, 304, 309.14	292, 304, 305.1–305.9, 327, 328
Organic disorders (other than alcoholism and drug)	290, 292, 293, 294 (except 294.3), 309.0, 309.2–309.9	290, 293, 294, 310
Affective disorders	296, 298.0, 300.4	296, 298.0, 300.4, 301.11, 301.13
Schizophrenia	295	295

disproportionate share hospital payments, cost sharing or enrollment fees collected from recipients or a third party, and administration and training costs.

Medicare—This is a nationwide health insurance program providing health insurance protection to people 65 years of age and over, people entitled to social security disability payments for 2 years or more, and people with end-stage renal disease, regardless of income. The program was enacted July 30, 1965, as Title XVIII, *Health Insurance for the Aged of the Social Security Act*, and became effective on July 1, 1966. It consists of two separate but coordinated programs, hospital insurance (Part A) and supplementary medical insurance (Part B). See related *Health expenditures, national; Health maintenance organization; Medicaid.*

Mental health disorder—The Center for Mental Health Services defines a mental health disorder as any of several disorders listed in the *International Classification of Diseases, Ninth Revision, Clinical Modification* (ICD–9–CM) or *Diagnostic and Statistical Manual of Mental Disorders, Third Edition* (DSM-IIIR). Table X shows diagnostic categories and code numbers for ICD–9–CM/DSM-IIIR and corresponding codes for the *International Classification of Diseases, Adapted for Use in the United States, Eighth Revision* (ICDA-8) and *Diagnostic and Statistical Manual of Mental Disorders, Second Edition* (DSM-II). See related *International Classification of Diseases, Clinical Modification.*

Mental health organization—The Center for Mental Health Services defines a mental health organization as an administratively distinct public or private agency or institution whose primary concern is the provision of direct mental health services to the mentally ill or emotionally disturbed. Excluded are private office-based practices of psychiatrists, psychologists, and other mental health providers; psychiatric services of all types of hospitals or outpatient clinics operated by Federal agencies other than the Department of Veterans Affairs (for example, Public Health Service, Indian Health Service, Department of Defense, and Bureau of Prisons); general hospitals that have no separate psychiatric services, but admit psychiatric patients to nonpsychiatric units; and psychiatric services of schools, colleges, halfway houses, community residential organizations, local and county jails, State prisons, and other human service providers. The major types of mental health organizations are described below.

Freestanding psychiatric outpatient clinics provide only outpatient services on either a regular or emergency basis. The medical responsibility for services is generally assumed by a psychiatrist.

General hospitals providing separate psychiatric services are non-Federal general hospitals that provide psychiatric services in either a separate psychiatric inpatient, outpatient, or partial hospitalization service with assigned staff and space.

Multiservice mental health organizations directly provide two or more of the program elements defined under Mental health service type and are not classifiable as a psychiatric hospital, general hospital, or a residential treatment center for emotionally disturbed children. (The classification of a psychiatric or general hospital or a residential treatment center for emotionally disturbed children takes precedence over a multiservice classification, even if two or more services are offered.)

Partial care organizations provide a program of ambulatory mental health services.

Private mental hospitals are operated by a sole proprietor, partnership, limited partnership, corporation, or nonprofit organization, primarily for the care of persons with mental disorders.

Psychiatric hospitals are hospitals primarily concerned with providing inpatient care and treatment for the mentally ill. Psychiatric inpatient units of Department of Veterans Affairs general hospitals and Department of Veterans Affairs neuropsychiatric hospitals are combined into the category Department of Veterans Affairs psychiatric hospitals because of their similarity in size, operation, and length of stay.

Residential treatment centers for emotionally disturbed children must meet all of the following criteria: (a) Not licensed as a psychiatric hospital and primary purpose is to provide individually planned mental health treatment services in conjunction with residential care; (b) Include a clinical program that is directed by a psychiatrist, psychologist, social worker, or psychiatric nurse with a graduate degree; (c) Serve children and youth primarily under the age of 18; and (d) Primary diagnosis for the majority of admissions is mental illness, classified as other than mental retardation, developmental disability, and substance-related disorders, according to DSM-II/ICDA-8 or DSM-IIIR/ICD-9-CM codes.

State and county mental hospitals are under the auspices of a State or county government or operated jointly by a State and county government.

See related *Addition; Mental health service type.*

Mental health service type—refers to the following kinds of mental health services:

Inpatient care is the provision of 24-hour mental health care in a mental health hospital setting.

Outpatient care is the provision of ambulatory mental health services for less than 3 hours at a single visit on an individual, group, or family basis, usually in a clinic or similar organization. Emergency care on a walk-in basis, as well as care provided by mobile teams who visit patients outside these organizations are included. "Hotline" services are excluded.

Partial care treatment is a planned program of mental health treatment services generally provided in visits of 3 or more hours to groups of patients. Included are treatment programs that emphasize intensive short-term therapy and rehabilitation; programs that focus on recreation, and/or occupational program activities, including sheltered workshops; and education and training programs, including special education classes, therapeutic nursery schools, and vocational training.

Residential treatment care is the provision of overnight mental health care in conjunction with an intensive treatment program in a setting other than a hospital. Facilities may offer care to emotionally disturbed children or mentally ill adults.

See related *Addition; Mental health organization.*

Metropolitan statistical area (MSA)—MSA's are defined by the U.S. Office of Management and Budget (OMB). The MSA standards are revised before each decennial Census. When Census data become available, the standards are applied to define the actual MSA's. An MSA is a county or group of contiguous counties that contains at least one city with a population of 50,000 or more or includes a Census Bureau-defined urbanized area of at least 50,000 with a metropolitan population of at least 100,000. In addition to the county containing the main city or urbanized area, an MSA may contain other counties that are metropolitan in character and are economically and socially integrated with the central counties. In New England, cities and towns, rather than counties, are used to define MSA's. For data from the National Health Interview Survey (NHIS) prior to 1995, metropolitan population is based on MSA's as defined by OMB in 1983 using the 1980 Census. Starting with the 1995 NHIS, metropolitan population is based on MSA's as defined by OMB in 1993 using the 1990 Census. For further information on MSA's, see U.S. Department of Commerce, Bureau of the Census, *State and Metropolitan Area Data Book*. See related *Urbanization*.

Multiservice mental health organizations—See *Mental health organization*.

National ambient air quality standards—The Federal Clean Air Act of 1970, amended in 1977 and 1990, required the Environmental Protection Agency (EPA) to establish National Ambient Air Quality Standards. EPA has set specific standards for each of six major pollutants: carbon monoxide, lead, nitrogen dioxide, ozone, sulfur dioxide, and particulate matter whose aerodynamic size is equal to or less than 10 microns (PM-10). Each pollutant standard represents a maximum concentration level (micrograms per cubic meter) that cannot be exceeded during a specified time interval. A county meets the national ambient air quality standards if none of the six pollutants exceed the standard during a 12-month period. See related *Particulate matter; Pollutant*.

Neonatal mortality rate—See *Rate: Death and related rates*.

Non-Federal physicians—See *Physician*.

Nonpatient revenue—Nonpatient revenues are those revenues received for which no direct patient care services are rendered. The most widely recognized source of nonpatient revenues is philanthropy. Philanthropic support may be direct from individuals or may be obtained through philanthropic fund raising organizations such as the United Way. Support may also be obtained from foundations or corporations. Philanthropic revenues may be designated for direct patient care use or may be contained in an endowment fund where only the current income may be tapped.

Nonprofit hospitals—See *Hospital*.

Notifiable disease—A notifiable disease is one that, when diagnosed, health providers are required, usually by law, to report to State or local public health

officials. Notifiable diseases are those of public interest by reason of their contagiousness, severity, or frequency.

Nursing care—The following definition of nursing care applies to data collected in National Nursing Home Surveys through 1977. Nursing care is the provision of any of the following services: application of dressings or bandages; bowel and bladder retraining; catheterization; enema; full bed bath; hypodermic, intramuscular, or intravenous injection; irrigation; nasal feeding; oxygen therapy; and temperature-pulse-respiration or blood pressure measurement. See related *Nursing home*.

Nursing care homes—See *Nursing home*.

Nursing home—In the Online Survey Certification and Reporting database, a nursing home is a facility that is certified and meets the Health Care Financing Administration's long-term care requirements for Medicare and Medicaid eligibility. In the National Master Facility Inventory and the National Nursing Home Survey, a nursing home is an establishment with three or more beds that provides nursing or personal care services to the aged, infirm, or chronically ill. The following definitions of nursing home types apply to data collected in National Nursing Home Surveys through 1977.

Nursing care homes must employ one or more full-time registered or licensed practical nurses and must provide nursing care to at least one-half the residents.

Personal care homes with nursing have some but fewer than one-half the residents receiving nursing care. In addition, such homes must employ one or more registered or licensed practical nurses or must provide administration of medications and treatments in accordance with physicians' orders, supervision of self-administered medications, or three or more personal services.

Personal care homes without nursing have no residents who are receiving nursing care. These homes provide administration of medications and treatments in accordance with physicians' orders, supervision of self-administered medications, or three or more personal services.

Domiciliary care homes primarily provide supervisory care but also provide one or two personal services.

Nursing homes are certified by the Medicare and/or Medicaid program. The following definitions of certification levels apply to data collected in National Nursing Home Surveys of 1973–74, 1977, and 1985.

Skilled nursing facilities provide the most intensive nursing care available outside of a hospital. Facilities certified by Medicare provide posthospital care to eligible Medicare enrollees. Facilities certified by Medicaid as skilled nursing facilities provide skilled nursing services on a daily basis to individuals eligible for Medicaid benefits.

Intermediate care facilities are certified by the Medicaid program to provide health-related services on a regular basis to Medicaid eligibles who do not require hospital or skilled nursing facility care but do require institutional care above the level of room and board.

Not certified facilities are not certified as providers of care by Medicare or Medicaid.
See related *Nursing care; Resident.*

Nursing home expenditures—See *Health expenditures, national.*

Occupancy rate—The American Hospital Association defines hospital occupancy rate as the average daily census divided by the average number of hospital beds during a reporting period. Average daily census is defined by the American Hospital Association as the average number of inpatients, excluding newborns, receiving care each day during a reporting period. The occupancy rate for facilities other than hospitals is calculated as the number of residents reported at the time of the interview divided by the number of beds reported. In the Online Survey Certification and Reporting database, occupancy is the total number of residents on the day of certification

inspection divided by the total number of beds on the day of certification.

Office—In the National Ambulatory Medical Care Survey, an office is any location for a physician's ambulatory practice other than hospitals, nursing homes, other extended care facilities, patients' homes, industrial clinics, college clinics, and family planning clinics. Offices in health maintenance organizations and private offices in hospitals are included. See related *Office visit; Outpatient visit; Physician.*

Office-based physician—See *Physician.*

Office visit—In the National Ambulatory Medical Care Survey, an office visit is any direct personal exchange between an ambulatory patient and a physician or members of his or her staff for the purposes of seeking care and rendering health services. See related *Outpatient visit.*

Operations—See *Procedure.*

Outpatient department—According to the National Hospital Ambulatory Medical Care Survey (NHAMCS), an outpatient department (OPD) is a hospital facility where nonurgent ambulatory medical care is provided. The following are examples of the types of OPD's excluded from the NHAMCS: ambulatory surgical centers, chemotherapy, employee health services, renal dialysis, methadone maintenance, and radiology. See related *Emergency department; Outpatient visit.*

Outpatient surgery—According to the American Hospital Association, outpatient surgery is performed on patients who do not remain in the hospital overnight and occurs in inpatient operating suites, outpatient surgery suites, or procedure rooms within an outpatient care facility. Outpatient surgery is a surgical operation, whether major or minor, performed in operating or procedure rooms. A surgical operation involving more than one surgical procedure is considered one surgical operation. See related *Ambulatory surgery; Procedure.*

Outpatient visit—The American Hospital Association defines outpatient visits as visits for receipt of medical, dental, or other services by patients who are not lodged in the hospital. Each appearance by an outpatient to each unit of the hospital is counted individually as an outpatient visit. In the National Hospital Ambulatory Medical Care Survey an outpatient department visit is a direct personal exchange between a patient and a physician or other health care provider working under the physician's supervision for the purpose of seeking care and receiving personal health services. See related *Emergency department visit; Outpatient department.*

Partial care organization—See *Mental health organization.*

Partial care treatment—See *Mental health service type.*

Particulate matter—Particulate matter is defined as particles of solid or liquid matter in the air, including nontoxic materials (soot, dust, and dirt) and toxic materials (for example, lead, asbestos, suspended sulfates, and nitrates). See related *National ambient air quality standards; Pollutant.*

Patient—A patient is a person who is formally admitted to the inpatient service of a hospital for observation, care, diagnosis, or treatment. See related *Admission; Average length of stay; Days of care; Discharge; Hospital.*

Percent change—See *Average annual rate of change.*

Perinatal mortality rate, ratio—See *Rate: Death and related rates.*

Personal care homes with or without nursing—See *Nursing home.*

Personal health care expenditures—See *Health expenditures, national.*

Physician—Physicians, through self-reporting, are classified by the American Medical Association and others as licensed doctors of medicine or osteopathy, as follows:

Active (or professionally active) physicians are currently practicing medicine for a minimum of 20 hours per week. Excluded are physicians who are

not practicing, practicing medicine less than 20 hours per week, have unknown addresses, or specialties not classified (when specialty information is presented).

Federal physicians are employed by the Federal Government; non-Federal or civilian physicians are not.

Hospital-based physicians spend the plurality of their time as salaried physicians in hospitals.

Office-based physicians spend the plurality of their time working in practices based in private offices.

Data for physicians are presented by type of education (doctors of medicine and doctors of osteopathy); place of education (U.S. medical graduates and international medical graduates); activity status (professionally active and inactive); employment setting (Federal and non-Federal); area of specialty; and geographic area. See related *Office; Physician specialty.*

Physician specialty—A physician specialty is any specific branch of medicine in which a physician may concentrate. Data are based on physician self-reports of their primary area of speciality. Physician data are broadly categorized into two general areas of practice: generalists and specialists.

Generalist physicians are synonymous with primary care generalists and only include physicians practicing in the general fields of family and general practice, general internal medicine, and general pediatrics. They specifically exclude primary care specialists.

Primary care specialists practice in the subspecialties of general and family practice, internal medicine, and pediatrics. The primary care subspecialties for family practice include geriatric medicine and sports medicine. Primary care subspecialties for internal medicine include diabetes, endocrinology and metabolism, hematology, hepatology, cardiac electrophysiology, infectious diseases, diagnostic laboratory immunology, geriatric medicine, sports medicine, nephrology, nutrition, medical oncology, and rheumatology. Primary care subspecialties for pediatrics include adolescent medicine, critical care pediatrics, neonatal-perinatal medicine, pediatric allergy, pediatric cardiology, pediatric endocrinology, pediatric pulmonology, pediatric emergency medicine, pediatric gastroenterology, pediatric hematology/oncology, diagnostic laboratory immunology, pediatric nephrology, pediatric rheumatology, and sports medicine.

Specialist physicians practice in the primary care specialties, in addition to all other specialist fields not included in the generalist definition. Specialist fields include allergy and immunology, aerospace medicine, anesthesiology, cardiovascular diseases, child and adolescent psychiatry, colon and rectal surgery, dermatology, diagnostic radiology, forensic pathology, gastroenterology, general surgery, medical genetics, neurology, nuclear medicine, neurological surgery, obstetrics and gynecology, occupational medicine, ophthalmology, orthopedic surgery, otolaryngology, psychiatry, public health and general preventive medicine, physical medicine and rehabilitation, plastic surgery, anatomic and clinical pathology, pulmonary diseases, radiation oncology, thoracic surgery, urology, addiction medicine, critical care medicine, legal medicine, and clinical pharmacology.
See related *Physician.*

Pollutant—A pollutant is any substance that renders the atmosphere or water foul or noxious to health. See related *National ambient air quality standards; Particulate matter.*

Population—The U.S. Bureau of the Census collects and publishes data on populations in the United States according to several different definitions. Various statistical systems then use the appropriate population for calculating rates.

Total population is the population of the United States, including all members of the Armed Forces living in foreign countries, Puerto Rico, Guam, and the U.S. Virgin Islands. Other Americans abroad (for example, civilian Federal employees and dependents of members of the Armed Forces or other Federal employees) are not included.

Resident population includes persons whose usual place of residence (that is, the place where one usually lives and sleeps) is in one of the 50 States or the District of Columbia. It includes members of the Armed Forces stationed in the United States and their families. It excludes international military, naval, and diplomatic personnel and their families located here and residing in embassies or similar quarters. Also excluded are international workers and international students in this country and Americans living abroad. The resident population is usually the denominator when calculating birth and death rates and incidence of disease. The resident population is also the denominator for selected population-based rates that use numerator data from the National Nursing Home Survey.

Civilian population is the resident population excluding members of the Armed Forces. However, families of members of the Armed Forces are included. This population is the denominator in rates calculated for the NCHS National Hospital Discharge Survey, the National Home and Hospice Care Survey, and the National Survey of Ambulatory Surgery.

Civilian noninstitutionalized population is the civilian population not residing in institutions. Institutions include correctional institutions, detention homes, and training schools for juvenile delinquents; homes for the aged and dependent (for example, nursing homes and convalescent homes); homes for dependent and neglected children; homes and schools for the mentally or physically handicapped; homes for unwed mothers; psychiatric, tuberculosis, and chronic disease hospitals; and residential treatment centers. Census Bureau estimates of the civilian noninstitutionalized population are used to calculate sample weights for the NCHS National Health Interview Survey, National Health and Nutrition Examination Survey, National Survey of Family Growth, National Ambulatory Medical

Care Survey, and the National Hospital Ambulatory Medical Care Survey.

Postneonatal mortality rate—See *Rate: Death and related rates.*

Poverty level—Poverty statistics are based on definitions originally developed by the Social Security Administration. These include a set of money income thresholds that vary by family size and composition. Families or individuals with income below their appropriate thresholds are classified as below the poverty level. These thresholds are updated annually by the U.S. Bureau of the Census to reflect changes in the Consumer Price Index for all urban consumers (CPI-U). For example, the average poverty threshold for a family of four was $16,400 in 1997 and $13,359 in 1990. For more information, see U.S. Bureau of the Census: *Money Income of Households, Families, and Persons in the United States, 1996.* Series P-60. Washington. U.S. Government Printing office. See related *Consumer Price Index; Family income.*

Preferred provider organization (PPO)—Health plan generally consisting of hospital and physician providers. The PPO provides health care services to plan members usually at discounted rates in return for expedited claims payment. Plan members can use PPO or non-PPO health care providers, however, financial incentives are built into the benefit structure to encourage utilization of PPO providers. See related *Managed care.*

Prevalence—Prevalence is the number of cases of a disease, infected persons, or persons with some other attribute present during a particular interval of time. It is often expressed as a rate (for example, the prevalence of diabetes per 1,000 persons during a year). See related *Incidence.*

Primary admission diagnosis—In the National Home and Hospice Care Survey the primary admission diagnosis is the first-listed diagnosis at admission on the patient's medical record as provided by the agency staff member most familiar with the care provided to the patient.

Primary care specialties—See *Physician specialty.*

Private expenditures—See *Health expenditures, national.*

Procedure—The National Hospital Discharge Survey (NHDS) and the National Survey of Ambulatory Surgery (NSAS) define a procedure as a surgical or nonsurgical operation, diagnostic procedure, or therapeutic procedure (such as respiratory therapy) recorded on the medical record of discharged patients. A maximum of four procedures per discharge in NHDS and up to six procedures per discharge in NSAS were recorded and coded to the *International Classification of Diseases, Ninth Revision, Clinical Modification.* Previous editions of *Health, United States* classified procedures into surgical and diagnostic and other nonsurgical procedures. The distinction between surgical and diagnostic and nonsurgical procedures has become less meaningful due to the development of minimally invasive and noninvasive surgery. Thus the practice of classifying procedures as surgical or diagnostic has been discontinued. See related *Ambulatory surgery; Outpatient surgery.*

Proprietary hospitals—See *Hospital.*

Psychiatric hospitals—See *Hospital; Mental health organization.*

Public expenditures—See *Health expenditures, national.*

Public health activities—Public health activities may include any of the following essential services of public health—surveillance, investigations, education, community mobilization, workforce training, research, and personal care services delivered or funded by governmental agencies.

Race—In 1977 the Office of Management and Budget (OMB) issued Race and Ethnic Standards for Federal Statistics and Administrative reporting in order to promote comparability of data among Federal data systems. The 1977 standards called for the Federal Government's data systems to classify individuals into the following four racial groups: American Indian or Alaska Native, Asian or Pacific Islander, black, and white. Depending on the data source, the classification by race was based on self-classification or on observation by an interviewer or other person filling out the questionnaire.

In 1997 new standards were announced for classification of individuals by race within the Federal Government's data systems (*Federal Register*, 62FR58781–58790). The 1997 standards have five racial groups: American Indian or Alaska Native, Asian, Black or African American, Native Hawaiian or other Pacific Islander, and White. These five categories are the minimum set for data on race for Federal statistics. The 1997 standards also offer an opportunity for respondents to select more than one of the five groups, leading to many possible multiple race

categories. As with the single race groups, data for the multiple race groups are to be reported when estimates meet agency requirements for reliability and confidentiality. The 1997 standards allow for observer or proxy identification of race but clearly state a preference for self-classification.

All Federal data systems are required to be compliant with the 1997 standards by 2003. Although some data systems already permit tabulation of race-specific estimates under the 1997 standards, most do not. In order to facilitate comparisons of race-specific estimates across the various data systems presented in *Health, United States*, the 1977 standard categories are used in all trend tables and charts. However, for illustration, two health statistics (cigarette

Table XI. Current cigarette smoking by persons 18 years of age and over, according to race and Hispanic origin under the 1977 and 1997 Standards for Federal data on race and ethnicity: United States, average annual 1993–95

1997 Standards	Sample size	Percent	Standard error	1977 Standards	Sample size	Percent	Standard error
Race:				Race:			
White only	46,228	25.2	0.26	White	46,664	25.3	0.26
Black or African American only	7,208	26.6	0.64	Black	7,334	26.5	0.63
American Indian or Alaska Native only	416	32.9	2.53	American Indian or Alaska Native	480	33.9	2.38
Asian only	1,370	15.0	1.19	Asian or Pacific Islander	1,411	15.5	1.22
Multiple race total	786	34.5	2.00				
Black or African American; White	83	*21.7	6.05				
American Indian or Alaska Native; White	461	40.0	2.58				
Race, any mention:							
White, any mention	46,882	25.3	0.26				
Black or African American, any mention	7,382	26.6	0.63				
American Indian or Alaska Native, any mention	965	36.3	1.71				
Asian, any mention	1,458	15.7	1.20				
Native Hawaiian or Other Pacific Islander, any mention	53	*17.5	5.10				
Hispanic origin and race:				Hispanic origin and race:			
Not Hispanic or Latino:				Non-Hispanic:			
White only	42,421	25.8	0.27	White	42,976	25.9	0.27
Black or African American only	7,053	26.7	0.65	Black	7,203	26.7	0.64
American Indian or Alaska Native only	358	33.5	2.69	American Indian or Alaska Native	407	35.4	2.53
Asian only	1,320	14.8	1.21	Asian or Pacific Islander	1,397	15.3	1.24
Multiple race total	687	35.6	2.15				
Hispanic or Latino	5,175	17.8	0.65	Hispanic	5,175	17.8	0.65

*Relative standard error 20–30 percent.

NOTES: The 1997 Standards for Federal data on race and ethnicity set five single race groups (White, Black, American Indian or Alaska Native, Asian, and Native Hawaiian or Other Pacific Islander) and allow respondents to report one or more race groups. Estimates for single race and multiple race groups not shown above do not meet standards for statistical reliability or confidentiality (relative standard error greater than 30 percent). Race groups under the 1997 Standards were based on the question, "What is the group or groups which represents _____ race?" For persons who selected multiple groups, race groups under the 1977 Standards were based on the additional question, "Which of those groups would you say best represents _____ race?" Race-specific estimates in this table were calculated after excluding respondents of other and unknown race. Other published race-specific estimates are based on files in which such responses have been edited. Percents are age adjusted to the year 2000 standard using three age groups: Under 18 years, 18–44 years, and 45–64 years of age. See Appendix II, Age adjustment.

SOURCE: Centers for Disease Control and Prevention, National Center for Health Statistics. National Health Interview Survey.

Table XII. Private health care coverage for persons under 65 years of age, according to race and Hispanic origin under the 1977 and 1997 Standards for Federal data on race and ethnicity: United States, average annual 1993–95

1997 Standards	Sample size	Percent	Standard error	1977 Standards	Sample size	Percent	Standard error
Race:				Race:			
White only	168,256	76.1	0.28	White	170,472	75.9	0.28
Black or African American only	30,048	53.5	0.63	Black	30,690	53.6	0.63
American Indian or Alaska Native only	2,003	44.2	1.97	American Indian or Alaska Native	2,316	43.5	1.85
Asian only	6,896	68.0	1.39	Asian or Pacific Islander	7,146	68.2	1.34
Native Hawaiian or Other Pacific Islander only	173	75.0	7.43				
Multiple race total	4,203	60.9	1.17				
Black or African American; White	686	59.5	3.21				
American Indian or Alaska Native; White	2,022	60.0	1.71				
Asian; White	590	71.9	3.39				
Native Hawaiian or Other Pacific Islander; White	56	59.2	10.65				
Race, any mention:							
White, any mention	171,817	75.8	0.28				
Black or African American, any mention	31,147	53.6	0.62				
American Indian or Alaska Native, any mention	4,365	52.4	1.40				
Asian, any mention	7,639	68.4	1.27				
Native Hawaiian or Other Pacific Islander, any mention	283	68.7	6.23				
Hispanic origin and race:				Hispanic origin and race:			
Not Hispanic or Latino:				Non-Hispanic:			
White only	146,109	78.9	0.27	White	149,057	78.6	0.27
Black or African American only	29,250	53.9	0.64	Black	29,877	54.0	0.63
American Indian or Alaska Native only	1,620	45.2	2.15	American Indian or Alaska Native	1,859	44.6	2.05
Asian only	6,623	68.2	1.43	Asian or Pacific Islander	6,999	68.4	1.40
Native Hawaiian or Other Pacific Islander only	145	76.4	7.79				
Multiple race total	3,365	62.6	1.18				
Hispanic or Latino	31,040	48.8	0.74	Hispanic	31,040	48.8	0.74

NOTES: The 1997 Standards for Federal data on race and ethnicity set five single race groups (White, Black, American Indian or Alaska Native, Asian, and Native Hawaiian or Other Pacific Islander) and allow respondents to report one or more race groups. Estimates for single race and multiple race groups not shown above do not meet standards for statistical reliability or confidentiality (relative standard error greater than 30 percent). Race groups under the 1997 Standards were based on the question, "What is the group or groups which represents ____ race?" For persons who selected multiple groups, race groups under the 1977 Standards were based on the additional question, "Which of those groups would you say best represents ____ race?" Race-specific estimates in this table were calculated after excluding respondents of other and unknown race. Other published race-specific estimates are based on files in which such responses have been edited. Percents are age adjusted to the year 2000 standard using three age groups: Under 18 years, 18–44 years, and 45–64 years of age. See Appendix II, Age adjustment.

SOURCE: Centers for Disease Control and Prevention, National Center for Health Statistics. National Health Interview Survey.

smoking and private health insurance coverage) based on data from the 1993–95 National Health Interview Survey have been tabulated by race and Hispanic origin using both the 1997 and 1977 standards (tables XI and XII). In these illustrations, three separate tabulations using the 1997 standards are shown: 1) Race: mutually exclusive race groups, including several multiple race combinations; 2) Race, any mention: race groups that are not mutually exclusive because each race category includes all persons who mention that race; and 3) Hispanic origin and race: detailed race and Hispanic origin with a multiple race total category. When applicable, comparison tabulations are shown for the 1977

standards. Under the 1997 standards the sample size in each race group declines slightly when compared with the 1977 standards because there are more race groups. There are few multiple race groups with sufficient numbers of observations to meet standards of statistical reliability. Tables XI and XII also illustrate changes in the terms used for specific groups in the 1997 standards. The race designation of Black was changed to Black or African American and the ethnicity designation of Hispanic was changed to Hispanic or Latino.

Additional information is provided in Appendix I under National Vital Statistics System. Also see related *Hispanic origin.*

Rate—A rate is a measure of some event, disease, or condition in relation to a unit of population, along with some specification of time. See related *Age adjustment; Population.*

■ *Birth and related rates*

Birth rate is calculated by dividing the number of live births in a population in a year by the midyear resident population. For census years, rates are based on unrounded census counts of the resident population, as of April 1. For the noncensus years of 1981–89 and 1991, rates are based on national estimates of the resident population, as of July 1, rounded to 1,000's. Population estimates for 5-year age groups are generated by summing unrounded population estimates before rounding to 1,000's. Starting in 1992 rates are based on unrounded national population estimates. Birth rates are expressed as the number of live births per 1,000 population. The rate may be restricted to births to women of specific age, race, marital status, or geographic location (specific rate), or it may be related to the entire population (crude rate). See related *Cohort fertility; Live birth.*

Fertility rate is the total number of live births, regardless of age of mother, per 1,000 women of reproductive age, 15–44 years.

■ *Death and related rates*

Death rate is calculated by dividing the number of deaths in a population in a year by the midyear resident population. For census years, rates are based on unrounded census counts of the resident population, as of April 1. For the noncensus years of 1981–89 and 1991, rates are based on national estimates of the resident population, as of July 1, rounded to 1,000's. Population estimates for 10-year age groups are generated by summing unrounded population estimates before rounding to 1,000's. Starting in 1992 rates are based on unrounded national population estimates. Rates for the Hispanic and non-Hispanic white populations in each year are based on unrounded State population estimates for States in the Hispanic

reporting area. Death rates are expressed as the number of deaths per 100,000 population. The rate may be restricted to deaths in specific age, race, sex, or geographic groups or from specific causes of death (specific rate) or it may be related to the entire population (crude rate).

Fetal death rate is the number of fetal deaths with stated or presumed gestation of 20 weeks or more divided by the sum of live births plus fetal deaths, stated per 1,000 live births plus fetal deaths. *Late fetal death rate* is the number of fetal deaths with stated or presumed gestation of 28 weeks or more divided by the sum of live births plus late fetal deaths, stated per 1,000 live births plus late fetal deaths. See related *Fetal death; Gestation.*

Infant mortality rate based on period files is calculated by dividing the number of infant deaths during a calendar year by the number of live births reported in the same year. It is expressed as the number of infant deaths per 1,000 live births. *Neonatal mortality rate* is the number of deaths of children under 28 days of age, per 1,000 live births. *Postneonatal mortality rate* is the number of deaths of children that occur between 28 days and 365 days after birth, per 1,000 live births. See related *Infant death.*

Birth cohort infant mortality rates are based on linked birth and infant death files. In contrast to period rates in which the births and infant deaths occur in the same period or calendar year, infant deaths comprising the numerator of a birth cohort rate may have occurred in the same year as, or in the year following the year of birth. The birth cohort infant mortality rate is expressed as the number of infant deaths per 1,000 live births. See related *Birth cohort.*

Perinatal relates to the period surrounding the birth event. Rates and ratios are based on events reported in a calendar year. *Perinatal mortality rate* is the sum of late fetal deaths plus infant deaths within 7 days of birth divided by the sum of live births plus late fetal deaths, stated per 1,000 live births plus late fetal deaths. *Perinatal mortality ratio* is the sum of late fetal deaths plus infant deaths within 7 days of birth divided by the number of live births, stated per 1,000 live births.

Maternal death is defined as the death of a woman while pregnant or within 42 days of termination of pregnancy, irrespective of the duration and the site of the pregnancy. Maternal death is one for which the certifying physician has designated a maternal condition as the underlying cause of death. Maternal conditions are those assigned to Complications of pregnancy, childbirth, and the puerperium, ICD-9 codes 630–676. (See related table V.) *Maternal mortality rate* is defined as the number of maternal deaths per 100,000 live births. The maternal mortality rate is a measure of the likelihood that a pregnant woman will die from maternal causes. The number of live births used in the denominator is a proxy for the population of pregnant women who are at risk of a maternal death.

Region—See *Geographic region and division.*

Registered hospitals—See *Hospital.*

Registered nursing education—Registered nursing data are shown by level of educational preparation. Baccalaureate education requires at least 4 years of college or university; associate degree programs are based in community colleges and are usually 2 years in length; and diploma programs are based in hospitals and are usually 3 years in length.

Registration area—The United States has separate registration areas for birth, death, marriage, and divorce statistics. In general, registration areas correspond to States and include two separate registration areas for the District of Columbia and New York City. All States have adopted laws that require the registration of births and deaths and the reporting of fetal deaths. It is believed that more than 99 percent of the births and deaths occurring in this country are registered.

The *death registration area* was established in 1900 with 10 States and the District of Columbia, and the *birth registration area* was established in 1915, also with 10 States and the District of Columbia. Both areas have covered the entire United States since 1933. Currently, Puerto Rico, U.S. Virgin Islands, and Guam comprise separate registration areas, although their data are not included in statistical tabulations of U.S. resident data. See related *Reporting area.*

Relative survival rate—The relative survival rate is the ratio of the observed survival rate for the patient group to the expected survival rate for persons in the general population similar to the patient group with respect to age, sex, race, and calendar year of observation. The 5-year relative survival rate is used to estimate the proportion of cancer patients potentially curable. Because over one-half of all cancers occur in persons 65 years of age and over, many of these individuals die of other causes with no evidence of recurrence of their cancer. Thus, because it is obtained by adjusting observed survival for the normal life expectancy of the general population of the same age, the relative survival rate is an estimate of the chance of surviving the effects of cancer.

Reporting area—In the National Vital Statistics System, the reporting area for such basic items on the birth and death certificates as age, race, and sex, is based on data from residents of all 50 States in the United States and the District of Columbia. The reporting area for selected items such as Hispanic origin, educational attainment, and marital status, is based on data from those States that require the item to be reported, whose data meet a minimum level of completeness (such as, 80 or 90 percent), and are considered to be sufficiently comparable to be used for analysis. In 1993–96 the reporting area for Hispanic origin of decedent on the death certificate included 49 States and the District of Columbia. See related *Registration area; National Vital Statistics System* in Appendix I.

Resident—In the Online Survey Certification and Reporting database, all residents in certified facilities are counted on the day of certification inspection. In the National Nursing Home Survey, a resident is a person on the roster of the nursing home as of the night before the survey. Included are all residents for whom beds are maintained even though they may be on overnight leave or in a hospital. See related *Nursing home.*

Resident population—See *Population.*

Residential treatment care—See *Mental health service type.*

Residential treatment centers for emotionally disturbed children—See *Mental health organization.*

Self-assessment of health—See *Health status, respondent-assessed.*

Short-stay hospitals—See *Hospital.*

Skilled nursing facilities—See *Nursing home.*

Smoker—See *Current smoker.*

Specialty hospitals—See *Hospital.*

State health agency—The agency or department within State government headed by the State or territorial health official. Generally, the State health agency is responsible for setting statewide public health priorities, carrying out national and State mandates, responding to public health hazards, and assuring access to health care for underserved State residents.

Substance abuse treatment clients—In the Substance Abuse and Mental Health Services Administration's Uniform Facilities Data Set substance abuse treatment clients have been admitted to treatment and have been seen on a scheduled appointment basis at least once in the month before the survey reference date or were inpatients on the survey reference date. Types of treatment include 24-hour detoxification, 24-hour rehabilitation or residential care, and outpatient care.

Surgical operations—See *Procedure.*

Surgical specialties—See *Physician specialty.*

Uninsured—See *Health insurance coverage.*

Urbanization—In this report death rates are presented according to level of urbanization of the decedent's county of residence. Metropolitan and nonmetropolitan counties are categorized into urbanization levels based on an NCHS-modification of the 1993 rural-urban continuum codes. The 1993 rural-urban continuum codes were developed by the Economic Research Service, U.S. Department of Agriculture using the 1993 U.S. Office of Management and Budget definition of metropolitan statistical areas (MSA's). The codes classify metropolitan counties by population size and level of urbanization and nonmetropolitan counties by level of urbanization and proximity to metropolitan areas. NCHS modified the 1993 rural-urban continuum codes to make the definition of core and fringe metropolitan counties comparable to the definitions used for the 1983 codes. For this report, the 10 categories of counties have been collapsed into 5 categories (a) core metropolitan counties contain the primary central city of an MSA with a 1990 population of 1 million or more; (b) fringe metropolitan counties are the noncore counties of an MSA with 1990 population of 1 million or more; (c) medium or small metropolitan counties are in MSA's with 1990 population under 1 million; (d) urban nonmetropolitan counties are not in MSA's and have 2,500 or more urban residents in 1990; and (e) rural counties are not in MSA's and have fewer than 2,500 urban residents in 1990. See related *Metropolitan statistical area (MSA).*

Usual source of care—Usual source of care was measured in the National Health Interview Survey (NHIS) in 1993 and 1994 by asking the respondent, "Is there a particular person or place that ____usually goes to when ____is sick or needs advice about ____health?" In the 1995 and 1996 NHIS, the respondent was asked, "Is there one doctor, person, or place that ____usually goes to when ____is sick or needs advice about ____health?" Starting in 1997 the respondent was asked, "Is there a place that ____usually goes when he/she is sick or you need advice about (his/her) health?" Persons who report the emergency department as their usual source of care are defined as having no usual source of care for the purposes of this report.

Wages and salaries—See *Employer costs for employee compensation.*

Years of potential life lost—Years of potential life lost (YPLL) is a measure of premature mortality.

Starting with *Health, United States, 1996–97*, YPLL is presented for persons under 75 years of age because the average life expectancy in the United States is over 75 years. YPLL-75 is calculated using the following eight age groups: under 1 year, 1–14 years, 15–24 years, 25–34 years, 35–44 years, 45–54 years, 55–64 years, 65–74 years. The number of deaths for each age group is multiplied by the years of life lost, calculated as the difference between age 75 years and the midpoint of the age group. For the eight age groups the midpoints are 0.5, 7.5, 19.5, 29.5, 39.5, 49.5, 59.5, and 69.5. For example, the death of a person 15–24 years of age counts as 55.5 years of life lost. Years of potential life lost is derived by summing years of life lost over all age groups. In *Health, United States, 1995* and earlier editions, YPLL was presented for persons under 65 years of age. For more information, see Centers for Disease Control. *MMWR*. Vol 35 no 25S, suppl. 1986.

Appendix III ....

Trend Tables With Additional Years of Data Available in Electronic Spreadsheet Files

Many of the trend tables in this report present data for extended time periods. Because of space limitations on the printed page, only selected years of data are shown to highlight major trends. For the tables listed below, additional years of data are available in electronic spreadsheet files that may be accessed through the Internet and on CD-ROM.

To access the files on the Internet, go to the FTP server on the NCHS homepage at www.cdc.gov/nchs and select "Data Warehouse" and *Health, United States*.

Spreadsheet files are also available on a CD-ROM entitled "Publications from the National Center for Health Statistics," featuring *Health, United States, 2000*, vol 1 no 6, 2000. The CD-ROM may be purchased from the Government Printing Office or the National Technical Information Service.

Table number	Table topic	Additional data years available
1	Resident population	1981–89,1991–96
2	Poverty	1986–89,1991–92
3	Fertility rates and birth rates	1981–84,1986–89,1991–93
5	Live births	1971–74,1976–79,1981–84,1986–89,1991–94
6	Prenatal care	1981–84,1986–89,1991
8	Teenage childbearing	1981–84,1986–89,1991
9	Nonmarital childbearing	1981–84,1986–89,1991
10	Maternal education	1981–84,1986–89,1991
11	Maternal smoking	1991
12	Low birthweight	1981–84,1986–89,1991
13	Low birthweight	1991
16	Abortions	1981–84,1986–88,89
17	Abortions	1981–84,1986–88,89
20	Infant mortality rates	1984,1985–89,1991
21	Infant mortality rates	1984,1985–89,1991
22	Infant mortality rates	1984,1986
23	Infant mortality rates	1981–84,1986–89,1991–94
28	Life expectancy	1975,1981–84
29	Age-adjusted death rates by State	1989–91,1992–94,1993–95,1994–96,1995–97
30	Age-adjusted death rates for selected causes	1991–94
31	Years of potential life lost	1985,1991–97
36	Death rates for all causes	1981–84,1986–89,1991–95
37	Diseases of heart	1981–84,1986–89,1991–94
38	Cerebrovascular diseases	1981–84,1986–89,1991–94
39	Malignant neoplasms	1981–84,1986–89,1991–94
40	Malignant neoplasms of trachea, bronchus, and lung	1981–84,1986–89, 1991–94
41	Malignant neoplasm of breast	1981–84,1986–89, 1991–94
42	Chronic obstructive pulmonary diseases	1981–84,1986–89,1991
43	Human immunodeficiency virus (HIV) infection	1988,1991
44	Maternal mortality	1981–84,1986–89, 1991–94
45	Motor vehicle-related injuries	1981–84,1986–89, 1991–94
46	Homicide	1981–84,1986–89, 1991–94
47	Suicide	1981–84,1986–89, 1991–94
48	Firearm-related injuries	1981–84,1986–87,1989,1991–93

Table number	Table topic	Additional data years available
49	Occupational diseases	1979,1981–84,1986–89
51	Occupational injuries	1981–84,1986–89
52	Notifiable diseases	1985,1988–89,1991–94
59	Cigarette smoking	1987–88,1991
60	Cigarette smoking	1987–88,1991
61	Cigarette smoking	1994–97
62	Use of selected substances	1982,1988
63	Use of selected substances	1981–84,1986–89
85	Ambulatory care visits	1997
87	Additions to mental health organizations	1986,1988
90	Discharges	1988–89,1993,1995
91	Discharges	1989,1994
92	Rates of discharges	1995
93	Discharges	1995
95	Hospital admissions	1991–94
100	Persons employed	1983–84,1986–89,1991–92
102	Physicians	1970,1980,1987,1989,1992–94
105	Staff in mental health organizations	1986,1988
109	Hospitals	1991–94
111	Community hospital beds	1985,1988–89,1995–97
112	Occupancy rates	1985,1988–89,1995–97
116	Consumer Price Index	1965,1975,1985
121	Employers' costs and health insurance	1992–93,1995–97
122	Hospital expenses	1991–92,1994
123	Nursing home average monthly charges	1964
124	Nursing home average monthly charges	1977
126	Funding for health research	1975,1984,1986–89,1991–92
131	Health maintenance organizations	1984,1986–87,1989,1991–92
136	Medicaid	1986–89,1991–94
137	Medicaid	1986–89,1991–94
138	Department of Veterans Affairs	1985,1988–89,1991–92
143	Medicare	1990,1995–96
146	Persons without health care coverage	1991

Index to Trend Tables

Index to Trend Tables ....

Index to Trend Tables ....

Index to Trend Tables ....

Index to Trend Tables ....

Index to Trend Tables ....